Managing Health Services Organizations and Systems

Fifth Edition

Managing Health Services Organizations and Systems

Fifth Edition

Beaufort B. Longest, Jr., Ph.D., FACHE
University of Pittsburgh

Kurt Darr, J.D., Sc.D., FACHE
The George Washington University

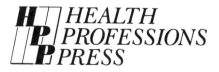
HEALTH
PROFESSIONS
PRESS

Baltimore • London • Sydney

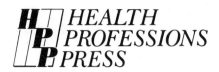
HEALTH
PROFESSIONS
PRESS

Health Professions Press, Inc.
Post Office Box 10624
Baltimore, Maryland 21285-0624

www.healthpropress.com

Typeset by BookMatters, Berkeley, California.
Manufactured in the United States of America by Maple-Vail Book Manufacturing Group,
York, Pennsylvania.

The information provided in this book is in no way meant to substitute for a medical practitioner's advice or expert opinion. This book is sold without warranties of any kind, express or implied, and the publisher and authors disclaim any liability, loss, or damage caused by the contents of this book.

Library of Congress Cataloging-in-Publication Data

Longest, Beaufort B.
  Managing health services organizations and systems / Beaufort B. Longest Jr., Kurt Darr. — 5th ed.
     p. ; cm.
  Includes bibliographical references and indexes.
  ISBN 978-1-932529-35-7 (cloth)
  1. Health facilities—Administration. I. Darr, Kurt. II. Title.
  [DNLM: 1. Health Facilities—organization & administration—United States. 2. Hospital
  Administration—United States. WX 150 L852m 2008]
RA971.R26 2009
362.1068—dc22   2008024147

Contents

PART II   MANAGING HEALTH SERVICES ORGANIZATIONS AND SYSTEMS

About the Authors

Beaufort B. Longest, Jr., Ph.D., FACHE, M. Allen Pond Professor and Director of the Health Policy Institute, Department of Health Policy & Management, Graduate School of Public Health, University of Pittsburgh, Pittsburgh, Pennsylvania 15261

Professor Longest holds a Ph.D. from Georgia State University. He is a fellow of the American College of Healthcare Executives and holds memberships in the Academy of Management, AcademyHealth, American Public Health Association, and the Association for Public Policy Analysis and Management. He is an elected member of the Beta Gamma Sigma Honor Society in Business as well as of the Delta Omega Honor Society in Public Health.

Professor Longest's research has led to numerous peer-reviewed articles published in respected national and international journals. He has authored or co-authored 10 books and 30 chapters. His current research and scholarship address corporate citizenship, policy making, and governance and management in healthcare settings. His work in these areas has underpinned his most recent books, *Managing Health Programs and Projects* and *Health Policymaking in the United States*.

Professor Longest consults with healthcare organizations and systems, universities, associations, and government agencies on health policy and management.

Kurt Darr, J.D., Sc.D., FACHE, Professor, Department of Health Services Management and Leadership, School of Public Health and Health Services, The George Washington University Medical Center, Washington, DC 20037

Dr. Darr is Professor of Hospital Administration in the Department of Health Services Management and Leadership and Professor of Health Care Sciences at The George Washington University. He holds the Doctor of Science from The Johns Hopkins University and the Master of Hospital Administration and Juris Doctor from the University of Minnesota.

Professor Darr completed his administrative residency at Rochester (Minnesota) Methodist Hospital and subsequently worked as an administrative associate at the Mayo Clinic. After being commissioned in the U.S. Navy, he served in administrative and educational assignments at St. Albans Naval Hospital and Bethesda Naval Hospital. He completed postdoctoral fellowships with the Department of Health and Human Services, the World Health Organization, and the Accrediting Commission on Education for Health Services Administration.

Professor Darr is a Fellow of the American College of Healthcare Executives, a member of the District of Columbia and Minnesota Bars, and serves as a mediator in the Superior Court of the District of Columbia. He serves on commissions and committees for various professional organizations, including The Joint Commission on Accreditation of Healthcare Organizations, the American College of Healthcare Executives, and the Commission on Accreditation of Healthcare Management Education. He is a voluntary consultant to several hospitals in the District of Columbia metropolitan area.

Professor Darr regularly presents seminars on health services ethics, hospital organization and management, quality improvement, and the application of the Deming method in health services. He is the author and editor of several books used in graduate health services administration programs and numerous articles on health services topics.

Preface

Leading health services organizations (HSOs) and health systems (HSs) are setting the benchmarks and establishing the best practice standards for the 21st century. They are simultaneously satisfying their customers, achieving quality and safety goals, and meeting cost objectives. The benchmarks of excellence in health services delivery are being established in organizations and systems that have excellent managers, as well as talented clinicians and dedicated governing bodies.

Our purpose in this 5th edition, as in previous editions, is to present information and insight that can help set the benchmarks of excellence in the management of health services. The book will be useful to two groups. It will assist students as they prepare for health services management careers through programs of formal study. It also has broad use as a new source of knowledge of applied management theory that is part of ongoing programs of professional development for current health services executives. We hope that both groups will find the book to be an important reference in their personal libraries.

As in previous editions, the primary focus is managing HSOs and HSs. This edition, however, gives much more attention to managing the increasingly important system of public health organizations and services. Hospitals and long-term care organizations continue to be prominent HSOs and are treated as such in this edition. Ambulatory care organizations, home health agencies, and managed care organizations, among other HSOs, are also covered. Whether HSOs operate as independent entities or align themselves into a variety of HSs, all face dynamic external environments—a mosaic of external forces that includes new rules, regulations, and technologies; changing demographic patterns; increased competition; public scrutiny; heightened consumer expectations; greater demands for accountability; and more constraints on resources. The interface between HSOs and HSs and their external environments is given added attention in this edition.

As in previous editions, we seek to present management theory in a way that demonstrates its widespread applicability to all types of HSOs and HSs. This objective is accomplished by using a process orientation that focuses on how managers manage. We examine management functions, concepts, and principles as well as managerial roles, skills, and competencies within the context of HSOs and HSs and their external environments. For nascent managers, we introduce terminology and concepts that will provide a foundation for lifelong learning and professional development. Experienced managers will find reinforcement of existing skills and experience, provision and application of new theory, and the application of traditional theory and concepts in new ways.

Managing in the unique environment that is health services requires attention to the managerial tools and techniques that are most useful in this environment. The thirteen chapters in this 5th edition of *Managing in Health Services Organizations and Systems* are an integrated whole that covers how management occurs in HSOs and HSs. The discussion questions and cases will stimulate thought and discussion of chapter content. It is our hope that the book will assist all who aspire to establish the new benchmarks of excellence in the extraordinarily complex and important process of delivering health services.

Acknowledgments

Professor Longest thanks Carolyn, whose presence in his life continues to make many things possible and doing them seem worthwhile. He extends appreciation to Judith R. Lave, Ph.D., Chair of the Department of Health Policy and Management; Donald S. Burke, M.D., Dean of the Graduate School of Public Health; and Arthur S. Levine, M.D., Senior Vice Chancellor for Health Sciences at the University of Pittsburgh, for encouraging and facilitating a work environment that is conducive to the scholarly endeavors of faculty members. He also wants to sincerely thank Linda Kalcevic for her tireless and professional efforts in helping make this book a reality.

Professor Darr is grateful to Anne for her unstinting support and for never once asking, "Isn't it done yet?" My department chair, Robert E. Burke, Ph.D., has been solidly supportive of my work on this 5th edition and I am pleased to acknowledge him. A book of this magnitude—even a revision—cannot be researched and written without help. Thanks are owed to my graduate assistant, Roulla Drego, who worked diligently, often under severe time constraints. It was a delight to work with her. Ms. Drego has all of the qualities to succeed in the health services field and I wish her the best in the future.

The authors wish to thank several people at Health Professions Press for their assistance with this book. Mary Magnus, Director of Publications; Amy Perkins, Marketing Manager; Erin Geoghegan, Senior Graphic Designer; and Louise Doucette, copyeditor, each in their own ways made important contributions. We are especially grateful to Cecilia González, Production Manager, for her untiring efforts to make the book as good as it could be. She saw us through the project with good cheer and much assistance. We also thank the publishers and authors who granted permission to reprint material to which they hold the copyright. We are grateful to those who have used previous editions of this book whose comments and critiques aided us in improving the 5th edition.

The authors respectfully acknowledge the contributions made by our coauthor on previous editions, Jonathon S. Rakich, Ph.D. Professor Rakich collaborated with us on *Managing Health Services Organizations and Systems* for over three decades. His participation and historic role in setting direction, selecting substance, and working effectively to achieve a high-quality textbook can be seen even in this 5th edition. We thank him.

Acronyms Used in Text

AA	associate of arts (degree)
AAAHC	Accreditation Association for Ambulatory Healthcare
AAHSA	American Association for Homes and Services for the Aging
AAMC	Association of American Medical Colleges
ABC	activity-based costing
ABMS	American Board of Medical Specialties
ACHE	American College of Healthcare Executives
ACS	American College of Surgeons
ADL	activity of daily living
ADR	alternative dispute resolution
AHA	American Hospital Association
AHCA	American Health Care Association
AHCPR	Agency for Health Care Policy and Research
AHRQ	Agency for Healthcare Research and Quality
AI	artificial intelligence
AIDS	acquired immunodeficiency syndrome
ALOS	average length of stay
AMA	American Medical Association
ANA	American Nurses Association
AOA	American Osteopathic Association
APACHE	acute physiology and chronic health evaluation
APC	ambulatory payment category
APG	ambulatory patient group
ASC	ambulatory surgery centers
BCG Matrix	Boston Consulting Group Matrix
BEAM	brain electrical activity mapping
BLS	Bureau of Labor Statistics
BSC	balanced scorecard
BSN	bachelor of science in nursing (degree)
CABG	coronary artery bypass grafting
CAD	computer-aided detection
CAHME	Commission on Accreditation of Healthcare Management Education
CAMH	Comprehensive Accreditation Manual for Hospitals
CAS	carotid artery stenting
CBO	Congressional Budget Office
CCU	cardiac care unit

CDSS	clinical decision support system
CEA	carotid endarterectomy
CEO	chief executive officer (president)
CEPH	Council on Education for Public Health
CFO	chief financial officer
CGE	continuing governance education
CHAP	Community Health Accreditation Program
CHC	community health center
CHIN	community health information network
CHIPS	Center for Healthcare Industry Performance Studies
CIO	chief information officer
CMO	chief medical officer
CMS	Centers for Medicare and Medicaid Services
CNA	certified nursing assistant
CNM	certified nurse midwife
CNO	chief nursing officer
CON	certificate of need
COO	chief operating officer
COP	conditions of participation
CPR	cardiopulmonary resuscitation
CQI	continuous quality improvement
CQO	chief quality officer
CRNA	certified registered nurse anesthetist
CPI	consumer price index
CSS	clinical support system
CT	computerized tomography
DBS	deep brain stimulation
DHHS	Department of Health and Human Services
DIC	diagnostic imaging centers
DNR	do not resuscitate
DO	doctor of osteopathy
DRG	diagnosis-related group
EAP	employee assistance program
ECHO	echocardiogram
ED	emergency department
EHR	electronic health record
EMR	electronic medical record
EMS	emergency medical services
EMT	emergency medical technician

EPC	evidence-based practice center
EPM	epidemiological planning model
FAA	Federal Aeronautics Administration
FC	fixed costs
FDA	Food and Drug Administration
FMEA	failure mode effects analysis
fMRI	functional magnetic resonance imaging
FQHC	Federally Qualified Health Centers
FTC	Federal Trade Commission
FTE	fulltime equivalent employee
GB	governing body
GDP	gross domestic product
GE	General Electric
GPO	group purchasing organization
GY	graduate year
HCFA	Health Care Financing Administration
HCQIA	Health Care Quality Improvement Act of 1986
HEDIS	Health Plan Employer Data and Information Set
HHA	home health agency
HHS	Department of Health and Human Services
HIPDB	Healthcare Integrity and Protection Data Bank
HIT	health information technology
HIV	human immunodeficiency virus
HME	home medical equipment
HMO	health maintenance organization
HR	human resources
HRET	Hospital Research and Educational Trust
HRM	human resources management
HS	health system
HSA	health systems agency
HSO	health services organization
ICF	intermediate care facility
ICRC	infant care review committee
ICU	intensive care unit
IDN	integrated delivery network
IDS	integrated delivery system
IEC	institutional ethics committee
IHIE	Indiana Health Information Exchange
IOR	interorganizational relationship

IPA	independent practice association
IRB	institutional review board
IRS	Internal Revenue Service
IS	information system
ISO	International Organization for Standardization
JCAHO	Joint Commission on Accreditation of Healthcare Organizations
JCC	joint conference committee
KQC	key quality characteristic
KPV	key process variable
LAN	local area network
LCL	lower control limit
LIP	licensed independent practitioner
LLC	limited liability company
LOS	length of stay
LPC	least preferred co-worker
LPN	licensed practical (vocational) nurse
LTCH	long-term care (extended stay) hospital
M&M	morbidity and mortality
MBNQA	Malcolm Baldrige National Quality Award
MBO	management by objectives
MCO	managed care organizations
MD	medical doctor
MDSS	management decision support system
MGMA	Medical Group Management Association
MICU	medical intensive care unit
MIS	management information systems
MRI	magnetic resonance imaging
MSI	magnetic source imaging
MSO	management services organization
MVS	multi-vendor servicing
NCQA	National Committee for Quality Assurance
NA	nursing assistant
NASA	National Aeronautics and Space Administration
NC	net contribution
NCHSRHCTA	National Center for Health Services Research and Health Care Technology Assessment
NCHCT	National Center for Health Care Technology
NCHL	National Center for Healthcare Leadership
NCVL	noninvasive cardiovascular laboratory

NF	nursing facility
NGC	National Guideline Clearinghouse
NHS	National Health Service (U.K.)
NICU	neonatal intensive care unit
NIH	National Institutes of Health
NLM	National Library of Medicine
NLN	National League for Nursing
NLNAC	National League for Nursing Accrediting Commission
NP	nurse practitioner
OBRA	Omnibus Budget Reconciliation Act of 1987 (PL 100-203)
ODS	organized delivery system
OPG	ocular plethysmograph
OR	operating room
OSHA	Occupational Safety and Health Administration
OT	occupational therapy
OTA	Office of Technology Assessment
PA	physician assistant
PAC	political action committee
PAF	performance assessment framework (U.K.)
PAS	physician-assisted suicide
PBT	proton beam therapy
PDCA	plan, do, check, act
PDSA	plan, do, study, act
PET	positron emission tomography
PGY	postgraduate year
PHO	physician-hospital organization
PI	productivity improvement
PICU	pediatric intensive care unit
PIT	process improvement team
PPO	preferred provider organization
PRO	peer review organization
PSDA	Patient Self Determination Act
PSO	professional staff organization
PSRO	professional standards review organization
PT	physical therapy
PTCA	percutaneous transluminal coronary angioplasty
PVR	pulse volume recording plethysmograph
PVS	persistent vegetative state
Q/PI	quality/productivity improvement

QA/I	quality assessment and improvement
QI	quality improvement
QIC	quality improvement council
QIO	quality improvement organization
QIT	quality improvement team
QMHCD	quality management for health care delivery
QWL	quality-of-work life
RBRVS	resource-based relative value scales
RDE	rule of double effect
RHIO	regional health information organization
RM	risk management
RN	registered nurse
RT	rehabilitation therapy
RUG	resource utilization group
SA	strategic alliance
SBU	strategic business unit
SCAP	service, consideration, access, and promotion
SHRM	strategic human resources management
SICU	surgical intensive care unit
SNF	skilled nursing facility
SPC	statistical process control
SPECT	single photon emission computerized tomography
SWOT	strengths/weaknesses/opportunities/threats
TC	total costs
TEAM	Technology Evaluation and Acquisition Methods
TEE	transesophageal echocardiography
TQM	total quality management
t-PA	tissue plasminogen activator
UCL	upper control limit
UR	utilization review
UPMC	University of Pittsburgh Medical Center
USPHS	United States Public Health Service
VC	variable costs
VNS	vagus nerve stimulation
VP	vice president
VPMA	vice president for medical affairs
WAN	wide-area network

*To those who manage health services organizations
and to those who aspire*

PART I

The Healthcare Setting

1

Healthcare in the United States

This first chapter describes the system of healthcare in the United States—the general environment in which managers of health services organizations (HSOs) and health systems (HSs) work. The chapter develops conceptual frameworks and presents information about healthcare resources that show their historical development, nature, and extent and the relationships among them. Resources include HSOs/HSs, programs, personnel, technology, and financing. Information about several types of HSOs—acute care hospitals, nursing facilities, ambulatory care organizations, hospice, managed care organizations (MCOs), and home health agencies—is provided in Chapter 2.

Data and information presented here describe the manager's environment. Successful managers have a comprehensive and accurate understanding of the world beyond their organizations; this includes a thorough understanding of trends and developments. The management model, Figure 5.8 in Chapter 5, shows this relationship and should be referenced as necessary. Data shown are drawn from private and public sources. It is important not only to understand the individual presentations, but also to appreciate their interactions.

Health expenditures in the United States in 2006 were about $2.2 trillion, which was 16% of gross domestic product (GDP), or more than $7,000 per capita.[1] Table 1.3 shows that actual numbers for 2002–2005 and projections to 2016 have a slower annual percentage change in the increase for health spending. Some of this slower rate of percentage growth is attributable to increases in GDP, which produce a larger denominator. These changes have halted the large upward trend of health expenditures as a percentage of GDP that had been observed since the 1960s.[2] Table 1.3 shows that expenditures are projected to increase from $2.1 trillion in 2006 to over $4.0 trillion in 2016, or about 20.0% of GDP. Growth in healthcare spending is projected to average 2.1 percentage points above the rate of GDP growth for 2005–2015.[3] Such huge sums suggest both the magnitude of the problems and the opportunities for HSO/HS managers.

Health and System Goals

Distinguishing the healthcare system from the health services system may seem a pedantic exercise, but health services managers must understand the connections between them.

Blum's model, shown in Figure 1.1, identifies factors affecting health. The relative size of the arrows shows the degree of their effects—medical care services (prevention, cure, care, rehabilitation) are much less important than environment and somewhat less important than heredity and lifestyles in affecting health (well-being). In explaining the model, Blum states that the "largest aggregate of forces resides in the person's environment. One's own behavior, in great part derived from one's experience with one's environment, is seen as the next largest force affecting health."[4] Effective managers understand the many influences on health status, both as factors that lead to episodes of illness and as effects on recovery and long-term absence of illness and minimization of disability. HSO/HS managers must have a broad view of illness and health. This requires looking beyond the organization. They must understand that, at best, the health services system has a limited effect and can provide only stopgap measures if negative influences on health undo what services delivery has done.

Blum suggests several goals for a health system:

- Prolonging life and preventing premature death
- Minimizing departures from physiological or functional norms by focusing attention on precursors of illness

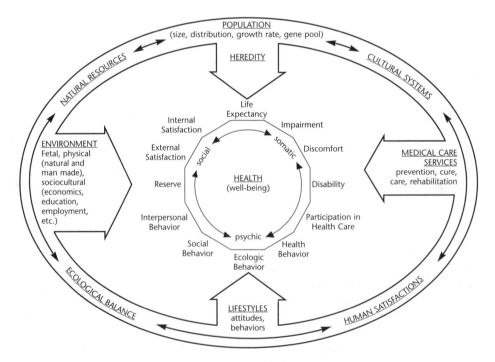

Figure 1.1.   The force-field and well-being paradigms of health. (From Blum, Henrik K. *Expanding Health Care Horizons: From General Systems Concept of Health to a National Health Policy,* 2nd ed., 37. Oakland, CA: Third Party Publishing, 1983; reprinted by permission.)

- Minimizing discomfort (illness)
- Minimizing disability (incapacity)
- Promoting high-level "wellness" or self-fulfillment
- Promoting high-level satisfaction with the environment
- Extending resistance to ill health and creating reserve capacity
- Increasing opportunities for consumers to participate in health matters[5]

These goals are part of the conceptual framework underlying the use of this book.

The Precede-Proceed planning model in Figure 1.2 is a more applied conceptualization of the relationships among activities that are part of health promotion planning and evaluation and that should be part of the efforts to deliver comprehensive healthcare.[6] Phase 1 is a social assessment that recognizes the relationships among health and various social issues by identifying a target population's social, economic, cultural, and other nonmedical concerns and goals. The epidemiological assessment in Phase 2 has the initial goal of identifying specific health goals or problems that may contribute to, or interact with, the social goals or problems noted in the social assessment of Phase 1. Phase 2 uses vital indicators such as morbidity, disability, mortality, and demographic patterns, as well as genetics and behavioral and environmental indicators of health problems. The health concerns needing amelioration are listed in rank order after the objectively appraised health problems identified in Phase 2 are compared with the subjectively appraised quality-of-life issues identified in Phase 1. The educational and ecological assessment in Phase 3 groups the factors associated with health concerns into predisposing factors, reinforcing factors, and enabling factors. The elements of these factors are sorted, categorized, and selected in terms of their greatest potential to change the behavioral and environmental targets generated in previous stages.

The administrative and policy assessment and intervention alignment in Phase 4 begins the interventions that lead to the Proceed portion of the model. This phase answers questions about what program components and interventions are needed and whether policy, organization, and resources are sufficient to make the program a reality. The result is the implementation in Phase 5. Phases 6, 7, and 8 are among the most important in the model. Here the program is evaluated in terms of

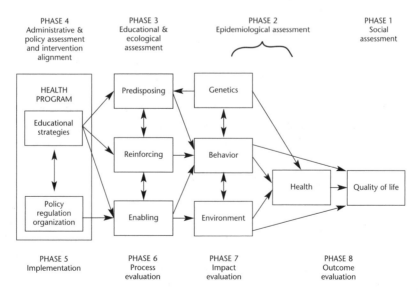

Figure 1.2. The model for health promotion planning and evaluation. (From *Health Program Planning: An Educational and Ecological Approach.* 4th ed. Lawrence W. Green and Marshall W. Kreuter. New York: McGraw-Hill, 2005, 10.) With permission of the McGraw-Hill Companies, Inc.

process, impact, and outcome. The evaluation criteria are linked to objectives defined in the corresponding steps of the Precede portion of the model. The increasing emphasis on health promotion and prevention makes the Precede-Proceed model a useful tool in planning and delivering comprehensive healthcare, especially in integrated delivery systems.

Lack of Synchrony

The wide geographic variation in rates of hospitalization and lengths of hospital stay by diagnosis has been known for decades. Similar geographic variation occurs in use of nursing facilities by Medicare beneficiaries.[7] The variation in hospital use is a true difference that cannot be explained by redefining or estimating the effect of variables such as age, gender, and climate. Even more puzzling are the large differences in rates of hospitalization and lengths of stay by diagnosis within geographic regions, and even within individual hospitals. The most plausible explanation is that physician practice patterns—physicians' clinical decisions—vary. It can be hypothesized that some rates of hospitalization and lengths of stay are more appropriate than others. This means that resource use beyond that appropriate has significant implications for HSOs/HSs striving to use resources judiciously.

Other data have shown significant differences between morbidity and mortality caused by a disease and the amount of hospitalization for that disease.[8] The lack of synchrony can be explained in various ways: hospitals are constrained by available technology; hospitalization may be inappropriate to treat the medical condition that causes death or limits activity; and some medical conditions require more attention to prevention, which is historically a general deficit of acute care hospitals. Achieving synchrony suggests that services provided by HSOs and their use are in harmony with health needs.

There are important distinctions between the need and the demand for health services. Need is measured by morbidity and mortality data and by disability that limits activity. Need is more objective than demand, but value judgments invariably underpin conclusions about need. Demand occurs when need (or perceived need) is converted into demand for services. As suggested, need and demand do not have a one-to-one relationship. Providers such as hospitals and physicians have a role in demand, as does the availability of third-party payment for services.

Demand for a particular service or treatment may be artificially low in a service area if, for instance, a hospital does not offer it and potential users must go elsewhere. Physicians' perspectives about whether a medical service is needed directly affect demand for it. From the consumers' perspective, need may not become demand, because they lack knowledge about a disease or because social or cultural mores dissuade them from seeking services or treatment. In addition, demand may be less than need because people lack financial resources or there are other access barriers. Further, some demand, such as that for cosmetic surgery, is subjective and varies by consumer. The relationships between need and demand must be considered as health services are planned. The ethical dimensions of need and demand are addressed in Chapter 4.

Processes That Produce Health Policy

The federal Constitution is the basic law of the United States. The federal system that it established arose after the American Revolution when the several sovereign states relinquished specific powers to a central government. The enumerated powers of the federal government are interpreted by the U.S. Supreme Court. Powers not delegated to the federal government are reserved to the states. This is important because of the states' police powers. Each state has a constitution that establishes its form of government. The right to petition government is found in the First Amendment to the federal Constitution. This guarantee of access to government and its processes has produced various nonpublic efforts to affect the legislative, regulatory, and judicial processes.

PUBLIC PROCESSES

Legislative Process

Statutes are enacted by state legislatures and the U.S. Congress. Comparable legislative activities are performed by local governments when ordinances are passed. The laws are binding, but they may be challenged in court if they violate constitutionally protected rights or were improperly enacted because of procedural irregularity. The legislative branch relies on the executive branch to implement and enforce the laws.

Paradigmatic of these processes is the process that occurs in the U.S. Congress. The basic legislative process in the Senate and House of Representatives is the same. The majority political party controls committee and subcommittee membership and determines legislative priorities. Bills related to healthcare introduced in either house are referred to committees or subcommittees and may be amended at various points, including in committee or subcommittee, on the floor, or in conference between the houses. During the legislative process, or to learn more about problems before drafting bills, committees or subcommittees may hold hearings in which testimony about a problem or issue is heard. Individual managers or governing body members of HSOs/HSs rarely participate in the legislative process. Testimony, drafts of bills, and other input are provided by professional or trade associations, either by their staffs or through hired lobbyists. A bill approved by the Senate and the House and signed by the president becomes law.

Implementing Law—Regulations

Laws are implemented by regulations issued by executive departments and agencies and independent regulatory bodies such as the Federal Trade Commission (FTC). This process is governed by the Administrative Procedure Act of 1946, as amended.[9] Requirements include notice of proposed rule making, proposed regulations, and final regulations. The steps before final regulations are issued permit interested parties to comment on provisions. Interim regulations that test the effect of proposed regulations may be issued before final regulations can be drafted and approved.

During the time for public comment, individual HSOs/HSs and their trade associations and lobbyists seek to affect the content of final regulations. It is most cost-effective to influence the process at this point. The record of HSOs/HSs and their trade associations is mixed. Lobbying by provider groups moderated the Medicare fraud and abuse regulations. Conversely, the National Labor Relations Board did not accept the position of hospitals during rule making regarding the definition of bargaining units.

Results of the implementation process appear in the *Federal Register,* which is published each working day. Final regulations are compiled in the *Code of Federal Regulations*.

Multiple Functions of the Regulatory Process

Implementation and enforcement of federal laws are accomplished by executive branch departments and agencies and by independent regulatory bodies, all of which were established by Congress. The regulatory process melds legislative, executive, and judicial functions.

Drafting and promulgating regulations (rule making) give executive departments and agencies and independent regulatory bodies quasi-legislative authority.[10] The basic law's specificity determines the latitude for interpretation in the rule-making process. The regulations reflect the law and congressional intent and have general (prospective) application.

Executive departments and agencies and independent regulatory bodies have quasi-executive powers because they have authority to enforce the regulations. Compliance is achieved by the bringing of complaints, issuing of directives such as cease-and-desist orders, and levying of fines, all of which can occur pending a decision in the agency's hearing and review process or prior to a hearing in an emergency. Executive departments and agencies and independent regulatory bodies have quasi-judicial powers because they judge compliance in hearings and reviews that are held before their hearing officers or administrative law judges. Such officials have a degree of independence because they are appointed for specific terms by the president and can be removed only for cause.

Challenging a regulatory decision by engaging in the administrative hearing and review process is time-consuming and expensive. Legal counsel who are expert in the law being disputed, as well as in administrative law, are needed to work with retainer or in-house corporate counsel. As a practical matter, small HSOs/HSs have little choice but to comply with a regulation or to simply accept an adverse administrative ruling without appeal to the courts. Legal challenges are costly and usually can be undertaken only by a large HSO/HS or association. This may change, however, because some federal laws permit successful challengers to recover costs.

An important development beginning in the late 20th century is the increasing complexity and significance of administrative law and the rule-making processes. Some political scientists argue that bureaucracies are a de facto fourth branch of federal government. Generally, the parties must exhaust the administrative review process before appeal to the federal courts is allowed.

JUDICIAL PROCESS

Space does not permit full discussion of various courts and their jurisdictions and authority. Suffice it to say that state and federal court systems are similar. Both have trial courts (county and district courts, respectively), intermediate courts (appeals courts), and supreme courts. Some states reverse use of the terms *supreme* and *appeals*. *Judge* is the title for jurists in courts other than the highest state and federal courts; *justice* is the title for members of state supreme courts and the Supreme Court of the United States. Typically, governors nominate state judges and justices, who are ratified by the state senates. Some states elect judges and justices, although the election of judges is more common. Elected jurists typically serve terms of 10 or 15 years. Federal court judges and justices are nominated by the president and confirmed by the Senate. They serve for life.

Appointment insulates the judiciary somewhat from politics, and this results in more predictable and consistent court-made law. Judges and justices appointed by governors or presidents likely will have compatible political philosophies; the history of the U.S. Supreme Court shows some notable exceptions, however. The need for legislative confirmation and the almost universal review of nominees by bar committees usually result in appointment of competent and ethical members of the judiciary.

The Courts

HSOs/HSs are often involved in state and federal courts, as plaintiffs (those bringing civil legal action) or defendants (those against whom civil legal action is taken). In addition, when a case is heard by an appeals court, an individual or association may submit legal briefs as a friend of the court, or *amicus curiae*. The briefs bring to a court's attention legal precedents and other information from that group's perspective.

Stare Decisis and *Res Judicata*

Two legal doctrines make courts a source of formal law. *Stare decisis* is Latin meaning that courts will stand by precedent and not disturb a settled point.[11] Intrinsic to a stable society is that the law is fixed, definite, and known and that courts and litigants are guided by previous cases with similar facts. Whimsical changes and uncertainty must not result from judge-made law or legislative enactments. Nevertheless, precedents are sometimes overturned.

The second doctrine is reflected in the Latin phrase *res judicata,* which means that a matter has been judged or a thing has been judicially acted on or decided.[12] Thus, rehearing will occur only if there is a substantial problem in the original judgment because of factual error, misrepresentation, or fraud or if significant new information becomes available. *Res judicata* adds stability and predictability to the law because a case is rarely reopened after appeals are exhausted.

EXECUTIVE ORDERS

Formal law results from executive orders issued by the president through the executive branch of the federal government. Authority for some executive orders, such as the president's role as commander-in-chief of the armed forces, is derived from the U.S. Constitution. Decisions arising from treaties result in executive orders. Another example is delegation of authority by Congress to the president to act in special circumstances, such as emergencies. An executive order that declares a disaster will enable an HSO/HS to qualify for federal assistance.

PRIVATE PROCESSES

Influence of HSOs/HSs

Healthcare became highly politicized after massive federal financing of health services began in the mid-1960s with enactment of Medicare and Medicaid. The legislative and regulatory processes affecting health services were increasingly subject to the influence of lobbyists, political action committees (PACs), and other interest groups, all seeking to ensure that their concerns became known. For HSOs/HSs and their trade associations, participating in federal and state government processes that affected them was a matter of survival.

In the management model in Figure 5.8, the change loop (number 6) suggests that HSOs/HSs affect their external environment, even as they are affected by it. This occurs when they advocate a position or support a trade association or PAC. Another effect results from bringing a lawsuit.

Trade Associations and Interested Parties

Washington, D.C., and environs are home to thousands of trade associations; among them are many from healthcare. Physical proximity to policy makers and the bureaucrats who develop and enforce federal laws and regulations is considered an advantage. In addition to major associations, there are hundreds of narrowly focused special interest groups. At best, trade associations and interested parties provide information that enhances results of legislative and regulatory processes. HSOs/HSs and their associations seek to further their own interests, but their quasi-public role means that their interests have much in common with the public's.

Associations and interested parties make their positions known at various points in the legislative and regulatory processes. The myriad bills and their often complex subject matter minimize the depth of decision makers' knowledge. An essential role of lobbyists is providing them with information that otherwise is unavailable, as well as analyzing the intended and unintended consequences of legislation being considered. Interactions with lobbyists occur in private, which is not to suggest illegal or immoral acts. Legislators and their staffs know that lobbyists will present information most advantageously for the party that they represent. A cardinal rule among lobbyists is that truthfulness is essential. Lobbyists caught lying or purposefully misleading decision makers or staff irretrievably lose the credibility that is their greatest asset. The obvious bears repeating: There will always be dishonest legislators whose vote can be bought and special interests who try to do more than express a viewpoint and make a convincing argument. Despite occasional publicity to the contrary, such ethical and legal lapses are the exception.

▬ A Brief History of Health Services in the United States ▬▬▬▬

Figure 1.3 shows trends in U.S. health services since 1945. It provides a useful context to understand the evolution and current status of healthcare and health services.

TECHNOLOGY

The importance of ensuring the purity of food and water was shown during the "great sanitary awakening" that occurred in the mid-19th century. One result was the universality of local and state health departments. At about the same time, the work of scientists such as Pasteur, Lister, and Koch resulted, first, in antisepsis and, later, asepsis. In addition, medical technology such as radiographs, inhalation anesthesia, blood typing, and improved clinical laboratories in the late 19th century permitted efficacious surgical interventions with greatly reduced morbidity and mortality. Making these scientific advances available to the public required an organization, specialized staff, and effective systems. Hospitals were the obvious answer.

It was common for hospitals to be sponsored by private, not-for-profit corporations that had been formed by religious groups, concerned citizens, or wealthy benefactors; local governments sponsored others. In addition, many small "hospitals" were established as for-profit corporations, often by individual physicians who needed a place to care for patients following surgery. Long-term care facilities were rare because extended families cared for one another. People with mental illnesses were isolated from society in facilities owned almost exclusively by state governments. Effective, large-scale treatment for them did not occur until after World War II through use of psychoactive drugs. Another type of HSO sponsored by local and state governments was the public health department. Chapter 3 details the role of technology in contemporary health services.

MORTALITY AND MORBIDITY

Table 1.1 shows male and female age-adjusted death rates by causes of death since 1970, with projections to 2020. Heart disease and cancer continue to be the leading causes of death. Notably, age-adjusted cancer death rates have increased since 1970 and are projected to continue increasing well into the 21st century before beginning to decline. Vascular disease includes stroke, which has been the third-leading cause of death historically.

Except for tuberculosis, the incidence of which declined rapidly at the end of the 19th century mainly because of improved nutrition and housing, and leprosy, which has never been a major medical problem in the United States, there were few chronic diseases before the 20th century. Primarily, people died of acute gastrointestinal and respiratory tract infections, such as pneumonia, that usually occurred before they could develop chronic diseases. Many communicable health problems common in the mid-19th century were solved through preventive measures taken by health departments. Pure food and water and improved sanitation were major contributors to decreased morbidity and mortality. The greatest influence on public health in the United States came from work done in England. Local public health departments were established in the early 19th century, with Baltimore, MD, and Charleston, SC, among the first.[13]

Causes of mortality and morbidity in the mid-20th century were much less amenable to easy prevention or inexpensive treatment, and the resulting increased emphases on acute services substantially increased costs. Table 1.1 shows overall age-adjusted mortality rates steadily declining well into the 21st century. This means increased longevity and a greater likelihood of chronic diseases, which are almost certain to increase total healthcare costs. Figure 1.1 shows a link between lifestyle and medical problems. Many types of prevention require changes in behavior. Efforts to effect these changes raise issues of individual choice and liberty rights, which are much more complex than purifying water and

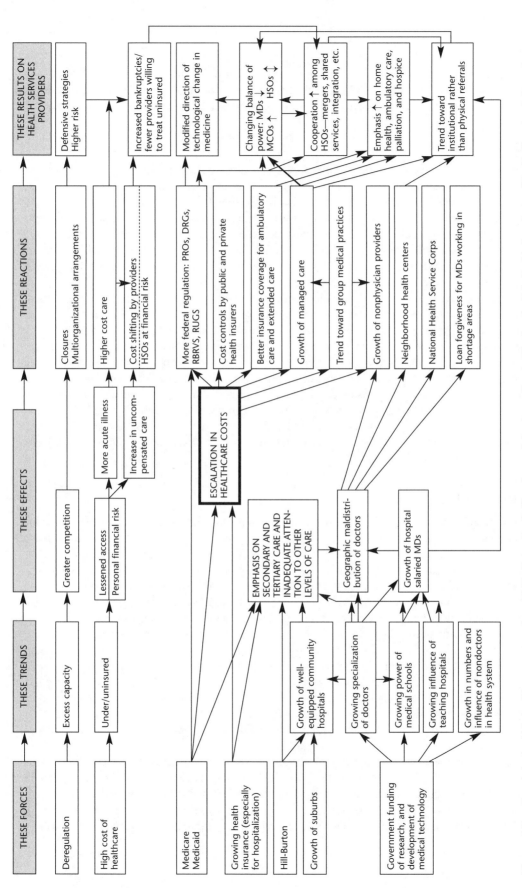

Figure 1.3. Trends in the U.S. healthcare system since 1945. (From Cambridge Research Institute. *Trends Affecting the U.S. Health Care System* [Health Planning Information Series], 409. Washington, DC: Human Resources Administration, 1976. Revised and updated by the authors, 2008.)

protecting food supplies. Modifying behavior raises questions such as these: What are the limits of government's efforts to force people to live healthy lives? What is society's obligation to treat those whose illnesses are a direct result of engaging in activities known to be unhealthy or to result in injury?

SOCIAL WELFARE

A major shift in the locus of responsibility for social welfare occurred with the Social Security Act of 1935,[14] whose enactment resulted from the Great Depression's catastrophic economic and social problems. To the extent that government was involved in social welfare before 1935, it was provided at the local and state levels. City or county governments might own a "poor farm," for example, where needy people could live and work until they could regain their independence. Since 1935, there has been a massive shift of perceived and actual responsibility for social welfare from state and local levels to the federal government. This accretion continued virtually uninterrupted until revenue sharing and other federal programs were developed in the 1970s and 1980s.

Federal government–sponsored national health insurance programs, ranging in scope from all-encompassing to modest, were seriously considered in the late 1940s and late 1960s and again in the early 1990s. Various factors made them unattractive: lack of voter interest because of their cost and the fear of government control, widely available employer-provided health insurance, and the presence of Medicare and Medicaid that covered millions of Americans. Organized medicine's opposition is often cited, but its role is overstated. The experience with Medicare and Medicaid from 1966—especially their rapidly rising costs—blunted the political will to universalize them.

In 2006, 12.1% of the population was age 65 or older; it is projected that by 2050, this proportion will grow to 20.0%.[15] These data suggest that there will be greatly increased demand for health services in geriatrics, chronic diseases, rehabilitation, and institutional long-term care. Unanswered is how these needs will be financed.

FEDERAL INITIATIVES

Major beneficiaries of early federal programs were not-for-profit acute care hospitals, including those operated by state and local governments. From 1946 to 1981, the Hill-Burton Act (Hospital Survey and Construction Act of 1946, PL 79-725)[16] provided more than $4 billion in grants, loans, and guaranteed loans in a federal-state matching program and aided nearly 6,900 hospitals and other health services facilities in more than 4,000 communities. Initially, new inpatient facilities were constructed; later, outpatient facilities were constructed or remodeled. In return for Hill-Burton assistance, organizations had to provide uncompensated services for varying lengths of time.[17] The legal processes that produced Hill-Burton and laws like it were discussed earlier in this chapter.

Another federal program provided generous funding for research activities. The National Institutes of Health (NIH) began with experimentation on cancer in the 1930s. In 2006, there were 20 institutes and 7 centers and related activities, such as the National Library of Medicine and the NIH Clinical Center.[18] In 2007, the NIH budget was $28.6 billion,[19] almost four times the $7.6 billion in 1990 and more than eight times the $3.4 billion in 1980 (for only nine institutes and related activities).[20] In 2005, NIH provided grants to more than 55,000 research projects in universities, medical schools, and independent research institutions.[21]

By way of context, an estimated $111 billion was spent on U.S. health research in 2005. Industry spent $61 billion (55%), including $35 billion (31%) from the pharmaceutical industry, $16 billion (15%) from the biotechnology industry, and $10 billion (9%) from the medical technology industry. Government spent $40 billion (36%); most of this was spent by NIH ($29 billion [26%]), and other federal agencies and state and local governments spent $12 billion (10%). The remaining

TABLE 1.1. FEMALE AND MALE AGE-ADJUSTED DEATH RATES BY CAUSE OF DEATH, SELECTED YEARS, PER 100,000

Year	Total	Heart disease	Cancer	Vascular disease	Violence	Respiratory disease	Infancy	Digestive disease	Diabetes mellitus	Cirrhosis (liver)	AIDS	Other
Female												
1970	803.6	308.4	141.0	144.9	45.6	38.5	24.7	19.0	21.2	10.3	0.0	50.0
1975	709.1	265.2	141.4	119.8	39.6	34.3	18.2	15.8	17.4	9.5	0.0	48.0
1980	668.1	250.1	146.0	92.1	36.0	37.0	14.5	16.8	15.1	8.8	0.0	51.7
1985	638.0	227.6	150.7	73.6	31.3	45.5	11.9	16.3	14.3	7.1	0.4	59.2
1990	620.9	206.8	153.6	61.3	30.2	52.5	10.3	15.9	13.8	6.2	3.5	66.7
1991	615.0	202.5	154.2	58.5	29.6	53.1	9.9	15.8	13.5	6.1	4.5	67.4
1992	609.5	198.4	154.4	55.9	28.9	53.6	9.5	15.7	13.2	6.0	5.5	68.2
1995	594.6	186.5	156.4	48.6	27.1	55.4	8.3	15.4	12.2	5.7	8.0	70.8
2000[a]	573.5	168.4	159.3	38.9	24.5	58.7	6.8	15.1	10.9	5.4	10.1	75.5
2005[a]	553.9	153.4	161.7	32.6	22.6	61.2	5.8	14.8	9.9	5.2	7.8	78.9
2010[a]	537.0	142.6	161.5	29.2	21.7	61.7	5.3	14.5	9.4	5.1	6.5	79.4
2015[a]	521.5	134.2	159.9	26.7	21.1	61.2	4.9	14.2	9.1	5.1	6.4	78.8
2020[a]	506.7	126.5	158.0	24.5	20.5	60.5	4.5	13.9	8.8	5.0	6.4	78.0
Male												
1970	1,359.5	554.3	221.1	187.5	126.0	93.3	31.5	29.0	19.9	22.2	0.0	74.7
1975	1,237.5	491.8	229.8	156.2	113.3	87.9	22.7	23.6	17.1	21.6	0.0	73.5
1980	1,165.1	454.1	240.6	119.8	108.6	88.4	17.8	23.5	15.6	19.2	0.0	77.6
1985	1,096.4	408.5	243.2	95.1	92.2	97.7	14.8	22.5	15.2	15.7	5.5	86.0
1990	1,055.0	360.7	246.2	80.0	88.1	101.4	12.5	21.1	15.3	14.4	26.1	89.2
1991	1,047.9	353.1	247.3	76.4	86.6	101.7	11.9	20.8	15.1	14.2	31.2	89.8
1992	1,040.9	345.6	248.5	72.9	85.0	102.0	11.4	20.5	14.8	13.9	35.8	90.5
1995	1,019.3	324.4	252.1	63.5	80.6	102.9	9.9	19.6	14.1	13.1	46.4	92.6
2000[a]	981.0	292.3	258.3	50.8	73.9	105.0	8.0	18.4	13.0	12.0	52.9	96.4
2005[a]	934.0	265.8	263.2	42.5	69.0	106.8	6.8	17.5	12.1	11.3	39.7	99.3
2010[a]	900.1	246.9	263.6	38.1	66.5	106.8	6.2	17.0	11.6	11.0	32.9	99.6
2015[a]	874.0	231.9	261.1	34.8	65.1	105.9	5.7	16.6	11.2	10.9	32.0	98.7
2020[a]	850.1	218.4	258.2	32.0	63.9	104.8	5.3	16.3	10.9	10.7	31.9	97.8

Source: Source Book of Health Insurance Data: 1997–1998, 157–158. Washington, DC: Health Insurance Association of America, 1998.

[a]Projected.

$10 billion (9%) was spent by universities, independent research institutes, voluntary health organizations, and foundations.[22]

Significant federal programs to educate more physicians, nurses, technicians, and managers were established and funded in the 1960s. It was clear to Congress that the knowledge produced by NIH and the hospitals built by Hill-Burton could improve health status only if members of the health professions were available in sufficient numbers.

Federal government has also built large numbers of Department of Veterans Affairs (DVA) hospitals and other HSOs to provide services to former military personnel. The DVA system is separate from the services provided to groups in special categories, including inmates in federal prisons, American Indian and Alaska Natives, and active-duty and retired military personnel and their dependents in U.S. Army, U.S. Navy, and U.S. Air Force health facilities.

In 1965, amendments[23] to the Social Security Act of 1935 obligated federal government to pay for health services under the newly enacted Medicare and Medicaid programs. Medicare is exclusively federal and pays for medical services provided to persons who have disabilities or are 65 or older. Originally, Medicare included only Part A, to pay for hospital inpatient services, and Part B, to pay for physicians' services. The Balanced Budget Act of 1997 (PL 105-33)[24] added Part C, which allows Medicare beneficiaries to choose from various health plans, including fee-for-service, coordinated care plans, provider service organizations, and medical savings accounts.[25] Part D was added to Medicare by the Medicare Prescription Drug, Improvement, and Modernization Act of 2003 (PL 108-173)[26] to establish a voluntary prescription drug benefit program.

Medicaid is a state-federal cost-sharing program. States determine eligibility. Federal government subsidizes a state's Medicaid program in various ratios. Medicaid requires that participating states offer a minimum set of benefits that includes inpatient and outpatient hospital services; physician, midwife, and certified nurse practitioner services; laboratory and x-ray services; nursing homes and home healthcare for individuals age 21 or older; early and periodic screening, diagnosis, and treatment for children under age 21; family planning services and supplies; and rural health clinic or federally qualified health center services. In addition to the basic benefits, states can receive federal matching funds for "optional" services, including prescription drugs, prosthetic devices, hearing aids, and dental care.[27] The open-ended cost-sharing commitment by federal government has proven to be largely uncontrollable (because limiting or reducing benefits is politically infeasible) and extremely expensive.

Meanwhile, federal legislators sought to rationalize health services.[28] The Comprehensive Health Planning and Public Health Service Amendments Act of 1966 (PL 89-749) was the first attempt. It enhanced the modest planning requirements in Hill-Burton by encouraging voluntary planning and use of planning processes and techniques. This legislation was amplified and expanded in the National Health Planning and Resources Development Act of 1974 (PL 93-641), which increased the control that planning agencies had over expansion of hospitals and services in an effort to regulate the supply of services. Monitoring the use and quality of services provided under Medicare and Medicaid programs was included in the Social Security Amendments of 1972 (PL 92-603) that established professional standards review organizations (PSROs). Political changes caused reassessment of planning and PSROs. Federal support of planning ended. PSROs were replaced by peer review organizations (PROs), which are discussed later in this chapter.

Such regulatory controls were thought essential to slow the rapid increases in healthcare costs. In general, however, they proved ineffective. With the exception of just 4 years between 1969 and 1996, the medical-care-items component of the consumer price index (CPI) had the highest rates of increase, usually by wide margins. In several years, the average annual percentage changes for hospital services were two to three times the annual percentage changes for all items measured by the CPI.[29] Healthcare costs are discussed in more detail later in this chapter.

The Tax Equity and Fiscal Responsibility Act of 1982 (PL 97-248) and the Social Security Amendments of 1983 (PL 98-21) established a prospective payment system to address the problem of cost increases in hospitals.[30] Medicare reimbursement is determined prospectively and is based on diagnosis-related groups (DRGs), which tie the payment from the federal government for Medicare patients to a hospital's case mix. Since the mid-1970s, the states have been concerned about rising health services costs. Certificate of need (CON) and rate review laws were passed to control costs. In addition, many states have reduced reimbursement for Medicaid beneficiaries to the point that service providers typically incur losses.

These federal legislative initiatives forced hospitals and other providers, such as nursing facilities, to become more efficient. Providers cannot control their environments, however. In addition, they may have to provide significant levels of uncompensated care. Under such circumstances, providers—especially hospitals—can survive only if they find other revenue sources. Previously, unpaid costs were shifted to Blue Cross, commercial insurance companies, and private-pay patients. Third-party payers became unwilling to bear these shifted costs. This left only private-pay patients—a group too small to make up the difference. Beyond the issue of fairness, cost shifting is a major political issue, especially with regard to the uninsured and the costs of medical education. To protect themselves financially, hospitals and other HSOs are developing new organizational entities and relationships through corporate restructuring, joint ventures, and participation in health systems. The result is a mix of not-for-profit and for-profit organizations that, it is hoped, will produce an enhanced revenue stream to offset deficits. These developments are discussed in Chapter 2.

MCOs, the most common of which is the health maintenance organization (HMO), have helped moderate the rate of increase in healthcare costs. Even MCOs have been unable to prevent increases in healthcare costs, however. Evidence for this includes a need for MCOs to recoup losses, the higher costs of prescription drugs, the difficulty of wresting additional price concessions from physicians and hospitals, and the fact that all the one-time savings that resulted from employees' changing to managed care have been realized. HMO costs are estimated to be growing as fast as, or faster than, the costs of traditional health insurance.[31] In addition, anecdotes asserting that economics drive certain physician decision making may be overstated, as seen when equalizing payments to physicians for caesarean sections and vaginal deliveries did not decrease the number of caesarean sections. The opportunity costs of waiting out a difficult labor, the fear of malpractice suits, and the impact of a bad outcome on self-respect, reputation, and long-term profits may be more important in caesarean decisions than current fees.[32]

Other Western Systems

By comparison, Western Europe, notably Germany and England, had government involvement in financing health services much earlier than did the United States. In 1883, Chancellor Otto von Bismarck achieved passage of a social insurance scheme, including a health services component, for certain working-class Germans. In 1911, England adopted a national health insurance program, and in 1948, the United Kingdom established the National Health Service, which included government ownership of the health services system. Generally, Western European and Canadian healthcare systems have much more governmental control and financing than does the United States.

It is noteworthy that in the past, many of these countries experienced inflation in health services costs similar to that in the United States, despite greater government involvement in planning and financing. However, since about 1985, U.S. increases have been much higher than those in all other countries.[33] Countries whose public budgets allocate expenditures for health services prospectively spend substantially less than does the United States. In 2004, as a percentage of GDP, the United States spent 15.3% ($6,100 per capita), Germany spent 10.9% ($3,005 per capita), Canada spent 9.9% ($3,165 per capita), and the United Kingdom spent 8.3% ($2,545 per capita).[34] One reason for this difference is that the United Kingdom and Canada spend much less on technology. Furthermore, elective and nonemergent procedures may be available only after long waiting periods, known as *queues*.

An important difference in expenditures for health in various countries is the source of funds. In 2000, public sources in the United States accounted for spending of 5.8% of GDP. This is virtually identical to public spending in Italy, Japan, and the United Kingdom (5.9% each) and very similar to that in Canada (6.5%). It is the private health funding that distinguishes these comparison countries from the United States. In 2000, private health spending as a percentage of total health spending was 26.3% in Italy, 23.3% in Japan, and 19.0% in the United Kingdom. In the United States, however, private spending for health was 55.7%.[35]

Structure of the Health Services System

Various types of HSOs are found in the private (owned by individuals or groups) and public (owned by government) sectors. HSOs may be institutions—the most important and numerous are hospitals and nursing facilities—or they may be agencies and programs such as public health departments and visiting nurse associations. Information about selected HSOs is found in Chapter 2. Various HSOs are aggregated into health systems for greater efficiency and to provide a seamless web of services.

In this regard, they are orienting their activities toward the health of populations and communities. HSOs depend on their environments (see Figure 5.8). The range of health services delivery and various providers is shown in Figure 1.4.

One way HSOs/HSs can improve their focus on populations and communities is to develop community care networks, which have the following objectives: increasing access and coverage, enhancing accountability to the community, imbuing the healthcare system with a community health focus, improving coordination among the many parts of the healthcare system, and using healthcare resources more efficiently. Participants include insurers, business alliances, schools, churches, social services agencies, public health departments, local governments, and community-based organizations, in addition to health systems, hospitals, clinics, and physician groups. An estimated 26% of hospitals participated in community care networks in the late 1990s.[36]

Health departments can and should take a leading role in coordinating disparate providers and minimizing political and competitive issues to deliver integrated and comprehensive health services to the community.[37] Delivery of integrated services is discussed in Chapter 2, and community health information networks are discussed in Chapter 3.

Preventive care is an essential part of meeting the needs of a population. It comprises two parts, education and prevention. Health education is a long-standing part of general education in elementary and high schools. It is part of health services delivery, too. Prevention has three parts: primary, secondary, and tertiary. Primary prevention is prevention of disease or injury. Examples include improved design of roadways, school education programs about tobacco use and substance abuse, and immunizing against poliomyelitis or measles. Secondary prevention slows or blocks progression of a disease or injury from an impairment to a disability. Using the Papanicolaou smear (Pap test) to identify early cellular changes that are precursors of cervical cancer is a type of secondary prevention. If impairment has already occurred, disability (or death) may be prevented through early intervention. Treating certain streptococcal infections with penicillin can prevent the occasional development of rheumatic fever and serious heart disease. Early detection and treatment of high blood pressure reduces the probability of heart attack or stroke. Tertiary prevention blocks or retards progression of a disability to a state of dependence. Early detection and effective management of diabetes can prevent some dependencies associated with the disease, or at least slow progression. Prompt medical care followed by rehabilitation can limit damage caused by a cerebrovascular accident (stroke); damage from heart attacks can be limited in the same way. Good vehicular design can reduce the dependency that might otherwise result from an accident.[38] HSOs such as state and local public health departments have programs at all three levels of prevention. Hospitals and nursing facilities are more likely to engage in secondary and tertiary prevention than primary prevention.

Figure 1.4 shows that primary care is delivered in various settings—most common are physicians' offices, clinics, and the outpatient units of acute care hospitals. Primary care is routine care; part of its work is primary prevention, but primary care may also be part of secondary and tertiary prevention.[39] In addition, acute care hospitals provide secondary and tertiary acute care services through emergency treatment and inpatient services. Restorative care (rehabilitation) may be provided in acute care hospitals. It is also available in specialized hospitals, nursing facilities, and in the home through home healthcare. Continuing care is available in settings such as the home, nursing facilities, and hospice.

Holistic, alternative, and complementary medicine are similar concepts that greatly broaden the theories about disease prevention, causation, and treatment. They focus on nontraditional medicine, with special emphasis on self-help and on interventions less dramatic than chemicals and surgery, and they stress health promotion and prevention. Such measures are, increasingly, adjuncts to allopathy—traditional Western medicine that emphasizes dramatic interventions such as chemicals and surgery to return the body to normal functioning.[40] Use of nontraditional medicine will significantly affect HSOs, physician (allopathic) practice, and healthcare financing. It is likely that using alternative sources will only shift where payment is made and not reduce costs to the system. In fact, costs may

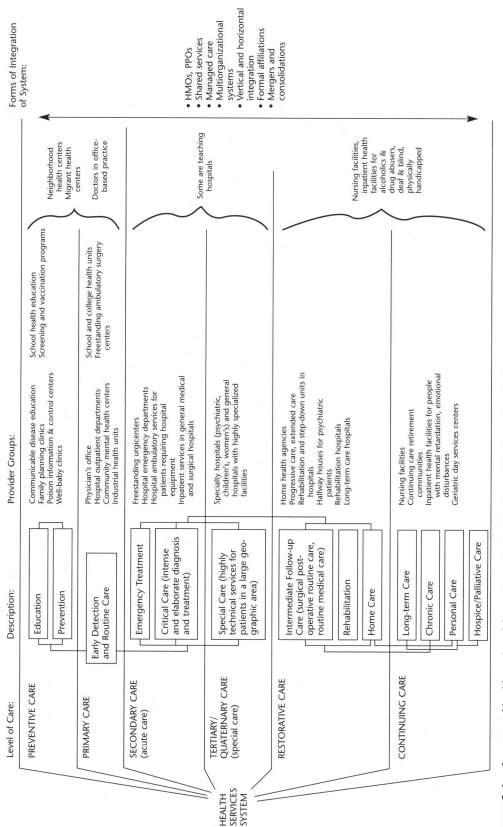

Figure 1.4. Spectrum of health services delivery. (From Cambridge Research Institute. *Trends Affecting the U.S. Health Care System* [Health Planning Information Series], 262. Washington, DC: Human Resources Administration, 1976. Revised and updated by the authors, 2008.)

Level of Care:

Description:

Provider Groups:

Forms of Integration of System:

PREVENTIVE CARE

Education

Prevention

Communicable disease education
Family planning clinics
Poison information & control centers
Well-baby clinics

School health education
Screening and vaccination programs

Neighborhood health centers
Migrant health centers

PRIMARY CARE

Early Detection and Routine Care

Physician's office
Hospital outpatient departments
Community mental health centers
Industrial health units

School and college health units
Freestanding ambulatory surgery centers

Doctors in office-based practice

SECONDARY CARE (acute care)

Emergency Treatment

Critical Care (intense and elaborate diagnosis and treatment)

Freestanding urgicenters
Hospital emergency departments
Hospital ambulatory services for patients requiring hospital equipment
Inpatient services in general medical and surgical hospitals

Some are teaching hospitals

TERTIARY/ QUATERNARY CARE (special care)

Special Care (highly technical services for patients in a large geographic area)

Specialty hospitals (psychiatric, children's, women's) and general hospitals with highly specialized facilities

RESTORATIVE CARE

Intermediate Follow-up Care (surgical post-operative routine care, routine medical care)

Rehabilitation

Home Care

Home health agencies
Progressive care, extended care
Rehabilitation and step-down units in hospitals
Halfway houses for psychiatric patients
Rehabilitation hospitals
Long-term care hospitals

CONTINUING CARE

Long-term Care

Chronic Care

Personal Care

Hospice/Palliative Care

Nursing facilities
Continuing care retirement communities
Inpatient health facilities for people with mental retardation, emotional disturbances
Geriatric day services centers

Nursing facilities, inpatient health facilities for alcoholics & drug abusers, deaf & blind, physically handicapped

HEALTH SERVICES SYSTEM

• HMOs, PPOs
• Shared services
• Managed care
• Multiorganizational systems
• Vertical and horizontal integration
• Formal affiliations
• Mergers and consolidations

increase, at least in proportion to increases in the alternate sources of care. Issues of third-party coverage and payment and effects on total costs and delivery of care are only beginning to be addressed.

Most physician-patient interactions occur in physician offices. In 2003, over 900 million physician-patient interactions occurred in physicians' offices; another 114 million occurred in hospital outpatient clinics, emergency departments (EDs), and other hospital locations.[41] Despite increasing numbers of physicians employed by HSOs, most physicians remain self-employed entrepreneurs who may share a receptionist, billing services, patient coverage, and perhaps diagnostic equipment with other physicians, or they may be in a partnership or may be "employees" of a physician (professional) corporation such as a multi- or single-specialty group practice. A physician office practice is not considered an HSO unless it is part of a clinic or group practice.

▬ Classification and Types of HSOs

PROFIT OR NOT FOR PROFIT

HSOs/HSs may be classified as profit seeking (for profit or investor owned) or not for profit. The former pay the owners (investors) a return on investment. In the latter, any excess of income over expense is not available to any person or corporation and is used by the HSO/HS to enhance the content or quality of health services or to reduce charges. Government-sponsored HSOs/HSs are not for profit, even though they are publicly owned, while privately owned corporations may be for profit or not for profit.

For-profit and not-for-profit HSOs/HSs can be converted to the opposite status. This is done for tax and other strategic reasons. Conversion of for-profit HSOs/HSs to not-for-profit status typically results in provision of more uncompensated care in the service areas, but it simultaneously decreases property tax revenue to local jurisdictions. Conversely, changing not-for-profit HSOs/HSs to for-profit status raises issues such as valuation of assets, charitable mission, private inurement, and the mission and activities of the charitable foundation usually established with proceeds of the sale.

OWNERSHIP

Another way to classify HSOs/HSs is by ownership. In addition to being privately owned, as are groups that are sectarian or nonsectarian and not for profit or investor owned, many HSOs/HSs are owned by a government (public) entity. Government-owned hospitals are classified as not for profit. Cities or counties establish, fund, and control public health departments. They also own acute care hospitals, some of which are financed by special tax entities. HSOs/HSs owned by state governments include health departments and psychiatric hospitals or HSOs for people with mental disabilities. Many states own academic health (medical) centers, which are often university-affiliated teaching hospitals that treat acute illness, conduct research, and educate those in the health occupations.

Federal government has a long history of involvement in financing. To a lesser extent, it has delivered preventive, acute, and long-term health services to special groups. U.S. Public Health Service (USPHS) hospitals were established in the late 18th century to care for merchant seamen. USPHS hospitals that treated general acute care patients operated until 1981, when the few remaining hospitals closed or were converted to other uses. The only facility in the United States devoted to Hansen's disease (leprosy) is the National Hansen's Disease Clinical Center at the Ochsner Medical Center in Baton Rouge, LA.[42]

In 2007, the Indian Health Service, an agency of the Department of Health and Human Services (DHHS), operated 33 hospitals, 54 health centers, and 38 health stations. In addition, through self-determination contracts, American Indian and Alaska Native corporations administer 15 hospitals, 229 health centers, 116 health stations, and 162 Alaska village clinics.[43]

In 2006, DVA operated 156 medical centers (hospitals), 877 outpatient clinics, 136 nursing homes, 43 residential rehabilitation treatment programs, 207 readjustment counseling centers, 57 veterans benefits regional offices, and 122 national cemeteries.[44] In addition, acute care hospitals and clinics operated by the U.S. Army, Navy, and Air Force serve active-duty and retired military personnel and their dependents.

LENGTH OF PATIENT STAY

A third way to classify HSOs is by the length of time care is provided. A general dichotomy divides HSOs by whether services are provided to inpatients—those treated 24 hours or longer—or to outpatients—those treated for less than 24 hours. Outpatient (ambulatory) services are provided in hospital EDs and clinics, physicians' offices, and freestanding HSOs such as surgery centers and imaging centers. Home health services are a unique blend of inpatient and outpatient services because care is provided in patients' homes over months or years. Hospice care is also a blend of inpatient care and care delivered in patients' homes. Hospice is available to the terminally ill—typically those who have less than 6 months to live. Chapter 2 discusses several types of HSOs in detail.

HSOs that provide inpatient care are divided into short term (acute) and long term. The American Hospital Association (AHA) defines a short-term hospital as one in which the average length of stay (ALOS) is less than 30 days; a long-term hospital has patient stays that average 30 days or longer. The ALOS in community (short-term [acute care]) hospitals has declined steadily from 7.6 days in 1981 to 5.6 days in 2005.[45]

In the continuum of care measured by length of stay (LOS), long-term care hospitals (LTCHs) are sited between acute care hospitals and nursing facilities. LTCHs provide extended medical and rehabilitative services to patients who are clinically complex because of multiple acute or chronic conditions. Federal regulations define LTCHs as hospitals whose ALOS is greater than 25 days.[46]

Further along the LOS continuum are nursing facilities (NFs). NFs typically treat only inpatients, who are known as residents. Some rehabilitation services may be provided, but the level of care provided is typically custodial. The LOS in an NF is measured in months or years.

ROLE IN THE HEALTH SERVICES SYSTEM

A fourth way to classify HSOs/HSs is by their role in delivery of services. Health or health-related services may be provided in public health department screening programs, in family planning and substance abuse treatment centers, or through sanitation efforts that protect food and water. There are thousands of privately and publicly owned and operated emergency medical units, such as rescue squads and ambulance services, often organized into emergency medical services systems. In addition, there are programs more oriented to social welfare activities; some only raise funds, others deliver specialized services. Depending on their activities, they may or may not be considered HSOs. The total number of HSOs in the United States is in the tens of thousands; Chapter 2 describes the history, numbers, functions, and organization of several types.

UNIQUE INSTITUTIONAL PROVIDERS

In addition to inpatient HSOs such as hospitals and nursing facilities, many other types of inpatient facilities provide health and health-related services. Data about them are sparse. They include residential facilities or schools for special groups such as blind or deaf people, people with emotional or physical disabilities, people with mental disabilities, dependent children, unwed mothers, alcoholics, drug abusers, and people with multiple physical and mental disorders.

In 2005, for example, there were 100,650 individuals with intellectual disabilities, developmental disabilities, or both who received training and support in 6,441 facilities;[47] this is a substantial decline in the number of similar individuals and facilities reported 2 decades earlier.[48] Privately operated facilities numbered 5,492, accounted for 85% of all facilities, and served 69% of clients. Thirty-one percent of clients resided in 937 state-owned/operated facilities. A few clients were served by city-, county-, or town-based facilities. The trend has been away from care in large state-run institutions toward smaller, privately operated facilities with fewer than 15 beds.[49]

Community services may reduce the need for long-term inpatient care for patients of all types. Examples of community services include diagnostic and evaluation clinics, day care centers, early childhood education facilities, rehabilitation programs, and summer camps and recreational facilities. All offer alternatives to institutional placement. Community-sponsored educational services are provided by local school districts directed by state special education programs. Developmental disability programs are typically operated at local levels with state funding.

MENTAL HEALTH ORGANIZATIONS

Mental health organizations are defined as HSOs that primarily provide mental health services to people with mental illness or emotional disturbances. Included are public or private psychiatric hospitals, psychiatric services in general acute care hospitals, outpatient psychiatric clinics, and mental health day/night facilities. Since 1955, the locus of delivering mental health services has changed remarkably. In the mid-1950s, state and county mental hospitals accounted for 77% of inpatient services; 23% were outpatient. By 1975, a reversal had occurred and 76% of mental health services were outpatient.[50] Inpatient treatment continues to be a major type of care. There were 3,319 inpatient and residential mental health organizations with more than 211,000 beds in 2002.[51]

TEACHING HOSPITALS

In 2006, 500 hospitals participated in graduate medical education, as defined by the Council of Teaching Hospitals and Health Systems,[52] a decline of 800 since 1990.[53] They fall under the general rubric of teaching hospital and offer a wide range of secondary, tertiary, and some quaternary medical services. These 500, plus a large number of other hospitals, participate in training a wide variety of students in the health occupations. Many teaching hospitals are part of a medical center complex that includes a medical school. Those having no medical school are likely affiliated with one. Prominence in medical education, plus their research and resulting publications in the medical and scientific literature, make teaching hospitals a vital resource in healthcare.

A unique HSO that fits into more than one of the categories described earlier merits special mention. The premier institution among all HSOs is the academic health (medical) center hospital, which is a subset of teaching hospitals. An academic health center hospital is one in which a majority of the chiefs of service at the hospital chair the academic departments in a medical school. In 2007, there were 133 academic health center hospitals.[54]

▓ Local, State, and Federal Regulation of HSOs/HSs ▓▓▓▓▓▓▓▓

When the original states delegated specific powers to a national government and ratified the U.S. Constitution, they retained a wide range of authority traditionally held by the sovereign. These are known as the *police powers,* generally defined as the authority to protect the public's health, safety, order, and welfare. State laws and regulations implement the police powers, many of which may be delegated to, or shared with, local governments. It is common for state departments of health to regulate licensure of HSOs, for example. The typical regulatory authority delegated to local governments, reflected in city and county ordinances and exercised by local health departments, includes food, fire, radiation, and environmental safety; air and water quality; waste and trash disposal; sanitation and pest control; and workplace hazards. These areas affect HSOs.

LICENSURE AND REGULATION

HSOs/HSs are subject to state laws and local ordinances, an important dimension of which is the group of inspections linked to licensure for specific types of HSOs. States may accept accreditation by a private organization in lieu of some types of regulation. For example, accreditation by The Joint Commission on Accreditation of Healthcare Organizations (The Joint Commission) is recognized for hospital licensure by 48 states. Similarly, many states recognize The Joint Commission's accreditation throughout the range of its accreditation programs.[55]

State and local government regulation focuses on physical plant and safety and pays scant attention to clinical quality issues in patient care. The *Fire Prevention Code, National Fuel Gas Code, National Electrical Code,* and *Life Safety Code* published by the National Fire Protection Association, an international, not-for-profit organization, are prominent sources of environmental standards used by state and local government in regulating HSOs.[56]

CONDITIONS OF PARTICIPATION

The 1965 Medicare law (1965 amendments to the Social Security Act of 1935) stated that Joint Commission–accredited hospitals were in "deemed" status (eligible) for purposes of reimbursement. In response to concerns about delegating government authority to a private group, the DHHS promulgated the "conditions of participation" (COPs) in 1966.[57] Federal legislation in 1972 mandated oversight of Joint Commission accreditation and review of accredited hospitals on the basis of random sampling or complaints. Originally, COPs emphasized physical plant and safety (e.g., the *Life Safety Code*) and minimized attention to the content and processes of clinical practice and organization; The Joint Commission emphases were the opposite. The two programs have evolved toward each other; COPs changed the most. Private accrediting groups such as the Community Health Accreditation Program (CHAP) and American Osteopathic Association (AOA) have achieved "deemed" status as well. HSOs not in "deemed" status must meet the applicable COPs if they are to receive payments from federal programs.

PLANNING AND RATE REGULATION

Much of what happens in the states is stimulated by federal government, and because hospitals consume disproportionate resources, policy makers have given them a great deal of attention. The Hill-Burton Act of 1946 included statewide planning for hospital services. The Comprehensive Health Planning and Public Health Service Amendments Act of 1966[58] encouraged use of planning methodologies to allocate resources, improve access, and contain costs. In the late 1960s, states began enacting laws to control health services costs. A special concern was Medicaid, whose funding they shared. The laws used rate review to control capital expenditures and costs of health services. New York and Maryland were among the first to enact capital expenditure review. Other states were prompted by the Social Security Amendments of 1972 (PL 92-603),[59] which established PSROs to review the quantity and quality of care for Medicare patients in hospitals. PSROs complemented the planning laws by controlling use of health services to reduce costs. Section 1122 required capital expenditure review to enhance planning agency control.

The National Health Planning and Resources Development Act of 1974 (PL 93-641)[60] required states to establish a health planning and development agency and a network of health systems agencies (HSAs). HSAs superseded the areawide health planning agencies ("b" agencies) required by the

1966 law. Planning laws sought to control costs by focusing on the supply of services. CON (certificate of need) laws required HSOs/HSs to have approval for a new service or construction or a renovation project exceeding a certain cost, usually several hundred thousand dollars. The purpose was to ration the supply of health services by controlling capital expenditures and preventing unneeded expansion. Critics of CON argued that this artificial limitation on the supply of services caused inflation. In the late 1970s, criticism about the usefulness of mandated planning grew. The antiregulatory mood in health services fit with the movement toward deregulation elsewhere in the economy. In 1987, the National Health Planning and Resources Development Act was repealed.[61] In the years since, states have scaled back their involvement in planning. In 2007, the District of Columbia and 35 states had CON laws; Maine's were the most restrictive, with review of 25 types of services. Ohio's were the least restrictive, with a review of only 2 types of service.[62]

In addition to CON, states began enacting health services rate review (cost review) laws. By 1983, mandatory programs had been enacted in six states,[63] and there were more than 20 voluntary programs. By regulating how much HSOs (primarily hospitals) charged or were paid, the states were treating them as public utilities. States with rates of increase in health services costs below the national average were exempt from the federal DRG system for Medicare patients. In the mid-1980s, exempt states included New York, New Jersey, Maryland, and Massachusetts.[64] By 2008, only Maryland was exempt. Since 1971, Maryland has had a highly regulated, all-payer system to pay for hospital-based inpatient and outpatient care. The system allows only limited discounts; this inhibits Maryland hospitals' ability to compete, especially in border areas.

UR, PSROs, AND PROs[65]

Utilization review (UR) was a mandated part of hospital participation in the original Medicare law. Hospitals had to certify the necessity of admission, continued stay, and professional services rendered to Medicare beneficiaries. Review was delegated to hospitals. Rapid Medicare cost increases in the late 1960s showed that hospital-based UR was ineffective. Consequently, PSROs were mandated by the Social Security Amendments of 1972 (PL 92-603)[66] as federally funded physician organizations responsible for ensuring the appropriateness, medical necessity, and quality of care furnished to Medicare beneficiaries. As with UR, emphasis in the PSRO program was on hospital review. The three functions of PSRO were admission and continued-stay review, quality assurance, and profile analysis (patterns of care).

Ten years later, PSROs had neither proved cost effective nor significantly improved quality. As a remedy, Congress established professional review organizations (PROs) as part of the Tax Equity and Fiscal Responsibility Act of 1982.[67] PROs were outcome rather than process and structure oriented, and outcomes were measured against performance standards. The core of PRO activities was to deny Medicare payment for medically unnecessary care, care rendered in an inappropriate setting, or care of substandard quality. PROs also educated problem providers, reviewed 100% of problem cases, and exerted peer pressure, and if correction was not achieved or if a gross and flagrant quality problem occurred, PROs recommended excluding the provider from Medicare.

Since the inception of PROs, their work has expanded to include all federal payments for medical services, including those in physicians' offices. A major initiative in the early 1990s was implementing a uniform clinical data set that enabled PROs to consistently select cases that required review. This database allowed epidemiological studies and inter-PRO comparisons. Critics of PROs have noted that few physicians and hospitals have been disciplined. The inspector general of the DHHS estimated that, beyond the few sanctions against providers, far more hospital admissions were inappropriate than were found by PROs.[68]

In 2001, PROs were officially renamed quality improvement organizations (QIOs). Like PROs, the QIOs provide their services under contract with the Centers for Medicare and Medicaid

Services (CMS), formerly the Health Care Financing Administration (HCFA), which is part of the DHHS. The name change is largely symbolic, however, and although QIOs have been charged with quality improvement initiatives in numerous clinical areas and across healthcare settings, there have been no published assessments of whether hospitals believe QIO interventions are improving the quality of care.[69] In 2007, there were 53 QIOs operational in the United States.[70]

Other Regulators of HSOs/HSs

In addition to the CMS, a multitude of federal regulators affect HSOs/HSs. Their activities are based on authority in the U.S. Constitution, as interpreted by the U.S. Supreme Court, to regulate interstate commerce and to provide for the general welfare. Regulators include independent agencies and various other executive branch departments and bureaus. The Department of Justice and the FTC enforce the Sherman Antitrust Act (1890)[71] and the Clayton Act (1914)[72] and their various amendments prohibiting anticompetitive practices. The National Labor Relations Board applies provisions of the National Labor Relations Act (1935)[73] and its amendments to the process of union organizing and collective bargaining. The Occupational Safety and Health Administration enforces provisions of the Occupational Safety and Health Act (1970)[74] to safeguard the work environment. The Food and Drug Administration enforces provisions of the Food, Drug, and Cosmetic Act of 1906[75] and its amendments and regulates drugs and medical devices. The Securities and Exchange Commission enforces the Securities Exchange Act of 1934, as amended,[76] and affects how investor-owned HSOs/HSs market, sell, and trade stock. The Nuclear Regulatory Commission enforces provisions of the Atomic Energy Act (1954)[77] and regulates and licenses the nuclear industry, thus regulating hazards arising from storage, handling, and transportation of radioactive materials. The Equal Employment Opportunity Commission enforces the Equal Pay Act of 1963,[78] Title VII of the Civil Rights Act of 1964,[79] and the Age Discrimination in Employment Act of 1967,[80] among others, and investigates complaints about treatment of employees and prospective employees. The Bureau of Alcohol, Tobacco, Firearms and Explosives of the Justice Department enforces the alcohol and tobacco tax provisions of the Internal Revenue Code[81] and the Alcohol Administration Act of 1935[82] and regulates the use of tax-free alcohol. It is noteworthy that many federal regulatory, review, and control activities have applied to HSOs only since the early 1970s.

Accreditation in Healthcare

ACCREDITORS OF HSOs/HSs

The Joint Commission on Accreditation of Healthcare Organizations

No voluntary, private organization has affected HSOs, especially hospitals, as has The Joint Commission. Its lineage can be traced to the "Hospital Standardization" program established by the American College of Surgeons (ACS), which began surveying hospitals in 1918. ACS single-handedly worked to improve hospital-based medical practice until 1951. Its director during most of its formative period was Malcolm T. MacEachern, a physician and health services leader, whose book, *Hospital Organization and Management*,[83] is a classic in the field. The Joint Commission was formed in 1951 and began accrediting hospitals in 1953. As noted earlier, accreditation became much more important with designation of "deemed" status in the 1965 Medicare law.

Since 1951, The Joint Commission has expanded its accreditation services far beyond hospitals. It accredits nine types of providers: ambulatory care, assisted living, behavioral healthcare, critical access hospitals, home care, hospitals, laboratory services, long-term care, and office-based surgery.[84] Accreditation of networks (MCOs, managed behavioral healthcare organizations, and preferred provider organizations) ended in 2006.[85] Each accreditation program has its own set of standards. Surveys of common standards such as physical plant, licensure, and corporate bylaws in multiprogram HSOs are combined to minimize duplication. Almost all hospitals are Joint Commission accredited. In 2006, there were 4,280 hospitals and 315 critical access hospitals accredited by The Joint Commission.[86]

The Joint Commission accreditation has the following benefits:

- Strengthens community confidence in the quality and safety of care, treatment, and service
- Provides a competitive edge in the marketplace
- Improves risk management and risk reduction
- Helps organize and strengthen patient safety efforts
- Provides education on good practice to improve business operations
- Provides professional advice and counsel, enhancing staff education
- Provides a customized, intensive process of review grounded in the unique mission of the organization
- Enhances staff recruitment and development
- Provides deeming authority for Medicare certification
- Is recognized by insurers and other third parties
- May reduce liability insurance costs
- Proves a framework for organizational structure and management
- May fulfill regulatory requirements in select states[87]

Accreditation by The Joint Commission establishes the HSO's community and professional credibility. HSOs that meet The Joint Commission's requirements for accreditation fulfill the standards for patient safety, provide education on good practice to improve business operations, and hold a competitive edge in the marketplace. These HSOs maintain a framework for organizational structure and management that improves quality of care and patient safety.

The Joint Commission will continue to be a major force in developing performance expectations for HSOs. Even those HSOs that choose not to be accredited by The Joint Commission will benefit from considering its standards in developing and managing their programs. The Joint Commission emphasizes outcomes and continuous quality improvement, the theory and application of which are described in Chapter 7. The Joint Commission will remain viable only if its standards are state of the art, if HSOs and the public value accreditation, and if the survey is worth the thousands of dollars that it costs. In their evolution, the COPs developed by CMS pose a substantial risk to the continued need for The Joint Commission. In addition, competing private specialty and programmatic accreditation efforts, several of which are described later, will almost certainly challenge The Joint Commission's preeminent position as "the" accrediting body.

American Osteopathic Association

Osteopathic hospitals may be accredited by the AOA as well as by The Joint Commission. AOA's Bureau of Healthcare Facilities Accreditation accredits acute care hospitals, mental health centers, substance abuse centers, and physical rehabilitation centers. CMS recognizes AOA accreditation as granting "deemed" status.[88] In 2006, AOA accredited 193 healthcare facilities.[89]

Community Health Accreditation Program

CHAP specializes in home care and community health. CHAP is a subsidiary of the National League for Nursing and began accreditation activities in 1965.[90] It accredits community nursing centers, home healthcare aide services, home health organizations, infusion therapy services, home medical equipment, hospice, private duty nursing, public health organizations, and supplemental staffing services.[91] CHAP confers "deemed" status for home health.[92] CHAP standards emphasize organizational structure and function; quality of services and products; adequacy of human, financial, and physical resources; and long-term viability.[93]

International Organization for Standardization

The International Organization for Standardization (ISO) in Geneva is a nongovernmental organization that was established in 1947. ISO is a worldwide federation of national standards bodies from 130 countries. Its work results in international agreements published as international standards, to the obvious benefit of consumers. ISO registers the organizations that meet its standards. Although it does not "accredit," as that term is generally used, ISO registration has a similar effect.

ISO 9000 and ISO 14000 are families of generic management system standards that focus on processes and not directly on the results of process activities, even though what happens in the process affects the outcome. This means that they can be applied to any organization in any sector of activity, including HSOs. ISO 9000 is concerned primarily with quality management, which means that the features of a product or of services conform to customer requirements. ISO 14000 is primarily concerned with environmental management, which is what an organization does to minimize harmful effects on the environment caused by its activities.[94] Organizations or components of organizations that seek certification or registration using ISO 9000 or ISO 14000 standards are surveyed by independent, ISO-qualified auditors, not by ISO representatives.[95] The certification or registration is not officially recognized by ISO, even though its standards are used. ISO does not accredit organizations or components of organizations against its standards, as does The Joint Commission. HSOs are beginning to use the ISO 9000 and ISO 14000 families of standards; Chapter 7 discusses their application.

National Committee for Quality Assurance

The National Committee for Quality Assurance (NCQA) began accrediting health plans in 1991. More than 500 of the nation's MCOs (covering 33% of all MCO enrollees) participate in NCQA's review of healthcare quality.[96] Of these, about 430 were accredited by NCQA in 2007.[97] In 1992, NCQA began developing the Health Plan Employer Data and Information Set, which is widely used by employers and HMOs in judging and comparing quality. As part of accreditation, NCQA requires health plans to submit audited results of clinical quality and consumer survey measures. Clinical quality includes childhood and adolescent immunization status, breast cancer and cervical cancer screening, advice to smokers to quit, and postpartum checkups. Examples of consumer survey measures are giving care quickly, having doctors who communicate, having courteous and helpful office staff, giving needed care, claims processing, and customer service. Most health plans offer several different types of products, such as a Medicare plan, a Medicaid plan, an HMO, and a point-of-service plan; NCQA reports on these products separately.[98]

EDUCATIONAL ACCREDITORS

The quality of didactic and clinical programs that educate health services professionals is ensured by various accreditors. Typically, accreditors have boards (policy-making bodies) composed of representatives from professional groups in their fields.

Managers

Programs for a master's level education of health services managers are accredited by the Commission on Accreditation of Healthcare Management Education (CAHME). The CAHME comprises representatives from professional associations in the healthcare field. In 2007, CAHME accredited 70 graduate programs in North America. Of those, 3 are in Canada.[99] The accreditation process is similar to The Joint Commission's.

The Council on Education for Public Health (CEPH) accredits schools of public health and graduate public health programs. CEPH is composed of representatives from various groups in public health. In 2007, CEPH accredited 39 graduate schools of public health and 69 graduate public health programs.[100]

Physicians

Medical school and postgraduate medical education are accredited by various groups, most of them connected to the American Medical Association (AMA). The Council for Medical Affairs provides policy development and review activities. The Liaison Committee on Medical Education, the Accreditation Council for Graduate Medical Education, and the Accreditation Council for Continuing Medical Education accredit various levels of medical training and education. Continuing medical education has received increasing emphasis.

Nurses

Since 1917, the National League for Nursing has been a strong force in nursing education.[101] The National League for Nursing Accrediting Commission (NLNAC) accredits registered nurse (RN) programs for master's, bachelor's, and associate's degrees and diplomas. In 2006, NLNAC accredited 1,191 of the 1,589 basic RN programs in the United States, including 259 baccalaureate, 617 associate, and 59 diploma programs.[102]

Medical Specialization

Medical specialization for allopathic physicians did not occur in the United States until the early 20th century. The American Board of Ophthalmology, incorporated in 1917, was the first certifying board; the American Board of Medical Genetics was approved in 1991. Each board offers at least one general certification of specialization; most recognize subspecialization. In 2007, the 24 specialty boards in allopathic medicine and surgery that were members of the American Board of Medical Specialties (ABMS) certified more than 130 specialties and subspecialties.[103] Specialty boards are vital in certifying training and in monitoring the continued competence of physicians in specialties. Through member boards, the ABMS is significant in undergraduate, postgraduate, and continuing medical education. Specialty boards include representatives of the associations organized for that specialty.

The Accreditation Council for Graduate Medical Education accredits residencies, but the content of residency education is largely determined by each medical specialty board's residency review committee. The Accreditation Council for Continuing Medical Education accredits the continuing medical education programs required by specialty boards for continued certification. The most recent iteration of medical specialty recertification is known as *maintenance of certification*. Developed by ABMS and the member boards, maintenance of certification is a program of continuous professional development that is used as a formal means of measuring a physician's continuing competency in a specialty or subspecialty.[104] About 90% of licensed physicians are board certified by an ABMS board.[105]

HSOs and HSs must be vigilant about board certification. There are scores of self-designated medical specialty boards with no ABMS recognition. Some states have sought to protect the public by regulating use of the terms *board certification* and *board certified*.[106] A proliferation of "boards" diminishes the public's ability to identify practitioners who have earned significant, accepted formal recognition of skills in a specialty.

Neither licensure nor board certification entitles a physician to clinical privileges in an HSO. Licensure is more basic—lawful medical practice is impossible without it; specialty certification is only one indicator of competence. The HSO has an independent ethical and legal duty to determine competence initially and to continually monitor the care delivered in it by licensed independent practitioners, whether or not they are board certified. The credentialing process is detailed in Chapter 2.

Education and Regulation of Health Services Managers

EDUCATION

Hospital administration was identified as a distinct educational discipline when the University of Chicago established the first professional master's program in 1934. This followed founding of the American College of Hospital Administrators, now the American College of Healthcare Executives (ACHE) in 1933. Graduate and undergraduate programs exist or are being developed worldwide. It is estimated that North American master's programs have more than 40,000 graduates.

To meet the demands of a complex environment, education for health services managers is eclectic, with an emphasis on generic management education. Some programs offer specialty preparation in hospital, nursing facility, or ambulatory services management. The didactic portion for accredited programs is at least 2 academic years, or 4 semesters. A field experience requirement is common; some programs require a 1-year, full-time residency to allow application of the academic preparation under the guidance of an on-site preceptor.

The curricula of accredited master's programs must include areas such as epidemiology; health policy; organizational development and behavior; human resources; information systems; legal principles; governance; written, verbal, and interpersonal skills; quantitative methods; financial management; economics; marketing; ethics; strategy formulation and implementation; and quality improvement.[107] Professional master's programs in health services management use various titles and are found in a number of different academic settings.

As with graduate programs, rapid growth in the number of undergraduate programs that prepare health services management personnel occurred in the late 1960s and early 1970s. There are 61 undergraduate programs affiliated with the Association of University Programs in Health Administration.[108] There are scores of other programs in the United States, in addition to which there are health services curricula of various types. Foci of the two levels of education are different. Master's programs prepare graduates to become senior-level line or staff managers; baccalaureate programs train supervisors or department managers. Coordinating graduate and undergraduate programs is a continuing challenge.

REGULATION

In 2007, no state required licenses for hospital administrators; all states licensed nursing facility administrators. Managers in other types of HSOs/HSs are rarely licensed. Regulation occurs when problems in an industry show that self-regulation and self-discipline have been ineffective.

Health Services Workers

In 2007, almost 13 million people were employed by healthcare providers such as ambulatory healthcare services, physicians' offices, outpatient care centers, home health services, hospitals, residential care facilities, and nursing facilities.[109] Table 1.2 shows the numbers in healthcare practitioner and technical occupations in the United States in 2006. Most individuals in the occupations listed are employed by healthcare providers and are counted in the 13 million noted above. Some, however, such as physicians, dentists, optometrists, and podiatrists, are predominantly self-employed or employed by organizations owned or controlled by them. To be meaningful, time series comparisons of the numbers in various healthcare occupations should use ratios of their numbers compared with the U.S. population. Ratios do not take into consideration maldistribution of health-

TABLE 1.2.   NUMBERS OF HEALTHCARE PRACTITIONER AND TECHNICAL OCCUPATIONS
              (U.S., 2005)

	No.	U.S. No./100,000 population** 2005 Population: 296,507,061
Professional Specialty		
Physicians*	817,500	275.7
Dentists	96,350	32.5
Optometrists	24,220	8.2
Pharmacists	239,920	80.9
Podiatrists	9,020	3.0
Registered nurses	2,417,150	815.2
Social workers	61,270	20.7
Physical therapists	156,100	52.6
Respiratory therapists	99,330	33.5
Occupational therapists	88,570	29.9
Speech-language pathologists and audiologists	109,600	37.0
Dietitians and nutritionists	51,230	17.3
Service		
Nursing assistants and psychiatric aides	1,433,660	483.5
Home health aides	751,480	253.4
Medical assistants	409,570	138.1
Dental assistants	277,040	93.4
Physical therapy assistants	59,350	20.0
Technicians		
Licensed practical nurses	720,380	243.0
Clinical lab technologists and technicians	305,470	103.0
Radiologic technologists	190,180	64.1
Dental hygienists	166,380	56.1
Health information technicians	164,700	55.5
Psychiatric technicians	58,940	19.9
Surgical technologists	84,330	28.4
Emergency medical technicians	196,190	66.2
Dispensing opticians	65,190	22.0

Source: Occupational Employment and Wages, May 2006: Healthcare Practitioner and Technical Occupations. Bureau of Labor: U.S. Department of Labor. http://www.bls.gov/oes/current/oes_nat .htm#b29-0000. Retrieved August 20, 2007.

*Current Physician Workforce October 2006. Health Research and Services Administration Bureau of Health Professions. ftp://ftp.hrsa.gov/bhpr/workforce/PhysicianForecastingPaperfinal.pdf. Retrieved August 29, 2007. The number of physicians is defined as the number of active physicians under the age of 75.

**Annual Population Estimates 2000 to 2006. U.S. Census Bureau. http://www.census.gov/popest/ states/NST-ann-est.html. Retrieved August 29, 2007.

care providers, who tend to be concentrated in metropolitan and urban areas even to the point of surplus. The result is that rural and less populated areas are underserved.

Physician and nonphysician clinicians who may independently treat patients are known as licensed independent practitioners (LIPs). Regulation and education of LIPs are discussed later in this chapter. Many types of LIPs are likely to be competitors because they provide similar or overlapping services, which has largely unknown implications for the cost of health services. Quality and productivity are less of an issue, however. For example, nurse practitioners (NPs) and physician assistants (PAs) provide care of equivalent quality as they perform many of the tasks of primary care physicians.[110]

Most physicians and many other types of LIPs are self-employed private entrepreneurs, even though employment may provide a portion of their incomes. In contrast, non-LIPs, or dependent caregivers, are employed in the practices of LIPs or in HSOs such as nursing facilities or hospitals. Physicians in residencies are usually employed by their residency sites; their training status makes them unique and unlike employed physicians, however. These relationships are part of the context for human resources issues in HSOs/HSs.

PHYSICIANS

Allopathic medicine—the profession of the medical doctor (MD)—traces its lineage to Hippocrates (460–377 B.C.). It emerged as the dominant theory of treating disease at the beginning of the 20th century. As noted earlier, allopathy holds that interruptions of the body's normal functioning must be treated with significant interventions to restore normal bodily functioning (health). Development of the germ theory of disease causation and increasingly efficacious surgery in the late 19th century gave allopathy a scientific basis, which secured its place and dominance in Western medical practice. The increase in effective chemical therapies early in the 20th century enhanced its stature, as did the scientific knowledge developed throughout the 20th century.

Major competing theories of disease causation and cure in the mid- to late 19th century were naturopathy, homeopathy, osteopathy, and chiropractic. After being relegated to the fringe of medical practice, naturopathy and homeopathy have had a revival of interest, though they remain far from medicine's mainstream. Osteopathy has largely merged with allopathy. Chiropractic is more accepted than at any time in its history; nevertheless, orthodox medicine still considers it a manipulative therapy with no clear scientific basis.

Osteopathy evolved from the bonesetters of England, who practiced the craft of repositioning dislocated collar bones, cartilages, and other skeletal structures—work spurned by orthodox medicine.[111] The philosophy and science of osteopathic medicine were first described in 1874 by Andrew Taylor Still, a physician who founded the American School of Osteopathy in 1892. Osteopaths are educated in osteopathic medical schools and earn the doctor of osteopathy (DO) in an education that emphasizes structure and functioning of the musculoskeletal system and an appreciation for the body's ability to heal itself when it is in its normal functional relationship and has a favorable environment and nutrition.[112] Osteopathic healthcare emphasizes manipulative methods of detecting and correcting structural problems, but it also utilizes generally accepted conventional medical and surgical treatment. Osteopathic medical training is similar to that of allopathic medicine, and in most respects, osteopaths are the same as allopaths. Many osteopaths enter allopathic residency training programs and are licensed under the same state statutes.

Chiropractic, an offshoot of osteopathy, emphasizes manipulation to correct anatomical faults that cause functional disturbances in the body. It is uniquely American. Daniel David Palmer established the first school of chiropractic medicine in Iowa in 1895. Palmer's theories stressed the importance of minor spinal displacements, or subluxations, as chiropractors later called them. Subluxations are less severe than dislocations but cause nerve irritation that leads to disturbances of the nervous system and eventually to illness. According to Palmer, medical orthodoxy's mistake is that it treats disorders without understanding the source—the spinal column—and chiropractic can remedy that problem.[113]

Physician Numbers

Table 1.2 shows the physician workforce in 2005. U.S. population growth to 2020 is projected to be 14%, which is almost the same as the projected growth rate for full-time equivalent physicians. This means that the ratio of physicians to 100,000 population will remain relatively constant.[114] Even with an adequate ratio, however, the major unresolved problem, as noted above, has and will almost certainly continue to be a maldistribution of physician resources.

Predictions of physician shortages or surpluses have caused federal support of medical education to wax and wane for several decades. In addition to federal and state government support, income from hospitals and clinics, nongovernmental grants and contracts, and endowment and philanthropy have been important revenue sources for medical schools. In 2005–2006, tuition and fees contributed only 3% of revenues in *both* public and private medical schools. For both, the largest contributions came from practice plans (34% and 41%, respectively), state and local governments (12% and 8%, respectively), hospital or medical school programs (12% and 12%, respectively), and federal research grants and contracts (23% and 25%, respectively).[115] Out-of-state tuition at some public medical schools, like tuition at some private (nongovernmental) medical schools, exceeds $40,000 per year.[116] In 2006, more than 103,000 residents were in Accreditation Council for Graduate Medical Education–accredited and combined special programs. Those residents included 68,267 U.S. medical graduates, 28,149 international medical graduates, 6,569 DOs, and 382 Canadian medical graduates.[117]

Historically, it was generally believed that a ratio of two thirds primary care physicians to one third specialists was desirable. In 1970, 40.9% of physicians were in primary care, defined by the AMA to include the general specialties of family medicine, general practice, internal medicine, obstetrics and gynecology, and pediatrics.[118] Federal legislation in the 1970s sought to redress the imbalance between primary care and specialists. Impetus was added to efforts to reduce emphasis on specialization when specialty societies and boards reconsidered the number of residencies to be offered in the various specialties. Third-party payers, including federal government, MCOs, and HMOs, also decided to de-emphasize specialists. Regardless, by 1996, only 34.0% of physicians were classified as primary care practitioners.[119] It was not until the late 1990s that efforts to increase the number of primary care physicians began to succeed. By 2003, 40.8% of physicians were in primary care, a percentage virtually identical to that in 1970.[120] Even as the ratio of primary care physicians increased, there were signs that specialists had become too few, however.

Driven by lack of attention to a need for specialists in delivery settings and by consumer demand for specialist services, the almost exclusive emphasis on primary care physicians subsided. Specialist physicians were once again in demand by the end of the 1990s.[121] Such cycles will recur as more private and public efforts are made to "manage" delivery of services and the uses and availability of various types of clinical providers. Focusing on numbers ignores the geographic maldistribution of physicians and nonphysician clinicians. It appears that the latter are no more interested in underserved areas—usually inner city and rural communities—than are physicians.[122]

NONPHYSICIAN CLINICIANS

Of concern, too, is that numbers of nonphysician caregivers will increase to meet needs. The 2004 National Sample Survey of Registered Nurses showed an increase—from 196,000 in 2000 to 240,461 in 2004—in nurses who had completed additional courses and training to become advanced practice nurses, such as clinical nurse specialists, nurse practitioners, nurse midwives, and nurse anesthetists.[123] The greatest growth is projected among nonphysician clinicians who provide primary care services, and the greatest concentration will occur in states that already have an abundance of physicians.[124]

This growth in nonphysician practitioners is occurring even as it is generally agreed that the United States has too few physicians. The Association of American Medical Colleges (AAMC) is seeking to increase medical school enrollment by 30% in the next 10 years.[125] As recently as the early 1990s, the AAMC projected a potential oversupply of physicians by the beginning of the third millennium. A physician shortage suggests potential problems for HSO/HS managers, while concomitantly creating opportunities.

Regulation and Education of Selected Health Occupations

LICENSURE, CERTIFICATION, AND REGISTRATION

Licensing of the healthcare occupations is ubiquitous. All states and the District of Columbia require physicians (MDs and DOs) and RNs, licensed practical (vocational) nurses (LPNs), and nurse practitioners to take licensing examinations after completing the appropriate educational programs at accredited educational institutions.[126] There is wide variation beyond these groups, however. The trend is toward greater regulation of the health occupations.[127] For example, the Omnibus Budget Reconciliation Act of 1987 (PL 100-203; commonly known as OBRA '87) required states to register nursing assistants.

Licensure, registration, and certification have important distinctions:

Licensure: Approval granted by government that allows someone to engage in an occupation after a finding that the applicant has achieved minimum competency. Licensing is a state function under the police powers. Physicians and dentists are always licensed, for example. Physicians and osteopaths are the only LIPs granted an unlimited license.

Registration: Listing of qualified individuals on an official roster maintained by a government or nongovernment body. States may require registration for someone to engage in a health occupation. If so, registration has the effect of licensure. Persons who are registered may use that designation. Registered nurses and registered dietitians are examples.

Certification: Process by which a nongovernment agency or association grants recognition to someone who meets its qualifications. States may require certification for someone to engage in a health occupation, thus giving certification the effect of licensure. Nurse-midwives are certified, for example.

In terms of regulation, nonphysician health services workers may generally be divided into two groups: LIPs, who are licensed to treat patients independently, and those who may or may not be licensed but who are dependent on an LIP's orders before they can deliver health services. Non-physician LIPs have state licenses that limit their practice to certain parts of the body or specific medical problems; optometrists, podiatrists, dentists, and chiropractors are examples. In many states, nurse midwives and some types of NPs are LIPs. Some states allow RNs without specialty training to perform specified examinations and procedures. Applying the general principle of independent-versus-dependent practice is complicated because acute care hospitals and many other types of HSOs further limit the scope of practice of health services workers (even of physicians) to clinical activities in which they have demonstrated current competence. Similarly, HSOs may limit the licenses of nonphysician LIPs to activities ordered or supervised by physicians.

Dependent caregivers may or may not be licensed, registered, or certified, but they provide services only on receiving an order from an LIP. Distinctions beyond this are blurred. Dependent caregivers include medical technologists, pharmacists, radiographers, LPNs, and nursing assistants. RNs and pharmacists use *registered* as a synonym for *licensed*. Dietitians are registered by a private association and are licensed or statutorily certified or registered in a number of states.[128]

Certification is a process of approval involving a professional association and oftentimes the AMA. Certificates are issued to those who pass an examination, the eligibility for which requires specified academic preparation. A confusing aspect of the process is that sometimes the certificate is issued by a body that uses the title *registry*. Often, a group of specialty physicians also certifies.

For example, the American Society of Clinical Pathologists certifies medical technologists through its board of registry.[129] Those who are unable to meet the private certifying group's standards are likely to be unemployable in HSOs; thus certification has the effect of licensure. Concomitantly, someone certified who does not continue to meet the group's standards loses certification, and employment is likely forfeited.

EDUCATION OF CLINICIANS

Physicians

The most important modern effort to improve allopathic medical education occurred in 1910 when Abraham Flexner's study of medical education in the United States detailed its weaknesses. As a result, the science curriculum was enhanced, the didactic portion was lengthened, and the clinical component was strengthened. Weak allopathic medical schools failed when they could not meet the more stringent standards.

In 1950 there were 79 U.S. allopathic medical schools, by 1970 there were 103, and by 1990 there were 126.[130] In 2006, there were 125 accredited allopathic medical schools[131] with 69,167 students[132] and 15,952 graduates.[133] Medical schools are accredited by the Liaison Committee on Medical Education, whose members include medical educators and administrators, practicing physicians, public members, and medical students.[134] In 2005, there were 119,000 faculty[135] involved in educating more than 170,000 medical students and residents.[136] In 2005, Canada's 16 accredited medical schools (none osteopathic) graduated 1,876 MDs.[137]

DOs are educated in 23 AOA-accredited colleges of osteopathic medicine, with 13,406 students in 2005. DOs may be board certified in 85 general medical specialties in addition to various subspecialties. In 2005 there were more than 52,000 DOs in the United States.[138]

Postgraduate Education. Following graduation from medical school with either a 4-year postbaccalaureate education or, less often, a 6- or 7-year combined baccalaureate-MD, the new allopathic physician begins a residency.

Historically, *intern* was a designation for medical school graduates who were in the first year of post-MD clinical training. *Resident* is the correct title, however; *intern* has not been used officially for allopaths in training since 1975.[139] Residents are designated by postgraduate year (PGY) or graduate year (GY). For example, a PGY-2 has had 1 year of clinical experience after medical school and is in the second. Clinical activities of residents are supervised by more senior residents, fellows (postresidency physicians in training), and teaching faculty (physicians) who have faculty appointments through a medical school or are active staff at the HSO, which is usually a hospital. Residencies are accredited by the Accreditation Council for Graduate Medical Education, which is composed of professional associations in the medical field.

Each specialty has a residency review committee that sets standards for specialty training and accredits the program. The specialty determines the number of PGYs and the specific clinical content of those years so that the program may be accredited and provide the basis for eligibility to be certified in that specialty. For example, anesthesiology requires 1 year of general residency, completion of an accredited anesthesiology residency, and at least 2 years in private practice;[140] family medicine requires 3 years of postgraduate training in an accredited family practice residency;[141] neurological surgery requires 1 year in an accredited general residency and 5 years of advanced specialty training in an accredited neurological surgery residency.[142]

In 2007, VA medical centers had affiliations with 107 of 125 allopathic medical schools and 15 of 25 osteopathic medical schools. Each year, about a third of the 100,000 U.S. medical residents rotate through a VA clinical training site. In addition, the VA has more than 5,000 affiliations with associated health professions training programs.[143] About 70% of VHA staff physicians have medical school faculty appointments, and about 10% of medical residents training in the United States are funded by the DVA.[144] It has been estimated that more than half of practicing physicians have received some part of their professional training in a DVA medical center.[145]

Licensure. U.S. and Canadian medical graduates are licensed in most states after passing the U.S. Medical Licensing Examination and completing 1 year of residency. Several states require 2 years of residency; a few require 3 years.[146] In addition, all states and the District of Columbia require physicians to complete continuing medical education credits to remain licensed.[147] State licenses are unlimited in terms of the medical activities that physicians may undertake. Thus, physicians may legally prescribe all medications (except some narcotics and experimental drugs) and perform all medical and surgical activities. It is only in HSOs that the scope of this otherwise unlimited right to practice medicine is modified.

Limiting practice activities to those consistent with demonstrated current competence is especially important in acute care hospitals because of the acuity of illnesses and the significant treatments provided. Protecting patients by ensuring the competence of physicians and other LIPs, such as podiatrists and clinical psychologists, is vital in all HSOs, however. Protection is achieved through the credentialing process, which includes a review of didactic and clinical experience, licensure, specialty certification, and health status, among other aspects. Periodic review of clinical performance is part of the recredentialing process that is necessary for the practitioner to continue to have privileges in an HSO. Credentialing and recredentialing are detailed in Chapter 2. State medical boards have been criticized for being insufficiently aggressive in disciplining physicians with problems related to their professional activities.[148] This continuing problem[149] is addressed further in Chapter 4.

Nonphysician Caregivers

Nowhere is there greater fragmentation and specialization of work than in HSOs. Apparently, each new technology requires a new category of technical expertise. In the early years of modern medicine, physicians usually worked without resort to other types of caregivers. Support became necessary, however, and some physician activities were performed by technicians. Nurses are the earliest example; sonographers are among the most recent.

Changes in staffing needs will continue as old technologies evolve and others are introduced. The use of roentgen rays (x-rays), which were discovered by Wilhelm Roentgen in 1895, is instructive. Roentgenology became radiology, which bifurcated into diagnostic radiology and therapeutic radiology. Diagnostic radiology has added computers, analysis of cellular emissions, and use of sound waves and has become known as diagnostic imaging. Similarly, therapeutic radiology now includes linear accelerators added to x-ray equipment, and use of radioactive sources spawned the specialty of nuclear medicine. Specialized staff are needed to deliver this state-of-the-art, high-technology medicine.

Podiatrists

Podiatrists are LIPs who provide services in offices, clinics, and hospitals. Podiatrists employed by HSOs or part of their attending staffs should be subject to a credentialing process; credentialing is required in hospitals.

Podiatry is the branch of the healing arts and sciences that treats the foot and its related or governing structures by medical, surgical, or other means. Applicants to the seven colleges of podiatric medicine in the United States should hold a baccalaureate, but exceptions are made. The first 2 years of instruction emphasize basic medical sciences, such as anatomy, physiology, microbiology, biochemistry, pharmacology, and pathology. The second 2 years emphasize clinical sciences, including general diagnosis, therapeutics, surgery, anesthesia, and operative podiatric medicine. Graduates are awarded the doctor of podiatric medicine degree. Most graduates complete a residency of 1 to 4 years. Podiatrists are licensed in all states. The American Podiatric Medical Association has approved two specialty boards; they certify in primary care and orthopedics, or in surgery.[150] Table 1.2 shows 9,020 active podiatrists in 2005.

Nurses

Early recognition and increased stature of nursing were achieved largely through the efforts of Florence Nightingale, an Englishwoman who worked to improve nursing in the mid-19th century. Until then, secular nursing had a poor reputation. Dorothea Dix was an early nursing leader and educator in the United States. As education and professional standards improved and licensing was introduced in the United States, RNs became second only to physicians in numbers and importance on the patient care team. Nurse licensing began in the early 1900s and initially concentrated on state registration. In 1903, North Carolina nurses were the first to establish state registration, and only those found qualified by a board of examiners could be listed as registered nurses in a county and use the designation *RN*. Voluntary licensure has been superseded by mandatory licensure.[151] RNs may be LIPs, depending on specialty preparation.

Of the 2.91 million licensed RNs in 2004, it was estimated that 2.4 million were employed in nursing. The largest source of employment is acute care hospitals (56.2%), followed by ambulatory care settings (11.5%), community/public health settings (10.7%), nursing home/extended care facilities (6.3%), and schools (3.2%). Other employment is in nursing education and other health education, insurance claims/benefits, and occupational health.[152]

RNs are educated in programs of varying length in various educational settings: baccalaureate (4 years, university based, leading to a bachelor of science in nursing [BSN]), diploma (3 years, hospital based, leading to a diploma in nursing), and associate's degree (2 years, junior or community college based, leading to an associate of arts [AA]). Graduates of all three programs may be licensed (registered) as RNs. BSN preparation is the gold standard and is preferred by organized nursing. It is considered a superior preparation in the practice setting.

LPNs, sometimes known as licensed vocational nurses, are another type of nurse and are found in all types of HSOs. Other nursing personnel widely found in nursing facilities and hospitals are nursing assistants (NAs), who are sometimes called nurse aides. NAs must be registered and may be certified. Certification is required by CMS for NAs working in nursing facilities; they are then certified nursing assistants (CNAs). LPNs and NAs are clinically and usually administratively subordinate to the RN. Table 1.2 shows more than 700,000 employed LPNs in 2005.

In the late 1970s, the American Nurses Association (ANA) began an RN certification program that became the American Nurses Credentialing Center. In 2007, RNs could take various certification examinations, depending on educational preparation. Advanced practice nurses (NPs, clinical nurse specialists, and those in other advanced practice specialties) must have a master's degree and can be certified in various specialties. RNs with bachelor's or associate's degrees or diplomas in nursing may take certification examinations in areas such as gerontology, pediatrics, perinatology, community/public health, and nursing administration.[153] The 11,000 RNs certified by ANA in 1982[154] increased to 77,000 by 1991[155] and to 135,000 by 2006.[156]

Most states have categories of caregivers who become RNs first and then prepare in a specialty. NPs, for example, have independent practice authority in 21 states.[157] Some types of independent practice nurses are certified by private associations (e.g., certified registered nurse anesthetists [CRNAs], certified nurse midwives [CNMs]). A majority of states allow CRNAs to administer anesthesia without a physician's supervision. Use of CRNAs will increase because Medicare regulations no longer require an anesthesiologist's supervision.[158] CNMs are licensed as RNs, certified by the American College of Nurse-Midwives, and licensed in almost half the states as nurse midwives. Advanced practice nurses generally include NPs, clinical nurse specialists (CNSs), CRNAs, and CNMs, who are likely to be credentialed by HSOs, either as a group or individually. Such providers are LIPs.

HSO managers will be challenged to recruit and retain RNs, as well as use RN resources effectively.[159] Productivity is addressed in Chapter 10.

Pharmacists

The pharmacist is a type of nonphysician caregiver commonly found in HSOs, and always in hospitals. The profession of pharmacist emerged later than nurse. Historically, the pharmacist's role in the spectrum of care was narrow and primarily limited to dispensing medications. Recently, hospital pharmacists have emerged as active members of the clinical care team, monitoring medication use as well as advising physicians in prescribing and nurses in administering medications. Pharmacists are educated in 89 accredited colleges of pharmacy in the United States. The baccalaureate in pharmacy has been replaced by the doctor of pharmacy, which is earned in a 6-year program that includes 2 years of college and 4 years in pharmacy college. State licensure requires graduating from an accredited program, completing a variety of experiences in practice settings under the supervision of licensed pharmacists, and passing a state board examination. Pharmacists are not LIPs and dispense medications only on the orders of LIPs such as physicians, podiatrists, and dentists.[160] Table 1.2 shows that there were 239,920 pharmacists in the United States in 2005.[161]

Dietitians

A type of nonphysician caregiver almost always found in hospitals and nursing facilities is the clinical or therapeutic dietitian, who plans therapeutic menus in consultation with a physician. Dietitians also provide nutritional counseling. Like pharmacists, dietitians emerged later than nurses, and their role is narrower. Historically, dietitians have been registered by the American Dietetic Association. In the mid-1980s, states began licensing or certifying dietitians. In 2006, there were 30 states and the District of Columbia that licensed; 13 states had statutory certification; and 1 state registered dietitians, nutritionists, or both.[162] Minimum preparation to become a registered dietitian includes a baccalaureate; completing a minimum of 900 supervised practice hours of professional experience; and passing a national, written exam administered by the Commission on Dietetic Registration.[163] Table 1.2 shows 51,230 employed dietitians and nutritionists in 2005.

Technologists

Radiologic technologists include radiographers, cardiovascular-interventional technologists, sonographers, radiation therapists, mammographers, nuclear medicine technologists, computerized tomography technologists, magnetic resonance imaging technologists, dosimetrists, and quality management technologists.[164] The titles reflect job responsibilities and the extent of specialization. Radiologic technologists are trained in 2-year academic or nonacademic programs or 4-year programs leading to a baccalaureate. They become registered by passing one of several national certifying examinations. Most states have specific licensing laws.[165] Table 1.2 shows 190,180 employed radiologic technologists in 2005.

More than half of clinical laboratory or medical technologists are employed in hospitals. Typically, they hold a baccalaureate in medical technology or one of the life sciences. They perform various laboratory tests and may specialize in clinical chemistry, blood bank technology, cytotechnology, hematology, histology, microbiology, or immunology. Training is offered by colleges, universities, and hospitals. Technologists are certified by various groups, including the Board of Registry of the American Society of Clinical Pathologists and the American Medical Technologists. Many states require medical technologists to be licensed or registered.[166] Table 1.2 shows 305,470 employed clinical laboratory technologists and technicians in 2005. Both radiologic technologists and medical technologists are dependent nonphysician caregivers because they have no independent access to patients and perform services only in response to an LIP's order.

Physician Assistants

Another type of dependent caregiver common to HSOs is the PA, the concept for which originated in the 1960s and was based on the military medic or corpsman. Typically, PAs are trained in a 2-year general medical (primary care) curriculum, approximately half of which is devoted to clinical rotations in a wide range of inpatient and outpatient settings. A number of programs award baccalaureates, and there is a trend to award master's degrees. In 2007, more than 130 accredited programs educated PAs.[167] Historically, PAs worked under the direction or supervision of a physician, who was accountable for their activities. The trend is for PAs to be more independent, as reflected by the fact that more states are regulating PAs, who may be licensed, registered, or certified. The National Commission on Certification of Physician Assistants awards a certification used by the states to regulate PAs.[168] In 2006, more than 60,000 PAs were in active practice in the United States. Almost half are in primary care; in addition, they may specialize in orthopedics, emergency medicine, and cardiology. Almost all states allow physicians to delegate the authority to write prescriptions to the PAs they supervise. Most PAs practice in ambulatory care settings. About 36% are employed by hospitals, many as house staff. The demand for PAs is expected to increase.[169]

▬ Associations for Individuals and Organizations ▬▬▬▬▬▬▬▬

The health services field has numerous professional and trade associations for personal and institutional providers, both in generic groups and in an increasing number of subsets.

PROFESSIONAL ASSOCIATIONS FOR INDIVIDUALS

Managers

With more than 30,000 affiliates, the ACHE is the leading professional association for HSO/HS managers. It was established in 1933 as the American College of Hospital Administrators. Important categories of affiliation are member, diplomate, and fellow, which are separated by time and achievement requirements, including years in category and passing an examination. ACHE offers continuing education programs and publishes and enforces a code of ethics.

The Medical Group Management Association (MGMA) was established in 1926. It has almost 21,000 members, including administrators, CEOs, physicians in management, office managers, and others who manage medical offices and ambulatory care organizations. MGMA promotes patient-focused care; sets standards of professional performance; supports continued learning for professional growth; and promotes evidence-based clinical and managerial decision making, physician and administrator teamwork, service to the community and profession, integrity, collegiality, and respect for the individual.[170]

Examples of other professional groups include those for specialized managerial personnel in HSOs: the Academy of Medical Group Management, the American College of Mental Health Administrators, the American College of Health Care Administrators (of nursing facilities), the National Association of Healthcare Executives, and the College of Osteopathic Healthcare Executives. Some groups have levels of affiliation and advancement requirements. All provide a forum and educational activities to improve the content and quality of professional practice. The American Public Health Association does not focus on managers but has a broad membership of those in public health and other types of HSOs.

Physicians

Preeminent among physician groups is the AMA, established in 1847. In 2007, the AMA had about 250,000 members,[171] including physicians, medical students, and residents. In 1998, it had 290,917.[172] The AMA is synonymous with "organized medicine"; it has been both a conservative and a progressive force in healthcare. Conservatism is exemplified by historical opposition to government-sponsored health insurance and by resistance to salaried physician arrangements and innovations such as HMOs, which were seen as infringing on professional independence and total commitment to patients. The AMA has been a progressive force by embracing programs such as Medicare (once enacted) and by encouraging federal expenditures for basic and applied research and medical and paramedical education. Its involvement in establishing standards for medical education and licensure has contributed significantly to the unequaled standards of American medicine. The AMA publishes and enforces a code of ethics.

There are many other associations for physicians. The National Medical Association represents more than 30,000 African American physicians and has goals similar to the AMA's.[173] In addition, medicine has numerous professional associations, called "colleges" or "academies," whose memberships are based on medical specialties. Among the most prominent are the American College of Physicians and the ACS. Affiliates are known as "fellow" or "diplomate." These associations represent the interests of affiliates and assist them in continuing education.

Nonphysician Providers

The list of associations for individuals is almost endless. Each new type of provider considers it necessary to have a professional association to focus common interests. Some are old; the ANA was established in 1896.[174] Other examples of nonphysician provider groups include the American Dental Association, the American Podiatry Association, the American Psychological Association, the Association of Operating Room Nurses, the National Association of Social Workers, the American Pharmaceutical Association, the National Federation of Licensed Practical Nurses, and the American Academy of Physician Assistants. The hundreds of professional associations for organizational and personal providers and managers suggest the level of specialization and fragmentation in the healthcare field.

ASSOCIATIONS FOR HSOs/HSs

American Hospital Association

With approximately 5,000 institutional members, the AHA is the most prominent association for hospitals.[175] Founded in 1898, AHA educates and represents its members. It is a focal point for hospital participation in the political process, a key element of which is lobbying federal government. In 1991, AHA's executive offices were moved to Washington, D.C. Other activities remain in Chicago.

Federation of American Health Systems

The Federation of American Health Systems (FAHS) is the investor-owned counterpart to AHA. Established in 1966, it had 1,100 members in 2007. It monitors health legislation, regulatory and reimbursement matters, and developments in the healthcare industry at the state and national levels. In addition, FAHS compiles statistics on the investor-owned hospital industry.[176]

Other Hospital Associations

The Catholic Health Association of the United States (CHA) represents a subset of hospitals with sectarian ownership and interests. CHA had over 2,000 members in 2007.[177] In addition to national hospital associations, there are regional and state hospital associations that link hospitals to geographical or state communities of interest. State hospital associations gained importance as states became more involved in regulating hospitals.

American Health Care Association

Founded in 1949, the American Health Care Association (AHCA) is a federation of 50 state health organizations that represent more than 10,000 not-for-profit and for-profit nursing, assisted-living, and subacute care providers. AHCA's objectives are to improve standards of service and administration of member nursing homes; to secure and merit public and official recognition and approval of the work of nursing homes; and to adopt and promote programs of education, legislation, better understanding, and mutual cooperation.[178]

American Association of Homes and Services for the Aging

The American Association of Homes and Services for the Aging (AAHSA) is the trade association of not-for-profit adult day services, home health services, community services, senior housing, assisted living residences, continuing care retirement communities, and nursing homes. It had 5,700 members in 2007.[179] AAHSA lobbies Congress and federal agencies on members' behalf; certifies practitioners and facilities; and offers conferences, programs, and publications. Members may participate in group purchasing and insurance programs.[180]

America's Health Insurance Plans

America's Health Insurance Plans (AHIP) is the successor organization to the American Association of Health Plans, which was established in 1996 when the Group Health Association of America and the American Managed Care and Review Association merged.[181] With 1,300 members, AHIP is a trade association for organizations that provide health insurance coverage to more than 200 million Americans. AHIP represents members in state and federal legislative and regulatory matters and in matters involving the media, consumers, and employers. It provides information to stakeholders and conducts education, research, and quality assurance.[182]

Paying for Health Services

EXPENDITURE TRENDS

As noted above, the percentage of this country's GDP devoted to health expenditures has increased steadily since the 1960s—an interesting juxtaposition to the passage of Medicare and Medicaid. Also as noted above, national health expenditures in 2006 consumed 16% of GDP, or about $2.2 trillion. CMS projects that health will consume $2.8 trillion, or 17.2% of GDP, by 2010 and $4.1 trillion, or 19.6% of GDP, by 2016.[183]

The period of rapid inflation occurred soon after the passage of Medicare and Medicaid in 1965; this demand–pull stimulation is a likely cause of the initial and continuing cost increases. In turn, these significant increases have been the stimulus for state and federal efforts to control health costs, or at least limit what they will pay.

Table 1.3 shows that, except for professional services (a category that has several elements), hospitals consume the largest amount of health expenditures. This has resulted in hospitals' bearing the brunt of state and federal efforts to control costs. The perspective of regulators and politicians seems to be that hospitals are badly managed and that excessive use of high technology, expensive tests, and treatments is a major source of the cost increases. Less time spent in hospitals has been posited as the best means of reducing costs; thus there has been great emphasis on reducing admission rates and average lengths of stay. It has been suggested, however, that a policy of "single-mindedly emptying hospitals not only does not save any money, it might even add to total national health spending."[184] More recently, rapid increases in Medicaid costs, both general costs and those for subacute and postacute services such as nursing facilities and home health, are likely to redirect and broaden cost-control efforts.

SOURCES AND USES OF FUNDS IN HEALTHCARE

As shown in Table 1.3, "personal healthcare" expenditures follow a similar trend of dramatic annual increases. In 2005, these expenditures total $1.7 trillion, compared with $1.2 trillion in 2001. It is forecast that by 2016, personal healthcare expenditures will total over $3.4 trillion. Table 1.3 shows other uses of funds expended on health from 2001 to 2005, with projections to 2016. Private non-governmental sources continue to provide almost 60% of personal healthcare expenditures.[185] As noted above, it is the willingness and ability of the American public (unlike those in systems in which private expenditures are illegal or purchasing power is limited) to spend personal funds on healthcare that makes expenditures high compared with other countries. Simultaneously, it shows the importance of freedom of choice in the United States.

The pie chart that is Figure 1.5 shows the sources and expenditures of the U.S. healthcare dollar for 2005. It is notable that, despite the significant growth of public expenditures since the enactment of Medicare in 1965, private sources provided almost 55% of funds in 2005. In terms of how the healthcare dollar is spent, hospital care expenditures predominate by consuming over 30% of funds.

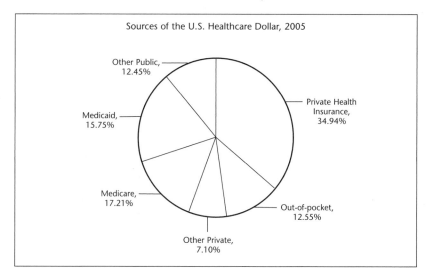

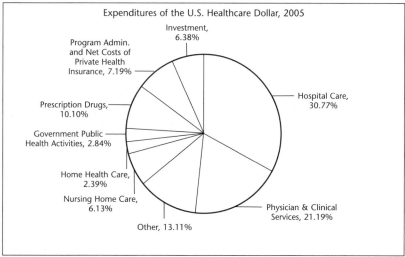

Figure 1.5. The U.S. Healthcare Dollar, 2005. Catlin, A., Cowan, C., Heffler, S., Washington, B., and the National Health Expenditure Accounts Team. *National Health Spending in 2005: The Slowdown Continues. Health Affairs* January/February 2007 (26)1:142–153. Copyright 2007 by Project Hope/Health Affairs Journal. Reproduced with permission of Project Hope/Health Affairs Journal via Copyright Clearance Center.

TABLE 1.3.   NATIONAL HEALTH EXPENDITURE AMOUNTS,
            AND ANNUAL PERCENT CHANGE BY TYPE OF EXPENDITURE: CALENDAR YEARS 2001–2016[1]

Type of Expenditure	2001	2002	2003	2004	2005
National Health Expenditures	$1,469.6	$1,602.8	$1,733.4	$1,858.9	$1,987.7
Health Services and Supplies	1,376.2	1,498.8	1,621.7	1,738.9	1,860.9
Personal Health Care	1,239.0	1,341.2	1,446.3	1,551.3	1,661.4
Hospital Care	451.4	488.6	525.4	566.9	611.6
Professional Services	465.3	503.1	543.0	581.1	621.7
Physician and Clinical Services	313.2	337.9	366.7	393.7	421.2
Other Professional Services	42.8	45.6	49.0	52.6	56.7
Dental Services	67.5	73.3	76.9	81.5	86.6
Other Personal Health Care	41.9	46.3	50.4	53.3	57.2
Nursing Home and Home Health	133.7	139.9	148.5	157.7	169.3
Home Health Care	32.2	34.2	38.0	42.7	47.5
Nursing Home Care	101.5	105.7	110.5	115.0	121.9
Retail Outlet Sales of Medical Products	188.5	209.6	229.4	245.5	258.8
Prescription Drugs	138.6	157.9	174.6	189.7	200.7
Other Medical Products	49.9	51.6	54.7	55.9	58.1
Durable Medical Equipment	19.6	20.8	22.4	23.1	24.0
Other Non-Durable Medical Products	30.3	30.9	32.3	32.8	34.1
Program Administration and Net Cost of Private Health Insurance	90.4	105.2	122.6	135.2	143.0
Government Public Health Activities	46.8	52.4	52.8	52.5	56.6
Investment	93.4	104.0	111.7	119.9	126.8
Research[2]	28.8	32.5	35.8	38.3	40.0
Structures & Equipment	64.7	71.5	75.9	81.7	86.8
National Health Expenditures	—	9.1	8.1	7.2	6.9
Health Services and Supplies	—	8.9	8.2	7.2	7.0
Personal Health Care	—	8.3	7.8	7.3	7.1
Hospital Care	—	8.2	7.5	7.9	7.9
Professional Services	—	8.1	7.9	7.0	7.0
Physician and Clinical Services	—	7.9	8.5	7.4	7.0
Other Professional Services	—	6.6	7.5	7.4	7.8
Dental Services	—	8.6	4.8	6.0	6.3
Other Personal Health Care	—	10.6	8.7	5.7	7.3
Nursing Home and Home Health	—	4.7	6.1	6.2	7.3
Home Health Care	—	6.3	11.1	12.3	11.1
Nursing Home Care	—	4.1	4.5	4.1	6.0
Retail Outlet Sales of Medical Products	—	11.2	9.5	7.0	5.4
Prescription Drugs	—	14.0	10.6	8.6	5.8
Other Medical Products	—	3.3	6.1	2.1	3.9
Durable Medical Equipment	—	5.7	8.1	3.1	3.7
Other Non-Durable Medical Products	—	1.8	4.7	1.5	4.1
Program Administration and Net Cost of Private Health	—	16.4	16.6	10.3	5.7
Government Public Health Activities	—	11.9	0.8	−0.6	7.7
Investment	—	11.3	7.4	7.3	5.7
Research[2]	—	13.2	10.1	6.7	4.6
Structures & Equipment	—	10.5	6.2	7.6	6.3

[1]The health spending projections were based on the 2005 version of the National Health Expenditures (NHE) released in January 2007.
[2]Research and development expenditures of drug companies and other manufacturers and providers of medical equipment and supplies are excluded from research expenditures. These research expenditures are implicitly included in the expenditure class in which the product falls, in that they are covered by the payment received for that product.

Inflationary pressures in health expenditures have moderated since 2000, although with few exceptions, they continue to lead increases in the CPI.[186] Hospital services have had very significant cost increases since 1969. The contribution of physicians' services has been significant, too, but less than hospital services. Data such as these caught the attention of federal policy makers. DRGs, resource utilization groups (RUGs), and resource-based relative value scales (RBRVS), which will be discussed below, have been their response.

Historically, much of the cost of health services has been borne by employers, and many have been instrumental in forming strategic alliances to control them. Strategic alliances bring together hospitals, physicians, employers, organized labor, insurers, and sometimes government to collect and exchange data and discuss how to finance and deliver health services in a community. Strategic

				Projected						
2006	2007	2008	2009	2010	2011	2012	2013	2014	2015	2016
$2,122.5	$2,262.3	$2,420.0	$2,596.0	$2,776.4	$2,966.4	$3,173.4	$3,395.8	$3,628.6	$3,874.6	$4,136.9
1,987.7	2,118.9	2,267.3	2,432.2	2,600.8	2,778.1	2,971.2	3,178.8	3,396.3	3,625.7	3,869.9
1,769.2	1,885.3	2,016.6	2,161.2	2,312.9	2,472.6	2,643.7	2,826.8	3,020.9	3,227.9	3,449.4
651.8	697.5	747.2	802.7	860.9	922.3	988.2	1,058.0	1,130.2	1,206.7	1,287.8
662.8	703.9	753.2	806.9	862.3	918.9	978.5	1,041.8	1,109.0	1,179.3	1,253.2
447.0	474.2	506.2	541.4	577.1	612.9	650.4	690.0	731.7	774.9	819.9
60.9	64.9	69.1	73.4	78.0	82.7	87.6	92.9	98.6	104.6	111.0
92.8	98.6	104.9	111.6	118.4	125.5	132.6	140.0	147.7	155.4	163.4
62.0	66.2	73.0	80.5	88.8	97.9	107.8	118.9	131.0	144.4	159.0
179.4	190.0	201.5	213.7	226.1	239.2	253.3	268.5	284.8	302.6	322.0
53.4	57.9	62.7	67.7	72.7	78.1	83.7	89.8	96.3	103.3	111.1
126.1	132.1	138.8	146.1	153.4	161.2	169.6	178.7	188.5	199.2	210.9
275.2	293.9	314.7	337.9	363.6	392.1	423.7	458.5	496.9	539.3	586.4
213.7	229.5	247.6	268.3	291.5	317.5	346.5	378.6	414.2	453.6	497.5
61.5	64.3	67.1	69.5	72.2	74.6	77.2	79.9	82.8	85.7	88.9
25.2	26.3	27.4	28.2	29.4	30.5	31.8	33.2	34.6	36.1	37.6
36.3	38.0	39.7	41.3	42.8	44.1	45.4	46.7	48.2	49.7	51.3
156.8	167.4	179.8	194.9	206.2	217.9	233.5	251.0	267.0	281.5	295.7
61.7	66.2	70.9	76.1	81.7	87.6	94.1	101.0	108.3	116.2	124.8
134.8	143.4	152.8	163.8	175.6	188.3	202.2	217.0	232.3	248.9	267.0
41.7	43.9	46.3	49.1	52.1	55.5	59.1	63.0	66.9	70.9	75.0
93.1	99.5	106.4	114.7	123.5	132.8	143.1	154.0	165.4	178.0	191.9
6.8	6.6	6.6	7.0	7.3	6.9	6.8	7.0	7.0	6.9	6.8
6.8	6.6	6.6	7.0	7.3	6.9	6.8	7.0	7.0	6.8	6.8
6.5	6.6	6.6	7.0	7.2	7.0	6.9	6.9	6.9	6.9	6.9
6.6	7.0	7.0	7.1	7.4	7.2	7.1	7.1	7.1	6.8	6.8
6.6	6.2	6.2	7.0	7.1	6.9	6.6	6.5	6.5	6.5	6.3
6.1	6.1	6.1	6.7	7.0	6.6	6.2	6.1	6.1	6.0	5.9
7.3	6.6	6.6	6.4	6.3	6.3	6.0	6.0	6.0	6.1	6.1
7.2	6.2	6.2	6.3	6.4	6.1	6.0	5.6	5.6	5.5	5.2
8.5	6.8	6.8	10.3	10.3	10.2	10.2	10.2	10.2	10.2	10.2
6.0	5.9	5.9	6.0	6.1	5.8	5.8	5.9	6.0	6.1	6.2
12.5	8.6	8.6	8.2	7.9	7.5	7.4	7.3	7.3	7.2	7.3
3.4	4.8	4.8	5.1	5.2	5.0	5.1	5.2	5.4	5.5	5.7
6.4	6.8	6.8	7.1	7.3	7.6	7.8	8.1	8.2	8.4	8.5
6.5	7.4	7.4	7.9	8.4	8.6	8.9	9.1	9.3	9.4	9.5
6.0	4.6	4.6	4.3	3.6	3.8	3.4	3.4	3.5	3.6	3.6
5.3	4.2	4.2	4.2	3.0	4.1	4.0	4.2	4.3	4.2	4.2
6.5	4.8	4.8	4.4	4.0	3.5	3.0	2.9	3.0	3.1	3.1
9.6	6.8	6.8	7.4	8.4	5.8	5.6	7.2	7.5	6.4	5.4
9.1	7.2	7.2	7.1	7.4	7.3	7.3	7.3	7.3	7.3	7.3
6.3	6.4	6.4	6.5	7.2	7.2	7.2	7.4	7.3	7.1	7.1
4.3	5.2	5.2	5.5	5.9	6.2	6.5	6.6	6.5	6.2	6.0
7.2	6.9	6.9	6.9	7.8	7.7	7.6	7.7	7.6	7.4	7.6

NOTE: Numbers may not add to totals because of rounding

SOURCE: Centers for Medicare & Medicaid Services, Office of the Actuary. (http://www.cms.hhs.gov/NationalHealthExpend Data/downloads/proj2006.pdf). Retrieved July 23, 2007.

alliances are discussed in Chapter 11. Large increases in healthcare costs to employers have caused many of them to stop providing health insurance; narrow the range and content of health insurance product choices; and/or require employees to pay a larger share of costs through higher premiums, copays, and deductibles.

PRIVATE PAYMENT UNDER THE INSURANCE PRINCIPLE

The first insurer to write "sickness" insurance did so in 1847, but the insurance industry paid little attention to health insurance until after World War II. Contributing to this lack of interest was a perception that sickness and paying for treatment were too unpredictable to fit traditional actuarial concepts.

It was not until 1929 that Blue Cross showed it could be done. Blue Cross began when a group of school teachers made an agreement with Baylor Hospital in Dallas, TX, to provide hospital room and board and certain diagnostic services for a monthly fee. In 1932, the first city-wide plan was established with a group of hospitals in Sacramento, CA. The comparable plan for physicians' services became known as Blue Shield and was established in California in 1939. Hospitals fostered development of Blue Cross to enhance their patients' ability to pay the costs of hospitalization. After several mergers and reorganizations during the 1990s, by 2007, there were 39 Blue Cross and Blue Shield plans insuring more than 98 million people.[187]

Private health insurance coverage grew rapidly during the 1940s and 1950s. It received a boost during World War II, when wages and salaries were subjected to federal government controls but fringe benefits were not. Commercial carriers began writing substantial amounts of health insurance. By 1955, they had more insureds than Blue Cross. By 1981, more than 1,000 commercial insurance companies were writing health insurance in the United States.[188]

Most private insurance coverage comes through the employment relationship.[189] The number of people uninsured was estimated to be more than 47 million in 2005.[190] It is important to analyze the categories of people who are uninsured. Some uninsured people are self-pay; many choose not to pay for insurance through their employers or similar sources; most uninsured people would be medically indigent in a major illness. The estimate of uninsured people does not indicate how many cannot get care when it is needed. About 60% of Americans (more than 180 million) had private (nongovernmental) health insurance coverage in 2007.[191]

Historically, Blue Cross was a community-rated service plan; that is, all insureds in the same geographic area paid the same rate, Blue Cross paid providers pursuant to a contract. In contrast to service plans, indemnity insurance—the type usually written by commercial carriers—indemnifies (pays) the insured person a fixed amount for each diagnosis or treatment. A variation of indemnification is assignment—the insured person assigns the payment to the provider, who is paid directly. Service plan limits are expressed in days of care and services covered. Blue Shield paid participating physicians according to a fee schedule, which was payment in full and which had the effect of assignment. Nonparticipating physicians billed the patient, who was reimbursed per the fee schedule. Another difference between Blue Cross and Blue Shield and the commercial carriers is that, historically, the former were not-for-profit corporations that prided themselves on providing consumer-oriented coverage with low overhead costs for plan administration.

▬ Government Payment Schemes ▬▬▬▬▬▬▬▬▬▬▬▬▬▬▬▬▬▬▬▬▬

BACKGROUND

As noted, until 1965, federal government concentrated on providing the wherewithal to support private delivery of services. The advent of Medicare and Medicaid brought federal and state governments into direct financing of medical care. Historically and presently, federal programs provide services to veterans, military personnel, and Native Americans. State governments provide services for special health problems such as mental illness and disabilities and tuberculosis. States also operate general acute care hospitals that are part of academic health centers connected with state medical schools. Other HSOs, typically general acute care hospitals, are owned by local governments.

As noted, federal government has sought to control the increase in healthcare expenditures through programs such as PROs, DRGs, RUGs, and RBRVS. Also as noted, the states have used regulatory efforts such as CON and rate review through rate-setting commissions to control the increase in healthcare expenditures. In addition, most have sought to slow the growth of Medicaid costs by hospital preadmission screening, limiting hospital days, reducing what is paid for each day of care or each service, paying months (or years) after bills are submitted by HSOs and physicians, requiring beneficiaries to pay larger copayments for optional services, increasing eligibility (income) restrictions, and decreasing the range of services available. Oregon developed a priority list of services (based on a budget) for which its Medicaid program will pay.

For many services, Medicaid pays only a fraction of the costs incurred by HSOs to provide them. Reducing what Medicaid pays has ripple effects. Other payers must make up the difference through cost shifting if the HSO is to be financially viable. Government programs do not pay charges (the non-negotiated fee charged by the HSO), nor does Blue Cross. Commercial insurers are almost certain not to pay charges, and indemnity plans have always paid only a fixed fee to the beneficiary regardless of what the beneficiary is charged or pays. It is only the self-pay patients who pay charges. The small number of self-payers makes cross subsidies increasingly infeasible.

Cost shifting raises basic questions of fairness. Should any payer pay less than costs for services? Medicare is a case more politically difficult than Medicaid because Medicare is an exclusively federal program. Congress has been unwilling to cut benefits, although it has increased copayments and deductibles (e.g., Medicare Part A, hospitalization) and the insurance premium (e.g., Medicare Part B, physicians' services) several times since 1965. Medicare has been called uncontrollable because once beneficiaries are eligible, all services are available. Meaningful savings will occur only if benefit levels are controlled, which is politically unpalatable.

DIAGNOSIS-RELATED GROUPS

Initially, Medicare reimbursement for hospital services was based on costs; the lack of incentives to be efficient caused runaway cost increases. By the early 1980s, a direct means of cost control was instituted when the Tax Equity and Fiscal Responsibility Act of 1982[192] and the Social Security Amendments of 1983 (PL 98-21)[193] mandated a prospective payment system for Medicare using DRGs. The CMS administers Medicare and Medicaid and establishes and reviews DRG rates for each Medicare inpatient admission. Discharged Medicare patients are assigned to one or more of the 559 DRGs, based on diagnosis, surgery, patient age, discharge destination, and sex.[194] Each DRG's weight is based primarily on Medicare billing and cost data and reflects the relative cost, across all hospitals, of treating cases that are classified in that DRG.[195] Hospitals that can provide services at lower costs keep the difference. Those exceeding the DRG rate must recoup the difference elsewhere.

The change from cost-based reimbursement to payment according to rates prospectively determined by CMS has had and will continue to have major effects on hospitals. One is that hospitals "unbundled" (separated) postacute services such as subacute, recuperative, and rehabilitative care from the acute episode hospital stay. For example, hospital-based nursing facility beds were established to provide transitional care. Under prospective payment, hospitals must be certain that their average costs per DRG do not exceed CMS rates. Managers and physicians must collaborate to eliminate unnecessary tests and procedures and reduce LOS, and in general, hospitals must become more efficient. Initially, the DRG payment system applied only to Medicare patients, but state Medicaid programs, Blue Cross, and other third-party payers have adopted it for inpatient services. Similar, DRG-like prospective payment system methodologies are being used for nursing facilities and outpatient clinics as well.

RESOURCE UTILIZATION GROUPS

DRGs are applied to hospitalized Medicare beneficiaries. The classification system applied to long-term care puts nursing facility residents with similar resource needs (utilization) into groups. Initially, these groups were based on the ability of nursing facility residents to engage in activities of daily living, which are major explanatory factors in resource use. Since the mid-1980s, RUGs have undergone significant derivation and validation and have evolved through RUG-II, which was used to determine nursing facility payment for Medicaid in New York and Texas.[196] RUG-III was mandated for Medicare residents by the Balanced Budget Act of 1997.[197] The number of reimbursement levels based on resident condition and use of services was increased from 44 to 53 in 2005. RUG-III uses a daily rate based on the needs of individual residents, adjusted for local labor costs. The rate changes as the resident's condition changes.[198] As with other federal payment schemes, other payers are likely to adopt RUG-III in determining payments to nursing facilities.

AMBULATORY PATIENT GROUPS AND AMBULATORY PAYMENT CATEGORIES

Other providers of services have drawn the attention of lawmakers and regulators. Research in the late 1980s led to development of ambulatory patient groups (APGs), a system of codes that explains the amount and type of resources used in an ambulatory visit. The variety of outpatient services settings, wide variation in the reasons for outpatient care, and the high percentage of costs associated with ancillary services necessitated a classification scheme that could reflect the range of services rendered. As with DRGs, patients in each APG are assumed to have similarities in clinical characteristics, resource use, and costs. Also like DRGs, a primary APG or a significant procedure is subdivided into groups by body systems. Unlike with DRGs, variables for additional services are based on clinically similar classes, and multiple APGs can be applied per patient encounter. APGs will eventually encompass the full range of ambulatory settings, including same-day surgery units, hospital emergency rooms, and outpatient services. They will not address telephone contacts, home health visits, nursing facility care, or inpatient services.[199]

HCFA (now the CMS) adapted ambulatory payment categories (APCs) from APGs. APCs group thousands of procedure and diagnosis codes into more than 300 categories, with separate classifications for surgical, medical, and ancillary services. Each group includes clinically similar services that require comparable levels of resources. A relative weight based on median resource use is assigned to each classification. Payment for each APC is determined by multiplying the relative weight by a conversion factor, which is the average rate for all APC services.[200]

RESOURCE-BASED RELATIVE VALUE SCALE

In 1992, CMS's predecessor, HCFA, began implementing a fee schedule for physicians who participate in Medicare Part B, a change mandated by the Omnibus Budget Reconciliation Act of 1989 (PL 101-239, OBRA '89).[201] Previously, physician payment under Part B was based on usual, customary, and reasonable charges. Among the most important effects of charge-based payment was that procedure-based specialties such as surgery were more highly paid than specialties such as internal medicine that use cognitive skills (e.g., evaluation, management). The new schedule used a RBRVS that resulted in dramatic changes in physician payment patterns. The prospectively set reimbursement is based on the resources that are used to produce physician services and is divided into three components: physician work, practice expenses, and malpractice insurance.[202] Nonphysician practitioners whose services are paid under Medicare Part B will continue to have their fees tied to those of physicians, and their fees will move in the same direction.[203]

RBRVS increased reimbursement for family and general practice physicians by about 15%; payments to ophthalmologists and anesthesiologists declined the most (approximately 35%), but payments to other procedure-based specialists, such as surgeons, decreased as well.[204] Since RBRVS was introduced, the inexorable trend in physician's fees has been downward. In addition, to prevent physicians who have not signed a Medicare participation agreement (accepting Medicare as full payment for services [sometimes called assignment]) from balance-billing patients (i.e., billing patients for the difference between what Medicare pays and what the physician charges), the statute imposed a cap on the amount that a nonparticipating physician may balance-bill a Medicare beneficiary.[205]

Regulations developed pursuant to the Balanced Budget Act of 1997 allow physicians (and other healthcare practitioners) to opt out of Medicare and provide services through private contracts.

The federal application of RBRVS is only to Medicare. However, RBRVS is likely to be used by other third-party payers, as they have used RUGs and DRGs. The effect will be a major change in how physicians are paid. Other likely effects are that physicians employed in high-technology practices will generate less income for their employers; physicians will try to unbundle services and move more of them out of hospitals; physicians may seek to have lost income made up by hospitals; physicians may limit their willingness to treat Medicare beneficiaries; and adjustments in how physicians are paid in rural areas as compared with urban areas will make it easier for rural hospitals to attract physicians, thus increasing access to care for rural beneficiaries while potentially decreasing it for urban beneficiaries.[206]

SUMMARY

Incentives in DRGs, RUGs, and APG/APCs may lead to underuse of services and consequently to inappropriate treatment. The effect of DRGs is an incentive to discharge patients from hospitals as soon as possible. Early discharge has significant implications for home health agencies, nursing facilities, and hospitals, but most of all for the patients.

Incentives in RBRVS are to overuse services because physicians are paid for each treatment. Treatment by specialists is not necessarily more expensive. Such interventions may be more effective, with lower total cost than the same diagnosis treated by a family practitioner. A likely long-term effect of RBRVS is that changes in physician income will reconfigure the ratios of physicians by specialty.

▤ System Trends ▤

Significant efforts by state and federal governments to control their health services programs' costs will continue. Hospitals consume about one third of health expenditures.[207] Thus, they will continue to receive disproportionate attention from government and other third-party payers. The large component of fixed and semivariable costs will limit the savings that HSOs can achieve. Case-mix cost control through DRGs will cause hospitals to treat patients with the most remunerative diagnoses. There will be economic pressure to discharge patients quickly, perhaps earlier than sound practice warrants. In addition, treating the less ill with alternative regimens and in nonhospital HSOs leaves only the most ill in acute care hospitals. The result will be that costs per day of care will increase, thus putting even greater financial pressure on hospitals. Unless hospitals close beds, discontinue services, and reduce the number of employees, the cost per case and the total cost per hospitalization will rise.

Regulation was the watchword in the late 1960s and early 1970s. The competitive environment that emerged in the late 1970s and early 1980s has continued. Public and private payment sources are unwilling to subsidize the inefficient. The bankruptcies, mergers, and joint activities among HSOs/HSs that began in the 1980s have continued. Increasingly, hospitals will be connected to one another through shared services, group purchasing, and strategic alliances. As with politics, all healthcare delivery is local. HSs tend to be local or regional rather than national, a reality that is likely to continue. Predictions that the end of the 20th century would find U.S. healthcare provided by a few national hospital systems, some large unaffiliated facilities, and few small freestanding hospitals proved incorrect.

The widespread corporate restructuring undertaken by hospitals in the early 1980s was largely unsuccessful. Even as corporate restructuring protected and enhanced hospitals' assets and reimbursement and expanded their range of activities, it caused management to lose sight of the core business. Consequently, hospitals have divested themselves of noncore businesses and are again focusing on their original raison d'etre. Restructuring is addressed in Chapter 2.

Physicians have increasingly undertaken activities that compete with hospitals. As technology becomes more portable and as new medical interventions that don't require hospitalization are developed, hospitals will have sicker and sicker patients. The fragmentation and ultraspecialization of hospital clinical staff will continue. As a result, the problems of acquiring, retaining, and managing human resources and their appropriate roles in HSOs will be exacerbated in the future.

DISCUSSION QUESTIONS

1. What are the ramifications and implications for the health services system of the model developed by Blum? What are its strengths and weaknesses?
2. Select a disease problem and apply the Precede-Proceed model described in the chapter. How should HSO/HS governing bodies and managers use this model?
3. Describe and analyze the relationships among the various institutional and programmatic providers in the health services system.
4. Facilities and programs other than acute care hospitals are much more numerous and arguably have a greater effect on health status, but acute care hospitals remain the focus of attention. Why is this? What are the desirable and undesirable aspects of this attention from the standpoint of the acute care hospital provider and the consumer of health services?
5. Proliferation of the health professions continues unabated. What is desirable and undesirable about this fragmentation? If something should be done to slow or stop it, what should it be, and how can it be achieved?
6. Highlight the changes in reimbursement to HSOs that have occurred since 1965. What forces in the general environment were most important in causing these changes? Sketch and defend a scenario that suggests the likely developments in reimbursement during the early 21st century.
7. Federally supported state health planning has risen and fallen since the passage of Medicare and Medicaid. Identify the advantages and disadvantages of statewide or areawide health planning from the standpoints of providers *and* consumers.
8. Describe how licensure, registration, and certification are different. What are the advantages and disadvantages of each from the standpoints of providers and consumers? How do they facilitate *and* inhibit the availability of health services occupations?
9. Resources consumed by the health services system have soared since the late 1960s. What factors contributed to the increases? Identify actions that have been taken. What else might be done to control costs?
10. Identify the advantages and disadvantages of excess numbers of physicians and nonphysician clinicians from the perspective of health services managers. What are the advantages and disadvantages to society?

Case Study 1: Gourmand and Food—A Fable[208]

The people of Gourmand loved good food. They ate in good restaurants, donated money for cooking research, and instructed their government to safeguard all matters having to do with food. Long ago, the food industry had been in total chaos. There were many restaurants, some very small. Anyone could call himself or herself a chef or open a restaurant. In choosing a restaurant, one could never be sure that the meal would be good. A commission of distinguished chefs studied the situation and recommended that no one be allowed to touch food except for qualified chefs. "Food is too important to be left to amateurs," they said. Qualified chefs were licensed by the state, and there were severe penalties for anyone else who engaged in cooking. Certain exceptions were made for food preparation in the home, but those meals could be served only to the family. Furthermore, a qualified chef had to complete at least 21 years of training (including 4 years of college, 4 years of cooking school, and a 1-year apprenticeship). All cooking schools had to be first class.

These reforms did succeed in raising the quality of cooking, but a restaurant meal became substantially more expensive. A second commission observed that not everyone could afford to eat out. "No one," they said, "should be denied a good meal because of income." Furthermore, they argued that chefs should work toward the goal of giving everyone "complete physical and psychological satisfaction." The government declared that those people who could not afford to eat out should be allowed to do so as often as they liked, and the government would pay. For others, it was recommended that they organize themselves into groups and pay part of their income into a pool that would be used to pay the costs incurred by members in dining out. To ensure the greatest satisfaction, the groups were set up so that members could eat out anywhere and as often as they liked, their meals could be as elaborate as they desired, and they would have to pay nothing or only a small percentage of the cost. The cost of joining such prepaid dining clubs rose sharply.

Long before this, most restaurants had employed only one chef to prepare the food. A few restaurants had been more elaborate, with chefs specializing in roasting, fish, salads, sauces, and many other things. People had rarely gone to these elaborate restaurants because they had been so expensive. With the establishment of prepaid dining clubs, everyone wanted to eat at these fancy restaurants. At the same time, young chefs in school disdained going to cook in a small restaurant where they would have to cook everything. Specializing and cooking at a very fancy restaurant paid much better, and it was much more prestigious. Soon there were not enough chefs to keep the small restaurants open.

With prepaid clubs and free meals for the poor, many people started eating three-course meals at the elaborate restaurants. Then restaurants began to increase the number of courses, directing the chefs to "serve the best with no thought for the bill." (Eventually, a meal was served that had 317 courses.)

The costs of eating out rose faster and faster. A new government commission reported as follows:

1. Noting that licensed chefs were being used to peel potatoes and wash lettuce, the commission recommended that these tasks be handed over to licensed dishwashers (whose 3 years of dishwashing training included simple cooking courses) or to some new category of personnel.
2. Concluding that many licensed chefs were overworked, the commission recommended that cooking schools be expanded, that the length of training be shortened, and that applicants with lesser qualifications be admitted.
3. The commission also observed that chefs were unhappy because people seemed to be more concerned about the decor and service than about the food. (In a recent taste test, not only could one patron not tell the difference between a 1930 and a 1970 vintage, but he also could not distinguish between white and red wines. He explained that he always ordered the 1930 vintage because he knew that only a very good restaurant would stock such an expensive wine.)

The commission agreed that weighty problems faced the nation. They recommended that a national prepayment group be established, which everyone must join. They recommended that chefs continue to be paid on the basis of the number of dishes they prepared. They recommended that the Gourmandese be given the right to eat anywhere they chose and as elaborately as they chose and pay nothing.

These recommendations were adopted. Large numbers of people spent all of their time ordering incredibly elaborate meals. Kitchens became marvels of new, expensive equipment. All those who were not consuming restaurant food were in the kitchen preparing it. Because no one in Gourmand did anything except prepare or eat meals, the country collapsed.

QUESTIONS

1. Read and analyze the fable of Gourmand. How well does the allegory fit delivery of healthcare in the United States?
2. What is, and what should be, the role of the consumer in healthcare?

Case Study 2: Where's My Organ?

Organizations that support and encourage transplantation of human organs estimate that tens of thousands of people with end-stage renal disease, who are now maintained on dialysis, could resume a relatively normal life with a kidney transplant. The supply of cadaver kidneys, however, falls far short of demand. To encourage people to sign organ donor cards and to encourage families to consent to organ donation, a member of the U.S. House of Representatives introduced a bill to provide tax incentives for what is often called the "gift of life." Here, the gift is vascularized organs, including the heart, liver, pancreas, lungs, and kidneys.

Tax incentives would be twofold: a $25,000 deduction per organ in the individual's last taxable year, plus a $25,000 exclusion per organ from estate taxes. To qualify, the organ must be in a condition suitable for transplantation. The same tax incentives would be granted for donations by dependents as defined by the federal tax code. When introducing the bill, the representative stated, "Thus, a minor with significant income would reduce the family's tax liability with a posthumous donation that would benefit both the minor's loved ones and the loved ones of the recipient of the life-saving organ."

The representative noted, too, that enactment of his bill would result in significant cost savings to the federal government, which pays for the dialysis of people with end-stage renal disease under Medicare. Assuming a 50% income tax bracket and an average of two organs per taxpayer, the deductions for 10,000 donors would reduce tax collections by $250 million. Renal dialysis is projected to cost the federal government almost $12 billion by fiscal year 2015.

QUESTIONS

1. Identify the issues that this proposed legislation raises.
2. Choose to support or oppose the bill. Develop a set of arguments that justifies your position.
3. Develop an alternative proposal that would be more effective in encouraging organ donation.

Case Study 3: Dental Van Shenanigans[209]

Use of vans to take healthcare services to the medically underserved is common in rural areas and inner cities. One Midwestern city had a federally funded community health center (CHC) that provided some dental clinic services to the needy. The CHC was well qualified but was known for an aggressive management style and creating self-serving alliances. This questionable management style was seen by CHC managers as the most savvy and efficient path to financial success.

Unilaterally, the CHC developed a proposal for a van with two dental care areas to take primary care dental services to underserved inner-city school children. Then, the CHC worked behind the scenes at other local agencies to get some of their funds to support the van. The effort included colluding with board members from other agencies on matters of those board members' personal interests in exchange for the board members' putting financial support of the dental van on their organizations' meeting agendas. Of course, these differing interests or actual conflicts of interest were not disclosed when dental van support was included on the agendas. The staffs of the other agencies were not consulted in advance, because CHC management thought it was unlikely that those staffs would support allocating funds for the CHC's big public relations initiative.

One agency learned about the dental van and the CHC's effort to obtain some of their budget when the van appeared as an agenda item that was added at the last minute. The proposal did not pass, however, because the board members who had conspired with the CHC were unable to answer the other board members' questions about how support of the CHC's dental van furthered their agency's mission.

The dental van was badly needed in the community, but it was about to lose its funding. Only if the staff from the other agency argued in support of the CHC's effort would it pass. Supporting the dental van, however, required that the agency's staff overcome its anger that the CHC's efforts had been surreptitious and had sought to gain support in a devious manner.

QUESTIONS

1. Make the assumption that your agency's budget had funds available. Should your staff have spoken in support of the dental van project even though it was outside your agency's mission and it was put on the agenda through questionable means?
2. Competitiveness or a desire for preeminence and public relations advantage may cause agencies providing public health services to act unethically or dishonestly. What is the best way to work to improve public health when this occurs?
3. In many states, dentists provide services to the economically disadvantaged who qualify for Medicaid. How should the CHC respond to protests from area dentists that sending a dental van into the inner city will disrupt their existing dentist–patient relationships (and, incidentally, reduce their incomes)?

Notes

1. Centers for Medicare and Medicaid Services. "National Health Expenditure Projections 2005–2015, Forecast Summary and Selected Tables." *hhtp//www.cms.hhs.gov/NationalHealthExpendData/downloads/proj/2005.pdf,* retrieved October 29, 2006.
2. Health Care Financing Administration. "Highlights: National Health Expenditures, 1998." *http://www.hcfa.gov/stats/NHE-OAct/hilites.htm,* retrieved March 21, 2000.
3. Borger, Christine, Sheila Smith, Christopher Truffer, Sean Keehan, Andrea Sisko, John Poisal, and M. Kent Clemens. "Health Spending Projections Through 2015: Changes on the Horizon." *Health Affairs* 25:2 (February 2006): W61–W73.
4. Blum, Henrik L. *Expanding Health Care Horizons: From a General Systems Concept of Health to a National Health Policy,* 2nd ed., 34. Oakland, CA: Third Party Publishing, 1983.
5. Blum, Henrik L. *Planning for Health: Development and Application of Social Change Theory,* 96–100. New York: Human Sciences Press, 1974.
6. The discussion of the Precede-Proceed model for health planning and evaluation is adapted from

Lawrence W. Green and Marshall W. Kreuter. *Health Program Planning: An Educational and Ecological Approach,* 4th ed., 9–17. New York: McGraw Hill, 2004.

7. Health Care Financing Administration. "Trends in Medicare Skilled Nursing Facility Utilization: CYs 1967–1994." *Health Care Financing Review,* Statistical Supplement (1996): 64.

8. Data from the National Center for Health Statistics, 1987 and 1988; Thompson-Hoffman, Susan, and Inez Fitzgerald Storck. *Disability in the United States: A Portrait from National Data,* 37. New York: Springer-Verlag, 1991.

9. Administrative Procedure Act of 1946, 60 Stat. 993 (1946).

10. As recently as 1932, the U.S. Supreme Court held that the delegation of legislative authority by the Congress was unconstitutional. *United States v. Shreveport Grain and Elevator Company,* 287 U.S. 77 (1932).

11. *Black's Law Dictionary,* 6th ed., 1406. St. Paul, MN: West Publishing, 1990.

12. *Black's Law Dictionary,* 1305.

13. Pickett, George, and John J. Hanlon. *Public Health: Administration and Practice,* 9th ed., 28–32. St. Louis: Times Mirror/Mosby College Publishing, 1990.

14. The Social Security Act of 1935. Social Security Online. *http://www.ssa.gov/history/35act.html,* retrieved January 25, 2008.

15. U.S. Census Bureau. "2005 American Community Survey: American FactFinder by Age and Sex." *http://factfinder.census.gov/servlet/ACSSAFFPeople? submenuId=people 2& sse=on,* retrieved October 16, 2006.

16. Hospital Survey and Construction Act of 1946 (Hill-Burton Act), PL 79-725, 60 Stat. 1040 (1946).

17. Public Health Service. *Directory of Facilities Obligated to Provide Uncompensated Services, by State and City as of March 1, 1989,* I. Washington, DC: U.S. Department of Health and Human Services, 1989.

18. National Institutes of Health, "Institutes, Centers & Offices." Updated December 4, 2006. *http:www.nih.gov/icd/,* retrieved May 22, 2007.

19. U.S. Department of Health and Human Services. "FY 2007 Budget in Brief: Advancing the Health, Safety, and Well-Being of our People." *http://www.hhs.gov/budget/07budget/overview.html,* retrieved October 16, 2006.

20. National Institutes of Health. "Institutes and Offices." *http://www.nih.gov/icd/,* retrieved March 22, 1999.

21. National Institutes of Health. "National Awards (competing and noncompeting) by Fiscal Year and Funding Mechanism Fiscal Years 1994–2005." *http://grants1.nih.gov/grants/award/trends/fund9405 .htm,* retrieved October 30, 2006.

22. Kaiser Family Foundation. "How Changes in Medical Technology Affect Health Care Costs." *http:// www.kff.org/insurance/snapshot/chcm030807oth.cfm,* retrieved July 30, 2007.

23. Social Security Act Amendments (1965). Our Documents. *http://www.ourdocuments.gov/doc.php?flash =true&doc=99,* retrieved January 25, 2008.

24. Balanced Budget Act of 1997, PL 105-33, 111 Stat. 251 (1997).

25. Grimaldi, Paul L. "Medicare Part C Means More Choices." *Nursing Management* 28 (November 1997): 30.

26. Medicare Prescription Drug, Improvement, and Modernization Act of 2003, PL108-173. CMS Legislative Summary. April 2004. *http://www.cms.hhs.gov/MMAUpdate/downloads/PL108-173summary.pdf,* retrieved January 25, 2008

27. Kaiser Commission on Medicaid and the Uninsured. "The Medicaid Program at a Glance." March 2007. (Photocopy.)

28. Comprehensive Health Planning and Public Health Service Amendments Act of 1966, PL 89-749, 80 Stat. 1180 (1966); National Health Planning and Resources Development Act of 1974, PL 93-641, 88 Stat. 2225 (1974); Social Security Amendments of 1972, PL 92-603, 86 Stat. 1329 (1972).

29. Bureau of Labor Statistics. *Consumer Price Index, Average Annual Percentage Change, All Urban Consumers, 1969–1996.* Washington, DC: U.S. Department of Labor, 1997.

30. Tax Equity and Fiscal Responsibility Act of 1982, PL 97-248, 96 Stat. 324 (1982); Social Security Amendments of 1983, PL 98-21, 97 Stat. 65 (1983).

31. Hilzenrath, David S. "Health Benefits Costs' Jump Called Ominous: Easy HMO Savings Ending, Survey Suggests." *The Washington Post,* January 6, 1999, F3.

32. Agency for Health Care Policy and Research. "Equalizing Payments for Cesarean and Vaginal Deliveries Has Little Effect on Cesarean Rates." *Research Activities* 201 (February 1997): 2.

33. National Center for Health Statistics. *Health United States 1990,* 185. Washington, DC: U.S. Department of Health and Human Services, 1991.

34. Organisation for Economic Co-operation and Development. "OECD Health Data 2006—Country Notes" and press releases. *http://www.oecd.org/document/46/0,2340,en 2649 34631 34971438 1 1 1 1,00.html,* retrieved October 16, 2006.

35. Anderson, Gerard F., Uwe E. Reinhardt, Peter S. Hussey, and Varduhl Petrosyan. "It's the Prices, Stupid: Why the United States Is So Different from Other Countries." *Health Affairs* 22 (May/June 2003): 91–93.

36. Hageman, Winifred M., and Richard J. Bogue. "Layers of Leadership: The Challenges of Collaborative Governance." *Trustee* 51 (September 1998): 20.

37. Strenger, Ellen Weisman. "The Road to Wellville." *Trustee* 49 (May 1996): 20–25.

38. Pickett, George E., and John J. Hanlon. *Public Health Administration and Practice,* 9th ed., 83. St. Louis: Times Mirror/Mosby College Publishing, 1990.

39. Adding to confusion about *primary* is that many small acute care hospitals are known as primary care hospitals. This means that they offer a limited range of services, including normal deliveries and routine medical and surgical treatment. Patients needing significant interventions are transferred to secondary, tertiary, or quaternary care hospitals.

40. Seebach, Linda. "Alternative Therapy Eruption." *The Washington Times,* July 6, 1998, A14; Okie, Susan. "Widening the Medical Mainstream: More Americans Using 'Alternative' Therapies, Some Prove Effective." *The Washington Post,* November 11, 1998, A1.

41. "Visits to Physician Offices and Hospital Outpatient and Emergency Departments by Selected Characteristics: United States, Selected Years 1995–2003," 309. *ftp://ftp.cdc.gov/pub/Health Statistics/NCHS/Publications/Health US/hus05tables/05listtables.pdf,* retrieved October 30, 2006.

42. "National Hansen's Disease Program." *http:www.hrsa.gov/hansens/clinicalcenter.htm,* retrieved April 17, 2007.

43. Indian Health Service. "Fact Sheet." Washington, DC: IHS/OD/PAS, January 2007.

44. *Organizational Briefing Book*, 1. Washington, DC: Department of Veterans Affairs, May 2006.

45. American Hospital Association. "Trends Affecting Hospitals and Health Systems." April 2007. *http://www.aha.org.aha/trendwatch/2007/cb2007chapter3.ppt,* retrieved August 27, 2007.

46. Centers for Medicare and Medicaid Services. "Long Term Care Hospitals." *http://www.cms.hhs.gov/LongTermCareHospitalPPS/,* retrieved August 24, 2007; MedPac. "Chapter 5. Defining Long Term Care Hospitals." *Report to the Congress: New Approaches in Medicare. http://www.medpac.gov/publications/congressional_reports/June04_ch5.pdf,* retrieved August 27, 2007.

47. "Intermediate Care Facility for Persons with Mental Retardation and Developmental Disabilities (ICF MR/DD)." *http://www.ahca.org/research/icf/icf mrdd 0510.pdf,* retrieved October 29, 2006.

48. "Intermediate Care Facility for the Mentally Retarded (ICFs/MR)." *http://www.ahca.org/info/icf.htm,* retrieved March 5, 1999.

49. "Intermediate Care Facility for Persons with Mental Retardation and Developmental Disabilities (ICF MR/DD), Survey Report for Publicly Operated Facilities." *http://www.ahca.org/research/icf/public icf mrdd 0510.pdf,* retrieved October 30,2006.

50. Norback, Judith. *The Mental Health Yearbook/Directory 1979–80*, 200. New York: Van Nostrand Reinhold, 1979.

51. "Mental Health Organizations and Beds for 24-Hour Hospital and Residential Treatment According to Type of Organization: United States, Selected Years, 1986–2002." *ftp://ftp.cdc.gov/pub/HealthStatistics/NCHS/Publications/Health US/hus05tables/Table113.xls,* retrieved November 6, 2006.

52. Council of Teaching Hospitals and Health Systems. *COTH Activities and Member Services.* Washington, DC: Association of American Medical Colleges, April 13, 2007.

53. Council of Teaching Hospitals and Health Systems. *Council of Teaching Hospitals: Selected Activities Report—May 1990*, 1. Washington, DC: Association of American Medical Colleges, 1990.

54. Personal communication, Hirsh Alexander, Vice President of Education, Association of Academic Medical Centers, May 31, 2007.

55. The Joint Commission on Accreditation of Healthcare Organizations. "States Recognizing Accreditation/Certification by the Joint Commission." May 31, 2006. *http://www.jointcommission.org/NR/rdonlyres/788AAOBD-9B9A-4F42-B17E-5DEB6647B2FB/0/5_06deeming.pdf*, retrieved February 13, 2007.

56. National Fire Protection Association. "Overview." *http://www.nfpa.org/itemDetail.asp?categoryID =495&itemID=17991&URL=About%20US/Overview*, retrieved February 12, 2007.

57. "Hospital Conditions of Participation in Medicare." In *Medicare: A Strategy for Quality Assurance,* vol. 1, edited by Kathleen N. Lohr, 119–137. Washington, DC: Institute of Medicine, 1990. *http://books.nap .edu/openbook.php?record_id=1547&page=119,* retrieved January 27, 2008.

58. Hilleboe, H.E., A. Barkhuus, and W.C. Thomas. "Health Planning in the USA." In *Approaches to National Health Planning,* edited by H.E. Hilleboe, A. Barkhuus, and W.C. Thomas, 69–86. Geneva: World Health Organization, 1972. (Public Health Paper No. 46.) *http://www.popline.org/docs/0133/ 725576.html,* retrieved January 28, 2008.

59. Statement of Robert D. Reischauer, Deputy Director, Congressional Budget Office, before the Subcommittee on Oversight, Committee on Ways and Means, U.S. House of Representatives, June 27, 1979. *http://www.cbo.gov/ftpdoc.cfm?index=5226&type=0,* retrieved January 28, 2008.

60. Werlin, S.H, A. Walcott, and M. Joroff. "Implementing Formative Health Planning under PL 93-641." *New England Journal of Medicine* 295, 3 (September 23, 1976): 698–703.

61. O'Donnell, James W. "The Rise and Fall of Federal Support." *Provider* 13 (December 1987): 6.

62. National Conference of State Legislatures. "Certificate of Need: State Health Laws and Programs." *http://www.ncsl.org/programs/health/cert-need.htm,* retrieved July 23, 2007.

63. Cohen, Harold A. *Health Services Cost Review Commission.* Baltimore: Health Services Cost Review Commission, 1983.

64. Kent, Christina. "Twenty Years of Maryland Rate Regulation." *Medicine & Health* 45 (August 19, 1991): Perspectives insert.

65. Parts of this section are adapted from *History of Peer Review.* Washington, DC: Health Care Financing Administration. (Undated, unpublished report received December 1991.)

66. Statement of Robert D. Reischauer, Deputy Director, Congressional Budget Office, before the Subcommittee on Oversight, Committee on Ways and Means, U.S. House of Representatives, June 27, 1979. *http://www.cbo.gov/ftpdoc.cfm?index=5226&type=0,* retrieved January 28, 2008.

67. *Legislative Summaries.* Centers for Medicaid and Medicare Services. *http://www.cms.hhs.gov/Relevant Laws/LS/list.asp,* retrieved January 28, 2008.

68. Ready, Tinker. "PROs Under Assault by Government, Consumers." *Healthweek* 4 (February 12, 1990): 6, 44–45.

69. Bradley, Elizabeth H. "From Adversary to Partner: Have Quality Improvement Organizations Made the Transition Look Smart?" *Health Services Research* (April 2005): 2. *http://findarticles.com/p/articles/ mi_m4149/is_2_40/ai_n13720101/print,* retrieved July 16, 2007.

70. U.S. Department of Health and Human Services, Centers for Medicare & Medicaid Services. "Overview: Quality Improvement Organizations." *http://www.cms.hhs.gov/QualityImprovementOrgs/,* retrieved July 16, 2007.

71. "The Sherman Antitrust Act." The Washington Post Company, 1998. *http://www.washingtonpost.com/ wp-srv/washtech/longterm/antitrust/sherman.htm,* retrieved January 28, 2008.

72. The Clayton Antitrust Act (1914). *http://www.stolaf.edu/people/becker/antitrust/statutes/clayton.html,* retrieved January 28, 2008.

73. National Labor Relations Act. National Labor Relations Board. *http://www.nlrb.gov/about_us/overview/ national_labor_relations_act.aspx,* retrieved January 28, 2008.

74. The Occupational Safety and Health Act (1970[0]). U.S. Department of Labor. *http://www.osha.gov/ pls/oshaweb/owadisp.show_document?p_table=OSHACT&p_id=3355,* retrieved January 28, 2008.

75. *History of the FDA: The 1906 Food and Drugs Act and Its Enforcement.* U.S. Food and Drug Administration. *http://www.fda.gov/oc/history/historyoffda/section1.html,* retrieved January 28, 2008.

76. "Securities Exchange Act of 1934." In *Securities Lawyer's Deskbook.* The University of Cincinnati College of Law. *http://www.law.uc.edu/CCL/34Act/sec2.html,* retrieved January 28, 2008.

77. The Atomic Energy Act of 1954, PL 83-703, 68 Stat. 919 (1954). U.S. Nuclear Regulatory Commission. *http://www.nrc.gov/reading-rm/doc-collections/nuregs/staff/sr0980/ml022200075-vol1.pdf#pagemode =bookmarks&page=14,* retrieved January 28, 2008.

78. The Equal Pay Act of 1963. U.S. Equal Employment Opportunity Commission. *http://www.eeoc.gov/ policy/epa.html,* retrieved January 28, 2008.

79. Title VII of the Civil Rights Act of 1964. U.S. Equal Employment Opportunity Commission. *http://www.eeoc.gov/policy/vii.html,* retrieved January 28, 2008.

80. The Age Discrimination in Employment Act of 1967. U.S. Equal Employment Opportunity Commission. *http://www.eeoc.gov/policy/adea.html,* retrieved January 28, 2008.

81. *Tax Code, Regulations and Official Guidance.* U.S. Department of the Treasury. *http://www.irs.gov/tax pros/article/0,,id=98137,00.html,* retrieved January 28, 2008.

82. *Trade Practices Laws and Regulations.* Alcohol and Tobacco Tax and Trade Bureau. *http://www.ttb.gov/trade_practices/laws_regs_tp.shtml,* retrieved January 28, 2008.

83. MacEachern, Malcolm T. *Hospital Organization and Management,* 3rd ed. Chicago: Physicians' Record Co., 1957.

84. The Joint Commission. "Accreditation Programs: Accreditation Program Fast Track." *http://www.joint commission.org/AccreditationPrograms/,* retrieved January 26, 2007.

85. The Joint Commission. "Networks: Discontinuation of Accreditation Program." *http://www.jointcom mission.org/AccreditationPrograms/Networks/,* retrieved January 26, 2007.

86. Personal communication, Julie Walsh, Professional Relations and Speakers' Bureau Coordinator, The Joint Commission on Accreditation of Healthcare Organizations, May 16, 2007.

87. The Joint Commission. "Benefits of Joint Commission Accreditation." *http://www.jointcommission.org/HTBAC/benefits_accreditation.htm?HTTP__JCSEARC,* retrieved February 2, 2007.

88. American Osteopathic Association. "AOA Fact Sheet." January 1999.

89. DO-Online. "HFAP Accredited Hospitals." *https://www.do-online.org/index.cfm?PageID=acc_hfhosp,* retrieved January 26, 2007.

90. "What Is CHAP?" (Information sheet.). New York: Community Health Accreditation Program, Inc., 1998.

91. Community Health Accreditation Program, Inc. "Description of CHAP Accreditation Program." *http://www.chapinc.org/chapdesc.htm,* retrieved February 16, 1999.

92. Community Health Accreditation Program, Inc. "The Community Health Accreditation Program (CHAP) Seeks Deeming Authority for Hospice Programs." *http://www.chapinc.org/pressc-081298.htm,* retrieved February 16, 1999.

93. Community Health Accreditation Program, Inc. "Description of CHAP Accreditation Program." *http://www.chapinc.org/chapdesc.htm,* retrieved February 1, 1999.

94. "Generic Management System Standards." *http://www.iso.ch/9000e/generic.htm,* retrieved February 10, 1999; "ISO 9000 and ISO 14000 in Plain Language." *http://www.iso.ch/9000/plain.htm,* retrieved February 10, 1999.

95. "The Three-Headed 'Action' Beast: Certification, Registration, and Accreditation." *http://www.iso.ch/9000e/ation.htm,* retrieved February 10, 1999; "ISO Certificates Don't Exist." *http://www.iso.ch/9000e/dontexis.htm,* retrieved February 10, 1999.

96. National Committee for Quality Assurance. "The State of Health Care Quality 2006." *http://web.ncqa.org/tabid/447ItemId/743/Default.aspx,* retrieved July 20, 2007.

97. National Committee for Quality Assurance. "NCQA Health Plan Report Card." *http://hprc.ncqa.org/,* retrieved July 20, 2007.

98. National Committee for Quality Assurance. "Accreditation '99." *http://www.ncqa.org,* retrieved January 25, 1999.

99. Commission on Accreditation of Healthcare Management Education. "Accredited Programs: By Name." *http://www.cahme.org/,* retrieved May 31, 2007.

100. Council on Education for Public Health. "Schools of Public Health and Public Health Programs Accredited by the Council on Education for Public Health." *http://cf51dev5.i4a.com/files/public/s&plist3.S07.pdf,* retrieved July 23, 2007.

101. National League for Nursing. "National League for Nursing History." *http://www.nln.org/info-history.htm,* retrieved February 19, 1999.

102. National League for Nursing Accrediting Commission. "About NLNAC." *http://www.nlnac.org/About%20NLNAC/whatsnew.htm,* retrieved July 22, 2007; U.S. Department of Labor, Bureau of Labor Statistics. "Registered Nurses." *http://www.bls.gov/oco/pdf/ocos083.pdf,* retrieved July 23, 2007.

103. American Board of Medical Specialties. "Specialties & Subspecialties." *http://www.abms.org/Who_We_Help/Physicians/specialties.aspx,* retrieved April 14, 2007.

104. American Board of Medical Specialties. "Maintenance of Certification (MOC)." *http://www.abms.org/ About_Board_Certification/MOC.aspx*, retrieved April 14, 2007.

105. American Board of Medical Specialties. "Study Profiles Effective Doctor–Patient Communication Key Component of Specialty Certification." (News release.) *http://www.abms.org/News_and_Events/release _ABMS_Study_06_07.aspx*, retrieved July 23, 2007.

106. Texas State Board of Medical Examiners. Chapter 164: Physician Advertising. 22 TAC § 164.4. Proposed Rules. December 29, 2000. 25 TexReg 12887. *http://texinfo.library.unt.edu/texasregister/ pdf/2000/1229is.pdf*, retrieved July 23, 2007; Medical Board of California. "Physician Credentials/ Practice Specialties—Frequently Asked Questions." *http://www.medbd.ca.gov/Complaint_Info_FAQ _Specialties.htm#2*, retrieved August 20, 2007.

107. Commission on Accreditation of Healthcare Management Education. *Criteria for Accreditation April 2007. http://www.cahmeweb.org/Accreditation/OfficialCAHMECriteriaFall2008andBeyond.pdf*, retrieved July 13, 2007.

108. Association of University Programs in Health Administration. "List of Undergraduate-Level AUPHA Member Programs." *http://www.aupha.org/custom/directory/programs.cfm?progtype=Undergraduate*, retrieved May 31, 2007.

109. U.S. Department of Labor, Bureau of Labor Statistics. "Employees on Nonfarm Payrolls by Industry Sector and Selected Industry Detail." (Table B-1.) *http://www.bls.gov/news.release/empsit.t14.htm*, retrieved April 13, 2007.

110. Mundinger, Mary O. "Advanced-Practice Nursing—Good Medicine for Physicians?" *New England Journal of Medicine* 330 (January 20, 1994): 211–214; Scheffler, Richard M., Norman J. Waitzman, and John M. Hillman. "The Productivity of Physician Assistants and Nurse Practitioners and Health Work Force Policy in the Era of Managed Health Care." *Journal of Allied Health* 25 (Summer 1996): 207–217.

111. Inglis, Brian. *Fringe Medicine*, 94–102. London: Faber & Faber, 1964.

112. *AOA Fact Sheet*. Chicago: American Osteopathic Association, January 1999.

113. Inglis, *Fringe Medicine*, 102–105, 111–113.

114. U.S. Department of Health and Human Services, Health Resources and Services Administration, Bureau of Health Professions. *Physician Supply and Demand: Projections to 2020,* 12–13. October 2006. *ftp:// ftp.hrsa.gov/bhpr/workforce/PhysicianForecastingPaperfinal.pdf,* retrieved May 31, 2007.

115. *Annual Financial Questionnaire, FY2005.* Washington, DC: Association of American Medical Colleges, 2006.

116. Association of American Medical Colleges. "Tuition and Student Fees Reports." 2006. *http://services .aamc.org/tsfreports/report.cfm?select_control=PUB&year_of_study=2006* and *http://services.aamc .org/tsfreports/report.cfm?select_control=PRI&year_of_study=2006,* retrieved May 22, 2007.

117. Accreditation Council for Graduate Medical Education. *2005–2006 Annual Report. http://www.acgme .org/acWebsite/annRep/an_2005–06AnnRep.pdf,* retrieved July 13, 2007.

118. Randolph, Lillian. *Physician Characteristics and Distribution in the U.S.: 1997–1998,* 9. Chicago: American Medical Association, 1998.

119. Randolph, Lillian. *Physician Characteristics and Distribution in the U.S.: 1997–1998,* 9. Chicago: American Medical Association, 1998.

120. U.S. Bureau of Labor Statistics. "Physicians and Surgeons." *http://www.bls.gov/oco/pdf/ocos074.pdf,* retrieved July 31, 2007.

121. Weinstock, Matthew. "Specialists Are Back in Demand as 'Frenzy' for Primary Docs Subsides." *AHA News* 34 (September 7, 1998): 5.

122. Grumbach, Kevin, and Janet Coffman. "Physician and Nonphysician Clinicians: Complements or Competitors." *Journal of the American Medical Association* 280 (September 2, 1998): 825–826.

123. "Preliminary Findings: The Registered Nurse Population: National Sample Survey of Registered Nurses," 13. Washington, DC: U.S. Department of Health and Human Services, Health Resources and Services Administration, March 2004.

124. Cooper, Richard A., Prakash Laud, and Craig L. Dietrich. "Current and Projected Workforce of Nonphysician Clinicians." *Journal of the American Medical Association* 280 (September 2, 1998): 788–794.

125. *Annual Report 2006, 9.* Washington, DC: Association of American Medical Colleges.

126. Eisenberg, David M., Michael H. Cohen, Andrea Hrbek, Jonathan Grayzel, Maria I. Van Rompay, and

Richard A. Cooper. "Credentialing Complementary and Alternative Medical Procedures." *Annals of Internal Medicine* 136 (2002): 965–973.

127. Omnibus Budget Reconciliation Act of 1987, PL 100-203, 101 Stat. 1330 (1987); *Professional Credentialing Statutes,* 1. Chicago: American Hospital Association, 1990.

128. *Laws that Regulate Dietitians/Nutritionists.* Chicago: American Dietetic Association, 1999.

129. American Society of Clinical Pathologists. "About the ASCP." *http://www.ascp.org/general/about,* February 24, 1999.

130. *U.S. Medical School Finances: Part I and Part II, 1989–1990,* 2. Washington, DC: Association of American Medical Colleges, 1991.

131. Liaison Committee on Medical Education. *Overview: Accreditation and the LCME.* Revised January 31, 2006. *http://www.lcme.org/overview.htm,* retrieved June 1, 2007.

132. Association of American Medical Colleges. *FACTS: Applicants, Matriculants and Graduates—Total Enrollment by School and Sex, 2002–2006. http://www.aamc.org/data/facts/2006/factsenrl.htm,* retrieved June 1, 2007.

133. Association of American Medical Colleges. *FACTS: Applicants, Matriculants and Graduates—Total Graduates by School and Sex, 2002–2006. http://www.aamc.org/data/facts/2006/schoolgrads.htm,* retrieved June 1, 2007.

134. Liaison Committee on Medical Education. *Overview: Accreditation and the LCME.* Revised January 31, 2006. *http://www.lcme.org/overview.htm,* retrieved June 1, 2007.

135. Barzansky, Barbara, and Sylvia Etzel. "Educational Programs in U.S. Medical School, 2004–2005." *Journal of the American Medical Association* 294 (September 7, 2005): 1068.

136. Accreditation Council for Graduate Medical Education. *2005–2006 Annual Report. http://www.acgme.org/acWebsite/annRep/an_2005–06AnnRep.pdf,* retrieved July 13, 2007; Association of American Medical Colleges. *FACTS: Applicants, Matriculants and Graduates—Total Enrollment by School and Sex, 2002–2006. http://www.aamc.org/data/facts/2006/schoolgrads.htm,* retrieved June 1, 2007 and July 13, 2007.

137. "2006 Canadian Medical Education Statistics." (Table 36.) *MD Degrees Awarded by Canadian Universities by University Awarding Degree and Sex of Recipients, 2005 calendar year.* Ottawa, ON: The Association of Faculties of Medicine of Canada.

138. American Osteopathic Association. "AOA Annual Statistical Fact Sheet 2006." *https://www.do-online.org/pdf/ost factsheet.pdf,* retrieved November 5, 2006.

139. *Health Care Almanac,* 2nd ed., edited by Lorri A. Zipperer, 305. Chicago: American Medical Association, 1998.

140. American Board of Physician Specialty. "Eligibility Requirements for Anesthesiology." *http://www.abpsga.org/certification/anesthesiology/eligibility.html,* retrieved June 11, 2007.

141. American Board for Family Medicine. "Eligibility Requirements for Certification." *http://www.theabfm.org/cert/cert.aspx#,* retrieved June 11, 2007.

142. American Board of Neurological Surgery. "Primary Certification Process." *http://www.abns.org/content/primary_certification_process.asp#,* retrieved June 11, 2007.

143. Department of Veterans Affairs. "Minutes of the March 27, 2007, Meeting of the Department of Veterans Affairs Blue Ribbon Panel on VA–Medical School Affiliations." *http://www1.va.gov/advisory/docs/MinutesMedical School AffiliationsMarch-27-07.pdf,* retrieved June 11, 2007.

144. Panangala, Sidath Viranga. "CRS Report for Congress: Veterans' Medical Care FY 2006 Appropriations." *http://holt.house.gov/pdf/CRS on FY06 VHA budget.pdf,* retrieved October 29, 2006.

145. Logan, Jane, and Billie Jean Summers. "The 'New' VA." *Tennessee Nurse* 60 (June 1997): 14–15.

146. Federation of State Medical Boards. "State-Specific Requirements for Initial Licensure." *http://www.fsmb.org/usmle_eliinitial.html,* retrieved July 13, 2007.

147. American Medical Association. "AMA's State Medical Licensure Requirements and Statistics, 2006." *http://www.ama-assn.org/ama1/pub/upload/mm/455/licensurereq-06.pdf,* retrieved July 13, 2007.

148. Rich, Spencer. "Report Questions Discipline by State Medical Units." *The Washington Post,* June 3, 1990, A17.

149. Public Citizen Health Research Group. "Ranking of State Medical Board Disciplinary Actions in 1997." (Faxed personal communication, February 9, 1999.); Public Citizen Health Research Group. "Health Group Names 16,638 Questionable Doctors." *http://www.citizen.org/Press/pr-qd1.htm.*

150. American College of Podiatric Medicine. "Frequently Asked Questions." *http://www.aacpm.org/html/careerzone/cz3,* retrieved June 11, 2007.

151. Stanfield, Peggy S., and Y.H. Hui. *Introduction to the Health Professions,* 131. Boston: Jones & Bartlett, 1998.

152. U.S. Department of Health and Human Services, Health Resources and Services Administration. *The Registered Nurse Population: Findings from the March 2004 National Sample Survey of Registered Nurses. ftp://ftp.hrsa.gov/bhpr/workforce/0306rnss.pdf,* retrieved June 1, 2007.

153. American Nurses Credentialing Center. "ANCC Certification/Specialty Certification." *http://www.nurse credentialing.org/ancc/cert/PDFs/SpecialtyCat.pdf,* retrieved July 13, 2007.

154. *ANA Certification Catalogue.* Kansas City, MO: American Nurses Association, 1983.

155. *ANCC Certification.* (Pamphlet.) Kansas City, MO: American Nurses Credentialing Center, 1991.

156. "Frequently Asked Questions—about ANCC Certification." Revised October 31, 2006. *http://www .nursingworld.org/ancc/cert/certfaqs.html,* retrieved November 28, 2006.

157. MedPac. *Advising the Congress on Medicare Issues: Medicare Payment to Advanced Practice Nurses and Physician Assistants,* 20. June 2002. *http:www.medpac.gov/publications/congressional reports/jun 02NonPhysPay pdf,* retrieved November 5, 2006.

158. Jacobson, Nadine M. "Rule on Physician Supervision for Certified Nurse Anesthetists." *Policy, Politics, & Nursing.* May 2001. *http://ppn.sagepub.com/cgi/reprint/2/2/157.pdf,* retrieved November 14, 2006.

159. Greene, J. and A.M. Nordhaus-Bike, "Nurse Shortage: Where Have All the RNs Gone?" *Hospital & Health Networks* 75 (15–18): 78, 80.

160. U.S. Department of Labor, Bureau of Labor Statistics. "Pharmacists." (Occupational Outlook Handbook.) *http://www.bls/gov/oco/ocos079.htm,* retrieved November 14, 2006.

161. U.S. Department of Labor, Bureau of Labor Statistics. "Occupational Employment and Wages." May 2005. *http://www.bls.gov/oes/current/oes291051htm,* retrieved October 30, 2006.

162. Commission on Dietetic Registration. "Laws that Regulate Dietitians/Nutritionists, 2006." *http://www .cdrnet.org/certifications/licensure/index.htm,* retrieved July 13, 2007.

163. Commission on Dietetic Registration. *Who Is a Registered Dietitian (RD)? http://www.cdrnet.org/about/rddefinition.htm,* retrieved July 13, 2007.

164. American Society of Radiologic Technologists. "Who We Are." *http://www.asrt.org/content/About ASRT/WhoWeAre/Who_We_Are.aspx#Professional_Profile,* retrieved July 13, 2007.

165. American Society of Radiologic Technologists. "Who We Are—Frequently Asked Questions." *http://www.asrt.org/content/AboutASRT/WhoWeAre/Who_we_are_FAQ.aspx,* retrieved July 13, 2007.

166. U.S. Department of Labor, Bureau of Labor Statistics. Clinical Laboratory Technologists and Technicians. *http://www.bis.gov/oco/ocos096.htm,* retrieved July 13, 2007.

167. American Academy of Physician Assistants. "Information about PAs and the PA Profession." *http://www.aapa.org/geninfo1.html,* retrieved July 13, 2007.

168. U.S. Department of Labor. Bureau of Labor Statistics. "Physician Assistants, 2006." *http://www.bls.gov/oco/pdf/ocos081.pdf,* retrieved July 13, 2007.

169. American Academy of Physician Assistants. "2006 AAPA Physician Assistant Census Report." *http://www.aapa.org/research/06census-intro.html#highlight,* retrieved July 13, 2007.

170. Medical Group Management Association. "About MGMA." *http://www.mgma.com/about/,* retrieved July 16, 2007.

171. Personal communication. Katherine Hartwell, Medical Relations Associate, American Medical Association, Chicago. July 23, 2007.

172. Personal communication, American Medical Association, Chicago, February 16, 1999.

173. National Medical Association. "Why Join"? *http://www.nmanet.org/index.php/membership_sub/why_join/,* retrieved July 17, 2007.

174. *Encyclopedia of Associations,* Vol. 1, 33rd ed., edited by Christine Maurer and Tara E. Sheets, 1498. New York: Gale Research, 1998.

175. American Hospital Association, "AHA Member Center." *http://www.aha.org/aha/member-center/index.html,* retrieved July 23, 2007.

176. Personal communication, Melanie Delaney, Membership Director, Federation of American Health Systems, July 23, 2007.

177. Personal communication, Kim Hewitt, Director of Member Services, Catholic Health Association, July 23, 2007.

178. American Health Care Association. "Profile of the American Health Care Association." *http://www.ahca .org/about/profile.htm,* retrieved July 23, 2007.

179. "About AAHSA." *http://www.aahsa.org/about_aahsa/default.asp,* retrieved July 23, 2007.

180. "2006 Accomplishments." *AAHSA—The Power of Membership.* Washington, DC: American Association of Homes and Services for the Aging, 2007.

181. "The American Association of Health Plans." *http://www.aahp.org/services/home_page_links/home links/about_aahp.htm,* retrieved April 13, 1999.

182. America's Health Insurance Plans. "Who We Are." *http://www.ahip.org/content/default.aspx?bc=21/42,* retrieved July 27, 2007.

183. Centers for Medicare and Medicaid Services. "National Health Expenditure Projections 2006–2016." *http://www.cms.hhs.gov/NationalHealthExpendData/downloads/proj2006.pdf,* retrieved July 23, 2007.

184. Reinhardt, Uwe E. "Spending More Through 'Cost Control': Our Obsessive Quest to Gut the Hospital." *Health Affairs* 15 (Summer 1996): 145–154. Reinhardt argues that the incremental cost of convalescent days in a hospital is much less expensive than care provided by alternative sources such as home health. Thus, rather than reduce national healthcare costs, shifting care outside hospitals has actually added to the costs. It is noted that, despite major reductions in inpatient stays from 1980 to 1995, total U.S. health spending increased by more than 50%.

185. U.S. Department of Health and Human Services, Centers for Medicare and Medicaid Services. "National Expenditure Projections 2006–2016." *http:www.cms.hhs.gov/NationalHealthExpendData/downloads/ proj2006.pdf,* retrieved July 23, 2007.

186. U.S. Department of Labor, Bureau of Labor Statistics. "Consumer Price Index." *http://www.bls.gov/cpi/,* retrieved July 23, 2007.

187. Blue Cross Blue Shield. "History of Blue Cross Blue Shield." *http://www.bcbs.com/about/history/,* retrieved July 23, 2007.

188. Health Insurance Association of America. *Source Book of Health Insurance Data, 1982–83,* 7. Washington, DC: Health Insurance Association of America, 1982–83.

189. Lopes, Gregory. "Health Care Costs Outstrip Pay, Inflation." *The Washington Times,* September 27, 2006, C10.

190. Davis, Karen. "Uninsured in America: Problems and Possible Solutions." *BMJ* 334 (February 17, 2007): 346.

191. Davis, Karen, "Uninsured in America."

192. *Legislative Summaries.* Centers for Medicaid and Medicare Services. *http://www.cms.hhs.gov/Relevant Laws/LS/list.asp,* retrieved January 28, 2008.

193. *Summary of P.L. 98-21, (H.R. 1900), Social Security Amendments of 1983*—Signed on April 20, 1983. Social Security Online. *http://www.ssa.gov/history/1983amend.html,* retrieved January 28, 2008.

194. U.S. Department of Health and Human Services, Centers for Medicare and Medicaid Services. CMS DRG Version 23 10/01/05 to 09/30/06. *http://www.dhs.state.or.us/policy/healthplan/guides/hospital/ drg_tables/drg_v23.pdf,* retrieved July 16, 2007.

195. Health Care Financing Administration. "Medicare Provider Analysis and Review (MEDPAR)." *http:// www.hcfa.gov/stats/medpar.htm,* retrieved March 22, 1999.

196. Fries, Brant E., Gunnar Ljunggren, and Bengt Winblad. "International Comparison of Long-Term Care: The Need for Resident-Level Classification." *Journal of the American Geriatrics Society* 39 (January 1991): 12–13.

197. White, Chapin, Steven D. Pizer, and Alan J. White. "Assessing the RUG-III Resident Classification System for Skilled Nursing Facilities." *Health Care Financing Review* (Winter 2002).

198. CMS Office of Public Affairs. "Proposed Nursing Home Payment Reforms Increase Accuracy, Predictability of Payment." May 13, 2005. *http://www.cms.hhs.gov/apps/media/press/release.asp?Counter =1461,* retrieved July 16, 2007.

199. HealthIQ. "IQToolkit™ Glossary: Definition for APG—Ambulatory Patient Groups." *http://www .healthiq.com/HealthcareResources/glossary/G25.htm,* retrieved March 30, 1999.

200. U.S. Department of Health and Human Services, Centers for Medicare and Medicaid Services. *Program*

Memorandum: Intermediaries Transmittal A-02-074, 3. August 7, 2002. *http://www.cms.hhs.gov/hospital outpatientpps/downloads/a02074.pdf,* retrieved July 16, 2007.

201. Omnibus Budget Reconciliation Act of 1989, PL 101-239, 103 Stat. 2106 (1989).

202. Inlander, Charles B., and Michael A. Donio. *Medicare Made Easy,* 111. Allentown, PA: People's Medical Society, 1997.

203. Grimaldi, Paul L. "RBRVS: How New Physician Fee Schedule Will Work." *Health Care Financial Management* 45 (September 1991): 74.

204. "Has HCFA 'Broken Faith' with MD Fee Schedule?" *Medical Staff Leader* 20 (August 1991): 8.

205. Grimaldi, Paul L. "RBRVS: How New Physician Fee Schedule Will Work," 74.

206. Koska, Mary T. "Hospitals: Begin Strategic Planning for RBRVS." *Hospitals* 65 (February 20, 1991): 28–30.

207. U.S. Department of Health and Human Services, Centers for Medicare and Medicaid Services. "National Health Expenditure Projections 2006–2016." *http://www.cms.hhs.gov/NationalHealthExpendData/downloads/proj2006.pdf,* retrieved July 23, 2007.

208. From Lave, Judith R., and Lester B. Lave. "Health Care: Part I." *Law and Contemporary Problems,* 35. (Spring 1970); reprinted by permission. Copyright 1970, 1971 by Duke University.

209. Written by Gary E. Crum, Ph.D., M.P.H., Executive Director, Graduate Medical Education Consortium, The University of Virginia at Wise, (Past Director, Northern Kentucky Health Department). Used with permission.

2

Types and Structures of Health Services Organizations and Health Systems

This chapter describes the organizational structures of common types of health services organizations (HSOs), including acute care hospitals, nursing facilities, ambulatory care organizations, hospice, managed care organizations, and home health agencies. HSOs may be freestanding or part of health systems (HSs), which are also described. The chapter begins with background information about three key components of HSO/HS organizational structures: governing bodies (GBs), chief executive officers (CEOs), and professional staff organizations (PSOs). With some variation across types, HSOs/HSs are characterized by this triad of key organizational components.

▬ The Triad of Key Organizational Components ▬▬▬▬▬▬

Although use of the term *triad* (group of three) to refer to the GB, CEO, and PSO components of HSOs/HSs is archaic, the concept of the triad remains relevant. Fundamentally, as Weber suggested in a classic formulation made decades ago, organizations must prevent the idiosyncrasies of individuals from interfering with their ability to accomplish specific tasks.[1] This end is achieved by establishing a bureaucracy in which each person has a place and a set of tasks. The pyramid of the typical bureaucratic organizational structure is shown in Figure 2.1. This structure is based on a chain of command that delegates authority and responsibility downward. Historically, larger HSOs were structured as bureaucracies; in this regard, they have been joined by HSs as shown in Figure 2.2. The three components of the triad are described briefly below and then discussed more fully in subsequent sections of this chapter.

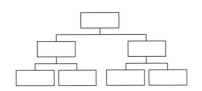

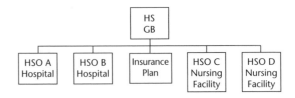

Figure 2.1. Typical bureaucratic pyramid.   **Figure 2.2.** Pyramidal organizational structure of HS.

GOVERNING BODY

Regardless of ownership, role, or other characteristics, all HSOs/HSs have a GB or its equivalent. These range from a GB as simple as one individual in a sole-proprietorship nursing facility, to an acute care hospital in an academic health (medical) center, to the GB of a large health system. The GB is the ultimate authority and decision maker for HSOs/HSs. It determines mission and evaluates progress toward accomplishing the mission. Among the GB's most important tasks is selecting and evaluating the CEO.

CHIEF EXECUTIVE OFFICER

Although titles vary, all HSOs/HSs have a CEO. As HSOs/HSs have adopted the accoutrements of business enterprise, they have tended to use corporate titles such as *president* and *executive vice president*. The GB selects and delegates authority to a CEO, who acts as its agent to organize inputs to achieve organizational missions and objectives. For many reasons, including legal relationships and the financial demands on healthcare organizations and systems, GBs currently are being held to a higher level of legal and public accountability, and this necessitates a close and effective working relationship between the CEO and GB. This relationship is extraordinarily varied and may range from having a CEO with great latitude in management decisions to having a CEO with little independence.

PROFESSIONAL STAFF ORGANIZATION

By definition, HSOs/HSs have clinical staff who deliver healthcare and health-related services. The makeup and organization of clinical staff vary markedly among HSOs/HSs, even within the same type. Broadly defined, clinical staff are all individuals who care for patients. Here, however, *clinical staff* refers to licensed independent practitioners (LIPs).[2] Increasingly, HSO/HS clinical staffs include nonphysician LIPs such as dentists, clinical psychologists, podiatrists, nurse midwives, and chiropractors. In acute care hospitals and some other types of HSOs/HSs, the clinical staff comprise a separate, unincorporated association with their own bylaws that organize these clinicians. This feature is unique and breaks the rigid mold of a true bureaucracy. In effect, there may be two pyramids in the structure, one for the professional staff organization and another for the rest of the organization. Previously, this dual pyramid was much clearer than it is now in most HSOs/HSs, but elements of it remain in the structures of some of these organizations and systems.

The association of clinical staff is commonly called the medical staff organization because historically it was composed almost exclusively of physicians. Increasingly, the term *professional staff organization* is more appropriate because it suggests the broad range of preparation and activities of members. Consequently, that term and the acronym *PSO* are used here.

PSO members provide services themselves or order other HSO/HS staff to do so. Relationships among PSO members depend on the setting and services being provided. In some HSOs/HSs, such as a physician group practice, the numbers of nonphysician providers may be equal to or greater than the number of physicians. The care in HSOs/HSs such as nursing homes is chronic and custodial. Here, only intermittent physician contact is necessary, because treatment is routine and given by other LIPs and non-LIP caregivers such as registered nurses (RNs), licensed practical nurses (LPNs), and certified nursing assistants, who are not part of the PSO. These caregivers are following either standing orders, approved prospectively by the chief medical officer (CMO) or the PSO and applied to all patients of that type, or LIP-determined individual treatment orders. The presence of a PSO increases organizational complexity greatly, but the HSO's/HS's work is impossible without its members.

In the sections that follow, important aspects of the roles and functions of GBs, CEOs, and PSOs are described in more detail. The highly complex relationships among the components of the triad in HSOs/HSs arise from factors that include the involvement of voluntary GB members in not-for-profit HSOs/HSs, lack of an employment relationship for most LIPs who provide medical treatment, and the technical and highly specialized functions of most staff.

Governing Body

The contemporary healthcare environment, as described in Chapter 1, is having a profound effect on GBs and continues to change them dramatically. James Rice describes critical shifts in the environments facing GBs as obstacles to financial vitality; population shifts and growing consumerism; physician challenges; quality and patient safety; new medical and information technologies; and public health, community collaborative, and health policy reform.[3] Members can no longer be chosen as a way to honor them or because they might make financial contributions. The pressures and need for GBs to be effective will increase, and this means recruiting people who understand health services, are prepared in business matters, and have backgrounds that are relevant to the HSO/HS. For example, it has been demonstrated that GBs that are engaged in the oversight of quality practices contribute to high performance on this dimension in their organizations.[4]

Suggested desirable personal characteristics of a trustee include capability in listening, consensus building, communicating, and leading, as well as ability to think outside the box.[5] GB members also need knowledge of finance, strategic and financial planning, community needs and assessment, medical and information technology, and real estate, among others. Of course, no member can be expected to be knowledgeable in all of these areas.

Other individual characteristics that are increasingly considered in selecting individuals for board membership include those that help boards reflect community demographics and exhibit greater cultural sensitivity. This means including on boards people who differ in age, race, ethnicity, religious affiliation, and gender. Indeed, in the quest for effective board members, consideration has been given to almost every conceivable physical or psychological characteristic, as well as to the full range of knowledge and capabilities acquired through education and experience, that might be relevant to an individual's performance on a board.[6]

RESPONSIBILITIES AND FUNCTIONS

GBs have extensive and demanding governance responsibilities, outlined in Table 2.1, along with associated activities. The first of these responsibilities—and perhaps the most complex of all their responsibilities—is to represent, advance, preserve, and balance the interests of the HSO's/HS's stakeholders.

TABLE 2.1.   KEY RESPONSIBILITIES AND ASSOCIATED ACTIVITIES OF HSO/HS GBs

Responsibilities	Associated activities
Representing, balancing, preserving, and advancing the interests of its various stakeholders in the entity	• Addressing needs of internal stakeholders such as employees, physicians, and volunteers • Addressing needs of external stakeholders such as consumers, regulators, and suppliers

Formulating organizational ends (vision, mission, and objectives)	• Assessing community needs
	• Planning and monitoring the implementation of the entity's
	  • mission, vision, and value statements
	  • goals and objectives

Ensuring suitable performance by the chief executive officer	• Selecting, evaluating, and retaining or dismissing the CEO • Balancing the relationship with the CEO so that the board governs and management manages
Ensuring acceptable quality of care and services	• Credentialing professional staff • Ensuring that procedures are in place for the assessment of the processes for, and the outcome of, care
Overseeing finances and financial performance	• Establishing financial objectives • Approving and monitoring the budget

Ensuring compliance with laws, regulations, and accreditation standards	• Making certain that management and the professional staff are in compliance with
	  • laws and regulations
	  • accreditation standards

Assisting with fund-raising	• Contributing to the entity • Facilitating contributions from the community
Advocating with the private and public sectors for the entity and field	• Advocating on behalf of the entity to private and public sectors • Advocating on behalf of the healthcare field
Governing in an effective and efficient manner	• Ensuring that bylaws, policies, and processes are appropriate • Evaluating board performance • Selecting new board members • Conducting board orientation and continuing governance education (CGE)

From Longest, Beaufort B., Jr., and Samuel A. Friede. "The Competent Board: Stitching Together Needed Skills and Knowledge." *Trustee* (February 2002): 16. Reprinted from *Trustee*, by permission, February 2002, Copyright 2002, by Health Forum, Inc.

The American Hospital Association's (AHA's) concept of GB responsibilities applies to all HSOs/HSs. The GB

1. Has the responsibility for organizing itself effectively, for establishing and following the policies and procedures necessary to discharge its responsibilities, and for adopting bylaws in accordance with legal requirements
2. Has the responsibility for selecting a qualified chief executive officer and for delegating to the chief executive officer the necessary authority to manage . . . effectively
3. Has the authority and responsibility for ensuring proper organization of the . . . [clinical] staff, and for monitoring the quality of care provided . . .
4. Has the authority and responsibility for monitoring and influencing public policies concerning the establishment and maintenance of appropriate external relationships
5. Has responsibility and authority, subject to the . . . charter, for determining . . . mission and for establishing a strategic plan, goals, objectives, and policies to achieve that mission
6. Is entrusted with resources . . . and with the proper development, utilization, and maintenance of those resources

7. Has the responsibility and authority for the organization, protection, and enhancement of . . . human resources
8. Is responsible for the provision of healthcare education and research programs that further the . . . mission[7]

In meeting these responsibilities, GBs perform many functions. They appoint CEOs and maintain effective relationships with them, establish missions and monitor progress toward accomplishing them, approve and monitor strategic plans and annual budgets, ensure the quality of care by approving quality goals and monitoring their accomplishment, and monitoring overall performance of the HSO/HS.[8] In addition, written bylaws, periodically reviewed and approved by the GB, set out the GB's organization and guide its activities.

COMPOSITION

Members of GBs capable of helping fulfill the responsibilities and carry out the functions noted above must possess considerable skills and knowledge.[9] In addition, they are likely to join GBs because their values are consistent with missions of the organizations whose boards they join.

An important contemporary development in GB composition is the addition of physicians to GBs. Historically, not-for-profit hospitals commonly excluded physicians from GB membership because they had potential conflicts of interest regarding resource allocation, capital equipment purchases, and quality of care. (Conflicts of interest are discussed in Chapter 4.) The contemporary view, however, encourages physician membership because it is generally believed that conflicts of interest are avoidable and that physicians bring vital clinical expertise to governance decisions. Research suggests that integrating physicians into management and governance enhances performance and helps align incentives,[10] and physicians are increasingly involved in governance in HSOs/HSs.[11]

GB members may be external or internal. External members are not employed by the HSO/HS, while internal members are. External members include those described earlier, such as community leaders. Internal members may include the CEO, chief operating officer (COO), CMO, and chief financial officer (CFO), as well as leaders of PSOs. The proportion of internal members is likely to grow as greater expertise is needed by GB members, although the probability of conflicts of interest increases.

COMMITTEES

Committees allow specialized, effective work when GBs are large. Boards range from a few members to more than 100 in HSOs/HSs, although boards of 10 to 20 members are most common.[12] GBs of not-for-profit HSOs/HSs tend to be much larger than those organized as for-profit corporations.

Standing committees of HSO/HS boards almost always include executive, audit, finance, quality, and nominations committees, and they often include others such as professional staff, ethics, human resources, strategic planning, public relations and development, investment, and capital equipment and expenditures. Committees on audit, ethics, and quality are more recent additions. Ad hoc (special) committees are established as needed.

Two committees are noteworthy. The executive committee is the most important because of its ongoing monitoring and reviewing, activities especially important when GBs are large or meet infrequently. The executive committee receives reports from other committees, oversees policy implementation, and provides interim decision making. The executive committee is chaired by the chair of the GB; membership usually includes chairs of standing committees. CEOs typically attend executive committee meetings.

The professional staff committee is responsible for the quality of clinical activities. It reviews

PSO recommendations on staff appointments, reappointments, and clinical activities (privileges) and the performance of PSO members to determine whether privileges should be modified. Both tasks rely heavily on assistance from the PSO, from GB members who are experts, or from consultants. The HSO's/HS's ethical and legal obligations to protect patients from substandard care are ultimately met through GB review and approval.

The critical need for the CEO and other senior-level managers, the PSO, and the GB to communicate and coordinate may be satisfied in several ways. The joint conference committee (JCC) can be a standing committee of the GB or the PSO. The JCC typically has three members from the GB and three from the PSO, with the CEO as a seventh member. Although the JCC has no line authority, it can play a major role in considering policy issues for the organization. Other means of coordinating GB–PSO–CEO activities include having members from each group on one another's committees and circulating copies of minutes and reports to other committees.

RELATIONSHIP TO THE CEO

The GB's responsibility to recruit, select, and evaluate the CEO has been noted. CEOs assemble and organize resources and develop the systems to carry out GB-approved programs and policies. CEOs also provide information to the GB so it can develop policy, monitor implementation, and oversee results.

The CEO's performance should be assessed annually by the GB; specific recommendations should result from this process. Performance should be measured against predetermined objectives mutually identified and accepted by the CEO and GB. GBs should not set objectives for CEOs without giving them sufficient authority and resources. A CEO performance appraisal form has been developed by Tyler and Biggs.[13] In addition, GBs can measure CEO performance (and that of other senior-level managers) by negative developments.

Employment contracts for CEOs and senior management are increasingly common in HSOs/HSs, a development that follows the pattern set elsewhere in the economy. These contracts set terms of employment, including severance. Many CEOs, especially of larger organizations or systems, have incentive employment contracts. Care must be exercised by GBs to be certain that CEO compensation complies with IRS requirements.[14]

CEOs walk a narrow line as they focus GB members' expertise and encourage interest, dedication, and enthusiasm but simultaneously dissuade direct participation in internal operations. When GB members intervene in operations, CEO authority is undercut, and subordinates are frustrated and confused—conditions unlikely to enhance effectiveness or efficiency. Interference is forestalled by GB job descriptions and clarification of roles and activities by GB member orientation and education.

CEOs should be present at GB meetings, as many are voting members. This raises the potential for conflicts of interest, just as when PSO members serve on the GB. Evaluation of the CEO raises the issue most starkly. The views of the CEO always should be considered, but GB membership gives the CEO a weight that may be at variance with objective assessment and the HSO's/HS's best interests. Problems are lessened if CEOs are absent when issues of self-interest are considered, a practice that reduces but does not eliminate potential conflicts of interest. In addition to membership, professional and personal ties between the CEO and GB members may give the CEO excessive influence, as well as lessen the objectivity of evaluations and decision making. Conversely, when the CEO is a voting member of the GB, two advantages are enhanced—communication and better coordination.

It also is important that the GB evaluate its own performance. First, it must demonstrate accountability for its actions and resource utilization. Discussions could begin by identifying how and where the GB adds value, beyond that contributed by management and staff. Once this is known, members can identify ways to use time, skills, and other resources more effectively to strengthen GB contributions. After selecting targets for improvement, the GB can identify criteria for monitoring progress and delineate steps to obtain and use feedback to ensure further improvement.[15]

▨ Chief Executive Officer ▨▨▨▨▨▨▨▨▨▨▨▨▨▨▨▨▨▨▨▨▨▨▨▨▨▨▨▨

The work of HSO/HS managers is unmatched elsewhere in society. They are responsible for organizations and systems that deliver unique personal services to ill or anxious people in complex settings, and often in emotionally charged circumstances. In addition, the relationships that HSOs/HSs have with professional staff through the PSO are unparalleled in other enterprises. CEOs' work must be accomplished in a highly competitive, economically demanding environment. Increasingly, HSOs/HSs are among the largest employers in their communities, which raises the expectations for their economic roles in communities.[16]

Historically, various titles were used for top-level managers in HSOs: *administrator, director, CEO, president,* and *superintendent.* This discussion uses *CEO,* a generic title applicable to HSOs/HSs of all types. There is no standard statement of a CEO's qualifications. Although directed to hospital CEOs, the Joint Commission on Accreditation of Healthcare Organizations (The Joint Commission) (www.jcaho.org) expectation is instructive, if general: "The chief executive officer is competent and has the education and experience required for the size, complexity, [and] mission of the hospital, and the scope of services it provides."[17] Similar requirements are found for other types of HSOs accredited by The Joint Commission.

The educational backgrounds for CEOs vary in terms of discipline or field, but they almost invariably involve graduate education. Increasingly, those leading HSOs/HSs are facilitating their senior-level managers in developing personalized plans of continuing education and selective experiences to enhance their capabilities and careers.[18]

Larger HSOs/HSs typically divide the CEO's role into two parts. The CEO is primarily involved in GB and external relations, as well as strategic planning, fund-raising, directing capital projects, and at times PSO relations. The COO is responsible for day-to-day operations and reports to the CEO. This division of responsibility helps meet increasingly complex demands.

Universally found in the large HSO/HS is a CFO and a CMO. The CFO is an extension of the concept of controllership, with additional responsibilities for reimbursement, capital financing, and investment. The CMO may be known as the medical director, chief of staff, or vice president for medical affairs and is responsible for PSO relations, credentialing and privileges, and quality of clinical care. Increasingly, large organizations or systems have a chief information officer (CIO), chief quality officer (CQO), and chief nursing officer (CNO)—responsible for information services, quality, and nursing, respectively. When these various chief officers are present in an executive suite, it is sometimes referred to as the "c-suite."

The presence of both a CEO and a COO is problematic if their spheres of authority and responsibility are ill defined. Confusion is certain if the CEO intervenes directly in matters for which the COO is responsible; unless there are emergencies, lines of authority and reporting relationships must be followed. The COO must be cognizant of GB reporting relationships so as not to bypass the CEO.

Below these senior-level managers are management layers that ultimately lead to staff who do the day-to-day work of the organization. The number of management layers in large health systems and major medical centers continues to decline, which is consistent with advice for "flattening" organizational structures from experts such as Peter Drucker.[19]

CEO RESPONSIBILITIES AND REQUIRED SKILLS AND KNOWLEDGE (COMPETENCIES)

The CEO's basic responsibility is effectively managing inputs (human resources, material, technology, information, and capital) to achieve the desired outputs that are the HSO's/HS's mission and objectives. Except in very small HSOs, the CEOs delegate tasks and authority to subordinate managers. The ultimate responsibility to design, change, and operate an effective management structure to achieve the mission and objectives is the CEO's, however, and cannot be delegated. It is the CEO whom the GB will hold accountable for organizational performance.

The CEO manages the entire entity. Management is defined and discussed more fully in Chapter 5 as a process composed of interrelated social and technical functions and activities (including roles) occurring in a formal organizational setting for the purpose of accomplishing predetermined objectives through utilization of human and other resources. To succeed at management, especially as HSOs/HSs continue their established trend toward larger, more complex structures, CEOs must possess and expand a substantial pool of skills and knowledge (competencies). For example, this continuing trend will require CEOs to have more competence in coalition building and negotiation as they establish strategic alliances and partnerships in providing health services and conducting other business activities. [20]

The work of managers in HSOs/HSs can be examined—as it is in detail in Chapter 5—from four perspectives: the functions that managers perform, the skills that they use in managing, the roles they play as managers, and the competencies (sets of knowledge and skills) required to manage effectively. Each perspective contributes to understanding management work, but overarching the functions, skills, and roles perspectives are clusters of knowledge and skill in using the knowledge (competencies). Increasingly, the professional field of health management is focusing on identifying and equipping managers and those who aspire to health management careers with vital managerial competencies. Although there may be some overlap among them, six rather distinct competencies are required for successful CEOs. The clusters of knowledge and skills that make up these competencies are 1) conceptual, 2) technical managerial/clinical, 3) interpersonal/collaborative, 4) political, 5) commercial, and 6) governance.[21] These competencies are described in detail in Chapter 5.

The National Center for Healthcare Leadership (NCHL) emphasizes competencies needed for good management.[22] The NCHL has developed a Healthcare Leadership Competency Model that features a comprehensive set of 26 technical and behavioral competencies that can be applied for senior-, middle-, and first-level managers in HSOs/HSs. This model also is described in detail in Chapter 5.

Effective GBs and CEOs are critical to performance in HSOs/HSs. However, members of the third component of the triad—the PSO—admit, diagnose, and treat patients. Their critical role in the structure of HSOs/HSs is discussed next.

Professional Staff Organization

It is crucial to understand that the LIPs who treat and order treatment for patients are the engine that drives an HSO/HS in its service delivery activities. No medical treatment can be rendered without express orders or standing orders that were approved prospectively. HSOs/HSs with PSOs have relationships that are not reflected by the conventional organizational pyramid shown in Figure 2.1. PSOs have bylaws, officers, a committee structure, and other characteristics that reflect the autonomy of physicians and other LIPs, who are often independent contractors in the HSO/HS. Even when salaried, LIPs exhibit a high degree of independence and may have more allegiance to their professions and one another than to the HSO/HS. Because of this independence and the technical content of clinical practice, GBs have historically exercised little direct control over PSOs, but this is changing.

INTEGRATING LIPS INTO MANAGEMENT

Individual LIPs, and the PSO as a whole, perform technical services that must be integrated into a total effort if the organization is to achieve its objectives. Non-LIP managers neither deliver clinical services nor judge quality independently. They must obtain the expert advice and technical assistance of LIPs to make informed judgments about individual and aggregate PSO practice.

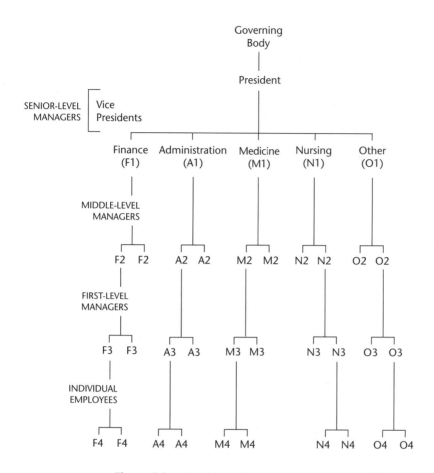

Figure 2.3. Template for the organization charts of HSOs.

Historically, PSO members have had little involvement in management. The exception has been clinical managers and PSO officers. In the past decade, however, the value of their participation has been recognized, and LIPs have become more involved in management decision making. Such interactions are good practice and are strongly recommended by accrediting bodies such as The Joint Commission.

PSO members can be integrated into an HSO's/HS's management structure in several ways: They may join PSO management and GB committees; managers may ask them for advice formally and informally; and those who manage clinical departments or units are part of the management team. Some aspects of such relationships in a single HSO are shown in Figure 2.3.

Clinical managers have a special place in an efficiently managed HSO/HS because even small PSOs are divided into departments or sections based on clinical interest. Although medical education and clinical practice teach physicians to think logically and to view problems systematically and consider their implications, these skills do not adequately prepare them as managers. Only competent clinical managers can further organizational objectives. Thus it is a matter of self-interest that the HSO/HS ensure their management competence. The presence of full- or part-time salaried clinical managers allows even more involvement in management. When clinicians and managers understand each other's problems, enhanced communication and organizational effectiveness result—all of which enable managers to align incentives to better deliver integrated, coordinated services successfully.[23]

SELF-GOVERNANCE

As evidence of the strong tradition of physician independence, PSOs continue to be largely self-governing. LIPs are part of the PSO whether they are salaried by the HSO/HS or are fee-for-service LIPs. The PSO's bylaws, which must be approved by the GB, are central to self-governance and identify officers, committees and their functions, categories of membership, the application process, the procedure for amending the bylaws, and a process for reviewing actions that are adverse to members. In addition, the PSO adopts rules and regulations that control clinical practice, which may be supplemented by even more detailed rules for clinical specialties, subspecialties, and departments.

OPEN OR CLOSED

The PSO may be open, closed, or a combination of the two. This concept is highly developed in acute care hospitals and systems but also affects other HSOs, such as nursing facilities and hospice. If a PSO is open, any qualified LIP (as defined in the PSO bylaws) is granted clinical privileges (with or without PSO membership) and may treat patients. If a PSO is closed, qualified LIPs (as defined in the PSO bylaws) may or may not be granted clinical privileges (with or without PSO membership), depending on the parameters put on the PSO by the PSO itself, as approved by the GB. Such parameters may include absolute size of the PSO or limits on the numbers in various specialties or types of LIPs. Many hospitals, for example, have a combination of an open and a closed PSO in that they close some clinical departments, such as anesthesia, clinical and anatomical laboratories, emergency medicine, and radiology, but grant privileges to any qualified surgeon or physician. Closing staffs, clinical departments, or both is justified on the grounds that doing so improves quality of patient care and enhances efficiency.

When departments are closed, the HSO usually has entered into an exclusive contract with an individual physician or provider group, which is known as a concessionaire. All LIPs who function under the terms of the contract must have clinical privileges that are consistent with their licenses and demonstrated current competencies.

COMMITTEES

In many ways, hospital GB and PSO committee structures are parallel. The PSO is led by an executive committee whose members usually include the chairs of standing committees. Like its GB counterpart, the executive committee acts for the PSO and coordinates its activities. It provides continuity and enhances communication between the PSO and CEO. Major activities of the executive committee include implementing PSO policies, receiving and acting on reports and recommendations from PSO committees, making recommendations on PSO membership and clinical privileges, monitoring quality of care, and taking corrective action, including discipline. Other functional areas that must be managed and for which there may be committees include

- *Credentials*—reviews qualifications of clinicians for PSO membership and recommends specific privileges to the executive committee; reviews continuing appropriateness of privileges
- *Surgical case review*—reviews justifications for surgery; checks relationship between pre- and postoperative diagnoses
- *Medical records*—checks for timely completion of medical records; reviews clinical usefulness and adequacy of record for quality of care
- *Pharmacy and therapeutics*—develops the formulary and monitors drug use and other therapeutics policies; may have special interest in antibiotics use

- *Utilization review*—reviews resource use in providing care, with special attention to length of stay and use of ancillary services
- *Quality assessment*—may be used instead of surgical case review and medical records committees, or may review pre- and postoperative reports, use of ancillary services such as radiology and laboratories, and conditions of patients on discharge to determine appropriateness of treatments. Increasingly, a PSO has a quality improvement committee that uses monitoring and assessment completed by its other committees to focus clinical process analysis and improvement activities. Continuous quality improvement is discussed in Chapter 7.

Other common committees are infection control, blood use, risk management and safety, disaster planning, bylaws, and nominating. The CEO or a designee should attend all PSO meetings, including its committee meetings and related functional activities.[24]

CLINICAL DEPARTMENTATION

The extent and type of clinical departmentation are determined by the HSO's/HS's size and activities. Nonhospital HSOs, such as health maintenance organizations (HMOs) and multispecialty group practices, have clinical departments. Nursing facilities and hospice have a medical director (or CMO) but are unlikely to have a PSO. Small hospitals have only departments of medicine and surgery in their PSOs. Larger hospitals and HSs typically add other specialties, such as obstetrics and gynecology, pediatrics, and family practice. Departmentation expands from there to include clinical specialties or subspecialties as separate departments or sections within departments.

Clinical department heads are elected by department members or are appointed by the CEO; in either case, they serve at the discretion of the GB. Clinical managers may be paid or unpaid, although larger units and greater demands increase the likelihood that clinical managers who are not already employees will be paid salaries. If specialization warrants, then divisions, sections, or both are established within departments. The upward chain of command goes to a physician, who is the CMO. Larger entities typically pay a salary to the CMO. Eventually, the line of authority reaches the GB. The CMO may report to the CEO, which is consistent with the accountability that the management structure should demand of the PSO. Contemporary HSOs/HSs are making special efforts to develop the management skills of physician managers and to develop physician leaders.[25]

CREDENTIALING

Credentialing LIPs is crucial to the quality of care and is done by the HSO/HS with the help of the PSO. One approach that is applicable in an HS is central credentials verification, with a multidisciplinary, uniform credentialing and privileging process carried out separately at each component HSO.[26] Credentialing is essential for physicians because, unlike other LIPs, their licenses are unlimited. Only through the credentialing process are physicians' activities in HSOs/HSs made consistent with their demonstrated current competencies. The activities allowed under the limited licenses of other LIPs may be narrowed even further by the HSO/HS. The same credentialing process can be used for all LIPs (including physicians), whether or not they are eligible to be members of the PSO.

Credentialing has two parts. The first is to determine the applicant's PSO membership category, if the LIP is eligible for membership. The second is assessing the LIP's demonstrated current competence to determine what the applicant will be allowed (credentialed) to do—this is known as delineating and granting clinical privileges. PSO membership (and category) and the clinical privileges the practitioner may have in the HSO/HS are separate. The two-part process applies to initial appointment and to reappointment, which are different. PSO bylaws determine the content of the process and include due process safeguards for the applicant or reapplicant.

The credentialing process usually is organized and monitored by the CEO or a designee. Completed application files are referred to the PSO for review by the specialty department and then the credentials committee; the credentials committee makes a recommendation to the PSO executive committee. The next level of review is by the CMO and the president of the PSO. Final approval of recommendations lies with the GB, through its committee structure.

Economic Credentialing

Under increasing financial pressures, HSOs/HSs have given more attention to judging LIPs by their economic performance as well as by their clinical performance. Physicians vary widely in the use of resources such as hospital admission and length of patient stay, diagnostic tests for outpatients, and types and durations of therapies. Decisions on such matters have major cost and revenue implications for HSOs. Patients should receive needed services—no more and no less. With few exceptions, such care is both high quality and efficient.

Judging economic performance, often called economic credentialing, means that, in addition to reviewing the quality of care, data are collected as to LIPs' economic effects on the HSO/HS. Two criteria are useful to assess how efficiently resources are used by LIPs: volume of referrals and practice patterns. The profiling that is necessary to undertake economic credentialing is possible because data systems enable HSOs/HSs to link cost and patient treatment information.[27] Economic credentialing is becoming commonplace.

Handling Impaired Clinicians

One area in which PSOs have a less than enviable record of self-governance is in handling impaired LIPs, especially physicians. It has been common for PSO members to band together to prevent patient and public scrutiny. This human tendency may cause HSOs/HSs to be less than rigorous in meeting ethical and legal duties to patients, and even to staff. However, organizations and systems are morally (and perhaps legally) obliged to try to rehabilitate all impaired staff, including LIPs, whenever possible.

All states now have formal programs focusing on rehabilitation and monitoring of physicians with psychoactive substance use disorders, as well as mental and physical illness.[28] Attention to this issue was increased in 1973, when the American Medical Association (AMA) issued a landmark policy paper through its Council on Mental Health, "The Sick Physician: Impairment by Psychiatric Disorders, Including Alcoholism and Drug Dependence."[29] The AMA acknowledged physician impairment and proposed model legislation that offered a therapeutic alternative to discipline, recognizing alcoholism and other drug addictions as illnesses. More recently, the AMA's Council on Ethical and Judicial Affairs provided additional guidance in the area of physician health in terms of how it affects physicians' professional activities, including patient care and trust in the profession.[30]

Its varied types and subtleties make impairment among caregivers difficult to detect and document. Impairment may be physical, mental, or both and may result from aging, disease, or chemical dependency. Perhaps as much as 15% of physicians are impaired due to drug and alcohol abuse.[31] A survey of physicians found that 8% had abused or been chemically dependent on alcohol or drugs during their lives.[32] Some physicians, such as anesthesiologists, appear to be at higher risk than others.[33] Similar estimates of impairment of all types have been made for nonphysician caregivers; one survey of nurses found that 10% were addicted to at least one controlled substance.[34]

This issue continues to receive attention by PSOs and, increasingly, by the GBs and CEOs of HSOs/HSs. Accountability mechanisms and authority that are available to CEOs and GBs are more clearly defined and used, and impairment is more likely to be identified through more sophisticated risk management activities, as discussed in Chapter 10.

PSO MEMBERSHIP

The process and substance of initial application for PSO membership must be thorough, detailed, and comprehensive. In 1984, The Joint Commission adopted a medical staff standard that allowed hospitals to extend PSO membership to LIPs other than physicians and dentists. The changes were especially important for podiatrists, clinical psychologists, nurse midwives, and chiropractors.

Applicants should provide basic information that is used in a screening process: demographic data; details on postsecondary, professional, and postgraduate education; certificates of specialty and professional memberships; licenses; information about previously successful and current challenges to licenses, certifications, registrations, and PSO memberships; voluntary or involuntary limitations, reductions, or losses of clinical privileges or licenses, certifications, or registrations; a statement of physical and mental health indicating that the applicant has no disability that is inconsistent with privileges being sought; an authorization allowing verification of information; and references.[35]

If the applicant meets the screening requirements, additional information is required: details of all malpractice actions in the previous 5 years and evidence of continuous malpractice insurance policy coverage to a limit set by the HSO/HS; a request for membership and privileges in the department in which the applicant desires to practice; a signed statement that the PSO bylaws and its rules and regulations have been read and will be met; and a statement that, if appointed, the applicant will provide, or provide for, the continuous care of patients for whom the applicant is responsible.

It is prudent to require photographs of applicants; these are sent to references to verify that applicants are who they claim to be. The national data bank established by the Health Care Quality Improvement Act of 1986 (PL 99-660)[36] (see Chapter 4) must be queried prior to both initial appointment and reappointment to determine whether there are adverse reports. Problems uncovered are investigated as necessary and can affect membership decisions.

The burden of proof is the applicant's. Applicants must complete the process to the HSO's/HS's satisfaction. Applicants must provide all information and documentation that the entity requires. The applicant may choose character references. It is imperative, however, that the entity choose which professional references to query, because this is the best way to obtain complete, objective information about clinical competence. Questions asked of references must be answered to the entity's satisfaction. No LIP should be allowed to undertake clinical activities until the application is complete in all respects and has been reviewed and approved.

The PSO may have several categories of membership. This is always true for acute care hospitals and systems of hospitals. Typically, these categories range from most involved (active) to least involved (honorary or emeritus). New members, except those in the consulting and honorary categories, often are given provisional appointments. This amounts to a probationary status and allows clinical performance to be monitored or reviewed.

Typically, reappointment to the PSO occurs every 2 years. Reappointment is similar to initial appointment but has one very important difference: During the preceding appointment, the HSO/HS has monitored and evaluated the LIP's performance. This information is used in decisions regarding membership category and clinical privileges to be granted, if any, in the next appointment cycle.

CLINICAL PRIVILEGES

Clinical privileges must be delineated (individually or by category) for all LIPs delivering care, whether or not they are PSO members. Prudence demands that clinical activities be limited to the skills and qualifications that LIPs can initially demonstrate and continue to justify. In addition, the HSO/HS must be able to support the LIPs' clinical activities.

By license, some LIPs are limited to performing specific clinical activities. For example, podiatrists are licensed to treat the foot and its related or governing structures by medical, surgical, or other means.[37] HSOs/HSs may restrict but may not expand what the state license allows LIPs to do.

Privilege delineation comprises two elements. The first is determining the specific content of clinical privileges. The second is ongoing and systematic review of care delivered, to determine whether changes in privileges, either increases or decreases, are justified. Clinical privileges should be specific to the entity. Each procedure/activity may be listed on the application or reapplication form, or there may be a general reference such as "internal medicine" with whatever limitations are appropriate for the level of qualification, such as board certification. The definition of a general term or category such as internal medicine must be found in the PSO bylaws or the PSO rules and regulations.

Clinical privileges for nonphysician LIPs are handled similarly, although the privileges are more likely to be listed specifically. It is common and desirable that any special relationships of non-physician LIPs to physicians be described in the granting of privileges or referenced in the PSO bylaws or the rules and regulations. Examples are nurse midwives, who practice with or are employed by obstetricians, and nurse anesthetists, who practice with or are employed by surgeons or anesthesiologists. Typically, privileges are granted on 2-year cycles or as accrediting bodies require.

Turf Conflicts

Conflicts as to what the various types of LIPs are allowed to do in HSOs/HSs result from profes-sionalism, economics, and technology. The egos of many professionals cause some groups to enhance their training, which may lead them to infringe on traditional clinical areas of other providers. The economics of reimbursement cause groups to gravitate toward more remunerative clinical activities.

Also, new diagnostic and therapeutic technology can be applied by several types of LIPs. HSOs/HSs must have a means by which LIPs claiming expertise in new procedures or clinical activities are reviewed and receive (or are denied) clinical privileges to perform them. Chapter 3 describes how technological developments blur the lines that traditionally separated medicine and surgery, medical and surgical specialties and subspecialties, and nonphysician LIPs. Such blurring causes turf conflicts that disrupt referral patterns and PSO relationships. The results can be negative for an HSO/HS with LIPs on its staff. The economic dimensions of turf conflicts for the HSO/HS include duplicating equipment, space, and staff to placate various LIPs, and the likelihood that dis-gruntled LIPs will sever their relationships with the HSO/HS and treat patients elsewhere.

PSO DISCIPLINARY ACTION

It may be necessary to take disciplinary action against an LIP with clinical privileges. Most often, such action results from minor infractions of the PSO bylaws or their subsidiary rules and regula-tions. Sometimes, HSO/HS policies are involved. Less frequently, the reason for disciplinary action is that the quality of care rendered by the practitioner is judged deficient. Regardless, it may be nec-essary to act to protect patients or find ways to encourage appropriate behavior, which almost always involves a recommendation by a PSO committee. Depending on the matter, it may be necessary for the GB to review and approve the recommendation.

A common problem is that LIPs do not complete medical records of discharged patients within the time limits that are set by the PSO rules and regulations. Such lapses diminish quality of care but usually pose no significant risk to patients. Verbal or written warnings are a typical first step in a dis-ciplinary process. A continuing problem might result in temporary suspension of admitting privi-leges, which means that elective admissions are prohibited. LIPs whose admitting privileges are suspended usually take immediate steps to make records current.

PSO bylaws usually identify a variety of disciplinary options. In order of increasing severity, they are mandatory continuing or special medical education, letter of admonition, supervision, suspension of admitting or clinical privileges or both, censure, reduction of privileges, and termination of privileges. The underlying motivation is to protect patients from deficient or inappropriate clinical treatment.

Depending on the disciplinary action, the affected LIP may be entitled to due process as set out in the PSO bylaws. If so, the PSO recommendation is reviewed, and the GB makes the final decision. In situations in which risk of imminent harm to patients exists, the CEO or another senior-level manager such as the CMO, acting for the GB, must take whatever action is necessary. The Health Care Quality Improvement Act of 1986 requires that actions that are adverse to clinical privileges for a period longer than 30 days must be reported to a national data bank.

Organizational Structures of Selected HSOs/HSs

The chapter has discussed the triad of key components of HSO/HS organizational structures: GBs, CEOs, and PSOs. As will be seen in subsequent sections, with some variation across the various types, many HSOs/HSs, especially the larger ones, are characterized by this triad of key organizational components.

The discussion focuses on the following HSOs/HSs: acute care hospitals, nursing facilities, ambulatory care organizations, hospice, managed care organizations (MCOs), home health agencies (HHAs), and health systems. These are the most common of the wide variety of types of HSOs/HSs found in the health services system. The Bureau of Labor Statistics (BLS) (www.bls.gov) tracks employment in the healthcare industry, the largest industry in the United States in terms of employment, employing about 13.5 million people, in nine industry segments:[38]

- *Hospitals.* Hospitals provide complete medical care, ranging from diagnostic services to surgery and continuous nursing care. Some hospitals specialize in treatment of the mentally ill, cancer patients, or children. Hospital-based care may be on an inpatient (overnight) or outpatient basis. The mix of workers needed varies, depending on the size, geographic location, goals, philosophy, funding, organization, and management style of the institution. As hospitals work to improve efficiency, care continues to shift from an inpatient to outpatient basis whenever possible. Many hospitals have expanded into long-term and home healthcare services, providing a wide range of care for the communities they serve.
- *Nursing and residential care facilities.* Nursing facilities provide inpatient nursing, rehabilitation, and health-related personal care to those who need continuous nursing care, but do not require hospital services. Nurse's aides provide the vast majority of direct care. Other facilities, such as convalescent homes, help patients who need less assistance. Residential care facilities provide around-the-clock social and personal care to children, the elderly, and others who have limited ability to care for themselves. Appropriate workers care for residents of assisted-living facilities, alcohol and drug rehabilitation centers, group homes, and halfway houses. Nursing and medical care, however, are not the main functions of establishments providing residential care, as they are in nursing facilities.
- *Offices of physicians.* About 37% of all healthcare establishments fall into this industry segment. Physicians and surgeons practice privately or in groups of practitioners who have the same or different specialties. Many physicians and surgeons prefer to join group practices because they afford backup coverage, reduce overhead expenses, and facilitate consultation with peers. Physicians and surgeons are increasingly working as salaried employees of group medical practices, clinics, or integrated health systems.
- *Offices of dentists.* About 1 out of every 5 healthcare establishments is a dentist's office. Most employ only a few workers, who provide general or specialized dental care, including dental surgery.

- *Home services*. Skilled nursing or medical care is sometimes provided in the home, under a physician's indirect supervision. Home healthcare services are provided mainly to the elderly. The development of in-home medical technologies, substantial cost savings, and patients' preference for care in the home have helped change this once-small segment of the industry into one of the fastest growing parts of the economy.
- *Offices of other health practitioners*. This segment of the industry includes the offices of chiropractors, optometrists, podiatrists, occupational and physical therapists, psychologists, audiologists, speech-language pathologists, dietitians, and other health practitioners. Demand for the services of this segment is related to the ability of patients to pay, either directly or through health insurance. Hospitals and nursing facilities may contract out for these services. This segment also includes the offices of practitioners of alternative medicine, such as acupuncturists, homeopaths, hypnotherapists, massage therapists, and naturopaths.
- *Outpatient care centers*. The diverse establishments in this group include kidney dialysis centers, outpatient mental health and substance abuse centers, health maintenance organization medical centers, and freestanding ambulatory surgical and emergency centers.
- *Other ambulatory healthcare services*. This relatively small industry segment includes ambulance and helicopter transport services, blood and organ banks, and other ambulatory healthcare services, such as pacemaker monitoring services and smoking cessation programs.
- *Medical and diagnostic laboratories*. Medical and diagnostic laboratories provide analytic or diagnostic services to the medical profession or directly to patients following a physician's prescription. Workers may analyze blood, take x-rays and computerized tomography scans, or perform other clinical tests. Medical and diagnostic laboratories provide the fewest . . . jobs in the healthcare industry.

Collectively, these nine segments total about 535,000 distinct organizations or, as the BLS refers to them, establishments. The vast majority of these establishments (approximately 76%) are offices of physicians, dentists, or other health practitioners. Hospitals and nursing and residential care facilities make up about 14% of establishments but employ about 63% of the total healthcare industry workforce.[39] The organizational structures of hospitals, nursing facilities, and systems of organizations are examined below, and other types of healthcare organizational structures are commented on briefly to give a sense of the variety of these structures. Before the actual structures are examined, however, HSOs/HSs as legal entities are discussed.

LEGAL STATUS OF HSOs/HSs

All HSOs/HSs are legal entities, although the forms of this status vary. Nongovernmental (privately owned) HSOs may be organized under state law as sole proprietorships, partnerships, corporations, or a new form—limited liability companies. HSs are invariably organized as corporations. Various types of HSOs/HSs are owned by state and local (county, city, or special tax district) governments and are established by enabling legislation, or they are incorporated like privately owned HSOs. Some HSOs/HSs are owned by the federal government; their legal status is based on federal legislation, and the states may not regulate them. Examples are Department of Veterans Affairs hospitals; U.S. Air Force, Army, and Navy hospitals; and U.S. Public Health Service clinics.

HSOs can exist as sole proprietorships, a form rarely used today, although they have no special legal status; the term simply describes a business owned by one person. A historical example was a for-profit nursing facility.

Partnerships are voluntary contracts between two or more persons to engage in commerce or business. Partnerships may be general or limited. Whether general partnerships have special legal status depends on state law. A common example of a general partnership is a physician group practice. *General* means that each partner is liable for the debts and errors of other partners. Limited partnerships have one or more general partners who are jointly and individually legally responsible for the partnership; the liability of *limited* partners is limited to the assets they have invested. Limited partnerships are commonly found in joint ventures between physicians and HSOs/HSs, such as imaging centers or ambulatory surgery centers. Limited liability partnerships are established with state approval.

Joint ventures are characterized by the presence of a contract or agreement and a legal entity through which participants pursue some activity in which they share costs, revenues, and control. Some joint ventures are organized as limited liability companies (LLCs). However, joint ventures involving HSOs/HSs and physician members of their clinical staff typically are limited partnerships, a different type of legal entity. The HSO/HS is the general partner, and physicians are limited partners. The general partner usually invests the bulk of the capital and usually is the managing partner. Limited partners invest far less capital, sometimes insignificant amounts, a fact that has caused problems with the Internal Revenue Service for some not-for-profit entities.

The primary reason to involve physicians in joint ventures, however, is not the capital they bring to the enterprise. It is the close ties and referrals they provide to the health services delivery activity, or in the case of a medical office building, physicians rent space from the limited partnership and locate their practices there. Bonding or tying independent contractor physicians into joint ventures may help HSOs/HSs improve profitability or market position, and perhaps physician relations.

In addition to joint ventures involving an entity and members of its professional staff, other joint ventures are undertaken between different entities. One example is a joint venture formed in 1996 between Columbia/HCA Healthcare Corporation, a for-profit entity, and the Arlington Health Foundation, a not-for-profit entity, to establish the for-profit Columbia Arlington Healthcare System LLC. The purpose of the joint venture was to manage several northern Virginia hospitals, including Arlington Hospital and Reston Hospital Center. This joint venture between entities with different tax-exempt statuses, however, dissolved in 1999 because the Internal Revenue Service questioned whether the Arlington Health Foundation could keep its charitable status while owning half of the for-profit joint venture.[40]

A common legal form for HSOs/HSs is the corporation, which the law recognizes as an artificial person. States allow physicians and other types of LIPs such as dentists, clinical psychologists, podiatrists, nurse midwives, and chiropractors to organize special types of corporations called professional corporations, which are designated as *PCs*. Some states use *limited (Ltd.)* to show the same status. On application and filing articles of incorporation, the state issues a charter that creates a corporation.

The LLC is a hybrid that uses partnership and corporate principles. It is favored for HSOs and in some HS relationships because it offers owners the same protection from personal liability as incorporating, while treating the owners as partners for federal and state income tax purposes.

Corporations may be organized as not-for-profit or for-profit entities. The advantages and disadvantages of each depend on the tax laws of the state where they are incorporated and on the purposes for which the corporation is organized. Corporate charters are amended on application to, and approval by, the state. A corporation must develop bylaws that include definitions and describe how it is organized to carry out its purposes—meetings, elections, GB composition, committees, officers, and roles of CEO and PSO, if any. Bylaws guide governance and senior management, together with the charter. They are the HSO's/HS's basic law, and all activities are subordinate to and must be consistent with them.

As legal entities, HSOs/HSs are largely regulated by states, although they are subject to federal regulation as well (discussed more fully in Chapter 4). States can delegate some regulatory power to local government, which regulates healthcare entities in the same way as other organizations that carry on similar functions, such as storing, preparing, and serving food. Specialized regulatory activities apply to some types of HSOs/HSs. An example is control, storage, and use of radioactive materials or disposal of hazardous waste. Federal laws affect some of these areas, and enforcement occurs through federal and state cooperation.

▪ Acute Care Hospitals

Hospitals have been present in various forms for millennia. Approximately 5,000 years ago, Greek temples were the first, but similar institutions existed in ancient Egyptian, Hindu, and Roman societies. These "hospitals" evolved from temples of worship and recuperation to almshouses and pesthouses and finally to places where advanced medical technologies are widely applied.

Hospital is derived from the Latin *hospitalis*. Although well regarded early in their history, hospitals in the Middle Ages and later had unsavory reputations and primarily served the poor. This reputation improved slowly, beginning in the middle of the 19th century. Until well into the 20th century, physicians provided charity care in hospitals but treated private (fee-for-service) patients at home. New medical technology made treatment in hospitals efficacious, especially with surgical intervention, and this focused attention on acute care hospitals. Treatment of private patients brought acute care hospitals prestige and wide acceptance. This evolution was well underway by the 1920s as acute care hospitals became differentiated and specialized to organize and deliver an expanding scope of services. Contemporary acute care hospitals are licensed and regulated by the states in which they are located.

Acute care hospitals serve various mixes of four major functions. Most important, they diagnose and treat the sick and injured; emphasis on other functions depends on their missions and objectives. A patient's medical condition determines the care received and, to some extent, the type of hospital where it is provided. Care and services can be delivered on an inpatient or outpatient basis.

A second function of acute care hospitals is preventing illness and promoting health. Examples include instructing patients about self-care after discharge, providing referrals to services such as home health, conducting disease screening, and holding childbirth education and smoking cessation classes.

A third function is educating people who will work in health services. HSOs/HSs train many different types of health services workers who need clinical experience to receive a state license or certification from a professional society. Having physicians in residencies and fellowships is a common example. Nursing assistants, medical social workers, and dietitians provide other examples. In addition, health services management education at both undergraduate and masters levels usually requires field experience.

A fourth function of acute care hospitals is research. Clinical trials for new drugs and devices are conducted in hospitals and other entities. Other types of research conducted in hospitals include assessing utilization of intensive care units and determining universal precautions for treating patients in emergency departments. One type of nonclinical research is for the purpose of improving hospital processes through quality improvement or other process improvement activities.

Hospitals have become involved in activities beyond traditional acute care—for example, home health services (58%), skilled nursing/long-term care (45%), and hospice (27%)—through diversification and involvement in HSs.[41]

HOSPITALS BY THE NUMBERS

By convention of common use, *community hospital* means an acute care hospital that treats the public for general medical and surgical problems. The title is used whether the hospital is organized as not for profit or for profit. A community hospital has permanent facilities (including inpatient beds) and continuous nursing services and provides diagnosis and treatment through an organized PSO for patients with a variety of surgical and nonsurgical conditions. This is in contrast to special hospitals, which admit only certain types of patients or those with specified illnesses or conditions.

From a peak of 7,174 hospitals of all types registered with the AHA in 1974, the number declined to 6,649 in 1990 to 6,021 in 1998, and to 5,759 in 2004.[42] This downward trend is likely

TABLE 2.2.   DISTRIBUTION OF COMMUNITY HOSPITALS BY BED SIZE IN **1980, 1990, 2000,** AND **2004**

No. of beds	No. of Hospitals				Percentage change (1990–2004)
	1980	1990	2000	2004	
	5,830	5,384	4,915	4,919	−8.6
6–24	259	226	288	352	+55.8
25–29	1,029	935	910	988	+5.7
50–99	1,462	1,263	1,055	1,028	−18.6
100–199	1,370	1,306	1,236	1,141	−12.6
200–299	715	739	656	621	−16.0
300–399	412	408	341	351	−14.0
400–499	266	222	182	185	−16.7
500+	317	285	247	253	−11.2

From American Hospital Association. *AHA Hospital Statistics 2006, and prior years.* Chicago: Health Forum LLC, an affiliate of the American Hospital Association.

to persist as ambulatory services continue to erode demand for in-patient beds. Almost half of existing community hospitals are under 100 beds in size, as shown in Table 2.2. These smaller hospitals tend to be isolated and need linkages to other hospitals through HSs.

Classification

Hospitals are classified by length of stay, type of control, and type of service. Length of stay is divided into short term and long term. *Acute* (of short duration or episodic) is a synonym for *short term*. *Chronic* (of long duration) is a synonym for *long term*. The AHA defines short-term hospitals as having an average length of stay (ALOS) of less than 30 days, and long-term hospitals as having an ALOS of 30 days or more. More than 90% of hospitals are short term. Community hospitals are acute care (short term). Rehabilitation and chronic disease hospitals are long term. Psychiatric hospitals are usually long term. Some acute care hospitals have long-term care units to treat psychiatric illnesses or to provide rehabilitation services.

Type of service denotes whether the hospital is "general" or "special." General hospitals provide a broad range of medical and surgical services, to which are often added obstetrics and gynecology; pediatrics; orthopedics; and eye, ear, nose, and throat services. *General* describes both acute and chronic care hospitals but usually applies to short-term hospitals. *Special* hospitals offer services in one medical or surgical specialty, such as pediatrics, obstetrics and gynecology, rehabilitation medicine, or psychiatry, or in a discrete surgical procedure, such as hernia repair.

A third classification scheme divides hospitals by type of control or ownership into not for profit, for profit (investor owned), or governmental (run by federal, state, or local governments or a hospital authority). Figure 2.4 shows various types of hospital ownership. In 2004, of the 5,759 AHA-registered hospitals in the United States, 4,919 were community hospitals (nonfederal short-term general and special hospitals), a decline from 5,384 in 1990. The 4,919 community hospitals included 2,967 nongovernmental not-for-profit (also called voluntary) hospitals with 568,000 beds, 835 investor-owned hospitals with 113,000 beds, and 1,117 hospitals owned by state or local governments with 128,000 beds. The difference between 5,759 and 4,919 (840) is federal and nonfederal psychiatric hospitals, federal general and special hospitals, nonfederal institutions for people with psychiatric problems, tuberculosis and other respiratory disease hospitals, and long-term general and special hospitals.[43]

The acute care hospital field has a strong tradition of voluntarism; ownership is predominantly not for profit.[44] During the late 19th and early 20th centuries, acute care hospitals became larger, more complex, and more costly. In addition to voluntarism, the increase in not-for-profit acute care hospitals resulted from favorable tax treatment and the federal Hill-Burton program (begun in 1946), which provided money for hospital construction, expansion, and refurbishment.

PRIVATE (NONGOVERNMENT) OWNERSHIP

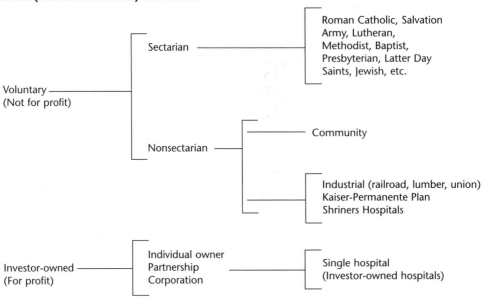

GOVERNMENT OWNERSHIP

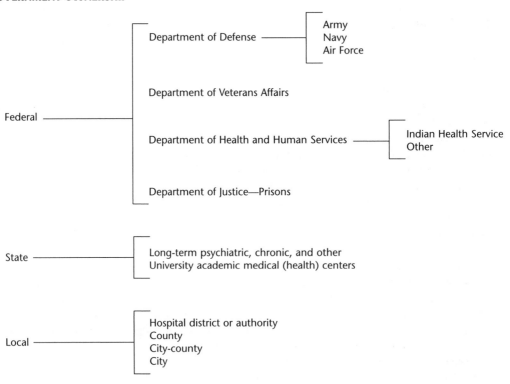

Figure 2.4. Hospital ownership.

Prior to the passage of Medicare in 1965, investor-owned acute care hospitals had become virtually nonexistent. After the passage of Medicare, investor ownership of community hospitals increased dramatically and stabilized in the 700–800 range.[45] In addition, investor-owned companies have management contracts with large numbers of hospitals.

Beginning in the 1980s and continuing to the present, several states blurred the traditional definition of acute care hospitals by licensing new types of HSOs. The postoperative (postacute) recovery center, sometimes called a medical inn or recovery care center, is neither a traditional acute care hospital nor an ambulatory HSO. These HSOs provide a lower-cost alternative to hospitalization when a patient has undergone outpatient surgery and may need observation for a short period. Some states also license a category of subacute facility whose level of service lies between an acute care hospital and a nursing facility. These extended-stay hospitals, or long-term care hospitals (LTCHs), are increasing in many locales.

ORGANIZATIONAL STRUCTURE OF ACUTE CARE HOSPITALS

The acute care hospital would be far less complex if it totally fit the usual organizational pyramid shown in Figure 2.1. However, its structure differs from the bureaucratic model of other types of large organizations. These differences are caused by the unusual relationships between the formal authority of position represented by the managerial hierarchy and the authority of knowledge possessed by members of the PSO. In the typical community hospital, PSO members do not fit into the organizational pyramid, as do staff who work for and are paid by the hospital. The LIPs who comprise the PSOs of acute care hospitals are usually not paid by the hospital, except for administrative work. As a result, the organizational pattern has traditionally been considered a "dual pyramid" with managerial and PSO hierarchies side by side. Some acute care hospitals, such as Department of Veterans Affairs hospitals and military hospitals, integrate the PSO into the organizational structure because in these situations the PSO's members are salaried. More contemporary hospital organizational structures do not emphasize this duality, although it still exists, albeit to a lesser degree. Adding the GB to the managerial hierarchy beginning with the CEO and the PSO completes the triad of key organizational components in hospitals. Figure 2.5 illustrates the organizational structure of a "typical" acute care hospital.

The hospital's GB is located organizationally atop the structure and has overall responsibility for and authority over the organization. GB members are driven by changes in the external environment, are increasingly scrutinized, and are under increasing pressure to perform well. There is a trend toward smaller, better qualified, and more active hospital GBs. Efforts to increase GB member competence have focused on specialized seminars and continuing education. Some hospitals think they will be better served by adopting the business enterprise model, in which directors are paid for their time and talent.

Acute care hospitals are complex organizations with several levels of management, beginning with the CEO. Figure 2.5 is the organizational chart of a community hospital that has reorganized into a small, vertically integrated healthcare system that includes a hospital, a physician-hospital organization (PHO), home health services, a nursing facility (part of senior services), and several joint ventures. The chart suggests the dual hierarchy described earlier.

The *medical staff,* the traditional name for members of the PSO, are shown as separate from the hospital. The senior vice president for medical affairs (or CMO) reports to the hospital president and has numerous responsibilities related to PSO functioning.

Departments and activities that provide direct patient care, clinical support, and administrative functions are identifiable from the titles. In addition, departments and units such as planning and marketing, development (fund-raising), and human resources perform a variety of essential staff functions. Numerous departments/units deliver clinical services: nursing, pharmacy, dietary ser-

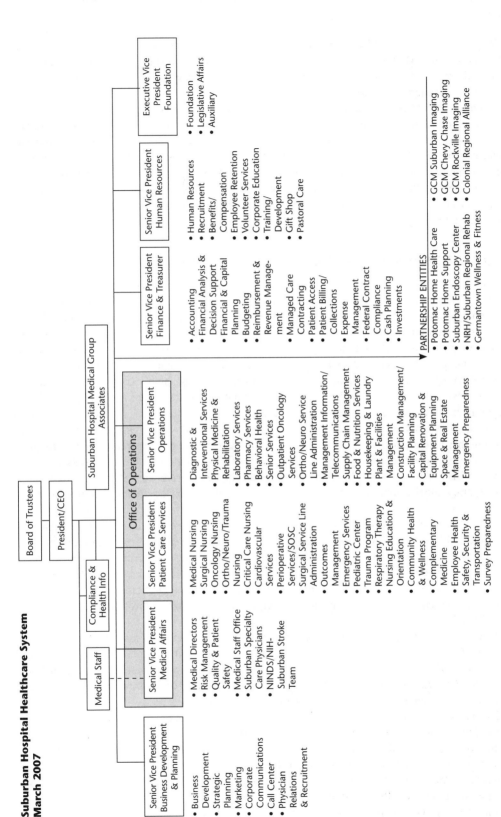

Figure 2.5. Organizational Chart of a Hospital. (Reprinted by permission of Suburban Hospital, Bethesda, MD; www.suburbanhospital.org)

vices, radiology, and laboratories are common. In addition, there is a wide variety of support departments, including housekeeping, maintenance, security, business office, and admitting. Figure 2.5 suggests the range and activity of these various departments/units.

The LIPs on the PSO, primarily its physicians, control all hospital admissions and, generally speaking, are key to a hospital's economic success. PSO members overwhelmingly are independent contractors, although some are salaried by the hospital. Accredited hospitals have a highly structured PSO, which reflects good practice. As noted earlier, hospital PSOs are largely self-governing. They have bylaws stating how the PSO is organized and detail officers, committees, and various processes, including appointment of members, credentialing, and discipline.

The CMO (the senior vice president for medical affairs in Figure 2.5) is central to effective coordination, communication, and management of the PSO. The CMO is usually employed full-time in larger hospitals and part-time in smaller hospitals. Smaller hospitals may have a volunteer CMO, often called the chief of staff. Other clinical managers include department chiefs or chiefs of service, who may be paid, depending on the demands on their time. Consistent with the bylaws, clinical managers have significant autonomy in managing their departments, but they are accountable to the CMO for clinical and administrative matters.

Generally, increasing physician participation in hospital management enhances effectiveness and efficiency and improves the quality of patient care. Similarly, physician involvement in governance appears to be beneficial and is increasingly popular in acute care hospitals.

Critical to good hospital performance is developing and maintaining an effective relationship among the GB, the CEO, and the PSO. Numerous means have been used, including adding physicians to GBs and appointing nonphysician GB members to PSO committees. This is a relatively easy and politically painless way to coordinate, but much effort, cooperation, and patience are required to develop policies and practices that simultaneously maintain the prerogatives of LIPs and the managerial integrity of the organization.

In the future, successful hospitals must compete for a declining amount of inpatient care and seize new opportunities. One strategy is to develop centers of excellence to diagnose and treat specific diseases; another is to focus on groups such as women or physical fitness and sports enthusiasts. These diagnostic and therapeutic services may be offered on either an inpatient or an outpatient basis, with strong financial incentives for the least-costly site. Such initiatives reflect a growing trend toward market segmentation and boutique medicine. Common, too, are joint risk taking or joint ventures between hospitals and their PSOs and efforts to provide advances in patient convenience and patient-centered care.

Chapter 3 describes the increasing portability of technology and suggests implications for hospitals. The most important implication is that PSO members will expand the nonhospital portion of their practices at the hospital's expense. Cooperating as well as competing with their PSOs puts hospitals in difficult positions. Extrapolating the trend of technological portability suggests significant changes for the inpatient portion of hospital services.[46]

The inpatient portion of acute care hospitals could become large intensive care units because only the most acutely ill patients will be hospitalized. This would change staff-to-patient ratios, and costs would increase, and the work of hospital CEOs and other managers, as well as that of GBs, would become even more complex.

Nursing Facilities

There is an extensive continuum of services for eldercare in the United States: adult day services, home health, community services, senior housing, assisted-living residences, continuing care retirement communities, and nursing facilities that serve older individuals with infirmities and other people needing skilled care.[47] Saint Helena (A.D. 250–330) is credited with establishing one of the first homes for older people *(gerokomion)*. "She was a wealthy, intelligent, Christian convert and mother of Constantine the Great. Like other early Christian 'nurses' who devoted their lives to the sick and needy, she gave direct care herself."[48] Many early American towns operated almshouses—or poorhouses, poor farms, or workhouses, as they were also known—for those who were "down on their luck" and who needed a sheltered environment. In the early 1900s, the affluent elderly lived in their own homes or in privately owned boarding houses, and church-sponsored homes for older Americans emerged.[49]

Enactment of Medicare and Medicaid in 1965 placed major emphasis on delivery of skilled nursing care in nursing facilities, increasing the average size of nursing facilities and the total number of nursing facility beds. Initially, federal regulations distinguished nursing facilities by the nursing care provided. Skilled nursing facilities (SNFs) provided the most nursing care. Intermediate care facilities (ICFs) provided nursing services in accordance with residents' needs and were available to help residents achieve and maintain the highest degree of function, self-care, and independence. The Nursing Home Reform Act, part of the Omnibus Budget Reconciliation Act of 1987 (PL 100-203),[50] eliminated the distinction between SNFs and ICFs; beginning in 1991, both were called nursing facilities. The Nursing Home Reform Act also addressed training, continuing education, levels of professional and nonprofessional staffing, quality of life, and residents' rights and made numerous other changes, most of which have been judged successful.[51]

Nursing facilities are licensed in all states and must meet applicable regulations and requirements. The Joint Commission has an accreditation program for nursing facilities, but they have no "deemed" status (as do accredited hospitals under Medicare), and accreditation does not relieve nursing facilities of federal Medicare certification inspections.

Currently, about 18,000 nursing facilities with more than 1.9 million beds serve approximately 1.6 million residents.[52] On average, nursing facilities have 106 beds. About 66% are owned for profit, 28% are not for profit, and 6% are government owned.[53] In 2003, 92% of nursing homes beds were dually certified for Medicare and Medicaid.[54]

Part A of Medicare covers long-term care services such as postoperative and post-hospitalization care, including rehabilitation. States provide Medicaid coverage to state residents who meet financial and medical eligibility requirements. Medicaid pays 66%, Medicare pays 12%, and private payment pays 22% of the total costs of nursing facility services.[55]

Medicare-certified nursing facilities have a wide range of staff. Most are part of the nursing service, including RNs, LPNs, and certified nursing assistants (CNAs). The Nursing Home Reform Act requires that any Medicare-certified nursing facility has an activities director and a dietitian. The ideal in developing an effective treatment milieu in a nursing facility is to have a multidisciplinary geriatrics team whose members have specialized expertise in such areas as gerontology, clinical pharmacology, dental/oral hygiene, medicine, nursing, nutrition support, ophthalmology, podiatry, surgery, psychiatry/psychology, rehabilitation therapy, physical therapy (PT), and occupational therapy (OT). Of course, only large nursing facilities will have all of these skills represented on staff, but smaller facilities can contract for them.

ORGANIZATIONAL STRUCTURE OF NURSING FACILITIES

Nursing facilities are organized into departments: clinical services, such as physician and dental care, nursing, rehabilitation (OT and PT), and speech-language pathology; clinical support services, such as laboratory, radiology, and pharmacy; and administrative services, such as housekeeping, laundry, and maintenance. The medical director (or CMO) provides direct clinical care and coordinates private physicians and the work of PSO committees in clinical areas.

Depending on their size, nursing facility organizational structures may be pyramidal (tall) with several levels of management, or they may be flat with few levels of management. Because most nursing facilities are small, they have few managers or levels of management between the adminis-

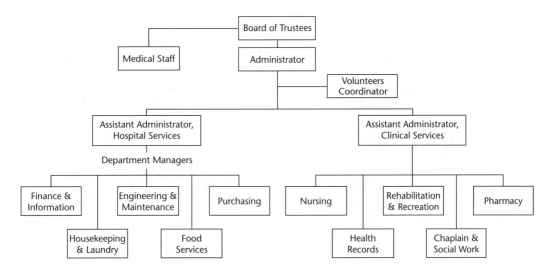

Figure 2.6. Organizational chart of a nursing home. Source: S.M. Shortell and A.D. Kaluzny: *Health Care Management Organization Design and Behavior, Fifth Edition,* 2006, p. 329. Reprinted with permission of Delmar Learning, a division of Thomson Learning (www.thomsonrights.com). Fax 800-730-2215.

trator (or CEO) and staff. A large nursing facility, however, may have several levels of managers between the administrator and staff. These managers perform the typical line and staff functions, such as general administration, financial management, and human resources management. An organizational chart for a large not-for-profit nursing facility is shown in Figure 2.6.

Nursing facilities have GBs performing functions very similar to those of acute care hospital GBs. Historically, small for-profit nursing facilities were sole proprietorships or partnerships, forms that are rare today. Frequently, now they are organized as for-profit corporations, with few directors, thus in effect combining governance and management functions. A larger for-profit or not-for-profit nursing facility is organized as a corporation and has a GB that is likely to be called the board of directors or board of trustees.

In addition to the CEO, other managers with special skills are present, as size and activities require. CEOs of nursing facilities that are part of an HS, especially those organized for profit, may have little independence from the system. Such systems centralize many functions, most prominently financial management. In addition, policies of all types are likely to be developed centrally and promulgated to the operating units.

All states require that nursing facilities have a licensed administrator of record. Most states use the national licensure examination governed by the National Association of Boards of Examiners for Long Term Care Administrators to test basic competencies of entry-level administrators.[56] The examination focuses on patient care, personnel management, financial management, marketing and public relations, physical resource management, laws, regulatory codes, and GBs.

A medical director (or CMO) is required by Medicare regulations and is good practice regardless. The CMO may be full- or part-time and ensures that medical services are coordinated and appropriate. In addition, the CMO is responsible for credentialing and privileging LIPs, ensuring compliance with regulations and disciplinary procedures, and reviewing and maintaining quality of care provided throughout the nursing facility.[57]

The PSOs of nursing facilities receiving federal funds must have written bylaws, rules, and regulations, just as do acute care hospital PSOs. The PSOs may be open or closed, as described earlier. Compared with hospitals, nursing facilities have far fewer LIPs. Use of standing orders allows clinical activities to occur without specific orders from physicians.

LIPs are credentialed, as described previously for acute care hospitals. Because most nursing facility care is chronic and does not rely on advanced clinical technologies, patients are perceived to be at low risk, so credentialing may be less demanding. However, nursing facilities should use the acute care hospital model and be rigorous in credentialing.

Residents may be admitted by any licensed physician. Residents whose physicians have privileges may be attended by them. These physician services are paid for by the resident, either directly or through a third-party payer, including Medicare and Medicaid as well as private insurance. The staff of larger nursing facilities may include salaried physicians who supplement the role of the resident's private physician and provide services as needed.

Pessimistic predictions of the future for nursing facilities suggest that inadequate reimbursement rates, costly demands of new federal regulations, and sicker residents may cause an economic crisis for them. Demographics support optimistic predictions, however, and suggest that rising demand for nursing facility beds and a more affluent elderly population are harbingers of a brighter future.

Maintaining adequate staffing levels will challenge nursing facilities, especially with respect to such technically skilled staff as RNs and PTs, who have been in chronically short supply. Recruiting and retaining less skilled employees such as CNAs may be a problem for many facilities as well. The American Association of Homes and Services for the Aging (AAHSA) (www.aahsa.org) observes that the future of services for the aging, including those offered in nursing facilities, may unfold in many different ways. AAHSA predicts that two variables will determine future developments: the level of funding of services, and the impact of major advances in medical or information technologies that can affect care for the elderly.

The demand for services for the elderly will increase as the U.S. population ages; this suggests strong future demand for nursing facilities. It is estimated that by 2020, approximately 52 million Americans, or more than 20% of the population, will be 65 or older. Of even greater importance in terms of care needs is that the number of people 80 or older is projected to double to 14 million by 2025.[58]

▬ Health Systems ▬

HSOs that are alike, such as groups of community hospitals or nursing facilities, can form horizontally integrated HSs. Alternatively, joining with dissimilar or other types of HSOs, they can form vertically integrated HSs. Both forms are illustrated in Figure 2.7.

Horizontal integration is the formation of lateral relationships among like entities performing at the same functional level. Its purpose is "to improve the degree to which resources are used efficiently and to increase purchasing power and marketing and management capacity."[59] Horizontal integration "occurs when two or more separate firms, producing either the same services or services that are close substitutes, join to become either a single firm or a strong interorganizational alliance."[60]

Vertical integration, in contrast, is "coordinating, linking or incorporating within a single organization activities or entities at different stages of a production process—in healthcare the processes of producing and delivering patient care. These activities or entities would otherwise be completely independent, or would interact through arm's-length transactions."[61] Figure 2.8 shows an actual HS with elements of vertical and horizontal integration.

Vertical integration can involve as few as two entities at different stages of the process of producing and delivering health services, or it may involve more entities at different stages. Although the terminology is not universally agreed on, the phrase *highly integrated HS* is increasingly reserved for situations in which an HS has integrated to the extent that it includes, through ownership or contract, at least three or more stages of health services delivery and at least one systemwide contract with a payer. The highly integrated HS either owns or contracts with three or more stages of health

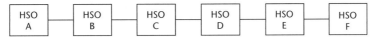

(A) Horizontally integrated HS. All HSOs in the HS perform at the same functional level: All are hospitals, nursing facilities, home health agencies, or the like.

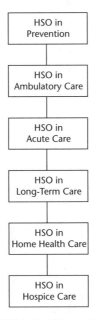

(B) Vertically integrated HS. The HSOs in the HS are performing at different functional levels: prevention, ambulatory care, and so forth.

Figure 2.7. Horizontally (A) and vertically (B) integrated HSs.

services delivery, including at least one acute care hospital; at least one physician component, such as a PHO or group practice; and at least one other stage, such as an HMO, nursing facility, home health agency, or surgery center. In addition, it has at least one systemwide contract with a payer, which can be an employer or employer coalition, a traditional insurer, an MCO, or a government entity.[62] Figure 2.9 shows the demographics of HSs, including the 331 highly integrated HSs in 2005.

Increasingly, integrated healthcare means highly integrated HSs. As might be expected, these HSs are difficult to establish and maintain. Satinsky identified eight key factors in the success of HSs by summarizing research that includes the views of consultants who have facilitated HS formation and of representatives of HSs.[63] A philosophical commitment to systems integration is a crucial factor. These factors are listed in Table 2.3, along with HSs that exemplify each. The CEOs and members of GBs who lead successful highly integrated HSs "have a vision that the whole [HS] is greater—and different from—the sum of its parts."[64]

The most highly integrated HSs combine under a unified approach, through either ownership or contractual relationships, all of the major components of the delivery system—physicians, hospitals, and other facilities, as shown in Figure 2.9, as well as health plan services. Most of the highly integrated HSs in existence and under formation "contract with multiple health plans without owning or being owned by any one."[65] Others, however, own health plans. For example, the University of Pittsburgh Medical Center (UPMC) (www.upmc.com) is a highly integrated healthcare delivery

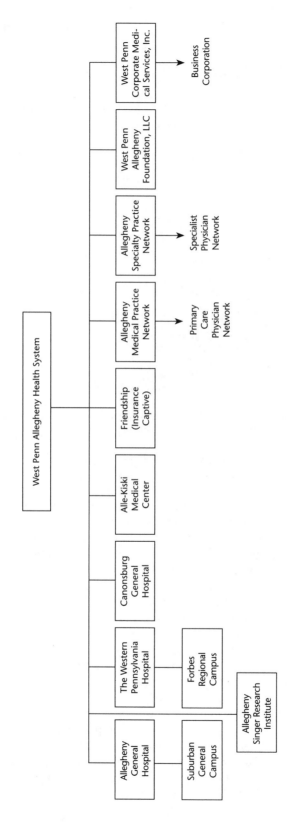

Figure 2.8. HS with vertical and horizontal elements of integration. (Reprinted with permission of West Penn Allegheny Health System, Pittsburgh, PA, 2007.)

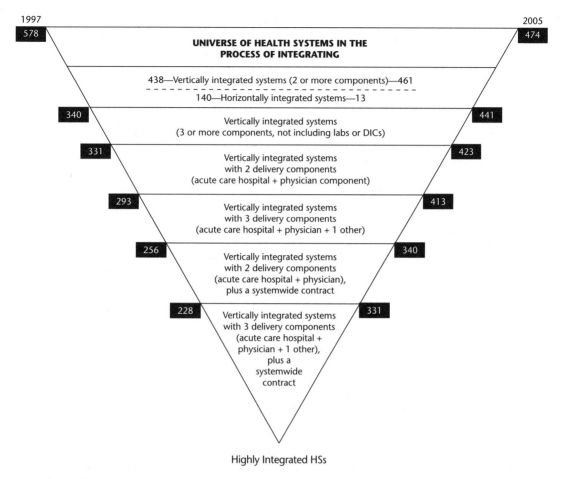

1997
578

2005
474

**UNIVERSE OF HEALTH SYSTEMS IN THE
PROCESS OF INTEGRATING**

438—Vertically integrated systems (2 or more components)—461
– –
140—Horizontally integrated systems—13

340

441

Vertically integrated systems
(3 or more components, not including labs or DICs)

331

423

Vertically integrated systems
with 2 delivery components
(acute care hospital + physician component)

293

413

Vertically integrated systems
with 3 delivery components
(acute care hospital + physician + 1 other)

256

340

Vertically integrated systems
with 2 delivery components
(acute care hospital + physician),
plus a systemwide contract

228

331

Vertically integrated systems
with 3 delivery components
(acute care hospital +
physician + 1 other),
plus a
systemwide
contract

Highly Integrated HSs

Figure 2.9.   HSs in the process of integrating. Adapted from Sanofi Aventis. *Managed Care Digest Series: eHospitals/Systems Digest for 2006.* Available at www.managedcaredigest.com/index.jsp. Accessed July 27, 2006. Bridgewater, NJ: Sanofi-Aventis. Used with permission from Sanofi-Aventis Managed Care Digest Series® Hospital/Systems Digest and Verispan LLC.

system primarily serving the region of western Pennsylvania through ownership of hospitals and other HSOs. The system also owns UPMC Health Plan, a managed care insurance company, as well as HMOs serving populations that are Medicaid and Medicare eligible.

Highly integrated HSs also are called integrated delivery systems (IDSs), organized delivery systems, or integrated delivery networks. Whatever the name, the highly integrated HSs are distinguished by the fact that each "provides or arranges to provide a coordinated continuum of services to a defined population and is willing to be held clinically and fiscally accountable for the outcomes and the health status of the population served."[66]

A critical aspect of HSs is that the establishment of formal linkages between or among HSOs can be made through ownership arrangements, or they can be based on contractual relationships, establishing what have come to be called virtual HSs.[67] This distinction also is termed ownership-based integration and contractual-based integration.[68]

HSs in which the component entities are linked through ownership or, alternatively, through contracts have led to use of the terms *health networks* (contractual linkages) and *health systems* (unified ownership of assets of linked HSOs).[69] A similar distinction between linked HSOs divides them again into two groups, one characterized as loosely coupled alliances that have two or more owners

TABLE 2.3.   KEY SUCCESS FACTORS IN HSS, WITH EXAMPLES

Success factor	HSs with proven track records
Philosophical commitment to systems integration	Advocate Health Care (IL); Henry Ford Health System (MI)
Clarity of purpose and vision	Baylor Health Care System (TX); Copley Health System (VT)
Strong physician leadership	Fairview Hospital and Healthcare Services (MN); Friendly Hills HealthCare Network (CA); Henry Ford Health System (MI); North Shore Medical Center (MA)
Alignment of financial incentives and rewards that recognize system performance	Samaritan Health System (AZ)
Customer focus on purchasers; enrollees; system components; legal, regulatory, and accrediting agencies; and communities	Appalachian Regional Healthcare (KY, VA, WV); Carolinas HealthCare System (NC, SC); Group Health Cooperative (WA); Laurel Health System (PA)
Information systems and technology that support systems goals and operations	Advocate Health Care (IL); Allina Health System (MN); Graduate Health System (NJ, PA)
Ongoing emphasis on quality improvement	Harvard Pilgrim Health Care (New England); Henry Ford Health System (MI); Lovelace Health Systems and Presbyterian Healthcare Services (NM)
Focus on creating market-driven value	Dartmouth-Hitchcock Health System–Northern Region (New England); Henry Ford Health System and Mercy Health Services (MI)

Adapted from Satinsky, Marjorie A. *The Foundation of Integrated Care: Facing the Challenges of Change*, 73. Chicago: American Hospital Publishing, by permission.

(corresponding to health networks) and the other as tightly coupled alliances that have single owners (corresponding to HSs).[70]

THE TRIAD IN HSs

As noted at the beginning of this chapter, almost all HSOs/HSs have some variation of the triad that refers to their CEO, GB, and PSO components. Beginning with the CEOs of HSs, this triad of key components is examined next, with emphasis on the specific aspects of the roles of these components in HSs.

CEOs

If the HS is to flourish, the CEO must be effective. To be effective, the system CEO must[71]

- Seek harmony in interactions within the HS
- Balance analysis (the examination of parts of the HS) with synthesis (seeing the parts as a whole)
- Focus on seeing the whole picture of the HS with all of its parts, large and small
- Emphasize patterns of change over time rather than static snapshots of activity or behavior
- Pursue root causes of performance problems to avoid symptomatic responses
- Focus on integration, interconnectedness, and interrelationships within the HS

Although managerial competencies are discussed more fully in Chapter 5, it is useful to note here that the important clusters of knowledge and skills that make up managerial competencies of CEOs are 1) conceptual, 2) technical managerial/clinical, 3) interpersonal/collaborative, 4) political, 5) commercial, and 6) governance. These competencies serve as a framework for the competencies needed by CEOs in HSs. Highlights of how the competencies pertain to managing in HSs are discussed in this section.[72]

The knowledge and skills that compose the conceptual competence needed by managers to envision the place and role of an HSO in the larger society should be magnified when applied to a complex HS. Two aspects of this competence are essential for the CEOs and other senior-level managers in HSs and are emphasized here. First, conceptual competence of system CEOs is necessary to visualize and understand both the HSOs within the HS and the place of the entire system in its larger context.

Second, compared with CEOs in HSOs, the CEOs of HSs must manage more complex organizational structures; such management includes a greater likelihood of sharing leadership responsibilities with physicians. As has been noted, "success in integrated healthcare absolutely requires physicians in leadership positions."[73] In relation to their PSOs, HSs are likely to continue to use pluralistic approaches to integrating physicians into the HS. They may use "combinations of owned physician groups, independent practice associations, physician hospital organizations, management services organizations and the like."[74]

Together with conceptual competence, CEOs in HSs need extensive technical managerial/clinical competence. They must possess both a high degree of clinical expertise and significant management expertise. When HSs include component organizations involved in diverse aspects of clinical care, clinical expertise is especially important and must be more expansive than for a single HSO.

Interpersonal/collaborative competence is very important in managing the component HSOs of HSs. It entails negotiating and maintaining multiparty organizational arrangements necessary for HSs to exist and succeed, as well as negotiating the various agreements and contracts that sustain these arrangements. A system CEO must convince senior managers of the component HSOs to view success in terms of the system's broader vision, values, and objectives. Interpersonal/collaborative competence is required of all CEOs, but it is especially important in managing interorganizational conflicts in HSs.

HS CEOs must possess political and commercial competencies to accurately assess the impact of public policies on their systems and to effectively influence policy making.[75] This is more difficult in HSs, in part because CEOs must interact with large numbers of policy decisions and numerous policy makers.

Commercial competence in identifying markets and positioning an HS in its markets is based on knowledge and associated skills. CEOs with adequate commercial competence can establish and operate successful value-creating situations involving economic exchanges between their systems and those that would purchase its services. The commercial success of an HS is often dependent upon the HS's ability to contract with health plans to provide a package of integrated services. Indeed, the ability to enter into such contracts is one of the principal motives in forming many HSs. As HSs are formed to deliver a continuum of health services under managed care contracts, the systems must develop the following attributes in order to enhance their likelihood of achieving commercial success:[76]

- Some level of clinical coordination, not just administrative or financial coordination, among organizations in the HS
- A focus by at least some HS actors, most likely primary care physicians, on performance of the HS as a whole
- Achievement of some level of physician integration (commitment of physicians to the HS), at least among primary care providers
- A focus on primary care and prevention
- An adequate service area and service breadth
- Development of sophisticated information systems
- A capacity to compete and improve on quality

Finally, governance competence is very important for CEOs who manage HSs. In many instances, these CEOs are GB members. As also noted earlier in this chapter, it is important for CEOs of HSs to possess governance competence, because it is so difficult to separate what occurs under the rubric of governance from what occurs in the context of strategic management. Consequently, CEOs must be knowledgeable about management and governance. In addition, system CEOs require governance competence so that they can assist their GBs in overall governance performance.

GBs

Understanding governance in HSs requires an appreciation of the fact that because HSs are wholes made up of parts, their governance involves three sets of issues: 1) issues of governance of the whole (the HS), 2) issues of governance of the various parts or component HSOs of the HS, and 3) issues that arise between the two levels of governance. The question of who governs what (or who controls what) is relatively straightforward in independent HSOs, but it is more complicated in HSs. In general, the more organizationally complex an HS is, the more complex its governance.

Centralized Versus Decentralized HS Governance Structures

The most basic governance issue in HSs is whether governance is centralized or decentralized.[77] The centralized governance structure model, sometimes referred to as a corporate or system board model, centralizes governance control in a single GB that exercises direct control over all of the component HSOs in the system. Figure 2.2 shows the structure of an HS with a centralized governance structure. Component HSOs in Figure 2.2 may have advisory bodies, but these bodies have no legal or fiduciary authority; there is only one GB for the HS with a centralized governance structure.

A second model, the decentralized governance structure, sometimes referred to as the parent holding company model, decentralizes governance control and shares it among the system GB and separate subordinate GBs at the level of component HSOs. "Probably the biggest single asset of this arrangement is that it provides the opportunity to push selected governance functions down to the level where they can be fulfilled with a greater sensitivity to the distinctive circumstances faced by system components."[78]

In a decentralized model (Figure 2.10), the parent or system GB retains defined authority over the subordinate GBs, perhaps including such areas as capital budgets, selection of CEOs, and sales of assets. The point is that governance responsibilities within the HS are divided and shared among the system-level and component-level GBs according to an agreed-on plan. A key responsibility of the system GB in a decentralized governance structure is oversight and coordination of subordinate GBs. This can be difficult to accomplish when the various GBs have differences in viewpoints or philosophies that create dynamic tension between them, often with the HS's CEO caught in the middle. For example, the parent GB may have a futuristic vision, whereas the subordinate GBs may focus more on day-to-day operational or financial concerns. These conflicts can occur even when some of the subordinate GB members serve on the HS's GB. CEOs may be able to avoid or minimize this conflict and the discontinuities it causes by insisting that their GBs help them develop a shared vision through the strategic plan.

In decentralized HSs, subordinate boards can be structured along organizational, regional, or functional lines.[79] In a decentralized HS that structures its subordinate boards organizationally, as shown in Figure 2.10, there is a system board, and each component HSO of the HS is overseen by its own GB. When subordinate boards are structured regionally, each subordinate board oversees a particular market or geographic region where the HS operates. When subordinate boards are structured functionally, each oversees groupings of system components that perform similar functions, such as physician groups, hospitals, and insurance companies. Figure 2.11 shows systems in which subordinate boards are structured regionally or functionally. Finally, Figure 2.12 illustrates a very complex governance structure in which an HS combines all three ways of structuring its subordinate boards. In this model, the HS board oversees a functional board (the insurance company board) as well as regional boards that, in turn, oversee organizational boards within the regions.

Orlikoff compares the advantages of the centralized and decentralized HS models as follows.[80]

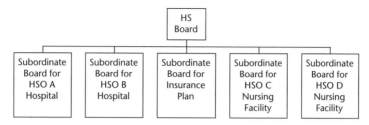

Figure 2.10. Decentralized governance structure.

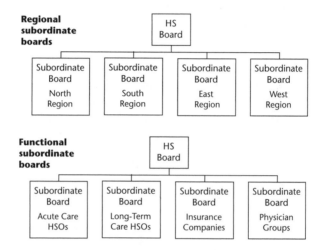

Figure 2.11. Decentralized governance structures with regional or functional subordinate boards.

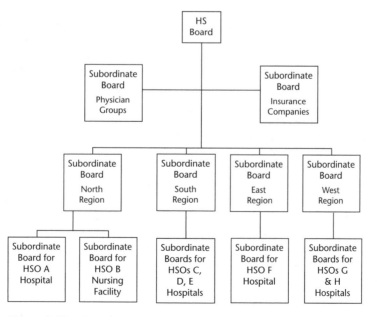

Figure 2.12. Complex governance structure combining organizational, regional, and functional bases of structuring subordinate boards.

In a centralized governance structure, decisions can be made more quickly; the time that CEOs must spend on governance interactions is minimized, and the system GB is encouraged to focus on strategic issues. Offsetting this, however, is the fact that a centralized governance structure limits the number of stakeholders that can serve on the GB. Advantages of the decentralized governance structure permit the system GB to push details to subordinate GBs; subordinate GBs may be closer to and can focus better on local community or HSO issues. In addition, decentralization permits a greater number of stakeholders to serve on an HS's GBs. Offsetting this, however, is the fact that multiple boards can contribute to confusion and conflict over roles and responsibilities and even lead to gridlock in extreme circumstances. Multiple boards can consume significant amounts of CEO time in GB interactions, and they may slow the decision-making process, especially if subordinate GBs insist on focusing on their interests at the expense of those of the HS. On this latter point, which is a common problem, Bader cited a recent example:

> Several years ago a California system of hospitals and physician enterprises confronted a jet-powered competitive market with a Model-T governance structure. The hospitals and physicians had joined up to gain system advantages. But, wary of losing control, individual-entity boards had retained enough power to put local interests ahead of system priorities. So the hospitals continued old habits of competing for patients instead of seeking system efficiencies and supporting investments to help the system as a whole vie for managed care business. "This multitude of local boards prohibited us from making planning or policy decisions on any reasonable basis that reflected all the areas we served," one board member says. Although the need to restructure governance was clear, there was one barrier: "The autonomy these boards felt was very important to them," the trustee says.[81]

Composition of the GB

Closely related to the issue of centralized versus decentralized governance structures in HSs is the issue of the composition of the GB, which can be composed of representative members, nonrepresentative members, or a combination.[82] Representative members of an HS's centralized corporate GB are selected because of their relationship to a particular component HSO of the system. Nonrepresentative members are not directly aligned with, nor do they represent the specific concerns of, any particular system component HSO. Most often, representative members of a system-level GB are the CEOs or members of the GBs of the component HSOs. Consequently, as the HS they govern grows, the size of the GB also grows, perhaps to an unmanageable size.

Governance Responsibilities in HSs

In addition to the fact that governance issues of control differ between HSs and single HSOs, various governance responsibilities are met differently. In both independent HSOs and HSs, those who govern have five responsibilities to which they must attend, albeit differently, if they are to fulfill their obligations to stakeholders, including the owners or shareholders in for-profit situations.[83]

First, GBs are responsible for formulating organizational ends. That is, they are responsible for establishing a vision for the HS, from which a mission and associated organizational objectives grow. As noted earlier in the discussion of the conceptual competence needed by CEOs of HSs, the missions of HSs differ from those of any of their component HSOs. In a highly integrated HS, for example, the mission emphasizes enhancing the health status of a defined population rather than reducing illness in individuals. Those who govern HSs must think very broadly and positively about health.

Second, GBs have a responsibility to ensure suitable performance from CEOs. The steps involved in fulfilling this responsibility typically include selecting the CEO, specifying performance expectations, and periodically appraising the CEO's actual performance.[84] This is not an easy task in an HS. As Ummel, reflecting on the difficulties faced by those who seek to build highly integrated HSs, noted, "it is obvious that the healthcare industry has not been through massive consolidation and restructuring before. Amateurish moves, setbacks, and missed opportunities are commonplace."[85] More than anything else, these difficulties reflect the fact that many CEOs and members of GBs of HSs are still on a learning curve about how to create highly integrated HSs.

Third, GBs are responsible, ultimately, for the quality of care that is provided. The legal responsibilities of GBs in this area are well established and involve them in such activities as credentialing members of the PSO; seeing that procedures to adequately address quality, utilization, and risk management issues are in place; and assessing both the process and the outcomes of healthcare, increasingly at the level of populations being served by HSs. Concern about the quality of care is a traditional imperative for those who govern HSOs. The emergence of HSs, however, affords GBs new opportunities and challenges in this area of governance responsibility. The integration of various providers along a continuum of care presents unprecedented opportunities for the application of new algorithms, guidelines, or pathways toward improved clinical outcomes, as well as new opportunities for improved service quality and levels of customer satisfaction among the populations served. The potential for such improvements remains embryonic in most HSs.

GBs also bear responsibility in a fourth area, the finances and financial performance of their HSs. Traditionally, this responsibility in independent HSOs includes such activities as establishing appropriate financial objectives; maintaining adequate controls over financial matters; and ensuring that the HSO's financial obligations, including investing its funds, are properly met. These aspects of financial performance responsibility continue in HSs, even as the responsibility expands into new areas.

Certain aspects of HSs' financial performance and financial responsibility on the part of those who govern are especially noteworthy. The HS is positioned to reap financial benefits of large-scale, unified selling when integration has developed to the point of single-signature contracting by an HS and when enough progress has been made in clinical outcomes management, continuum-of-care development, and lower cost structures for episodes of care. That is, the HS is positioned to garner more managed care contracts with insurers and other payers and to obtain such contracts under more favorable terms, such as multiyear agreements and fair rates.

As HSs develop and mature, they also may successfully pursue commercial and Medicare risk contracting; however, with the assumption of risks come significant opportunities for financial gain. The potential financial benefits inherent in unified selling opportunities and in risk contracting represent significant new opportunities—and challenges—in the area of GBs' responsibilities for financial performance.

The fifth area of GB responsibility is for self. That is, those who govern are responsible for doing so in an effective and efficient manner. Fulfilling this responsibility includes establishing and maintaining appropriate bylaws to guide the governance process, selecting GB members who can serve the HS and component HSOs well and seeing that they do, and ensuring that processes for evaluating GB performance and member development are in place and properly functioning. The differences here between independent HSOs and HSs are mostly those of scope and complexity, although, as noted earlier, when HSs have a number of boards, there are significant challenges involved in having them work together well.

PSOs

The information provided in the Professional Staff Organization section generally applies to HSOs and to HSs built from them. Some differences, however, do arise as LIPs relate to the more complex organizational structures of HSs. The relationships of LIPs as individuals and in PSOs as organized entities whose members are LIPs begin with the relationships that LIPs form among themselves. For example, individual physicians can form a group practice, which is "a formal association of three or more physicians, dentists, podiatrists, or other health professionals providing services, with income from the medical practice pooled and redistributed to the members of the group according to a pre-arranged plan."[86] In addition to group practices, physicians can form independent practice associations, which are legal entities "composed of physicians who have organized for the purpose of negotiating contracts to provide medical services."[87] They also can form a physician-owned management services organization (MSO), a "legal corporation formed to provide practice management services to physicians."[88]

In turn, LIPs, as individuals or groups, can be employed by, have their practices owned by, or contract with HSOs/HSs. The popularity of HSO/HS ownership of physician practices has been mixed, however, as Orlikoff and Totten noted:

> A fully integrated health system model is often achieved by purchasing physician practices (and subsequent employment of those physicians) or by establishing a staff-model health maintenance organization, or HMO. . . .This model promises the greatest opportunity for hospitals and physicians to respond together to the market, manage outcomes, and rationalize resource allocation. While doctors still tend to favor a degree of autonomy over total integration with hospitals, continuing market pressure for effective cost control and the ability to demonstrate quality and performance are moving hospitals and physicians closer together.
>
> Regardless of the relationship model selected, to be truly integrated, an integrated delivery system (IDS) must share risk and align incentives with its doctors.[89]

Other relationship models include MSOs formed by HSOs/HSs and physicians. These MSOs, in contrast to MSOs that are physician only, are typically based in the HSOs/HSs. The services that are provided to physicians by such MSOs typically include billing, information system acquisition and installation, staffing, staff training and development, managed care contract negotiation and compliance, and other office management functions.[90]

Physicians and a hospital within an HS can form a PHO, defined as a "legal entity formed by a hospital and a group of physicians to further mutual interests and to achieve market interests."[91] PHOs, by combining physicians and a hospital into a single entity, make it easier to obtain contracts with health plans, employers, or purchasing coalitions.[92]

MSOs and PHOs involving HSOs/HSs and physicians typically are organized as joint ventures. A joint venture is "a legal entity characterized by two or more parties who work on a project together, sharing profits, losses, and control."[93] Joint ventures between HSOs/HSs and members of their PSOs, including ventures in which they set up diagnostic imaging centers (DICs) or establish ambulatory surgery centers (ASCs), are commonplace.[94]

Ambulatory Health Services

Ambulatory care is delivered to people who go to a physician's office or another setting, such as an ASC, at a time and place they determine and who receive care and then return home. In addition, ambulatory services have been available for decades in the emergency departments and outpatient clinics of acute care hospitals. Chapter 3 describes how technology increasingly allows significant diagnostic and therapeutic services to be provided to outpatients. Americans made more than 1.1 billion visits to doctors' offices and hospital emergency and outpatient departments in 2004, up by 31% in the preceding 10 years.[95]

Medical group practices, ASCs, and DICs are examples of HSOs providing ambulatory health services.[96] There are approximately 12,000 group practices of five or more full-time equivalent physicians in the United States, more than 4,200 ASCs, and about 4,500 diagnostic imaging centers.[97] Each of these types of HSOs, and many other types providing ambulatory health services, have experienced phenomenal grown in the past decade.

Competition based on price and convenience is shifting the location of some ambulatory services. For example, walk-in clinics in retail stores, staffed primarily by nurse practitioners, are growing dramatically. The CEO of Take Care Health, which operates clinics in Walgreens and Rite Aid drugstores, predicts, "By the end of the decade, the number of clinics could grow . . . to 10,000."[98]

Ambulatory HSOs provide a wide range of services: comprehensive outpatient rehabilitation facilities, renal dialysis centers, abortion clinics, family planning clinics, podiatric surgery centers, oral surgery centers, birth centers, HMOs, general purpose (same-day) ASCs, eye surgery centers, and dermatology surgery centers.[99]

Making up a uniquely important type of ambulatory health services provider are the approximately 722 federally qualified health centers (FQHCs) in the United States. These nonprofit, consumer-directed HSOs provide services to the medically underserved and the uninsured. FQHCs include community health centers (CHCs), migrant health centers, healthcare for the homeless programs, public housing primary care programs, and urban Indian and tribal health centers.[100]

Many ambulatory health services operate as freestanding HSOs. Others exist as parts of HSs through an extraordinarily wide range of business affiliations, such as joint ventures, contractual relationships, and vertically and horizontally integrated systems that can result in establishing ambulatory HSOs.

The various types of ambulatory HSOs are like typical HSOs in organization, although the specifics vary widely. Figure 2.13 is the organizational chart of a FQHC. Ambulatory HSOs are almost always corporations that can be organized for profit or not for profit. Physicians are commonly involved as owners-investors, which suggests that many ambulatory HSOs will be organized for profit. Regardless of ownership, the GBs of ambulatory HSOs set policy and evaluate performance of management and, ultimately, the practitioners. GB composition and size are dependent on whether the ambulatory HSO is organized for profit or not for profit.

Ambulatory services HSOs typically have a CEO, whose title is likely to be *administrator, director,* or *clinic manager.* In addition to the competencies discussed earlier in this chapter for all HSO/HS managers, important skills and knowledge that ambulatory services managers should have include knowledge of health insurance product design, sales, and marketing skills.[101]

Ambulatory HSOs are likely to have flat organizational structures with few managerial levels, although larger organizations will have intermediate-level managers as required. These HSOs are unlikely to have the number of LIPs that would necessitate a PSO, as hospitals would. Other types of staff depend on the specific activities of the organization. Physician assistants, RNs, LPNs, nursing assistants, surgical assistants, laboratory technologists, and radiology technicians are common.

Licensure requirements for ambulatory HSOs vary widely; some must be licensed and affiliated with a hospital. For example, most but not all states require ASC licensure. The Joint Commission accreditation of ambulatory HSOs began in 1975 when it established the ambulatory health care accreditation program. This program is applicable to all types of freestanding ambulatory care facilities.[102] The Accreditation Association for Ambulatory Healthcare also accredits virtually every type of ambulatory care HSO.[103]

Ambulatory HSOs have become a major force in delivering health services and have challenged more traditional providers for market share. Improved and more portable technology, improved drugs, increasing competition between hospitals and their LIPs, and consumer awareness and eco-

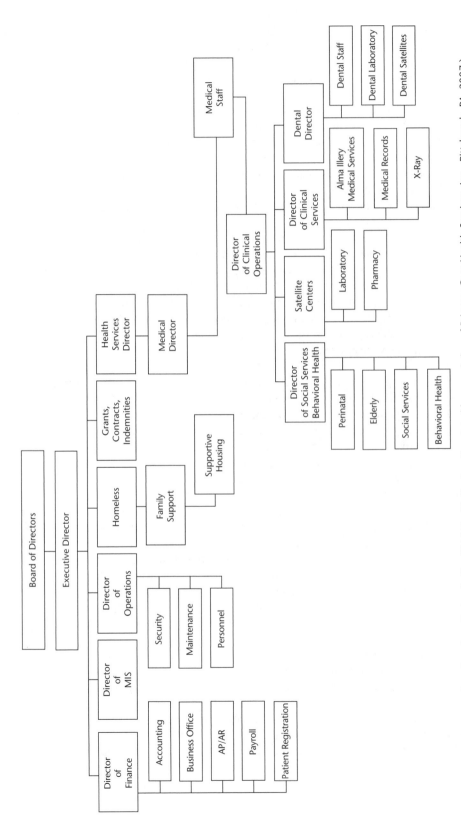

Figure 2.13. Organization chart for a Federally Qualified Health Center. (Reprinted by permission of Primary Care Health Services, Inc., Pittsburgh, PA, 2007.)

nomics are likely to mean continued strong growth in the number, range, and medical complexity of services that are offered in ambulatory HSOs.

Hospice

Hospice is described by the National Hospice and Palliative Care Organization as follows: Providing "quality, compassionate care for people facing a life-limiting illness or injury, hospice and palliative care involve a team-oriented approach to expert medical care, pain management, and emotional and spiritual support expressly tailored to the patient's needs and wishes. Support is provided to the patient's loved ones as well."[104] Hospice, as noted by the National Hospice Foundation[105] and others,[106]

- Focuses on caring, not curing, and in most cases, is provided in the person's home
- Increasingly is also provided in freestanding hospice centers, hospitals, and nursing homes and other long-term care facilities
- Is covered by Medicare, Medicaid, most private insurance plans, HMOs, and other managed care organizations

Beginning in England in the early 1960s, the modern hospice concept was stimulated by the unsatisfactory conventional treatment of people with terminal illnesses. The first U.S. hospice program was established in New Haven, CT, in 1974.[107] From that single program, the number of hospice programs grew to 3,650 in 2004, caring for more than 1 million patients.[108]

The interdisciplinary team concept has been integral to hospice from its beginning, and it continues to form the heart of how hospice programs operate[109] (Figure 2.14). Each member of the hospice interdisciplinary patient care team, including volunteers, contributes to meeting at least one aspect of patient and family needs.[110]

The Medicare hospice benefit, initiated in 1983, is covered under Medicare Part A (hospital insurance). More than 80% of people who use hospice are over the age of 65, entitling them to the set of services covered by the Medicare hospice benefit. "This benefit covers virtually all aspects of hospice care with little out-of-pocket expense to the patient or family. As a result, the financial burdens usually associated with caring for a terminally ill patient are virtually nonexistent."[111] Hospice services that are not reimbursed depend on community charitable support in the form of volunteers, who are an essential part of the hospice philosophy.[112]

States license hospice programs and establish requirements that must be met. Hospices must also comply with federal regulations in order to be certified for reimbursement under Medicare. They undergo periodic inspections from both federal and state regulators. Typically, hospice programs utilize the Standards of Practice for Hospice Programs developed by the National Hospice and Palliative Care Organization as a means of ensuring quality.[113]

ORGANIZATIONAL MODELS AND STRUCTURES OF HOSPICES

Hospice can be structured and offered in a variety of ways, although the typical organizational models are the following:[114]

1. *Hospital-based hospice units.* These are programs or departments of hospitals, sometimes called palliative care units.
2. *Hospital-based hospice teams.* Caregivers go to hospital units and to nursing facilities or chronic care hospitals. Hospice staff may coordinate all other services.

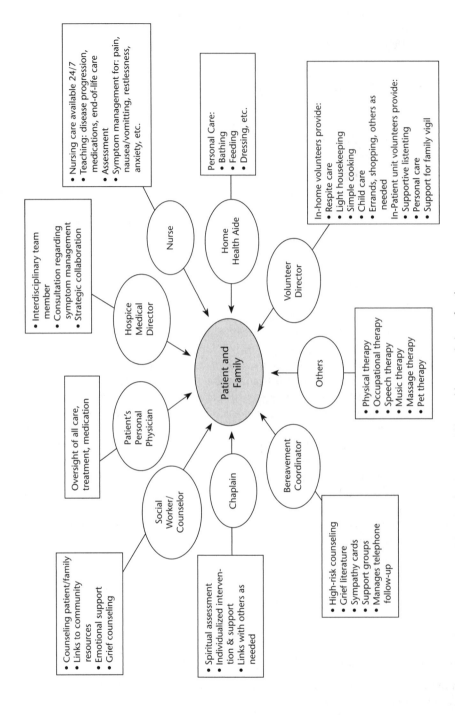

- Nursing care available 24/7
- Teaching: disease progression, medications, end-of-life care
- Assessment
- Symptom management for: pain, nausea/vomiting, restlessness, anxiety, etc.

Personal Care:
- Bathing
- Feeding
- Dressing, etc.

In-home volunteers provide:
- Respite care
- Light housekeeping
- Simple cooking
- Child care
- Errands, shopping, others as needed

In-Patient unit volunteers provide:
- Supportive listening
- Personal care
- Support for family vigil

- Interdisciplinary team member
- Consultation regarding symptom management
- Strategic collaboration

Oversight of all care, treatment, medication

- Physical therapy
- Occupational therapy
- Speech therapy
- Music therapy
- Massage therapy
- Pet therapy

- Counseling patient/family
- Links to community resources
- Emotional support
- Grief counseling

- Spiritual assessment
- Individualized intervention & support
- Links with others as needed

- High-risk counseling
- Grief literature
- Sympathy cards
- Support groups
- Manages telephone follow-up

Nurse

Home Health Aide

Volunteer Director

Hospice Medical Director

Patient's Personal Physician

Others

Patient and Family

Social Worker/ Counselor

Chaplain

Bereavement Coordinator

Figure 2.14. Model of Hospice Team. © 2006 Carolyn Longest, MA; used by permission of author.

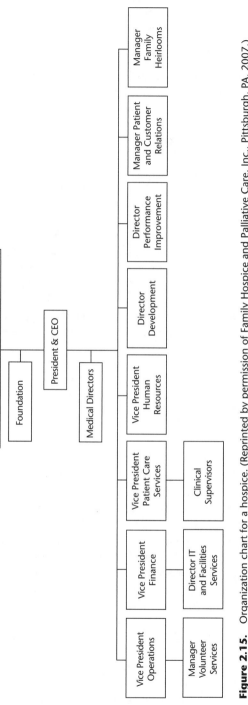

Figure 2.15. Organization chart for a hospice. (Reprinted by permission of Family Hospice and Palliative Care, Inc., Pittsburgh, PA, 2007.)

3. *Freestanding hospital-affiliated units.* Located in separate buildings, they are affiliated with specific hospitals, usually teaching hospitals.
4. *Home health agency–based hospice.* Sometimes known as hospice without walls, these programs care for people who stay at home and receive care from homemakers, clergy, volunteers, social workers, nurses, and physicians.
5. *Freestanding facilities.* St. Christopher's Hospice is the prototype of a hospice that provides the care and atmosphere needed for comfort and pain control but has no facilities for acute medical care. Figure 2.15 shows a freestanding hospice.

The freestanding hospice organizational structure is typically flat. Few managers or levels are needed, because the hospice tends to be small and there are fewer staff than in most types of HSOs/HSs. Below the director are a few supervisors and the staff. A large hospice has middle-level managers between the director and staff. These people perform the typical line and staff functions such as general administration, financial management, and human resources administration, with the latter especially concerned with recruiting and coordinating volunteers. Because reimbursement and patient services depend on staff providing direct services, hospice minimizes management staff.

The type of governance depends on whether the hospice is independent or dependent. An independent hospice, as shown in Figure 2.15, has a GB similar to that of other freestanding organizations. This means the GB has full authority and accountability and performs the generic governance functions described earlier. A dependent hospice may have a committee that provides guidance, or direction may simply be the responsibility of a member of the parent organization's management team. Typically, a hospice has a director, who may be a registered nurse, a social worker, or someone trained in management.

The growth of hospice programs has been dramatic. Given U.S. demographics and increasing acceptance of hospice for the terminally ill, these programs are likely to achieve continued growth well into the 21st century. Bereavement support and respite care are likely to be increasingly important services provided by hospice.

Home Health Agencies

Home health is provided to individuals and families in their places of residence. This care is intended to promote, maintain, or restore health and to maximize the level of independence while minimizing the effects of disability and illness.[115] The first sustained effort for home healthcare in the United States, except for that provided by families or privately employed caregivers, dates from 1893, when Lillian Wald established the Visiting Nurse Service of New York City as part of the Henry Street Settlement services to the poor. By 1909, she had persuaded the Metropolitan Life Insurance Company to begin covering home nursing care for policyholders in New York City. The pilot project was so successful that it was adopted in many communities by other insurance companies in the 1920s.[116]

In 1947, the first hospital-based home health program was established at Montefiore Hospital in the Bronx, New York, to serve patients newly discharged from hospitals. It expanded traditional home nursing care and used an interdisciplinary team that coordinated physicians, therapists, aides, and social workers.[117]

Contemporary home health is much more than skilled nursing services; it includes a wide array of services. HHAs are HSOs that primarily provide services including skilled nursing services by RNs and LPNs; PT, OT, and speech-language therapy; medical social work; and home health aide services. HHAs may offer home hospice, home-delivered meals, Lifeline® (telephone link with clients), and other supportive services. Services often use a multidisciplinary team approach and are commonly part of postacute hospital care. There are about 11,400 agencies serving approximately 1.5 million patients.[118]

To be Medicare certified, HHAs must provide part-time or intermittent skilled nursing services and at least one other therapeutic service—medical social work, OT, PT, speech-language therapy, or home health aide services. States that require HHA licensure may establish additional requirements concerning qualifying services.

Unskilled providers include home health aides, homemakers, chore workers, and personal care aides—in aggregate, one of the most costly parts of home health services. Other services may include medical supplies and equipment. Most providers use Medicare eligibility guidelines because a large percentage of their clients are Medicare beneficiaries. Many commercial insurance and managed care organizations have adopted the Medicare guidelines as well. Medicare regulations are becoming increasingly stringent and adding more requirements, such as licensing or certification for nonprofessional staff and limitations on using independent contractors, which increase costs and diminish the ability of smaller HHAs to deliver services, especially in rural areas.

Clients for skilled services are referred directly by, or with concurrence of, attending physicians, often through hospital discharge planners who identify a need for skilled services and assist with the referral. Hospitals are a major source of referrals of people needing home health.

HHAs also provide home medical equipment (HME) such as respiratory therapy equipment including oxygen, oxygen concentrators, and associated apparatuses; humidifiers; nebulizers; ventilators; and tracheostomy supplies. Durable medical equipment supplied by HHAs includes hospital beds, wheelchairs, bathroom aides, and walkers. Third-party payment for HME usually requires a physician's order, and the recipient is subject to qualification guidelines.

Most states license HHAs, in which case they must meet legal and regulatory requirements. As noted previously, only certified HHAs are eligible for Medicare reimbursement. The certification process is conducted for Medicare by state health departments. Two organizations accredit HHAs— The Joint Commission, which was discussed earlier, and the Community Health Accreditation Program (CHAP) (www.chapinc.org).

ORGANIZATIONAL STRUCTURES OF HHAs

HHAs can be organized in several ways; each arrangement has advantages and disadvantages. They may be independent organizations, incorporated either for profit or not for profit. They may be in a dependent relationship with another HSO such as an acute care hospital, either as a department or freestanding.

The organizational structure is likely to be flat, with a CEO, perhaps an associate, and department heads for various specialized activities such as skilled care (provided by RNs, LPNs, OTs, PTs, speech-language pathologists, and medical social services) and unskilled services (such as those provided by home health aides). The management team also will include staff with financial, accounting, billing, and information systems expertise. The presence of marketing staff, as well, reflects the increasing attention to marketing the HHA. Foci of marketing include insurers, employers, discharge planners, and case managers in acute care hospitals, as well as private physicians, all of whom are important sources of referrals, especially for home care agencies that are not hospital affiliated . Figure 2.16 presents an organizational chart for a freestanding HHA.

Not-for-profit HHAs that are not hospital affiliated have a separate GB. HHAs organized for profit may or may not have a GB. In either a sole proprietorship or a partnership, all decisions are made by the owner(s). Hospital-affiliated HHAs may be freestanding, in which case they have a separate GB. If integrated as a hospital department, the HHA may report through the hospital hierarchy to the hospital CEO and on to the GB. Vertically integrated HSs or diversified HSOs may have a variety of relationships with the HHA, including overlapping GB membership.

As is typical in small HSOs, small HHAs have few managers beyond the CEO, who uses a title such as *executive director* or *administrator*. In small HHAs, the CEO is usually responsible for oper-

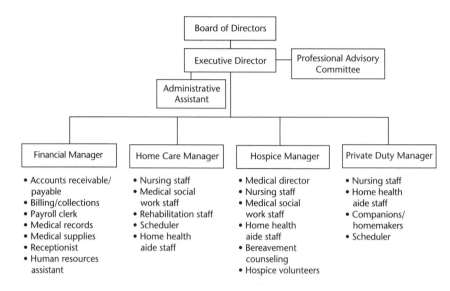

Figure 2.16. Organization chart of a freestanding home health agency.

ations and is also the clinical leader. Larger HHAs have a CEO educated in management, who may have a clinical background. Large HHAs have characteristics and scalar relationships similar to those of other large HSOs, and specialized functions are provided by staff; clinical coordinators, a financial officer, and marketing specialists are common. Special attention to financial management is important because of the distinct reimbursement and regulatory constraints governing home health.

Home health is very different from the services provided by most HSOs. It is unique because practitioners work without direct supervision at many individual sites. This necessitates specialized mechanisms to organize staff and ensure quality of care. HHAs have no PSO as such. Medicare-certified HHAs, however, must have a clinical director who is responsible for the clinical coordination of services. They also must have a group of professional personnel, often called the professional advisory committee, that is composed of at least one physician, one RN, and appropriate representation from other disciplines. This group's function is to establish and review annually the HHA's policies regarding scope of services, admission and discharge policies, medical supervision and plans of care, emergency care, clinical records, personnel qualifications, and program evaluation.

Despite the tumultuous reimbursement environment, the need for home health is almost certain to increase as the population ages. Significant involvement by hospitals and HSs in home health is likely to continue. Historically, home health was low technology and low cost; however, it has become a service filled with high-cost services under Medicare. Use of high-technology diagnostic and therapeutic activities in home healthcare seems almost limitless. Although high-technology services receive more attention, low-technology services, including companionship, housekeeping, respite care, transportation services, errand running, shopping, and general security services, also will be increasingly needed in the future.

▬ Managed Care ▬▬▬▬▬▬▬▬▬▬▬▬▬▬▬▬▬▬▬▬▬▬▬▬▬▬▬▬▬▬

The first "managed care" can be traced to HMOs, formerly called prepaid group practice plans. The term *health maintenance organization* was coined in the early 1970s and is reflected in the Health Maintenance Organization Act of 1973 (PL 93-222).[119] HMOs resulted from efforts to provide an alternative delivery system based on a unique philosophy about health services. The HMO philosophy stresses a close relationship between patients and physicians, as well as a financial arrangement and preventive measures (compared with the acute treatment emphasized by traditional insurance coverage), and provides incentives to both insureds and providers to minimize expensive inpatient (hospital) treatment. Prepaid group practice plans and early HMOs usually employed physicians who were paid a salary. Enrollees paid a fixed premium that covered all services.

A unique aspect of early HMOs was that, unlike conventional HSOs, HMOs grouped hospitals, physicians, and other health services staff and providers into an "organization"—more accurately, an arrangement—that provided a full range of medical services to an enrolled population for a fixed, prepaid fee. Thus an HMO may have been a set of contracts—a virtual HSO—or an actual organization. Its most distinguishing characteristic, compared with other delivery and financing arrangements, was the combination of health services delivery and financing in a single organizational arrangement. Most HMOs today view themselves as MCOs that offer an array of health plans and products, rather than as traditional, closed-ended HMOs.[120] Point-of-service (POS) plans are a contemporary variation in HMOs, in which an HMO plan is combined with a traditional insurance plan. The POS permits members to decide whether to stay within the HMO or go outside its restrictions to receive care under the traditional insurance. This arrangement permits members to obtain care "in or out of the network" established by the HMO.[121]

There were 465 licensed HMOs in 2004, down 3.3% from the prior year. Similarly, HMO enrollment declined 4.8% between 2003 and 2004, from 82.5 million to 78.6 million enrollees.[122] In 1998, there were about 76 million enrollees in 651 HMOs.[123]

TYPES OF MCOs

Twenty-five years ago, most people in the United States with health insurance had indemnity insurance coverage, which meant they could go to any physician, hospital, or other provider. The providers would bill for their services, and the insurance and the patient would each pay part of the bill. Now, however, more than half of all Americans who have health insurance are enrolled in some kind of MCO or plan, an organized way of both providing services and paying for them.[124] MCOs come in a variety of types.[125] MCOs in general and the primary types of MCOs—HMOs, preferred provider organizations (PPOs), and PSOs—are defined below:[126]

Managed care organizations. MCOs are entities that offer [an] HMO, PPO, or PSO plan, or a combination of them. They can be owned by national managed care firms, physician groups, hospitals, commercial health insurers, Blue Cross Blue Shield plans, community cooperatives, private investors, or other organizations, both for profit and not for profit.

Health maintenance organizations. HMOs offer comprehensive health services to members for a fixed monthly fee by contracting with or employing physicians, hospitals, and other health professionals to provide services on behalf of enrollees. Ownership runs a gamut from national managed care organizations to Blue Cross Blue Shield to independent ownership. There are four basic models of HMOs.

Staff-model. Physicians and other health services providers are salaried employees who work only for that HMO and generally care only for that HMO's patients. Care is usually delivered at sites owned by the HMO.

Group-model. The HMO contracts on an exclusive basis with a large physician practice to provide comprehensive services to HMO enrollees. The HMO and group practice are separate organizational entities. The HMO pays the group, which pays the physicians.

Independent practice association (IPA)–model. The HMO contracts with individual physicians or groups of physicians to treat patients in their offices. These physicians are usually organized as solo practitioners or small group practices. IPA physicians may treat nonplan patients.

Network-model. [An] HMO that uses several contracting methods is often called a network-model HMO. The HMO contracts with several larger multispecialty groups or IPAs, rather than individual physicians or small practices. These groups or IPAs treat nonplan patients.

Preferred provider organizations. PPOs are networks of hospitals, physicians, and other healthcare providers that provide services for a negotiated fee. PPOs are often sold as an option (also known as a rider) to a traditional insurance plan. PPOs do not assume the financial risk of the health benefits being offered; risk is often assumed by the sponsoring organization, such as an insurance company, third-party administrator, or self-insured employer. PPOs do not perform many customary HMO functions, such as underwriting, utilization management, and review of quality. (Shouldice argued that a better name for PPOs is preferred provider arrangements because they are brokered arrangements between providers and purchasers of health services, the terms and conditions of which are specified by contract.[127])

Provider sponsored organizations. PSOs are MCOs that are owned or controlled by healthcare providers. Many of the original HMOs were and are provider controlled. PSO is a term that is used to describe the emerging provider organizations that are formed to directly contract (direct contracting) with purchasers to deliver services. Unlike IPAs and other provider groups, PSOs assume insurance risk for beneficiaries. PSOs are formed by organizations such as IPAs, physician-hospital organizations (PHOs), and integrated delivery systems (IDSs).

No matter which type, all MCOs have the following six characteristics and functions:[128]

1. Establish arrangements with hospitals, physicians, and other LIPs to provide a defined set of health services to members
2. Establish criteria and develop processes for selecting and subsequently monitoring performance of LIPs
3. Establish processes to measure health services utilization, referral patterns of physicians, and measures of quality
4. Provide incentives for MCO members to utilize MCO-associated LIPs and HSOs, or require that they do
5. Provide incentives for MCO-associated LIPs and HSOs to encourage the appropriate use of health services resources
6. Provide and encourage utilization of programs and activities intended to improve the health status of MCO members

In spite of their shared characteristics, MCOs differ widely in how they pay providers, and most use several different types of reimbursement methods, even in the same market. Salaried physicians and other LIPs in staff-model HMOs are the easiest example. Hospitals may be paid by discounted fee-for-service, per diem, or per-case rates; DRGs; or capitation. HHAs are usually paid using a per-hour or per-visit fee schedule. DRGs are used exclusively for hospitals; other payment methods, such as discounted fee-for-service, can apply to all providers. PPOs use discounted fee-for-service arrangements almost exclusively.[129]

ORGANIZATIONAL STRUCTURES OF MCOs

MCOs are quite varied in how they are organized, although all are corporations organized for profit or not for profit. Both forms have GBs that set policy and evaluate overall performance. Figures 2.17 and 2.18 are sample organizational charts for an HMO and a PPO, respectively.

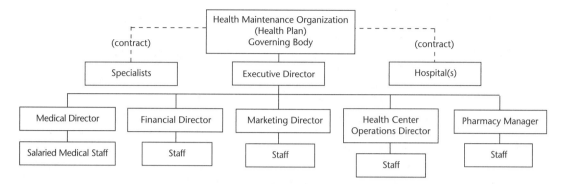

Figure 2.17. Organization structure of a staff-model HMO. Solid lines, direct lines of authority/accountability; dashed lines, contractual relationships between the HMO and another party. (From Shouldice, Robert G. *Introduction to Managed Care, 98.* Arlington, VA: Information Resources Press, 1991; reprinted by permission.)

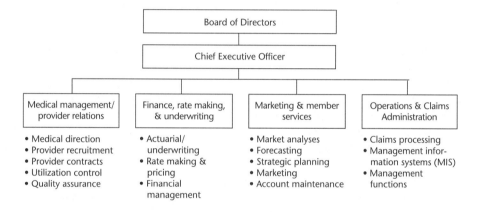

Figure 2.18. Typical PPO organization chart. (From Shouldice, Robert G. *Introduction to Managed Care, 69.* Arlington, VA: Information Resources Press, 1991; reprinted by permission.)

Managers include a CEO, whose title is likely to be *executive director* or *president.* It is not unusual to find CEOs of MCOs who are physicians, often with management training. Small MCOs are likely to have flat organizational structures with few management levels; those larger will have taller hierarchical structures.

Among the most important senior-level managers is the position of CMO, employed part- or full-time, with clinical and management responsibilities. Monitoring efficient use of medical and hospital services (utilization review) is a primary activity. Other activities include quality assurance, recruiting clinicians, credentialing, disciplinary action, and developing and implementing policies and procedures related to medical services. Also, the CMO plays a role in negotiating and managing provider contracts and in enrollee relations.

MCOs use various approaches to organizing the professional staff. They are unlikely to use the PSO model found in hospitals, however. The most tightly controlled approach is the staff-model HMO, in which physicians and other LIPs are screened and credentialed in a manner similar to that used in hospitals. The least controlled are MCOs with IPA characteristics. In the past, HMOs were unlikely to perform their own credentialing of LIPs, relying instead on the credentialing done by affiliated or nonaffiliated hospitals. The numerous disadvantages of this approach, including issues of liability, stimulated MCOs to begin credentialing. In addition, accreditors such as the National

Committee for Quality Assurance (NCQA) (www.ncqa.org) and The Joint Commission began to require credentialing by MCOs. Using information provided by the LIP applicant, the credentialing process is likely to include primary source verification: licensure and board certification status, medical education and training, drug-dispensing license, hospital-admitting privileges, malpractice history and insurance coverage, and any sanctions under the Medicare and Medicaid programs.

Relationships with physicians are established through employment contracts or service contracts, depending on the type of MCO. Such contractual relationships contrast with those used by hospitals, in which physicians are likely to not be employees, to use the hospital only to treat patients, and to have no financial relationship with it. The least complex contract is found in a staff-model HMO, in which the plan hires practitioner and support staff in all categories and is their employer. Employed nonphysician LIPs may have employment contracts that specify duties and compensation. Support staff are unlikely to have contracts and are considered employees at will.[130]

MCOs are accredited by the NCQA criteria, which are stringent and evolving. Since 2006, MCOs seeking accreditation are required to demonstrate that they provide their members with information to help them navigate the care system and that they have programs to promote wellness and manage complex conditions.[131] The Joint Commission also accredits MCOs as part of its ambulatory care accreditation program.

Despite their early presence in American health services and the boost given them by federal legislation, the overall number of HMOs has grown in some years and declined in others. Contributing factors include consumer hesitance to give up choice of physicians and physician reluctance to relinquish autonomy and fee-for-service payment. Major efforts by employers and, to a lesser extent, beneficiaries to control costs has kept pressure on maintaining and enhancing MCO options for providing and financing services.

MCOs have established their importance among providers, payers, and employers eager to control healthcare costs. Winners in the continuing managed care drama will be those organizations or plans—whatever their structure or acronym—that exhibit excellent management, are diversified, and can document delivery of high-quality care and services in a cost-efficient manner.

Public Health

The organizations described above are components of the health services delivery system, in which, to a great extent, individual patients and clients are cared for. In contrast, within the public health system there are many organizations, often units of the federal government, such as the Food and Drug Administration (www.fda.gov) or the Centers for Disease Control and Prevention (www.cdc.gov). States have health departments such as the Minnesota Department of Health (www.health.state.mn.us). Similarly, many cities, counties, and other local levels of government maintain more than 3,000 local health departments.[132] An example of a local unit is the Allegheny County (PA) Health Department (www.achd.net) depicted in Figure 2.19. This organizational chart of a county health department is an example showing that public health organizations share many of the organizational elements found in private health services delivery organizations.

BOARDS OF HEALTH

State and local health departments are governed by boards of health, usually appointed by the state or county chief executives. For example, Allegheny County has a nine-member governing board appointed by the county chief executive, subject to approval by the county council. Its members serve staggered 4-year terms. Key among this board's duties are to appoint and advise the county health director, who functions as the CEO.

Other duties of this board include formulating rules and regulations for the prevention of disease,

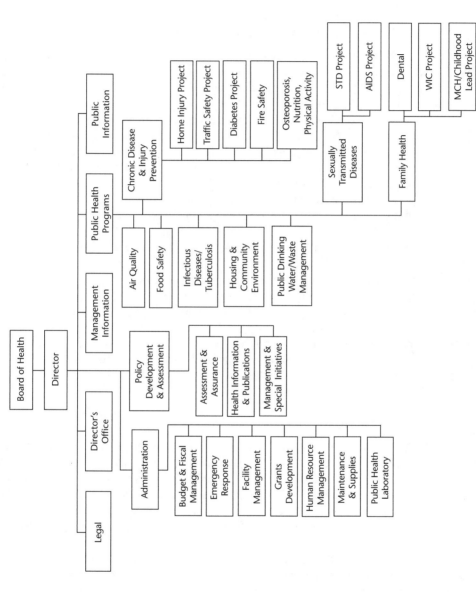

Figure 2.19. Allegheny County (PA) Health Department, 2007.

for the prevention and removal of conditions that constitute a menace to health, and for the promotion and preservation of the public health. This is consistent with general roles played by state and local public health organizations, preventing disease and injury, protecting against environmental hazards, promoting healthy behaviors, responding to disasters, and helping ensure access to health services.[133]

◼ The Ongoing Phenomenon of Corporate Diversification in HSOs/HSs

Several types of HSOs/HSs have been described above. However, none of these paradigmatic organizational structures of HSOs/HSs, or others, should be considered in a static state. All of them are evolving and changing in significant ways. An especially important and ubiquitous aspect of these changes is the result of diversification strategies of the organizations and systems (see Chapter 8). Since the mid-1980s, many HSOs/HSs have used diversification strategies to generate added revenue from new sources such as home care, primary care, and long-term care.

Diversification is a process through which HSOs/HSs add to existing product/service mixes, enter new markets with existing or new products/services, or both. It has been pursued almost without exception in the hope that new activities would provide income to offset declines in revenue from traditional sources, such as hospitals' inpatient activities. Revenue enhancement and profitability are the most important reasons to diversify, but there are other motives:[134]

- *Community service*—Healthcare needs might go unmet without HSO/HS diversification.
- *Innovation*—Being at the cutting edge of new products/services gives HSOs/HSs an advantage in identifying emerging business opportunities.
- *Risk management*—HSOs/HSs can minimize financial risk by spreading it among several activities and markets.
- *Professional staff relations*—Diversifying into services that the professional staff wants to provide or have available to patients, such as substance abuse treatment, is a way to improve relationships with them.

TYPES OF DIVERSIFICATION

There are two basic types of diversification: concentric and conglomerate. Concentric diversification is that in which different but related and complementary products/services are added to the HSO's/HS's existing set of products/services. Conglomerate diversification is that in which products/services that are unrelated to the HSO's/HS's principal business or core products/services are added to the portfolio. Almost all diversification by HSOs/HSs is concentric.

Concentric diversification in general entails developing or acquiring products/services to complement existing ones, expanding sales to current markets, and/or penetrating new markets. In pursuing such diversification, an HSO/HS typically remains close to its core competencies. Because health services involve unique competencies that often are protected by licensure and professional dominance and rarely are substitutable, it is not surprising that most diversification in HSOs/HSs is concentric. This proclivity for concentric diversification distinguishes HSOs/HSs from organizations elsewhere in the economy, where diversifying within present competencies may be less important.

Related or concentric diversification can be achieved through internal development or acquisition. Opportunities for product/service diversification by this means are limited only by the products/services that the diversifying HSO/HS does not offer. Prominent examples of product/service diversification by acute care hospitals include outpatient therapeutic services such as chemotherapy and radiation therapy, outpatient diagnostic services such as imaging, and outpatient health promotion services such as health screening and fitness centers. In addition, to expand their products/services, hospitals can add an array of inpatient services, including rehabilitation, psychiatric, obstetrical, pediatric, or trauma services.

Often, the objective of concentric diversification is to enter new markets for existing or new products/services. Many of the product/service diversifications noted previously allow this. For example, adding obstetrics or pediatrics may open new population groups to other hospital services. Services that target older adults, such as adult day services, home-delivered meals, home medical equipment, and in-home skilled nursing services, are examples of the opportunities that can be derived by serving a new population group.

Diversification in order to reach new markets often means establishing satellite primary care or urgent care centers to serve as sources of new customers, both for the new center and through referral to existing services. In this instance, vertical integration is coupled with diversification. Diversification also may include establishing new patient referral patterns for existing services to enhance market share. This widely used strategy is based on redefining markets, such as the flow of patient referrals, which in the past went almost exclusively from routine care to specialty care. This meant teaching hospitals were the prime beneficiaries. As consumers and payers become more price sensitive, however, such high-cost providers as teaching hospitals must refer routine cases to less-expensive settings. This is greatly facilitated when an HS is formed with teaching hospitals and community hospitals. HSOs/HSs that recognize this change and develop appropriate referral arrangements can expand markets for current and new products/services.

Although diversification continues to be a popular strategy for many HSOs/HSs, others have reconsidered some of their earlier restructuring activities and moved to simplify corporate structures and relationships. Reconsidering earlier diversification decisions may reflect a changed external environment, confused lines of authority that result from some arrangements, management that may have been ill prepared for the demands of a highly diversified structure, different views of mission and objectives among CEOs and members of GBs, high overhead costs, diversification into activities that did not support the HSO's/HS's original mission, risk to tax-exempt status, and damage to community image.[135] HSOs/HSs that simplify corporate structures—or resimplify them—do so because they see potential advantages, including[136]

- Reducing administrative expenses that come with multiple corporations and multiple GBs
- Cutting subsidiary losses in some cases
- Divesting businesses that no longer fit with the mission and strategies
- Permitting a stronger focus on the core business
- Avoiding challenges to tax-exempt status

Environmental Pressures to Change Types and Structures of HSOs/HSs

HSOs/HSs face unusually complex and dynamic external environments. This fact has influenced the types and structures of these organizations and systems, and it will continue to do so. Environmental pressures for continuing development and change in the types and structures of HSOs/HSs include[137]

- Changing demographic characteristics of the population being served with an increase in the proportion of elderly persons needing services
- Greater sophistication of the general public and consumers of health services in terms of their demands on the system

- Increasing range of services being provided outside of traditional hospitals including ambulatory care programs, home care, long-term care, community health centers, and so on
- Growing involvement with the community to address underlying health issues, such as teenage pregnancy, substance abuse, and violence
- Increasing competition among health services organizations providing similar services in the same geographic location to maximize their market share
- Increasing attempts by government at all levels to regulate the quantity and quality of services provided
- Changing systems of reimbursement to health services organizations to control costs
- Expanding private-sector involvement in health services organizations to augment services and control costs
- Increasing involvement of trustees, physicians, and other health professionals in the strategic planning and management of health services organizations
- Increasing attempts by external professional associations and accrediting bodies to set standards for professional conduct in health services organizations
- Increasing demand for outcome accountability and greater value
- Increasing focus on patient safety and quality of care by insurers and employee groups
- Rapidly developing medical technologies and proliferation of increasing specialized services
- Increased information demands, development of real-time information-processing systems to relate to the external environment, and growth of artificial intelligence systems

Among these challenges for HSOs/HSs, none is greater than the challenge of providing quality services with a high degree of patient safety. The Institute of Medicine concluded, "At its best, healthcare in the United States is superb. Unfortunately, it is often not at its best."[138] Serious and extensive problems in quality occur in all HSOs/HSs, as well as in public and private financing mechanisms.

1. **Beyond patient visits:** You will have the care you need when you need it . . . whenever you need it. You will find help in many forms, not just in face-to-face visits. You will find help on the Internet, on the telephone, from many sources, by many routes, in the form you want it.

2. **Individualization:** You will be known and respected as an individual. Your choices and preferences will be sought and honored. The usual system of care will meet most of your needs. When your needs are special, the care will adapt to meet you on your own terms.

3. **Control:** The care system will take control only if and when you freely give permission.

4. **Information:** You can know what you wish to know, when you wish to know it. Your medical record is yours to keep, to read, and to understand. The rule is: "Nothing about you is without you."

5. **Science:** You will have care based on the best available scientific knowledge. The system promises you excellence as its standard. Your care will not vary illogically from doctor to doctor or from place to place. The system will promise you all the care that can help you, and will help you avoid care that cannot help you.

6. **Safety:** Errors in care will not harm you. You will be safe in the care system.

7. **Transparency:** Your care will be confidential, but the care system will not keep secrets from you. You can know whatever you wish to know about the care that affects you and your loved ones.

8. **Anticipation:** Your care will anticipate your needs and will help you find the help you need. You will experience proactive help, not just reactions, to help you restore and maintain your health.

9. **Value:** Your care will not waste your time or money. You will benefit from constant innovations, which will increase the value of care to you.

10. **Cooperation:** Those who provide care will cooperate and coordinate their work fully with each other and with you. The walls between professions and institutions will crumble, so that your experiences will become seamless. You will never feel lost.

Figure 2.20. What patients/customers should expect of healthcare services. From the Committee on Quality of Health Care in America, Institute of Medicine, *Crossing the Quality Chasm: A New Health System for the 21st Century,* p. 63. Reprinted with permission from the National Academies Press, Washington, D.C. Copyright 2001, National Academy of Sciences.

There are significant difficulties in managing quality and safety. For example, a major study conducted in the British National Health Service finds that "the inertia built into established ways of working, and the effort needed to implement new work processes"[139] are among the important difficulties.

The Institute of Medicine, which has given a great deal of attention to the issue of quality and safety in healthcare, has developed a list of 10 things that patients/customers should be able to expect from providers of health services in any setting. Clearly an ideal to be pursued, these expectations, shown in Figure 2.20, suggest the magnitude of fully meeting the challenges of satisfying contemporary patients/customers regarding the quality and safety of their health services. The results of the pressures, especially in regard to quality and safety, will be a continued pattern of new and different types and structures.

DISCUSSION QUESTIONS

1. Identify the typical legal status of various types of HSOs. Why are HSOs overwhelmingly organized as corporations? (Refer to Chapter 4.)
2. Describe the generic roles and activities of the GB, management, and PSO triads in HSOs/HSs.
3. Most types of HSOs have physicians and other LIPs whose credentials are reviewed before their membership in the PSO is approved and clinical privileges are delineated. Describe the credentialing process. How does it differ for an acute care hospital, a nursing facility, and an independent practice association–model HMO? Why?
4. What are the functions of a general acute care hospital?
5. How does the typical general acute care hospital differ organizationally from the usual bureaucratic form? Why? Are these differences necessary?
6. How does the organizational structure of a nursing facility differ from that of a general acute care hospital? Relate these differences to the ease or difficulty of managing each.
7. How can relationships between members of the typical PSO (or physicians and other LIPs, if there is no PSO) and management be improved to enhance organizational effectiveness? Why is this important?
8. Federal reimbursement for medical services provided in several types of HSOs was referenced in this chapter. Identify why federal reimbursement is important and the implications it has for managing these HSOs.
9. What are the key roles of public health organizations?
10. Discuss governance in HSs.

Case Study 1: The Clinical Staff

You are the CEO of Bradley Hospital, a 400-bed voluntary, general acute care hospital. The recently elected president of the PSO has just told you that many members, but especially the physicians, are unhappy because they believe you are trying to control their activities. She stated, "We feel that hospital management should take care of the nonmedical areas and leave the practice of medicine where it belongs—in the hands of professionals."

QUESTIONS

1. How should you respond to the president of the PSO?
2. What arguments should you use to support your position?
3. Sketch an outline showing the appropriate relationship among the GB, CEO, and PSO.

▣ Case Study 2: The Role of the Healthcare Executive in a Change in Organizational Ownership or Control: Consolidations, Mergers, Acquisitions, Affiliations, Divestitures, or Closures[140]

STATEMENT OF THE ISSUE

Changes in organizational ownership or control present special challenges for healthcare executives. Executives must lead their organizations through the transition without self-serving motives. Perhaps most important is the challenge of community accountability—balancing the needs of the community for patient care and health improvement with the needs of the organization for adaptation.

POLICY POSITION

The American College of Healthcare Executives (ACHE) believes that CEOs, their boards, and members of their senior management teams should take a systematic approach to evaluating community health status and how the stakeholders might be affected by proposed changes to organization ownership or control. To this end, ACHE offers the following as a guide.

On an Ongoing Basis
- Listen to the community and identify its future health improvement requirements. This assessment should include an evaluation of current health status, available healthcare resources, and health improvement initiatives, as well as anticipated future needs.
- Ensure that a plan exists for providing care to the underserved in the community and for the continuation of other essential community services.

Before Considering a Change in Ownership or Control
- Identify your organization's values and goals.
- Understand any legal limitations of your organization's certificate of incorporation, articles of organization, charter, or other binding documents that may restrict consideration of alternatives.
- Establish a code of conduct and specific criteria that the board, management team and other staff, and medical staff can use to evaluate proposals regarding change of ownership or control. Consider severance agreements for selected executives who will lead these studies, to remove or lessen self-interest concerns related to loss of position and income.
- Conduct a study to assess various options for change that may be available to your organization and community. The study should examine your market and understand the changes that may affect your organization's ability to fulfill its vision and mission.

When Considering Specific Proposals Related to Change of Ownership or Control
- Assess the compatibility between your organization's values and philosophy and those of your potential partner.
- Identify financial incentives that may have an undue influence on the views of board members, executives, and others involved in proposing and evaluating any change in ownership or control.
- Disclose all conflicts of interest, offers of future employment or future remuneration, and other benefits related to the transaction.
- Evaluate proposals in terms of their likely impact on community healthcare and health status, organization mission and values, protection of the community's assets, and financial viability.

- Gain a thorough understanding of all the terms of the proposed transaction and of all collateral agreements.
- Develop and implement a communications plan that involves and informs all constituencies.

If the Decision Is Made to Proceed with a Change of Ownership or Control
- Obtain a valuation, by a party not involved in the transaction, of charitable assets being converted or restructured, to ensure that reasonable value is received or used in structuring the transaction.
- In a nonprofit setting, prohibit private inurement or personal financial gain by individuals involved in the transaction.
- Ensure that control and administration of any foundation or charitable trust that would be created by the transaction be distinct from the restructured healthcare organization and that the foundation or trust continues to serve a healthcare-related charitable purpose in the community.
- Require that any foundation or trust created provide regular reports to the community on its efforts to improve community health status.
- Explain to the community the issues related to the change in ownership or control, the decision-making process, and how the transaction will benefit the community.
- Provide an opportunity for comment by the public, including stakeholders, on the transaction before it becomes final.
- Make a public announcement at the earliest appropriate time.
- Inform the appropriate federal, state, and local officials of the terms of the transaction in accordance with their requirements.
- Develop and implement a restructuring plan that provides for fair treatment of all employees.

As consolidation and related activities continue in the healthcare field, organizations and their executives will be under increased scrutiny. Executives must demonstrate through their words and actions that their business decisions are guided by professional ethics and a commitment to improving community health status.

QUESTIONS

1. In addition to the roles of CEOs and other senior-level managers in HSOs/HSs during a change in organizational ownership or control, what roles do you think their GBs and PSOs should play?
2. Why is it important for senior-level managers in HSOs/HSs to have governance competence when they are involved in changes in organizational ownership?

■ Case Study 3: Public Health and the Health Services Delivery System

Most of the organizations described in this chapter are components of the health services delivery system primarily serving individual patients and clients. There are, however, more than 3,000 organizations in the United States that are included in the public health system. These organizations primarily focus on "fulfilling society's interest in ensuring conditions in which people can be healthy."[141] Public health organizations are concerned with populations of people, while health services delivery organizations and systems are concerned with the health of individuals and how their health can be enhanced by improvements in the health-related conditions in which they live.[142] Both groups of organizations seek to enhance and improve health, yet they seek this end in different ways and with little collaboration or cooperation between them, for the most part.

1. Why are HSOs/HSs in the personal health services and public health domains so different?
2. What are the implications of these differences for society?
3. How can their roles be more complementary?

Case Study 4: Board Effectiveness[143]

This questionnaire is designed to test whether GBs are hampered by some typical pitfalls that prevent board effectiveness. Read the statements and then, for each one, answer the two questions posed at the end.

1. Our board has representatives from various constituencies, such as our medical staff and subsidiary organizations, and the role of these board members is to represent the issues and interests of their community.
2. Our board agenda materials for each meeting include our organization's mission statement, and we refer to the mission frequently during our decision-making processes.
3. During board meetings, we spend the majority of our time reviewing what happened at committee meetings and approving the actions taken by our committees, and little time remains for discussion of strategic issues.
4. Our board's agenda materials consist primarily of management reports and committee minutes.
5. Our board has a clearly articulated process for removing dysfunctional board members.
6. Our board has performance standards that we use at least annually to review the performance of each board member.
7. Our trustees have a clear understanding of the roles of the board(s) and board committees of our organization, and little, if any, duplication exists among those boards and committees.
8. Job descriptions exist for each of our boards, for trustees, and for board officers.
9. Our board members understand the role of the board on which they serve and its relationship to management, the medical staff, and other physician organizations in our system.
10. All board members participate in an orientation and continuing education and evaluation process that not only introduces them to health care, their board, and the system of which it is a part but also identifies and explains the governance culture—the way we do things on our boards.

QUESTIONS

1. What pitfall (problem or issue) is this statement designed to identify?
2. What steps should be taken to ensure that the pitfall (problem or issue) does not arise and hamper board effectiveness?

Notes

1. Weber, Max. *The Theory of Social and Economic Organizations,* 151–157. Translated by A.M. Henderson and Talcott Parsons. New York: The Free Press, 1947.
2. The Joint Commission on Accreditation of Healthcare Organizations defines licensed independent prac-

titioner (LIP) as "any practitioner permitted by law and by the organization to provide care and services, without direction or supervision, within the scope of the practitioner license and consistent with individually assigned clinical responsibilities." Joint Commission on Accreditation of Healthcare Organizations. *2006 Comprehensive Accreditation Manual for Hospitals: The Official Handbook (CAMH).* Oakbrook, IL: Joint Commission Resources, Inc., 2006.

3. Rice, James A. *Environmental Scan: Trends and Responses for Great Governance 2005–2010.* San Diego: The Governance Institute, 2005.
4. Becker, Cinda. "Board, Quality Linked." *Modern Healthcare* (July 3/10, 2006): 18.
5. Bader, Barry S., and Sharon O'Malley. "Putting All the Pieces Together: The Complete Board Needs the Right Mix of Competencies." *Trustee* (March 2000): 7–10.
6. Longest, Beaufort B., Jr., and Samuel A. Friede. "The Competent Board: Stitching Together Needed Skills and Knowledge." *Trustee* (February 2002): 16–20.
7. American Hospital Association. *Role and Functions of the Hospital Governing Board*, 1–4. Chicago: American Hospital Association, 1990. This statement is unchanged as of July 2006.
8. Griffith, John R., and Kenneth E. White. *The Well-Managed Healthcare Organization*, 5th ed. Chicago: Health Administration Press, 2002.
9. Orlikoff, James E., and Mary K. Totten. *The Trustee Handbook for Healthcare Governance.* Chicago: American Hospital Publishing, Inc., 1998; Pointer, Dennis D., and James E. Orlikoff. *Board Work: Governing Healthcare Organizations.* San Francisco: Jossey-Bass, 1999.
10. Shortell, Stephen M., Robin R. Gillies, David A. Anderson, Karen Morgan Erickson, and John B. Mitchell. *Remaking Healthcare in America*, 2nd ed. San Francisco: Jossey-Bass, 2000.
11. Lister, Eric D. "Physicians in the Boardroom: Essential or Conflicted?" *Healthcare Executive* (July/August 2007): 61.
12. Griffith, John R., and Kenneth E. White. *The Well-Managed Healthcare Organization*, 5th ed. Chicago: Health Administration Press, 2002.
13. Tyler, J. Larry, and Errol Biggs. *Practical Governance.* Chicago: Health Administration Press, 2001.
14. Friede, Samuel A. "Paying for Performance: Executive Compensation Should Be Examined from Many Different Angles." *Modern Healthcare* (November 14, 2005): S6–S7; *Nonprofit Hospital Systems: Survey on Executive Compensation Policies and Practices.* Washington, DC: U.S. Government Accountability Office, June 30, 2006. (GAO-06-907R.)
15. American Hospital Association. "Better Boards and Beyond." *Hospitals & Health Networks* 71 (April 5, 1997): 80, 82, 84.
16. Longest, Beaufort B., Jr. "The Community Development Potential of Large Health Services Organization." *Community Development Journal* 41 (2006): 1, 89–103.
17. Joint Commission on Accreditation of Healthcare Organizations. *2006 Comprehensive Accreditation Manual for Hospitals: The Official Handbook (CAMH).* Oakbrook, IL: Joint Commission Resources, Inc., 2006.
18. Warden, Gail L., and John R. Griffith. "Ensuring Management Excellence in the Healthcare System." *Journal of Healthcare Management* 46, 4 (2001): 228–238.
19. Drucker, Peter F. "The Coming of the New Organization." *Harvard Business Review* 66 (January/February 1988): 45–53.
20. Shortell, Stephen M., and Arnold D. Kaluzny. "Creating and Managing the Future." In *Healthcare Management: Organization Design and Behavior*, 5th ed., edited by Stephen M. Shortell and Arnold D. Kaluzny, 488–521. Clifton Park, NY: Thomson Delmar Learning, 2006.
21. Longest, Beaufort B., Jr. "Managerial Competence at Senior Levels of Integrated Delivery Systems." *Journal of Healthcare Management* 43(2)(1998): 115–133.
22. *NCHL Healthcare Leadership Competency Model, version 2.0.* Developed by the National Center for Healthcare Leadership (NCHL) and Hay Group, Inc., © 2004 National Center for Healthcare Leadership. All rights reserved. Chicago: National Center for Healthcare Leadership, 2004.
23. Orlikoff, James E., and Mary K. Totten. "New Relationships with Physicians: An Overview for Trustees." *Trustee* 50 (July/August 1997): W1–W4.
24. Lambdin, Morris, and Kurt Darr. *Guidelines for Effectively Organizing the Professional Staff.* Baltimore: Health Professions Press, 1999.

25. Asplund, Jon. "Physician Relations." In *Leadership Report 1998: Key Issues Shaping the Future of Healthcare*, edited by Alden Solovy, 181–184. Chicago: American Hospital Publishing, 1998.

26. Lumb, Eileen W., and Roger M. Oskvig. "Multidisciplinary Credentialing and Privileging: A Unified Approach." *Journal of Nursing Care Quality* 12 (April 1998): 36–43.

27. Ewell, Charles M. "Economic Credentialing: Balancing Quality with Financial Reality." *Trustee* 44 (March 1991): 12.

28. American Medical Association. "Federation of State Physician Health Programs, History." *http://www .ama-assn.org/ama/pub/category/5706.html,* retrieved July 22, 2006.

29. Council on Mental Health, American Medical Association. "The Sick Physician: Impairment by Psychiatric Disorders, Including Alcoholism and Drug Dependence." *Journal of the American Medical Association* 223 (1973): 684–687.

30. Council on Ethical and Judicial Affairs, American Medical Association. "Physician Health and Wellness." In the Proceedings of the 2003 Interim Meeting of the AMA House of Delegates. *www.ama-assn .org/ama/pub/category/12552.html,* retrieved July 22, 2006.

31. Fugedy, James. "Should Hospitals Test Doctors for Drugs?" *The Washington Post*, July 16, 1991, Health 14.

32. Perignon, Maria-Caroline. "This Is Your Doc on Drugs." *The Wall Street Journal*, September 15, 1997, A20.

33. Montoya, Isaac D., Jerry W. Carlson, and Alan J. Richard. "An Analysis of Drug Abuse Policies in Teaching Hospitals." *Journal of Behavioral Health Services & Research* 26 (February 1999): 28–38.

34. Fiesta, J. "The Impaired Nurse: Who Is Liable?" *Nursing Management* 21, 10 (October 1990): 20, 22.

35. Lambdin, Morris, and Kurt Darr. *Guidelines for Effectively Organizing the Professional Staff.* Baltimore: Health Professions Press, 1999.

36. Health Care Quality Improvement Act of 1986, PL 99-660, 100 Stat. 3784 (1986).

37. American Podiatric Medical Association. "What Is Podiatry." *www.apma.org,* retrieved July 21, 2006.

38. Bureau of Labor Statistics, U.S. Department of Labor. "Nature of the Industry." *http://www.bls.gov/ oco/cg/cgs035.htm,* retrieved July 31, 2006.

39. Bureau of Labor Statistics, U.S. Department of Labor. "Nature of the Industry."

40. Hilzenrath, David S., and Michael D. Shear. "Hospital Alliance in N. Va. to End." *The Washington Post*, January 29, 1999, E01.

41. "What Hospitals Do." *AHA News* 35 (March 1, 1999): 6.

42. American Hospital Association. *AHA Hospital Statistics*. Chicago: Health Forum LLC (an American Hospital Association Company), various years.

43. American Hospital Association. *AHA Hospital Statistics,* 2006 ed. Chicago: Health Forum LLC (an American Hospital Association Company).

44. Schlesinger, Mark, and Bradford H. Gray. "How Nonprofits Matter in American Medicine, and What to Do About It." *Health Affairs* 25 (2006): w287–w303. (Published online June 20, 2006; 10.1377/ hlthaff.25.w287.)

45. American Hospital Association. *AHA Hospital Statistics,* 2006 ed. Chicago: Health Forum LLC (an American Hospital Association Company).

46. Berenson, Robert A., Thomas Bodenheimer, and Hongmai H. Pham. "Specialty-Service Lines: Salvos in the New Medical Arms Race." *Health Affairs,* Web Exclusive (July 25, 2006): W337–W343.

47. *Services for the Aging in America: Four Scenarios for the Next Decade.* Washington, DC: American Association of Homes and Services for the Aging, 2002.

48. Stryker, Ruth. "The History of Care for the Aged." In *Creative Long-Term Care Administration*, 4th ed, edited by George Kenneth Gordon, Leslie A. Grant, and Ruth Stryker, 6. Springfield, IL: Charles C Thomas, 2004.

49. Stryker, Ruth. "The History of Care for the Aged."

50. Omnibus Budget Reconciliation Act of 1987, PL 100-203, 101 Stat. 1330 (1987).

51. Marek, Karen Dorman, Marilyn J. Rantz, Claire M. Fagin, and Janet Wessel Krejci. "OBRA '87: Has It Resulted in Positive Change in Nursing Homes?" *Journal of Gerontological Nursing* 22 (December 1996): 32–40.

52. National Center for Health Statistics. "Fast Stats A-Z, Nursing Home Care." *http://www.cdc.gov/nchs/ fastats/nursingh.htm,* retrieved July 26, 2006.

53. Harrington, Charlene, Helen Carrillo, and Cassandra Crawford. Table 7, "Nursing, Facilities, Staffing, Residents, and Facility Deficiencies, 1997 Through 2003." Department of Social and Behavioral Sciences, University of California, San Francisco, August 2004. Based on the Online Survey, Certification, and Reporting System (OSCAR), Centers for Medicare and Medicaid Services, U.S. Department of Health and Human Services. *http://www.nccnhr.org/uploads/CHStateData04.pdf.*

54. Harrington, Charlene, Helen Carrillo, and Cassandra Crawford. Table 5, "Nursing, Facilities, Staffing, Residents, and Facility Deficiencies, 1997 Through 2003." Department of Social and Behavioral Sciences, University of California, San Francisco, August 2004. Based on the Online Survey, Certification, and Reporting system (OSCAR), Centers for Medicare and Medicaid Services, U.S. Department of Health and Human Services. *http://www.nccnhr.org/uploads/CHStateData04.pdf.*

55. Kaiser Family Foundation. "Distribution of Certified Nursing Facility Residents by Primary Payer Source, 2003." *www.statehealthfacts.org/cgi-bin/healthfacts.cgi,* retrieved July 26, 2006.

56. National Association of Boards of Examiners for Long Term Care Administrators. *http://www.nabweb .org/Home/default.aspx,* retrieved July 24, 2006.

57. Levinson, Monte J., and Jonathan Musher. "Current Role of the Medical Director in Community-Based Nursing Facilities." *Clinics in Geriatric Medicine* 11 (August 1995): 343–358.

58. Williams, T. Franklin, and Helena Temkin-Greener. "Older People, Dependency, and Trends in Supportive Care." In *The Future of Long-Term Care: Social and Policy Issues*, edited by Robert H. Binstock, Leighton E. Cluff, and Otto von Mering, 51–52. Baltimore: The Johns Hopkins University Press, 1996.

59. O'Leary, Margaret R. *Lexikon,* 366. Oakbrook Terrace, IL: Joint Commission on Accreditation of Healthcare Organizations, 1994.

60. Conrad, Douglas A., and Stephen M. Shortell. "Integrated Health Systems: Promise and Performance." *Frontiers of Health Services Management* 13 (Fall 1996): 3–40, p. 7.

61. Dowling, William L. "Strategic Alliances as a Structure for Integrated Delivery Systems." In *Partners for the Dance: Forming Strategic Alliances in Healthcare*, edited by Arnold D. Kaluzny, Howard S. Zuckerman, and Thomas C. Ricketts, III, 141. Chicago: Health Administration Press, 1995. For further discussion of vertical integration, see Douglas A. Conrad and William L. Dowling. "Vertical Integration in Health Services: Theory and Managerial Implications." *Healthcare Management Review* 14 (Fall 1990): 9–22.

62. Sanofi Aventis. *Managed Care Digest Series: eHospitals/Systems Digest for 2006. www.managedcare digest.com/index.jsp,* retrieved July 27, 2006.

63. Satinsky, Marjorie A. *The Foundations of Integrated Care: Facing the Challenges of Change.* Chicago: American Hospital Publishing, 1998.

64. Orlikoff, James E., and Mary K. Totten. "Systems Thinking in Governance" [workbook insert]. *Trustee* 52 (January 1999): 2.

65. Robinson, James C. "Physician-Hospital Integration and the Economic Theory of the Firm." *Medical Care Research and Review* 54 (March 1997): 3–24, p. 6.

66. Shortell, Stephen M., Robin R. Gillies, David A. Anderson, Karen Morgan Erickson, and John B. Mitchell. *Remaking Healthcare in America: Building Organized Delivery Systems*, 7. San Francisco: Jossey-Bass, 1996. Reaffirmed in Shortell, Stephen M., Robin R. Gillies, David A. Anderson, Karen Morgan Erickson, and John B. Mitchell. *Remaking Healthcare in America: The Evolution of Organized Delivery Systems*, 2nd ed. San Francisco: Jossey-Bass, 2000.

67. Robinson, James C., and Lawrence P. Casalino. "Vertical Integration and Organizational Networks in Healthcare." *Health Affairs* 15 (Spring 1996): 7–22.

68. Bazzoli, Gloria J., Stephen M. Shortell, Nicole Dubbs, Cheeling Chan, and Peter Kralovec. "A Taxonomy of Health Networks and Systems: Bringing Order Out of Chaos." *Health Services Research* 33 (February 1999): 1,683–1,717.

69. Bazzoli, Gloria J., Stephen M. Shortell, Nicole Dubbs, Cheeling Chan, and Peter Kralovec. "A Taxonomy of Health Networks and Systems: Bringing Order Out of Chaos." *Health Services Research* 33 (February 1999): 1,683–1,717.

70. Clement, Jan P., Michael J. McCue, Roice D. Luke, James D. Bramble, Louis F. Rossiter, Yasar A. Ozcan, and Chih-Wen Pai. "Strategic Hospital Alliances: Impact on Financial Performance." *Health Affairs* 16 (November/December 1997): 193–203.

71. Orlikoff, James E., and Mary K. Totten. "Systems Thinking in Governance." *Trustee* 52 (January 1999): workbook insert.

72. This discussion is adapted from Longest, Beaufort B., Jr. "Managerial Competence at Senior Levels of Integrated Delivery Systems." *Journal of Healthcare Management* 43 (March/April 1998): 115–135.

73. Coddington, Dean C., Keith D. Moore, and Elizabeth A. Fischer. "Physician Leaders in Integrated Delivery." *Medical Group Management Journal* 44, 5 (September/October 1997): 85–90, p. 90.

74. Shortell, Stephen M., Robin R. Gillies, David A. Anderson, Karen Morgan Erickson, and John B. Mitchell. *Remaking Healthcare in America*, 2nd ed., 68. San Francisco: Jossey-Bass, 2000.

75. Longest, Beaufort B., Jr. *Health Policymaking in the United States*, 4th ed. Chicago: Health Administration Press, 2006.

76. Zelman, Walter A. *The Changing Healthcare Marketplace: Private Ventures, Public Interests*. San Francisco: Jossey-Bass, 1996.

77. Pointer, Dennis D., Jeffrey A. Alexander, and Howard S. Zuckerman. "Loosening the Gordian Knot of Governance in Integrated Healthcare Delivery Systems." *Frontiers of Health Services Management* 11 (Spring 1995): 3–37.

78. Pointer, Alexander, and Zuckerman. "Loosening the Gordian Knot of Governance in Integrated Healthcare Delivery Systems," 17–18.

79. Orlikoff, James E. "Ensuring Board Effectiveness: It Could Be as Simple as Changing Your Board Structure." *Healthcare Executive* 13 (September/October 1998): 12–16.

80. Orlikoff. "Ensuring Board Effectiveness: It Could Be as Simple as Changing Your Board Structure."

81. Bader, Barry S. "Weight Loss: A Painless Approach to a Sleeker Governance Model." *Trustee* 56 (April 1997): 12–16, p. 14.

82. Pointer, Alexander, and Zuckerman. "Loosening the Gordian Knot of Governance in Integrated Healthcare Delivery Systems," 3–37.

83. Pointer, Alexander, and Zuckerman. "Loosening the Gordian Knot of Governance in Integrated Healthcare Delivery Systems," 3–37.

84. Charan, Ram. *Boards at Work: How Corporate Boards Create Competitive Advantage*, 151–178. San Francisco: Jossey-Bass, 1998.

85. Ummel, Stephen L. "Pursuing the Elusive Integrated Delivery Network." *Healthcare Forum Journal* 40 (March/April, 1997): 13–19, p. 13.

86. O'Leary, Margaret R. *Lexikon*, 337. Oakbrook Terrace, IL: Joint Commission on Accreditation of Healthcare Organizations, 1994.

87. Swayne, Linda M., W. Jack Duncan, and Peter M. Ginter. *Strategic Management of Healthcare Organizations,* 5th ed., 51. Malden, MA: Blackwell, 2006.

88. Swayne, Duncan, and Ginter, *Strategic Management of Healthcare Organizations*.

89. Orlikoff, James E., and Mary K. Totten, "New Relationships with Physicians: An Overview for Trustees." *Trustee* 50 (July/August 1997): workbook insert.

90. Orlikoff and Totten, "New Relationships with Physicians: An Overview for Trustees."

91. O'Leary. *Lexikon*.

92. Burns, Lawton R., and Darrell P. Thorpe. "Physician-Hospital Organizations: Strategy, Structure, and Conduct." In *Integrating the Practice of Medicine: A Decision Maker's Guide to Organizing and Managing Physician Services*, edited by Ronald B. Connors, ch. 17. Chicago: AHA Press, 1997.

93. O'Leary. *Lexikon*.

94. Blair, John D., Charles R. Slaton, and Grant T. Savage. "Hospital-Physician Joint Ventures: A Strategic Approach for Both Dimensions of Success." *Hospital & Health Services Administration* 35 (Spring 1990): 3–26.

95. Burt, Catharine W., Linda F. McCaig, and Elizabeth A. Rechtsteiner. *Ambulatory Medical Care Utilization Estimates for 2004*. Hyattsville, MD: National Center for Health Statistics, 2006. *http://www.cdc.gov/nchs/products/pubs/pubd/hestats/estimates2004/estimates04.htm,* retrieved July 25, 2006.

96. While this list is not exhaustive, the following types of ambulatory health services HSOs exist: ambulatory healthcare clinics, ambulatory surgery centers, birthing centers, college and university health centers, community health centers, dental group practices, diagnostic imaging centers, endoscopy centers, Health Maintenance Organizations (HMOs), Independent Physician Associations (IPAs), Indian health centers, lithotripsy centers, managed care organizations, multi-specialty group practices, office-based anesthesia organizations, occupational health centers, office-based surgery centers and practices, oral and

maxillofacial surgeons' offices, pain management centers, podiatrists' offices, radiation oncology centers, single-specialty group practices, surgical recovery centers, urgent or immediate care centers, and women's health centers.

97. Sanofi Aventis. *Managed Care Digest Series: eManaged Care Trends Digest for 2006. www.managedcaredigest.com/index.jsp,* retrieved July 29, 2006; Federated Ambulatory Surgery Association. "Frequently Asked Questions About Ambulatory Surgery Centers." *www.fasa.org/faqaboutasc.html,* retrieved July 29, 2006; U.S. Census Bureau. "NAICS 621512 - Diagnostic Imaging Centers." In *Statistics of U.S. Businesses: 2003. www.census.gov/epcd/susb/2003/us/US621512.HTM,* retrieved July 29, 2006.

98. Landro, Laura. "The New Force in Walk-In Clinics." *The Wall Street Journal,* July 26, 2006, D1–D2.

99. Duggar, Benjamin C. "Ambulatory Surgery Facilities: Definition and Identification." *Journal of Ambulatory Care Management* 13 (February 1990): 2–3.

100. National Conference of State Legislatures. "Federally Qualified Health Centers in the United States." *http://www.ncsl.org/programs/health/fqhc.htm,* retrieved July 29, 2006.

101. Hudak, Ronald P., Paul P. Brooke, Jr., Kenn Finstuen, and James Trounson. "Management Competencies for Medical Practice Executives: Skills, Knowledge and Abilities Required for the Future." *Journal of Health Administration Education* 15 (Fall 1997): 219–239.

102. Joint Commission on Accreditation of Healthcare Organizations. "Ambulatory Care." *www.jointcommission.org/AccreditationPrograms/AmbulatoryCare/ed_amb.htm,* retrieved July 29, 2006.

103. Accreditation Association for Ambulatory Healthcare. "Types of Organizations Accredited." *http://www.aaahc.org/eweb/dynamicpage.aspx?site=aaahc_site&webcode=types_accredited,* retrieved July 29, 2006.

104. National Hospice and Palliative Care Organization. "What Is Hospice?" *http://www.caringinfo.org/i4a/pages/index.cfm?pageid=3466,* retrieved July 30, 2006.

105. National Hospice Foundation. *http://www.nationalhospicefoundation.org/i4a/pages/index.cfm?pageid=1,* retrieved September 1, 2007.

106. Lynn, Joanne, Janice Lynch Schuster, and Andrea Kabcenell. *Improving Care for the End of Life.* New York: Oxford University Press, 2000.

107. Mor, Vincent, David S. Greer, and Robert Kastenbaum. "The Hospice Experiment: An Alternative in Terminal Care." In *The Hospice Experiment*, edited by Vincent Mor, David S. Greer, and Robert Kastenbaum, 11. Baltimore: The Johns Hopkins University Press, 1988.

108. National Hospice and Palliative Care Organization. "NHPCO's 2004 Facts and Figures." *http://www.nhpco.org/files/public/Facts_Figures_for2004data.pdf,* retrieved July 30, 2006.

109. Leland, June Y., and Ronald S. Schonwetter. "Advances in Hospice Care." *Clinics in Geriatric Medicine* 13 (May 1997): 381–401.

110. National Hospice and Palliative Care Organization. "What Is Hospice?"

111. National Hospice and Palliative Care Organization. "How Is Hospice Paid For?" *http://www.caringinfo.org/i4a/pages/index.cfm?pageid=3468,* retrieved July 30, 2006.

112. Gardia, Gary. "Hanging on to the Spirit of Hospice in the Midst of Bottom Line Management." *American Journal of Hospice & Palliative Care* 15 (January/February 1998): 7–9.

113. National Hospice and Palliative Care Organization. "Standards Committee." *http://www.nhpco.org/i4a/pages/Index.cfm?pageID=4707,* retrieved July 31, 2006.

114. Burnell, George M. *Final Choices: To Live or to Die in an Age of Medical Technology,* 281–282. New York: Plenum, 1993.

115. National Center for Health Statistics. "Home Health Definitions of Terms." *http://www.cdc.gov/nchs/about/major/nhhcsd/nhhcsdefhomehealth.htm,* retrieved July 31, 2006.

116. Mundinger, Mary O'Neil. *Home Care Controversy: Too Little, Too Late, Too Costly,* 37. Rockville, MD: Aspen Systems Corporation, 1983.

117. Lerman, Dan. "The Home Care Controversy." In *Home Care: Positioning the Hospital for the Future*, edited by Dan Lerman, 1. Chicago: American Hospital Publishing, 1987.

118. National Center for Health Statistics. "Current Patient Trends." *http://www.cdc.gov/nchs/about/major/nhhcsd/nhhcschart.htm,* retrieved July 31, 2006.

119. Health Maintenance Organization Act of 1973, PL 93-222, 87 Stat. 914 (1973).

120. Gabel, Jon, Heidi Whitmore, Chris Bergsten, and Lily Pan Grimm. "Growing Diversification in HMOs, 1988–1994." *Medical Care Research and Review* 54 (March 1997): 101–117.

121. Swayne, Duncan, and Ginter. *Strategic Management of Healthcare Organizations*, 52.

122. Sanofi Aventis. *Managed Care Digest Series: eManaged Care Trends Digest for 2006. www.managedcare digest.com/viewslides.do?page=/slides/2005hmo/Slides.jsp?SlideID=2,* retrieved August 1, 2006.

123. Sanofi Aventis. "HMO Summary and Trends." *Managed Care Digest Series: eHMO-PPO/Medicare-Medicaid Digest 2005. http://www.managedcaredigest.com/edigests/hm2005/HMOData.jsp,* retrieved August 1, 2006.

124. America's Health Insurance Plans. *Guide to Managed Care. http://www.ahip.org/content/default.aspx ?bc=41/329/353#overview,* retrieved August 2, 2006.

125. Kongstvedt, Peter R. *Essentials of Managed Healthcare*, 4th ed, 19–30. Gaithersburg, MD: Aspen Publishers, 2001.

126. Knight, Wendy. *Managed Care: What It Is and How It Works*, 24. Gaithersburg, MD: Aspen Publishers, 1998.

127. Shouldice, Robert G. *Introduction to Managed Care*, 2nd ed., 60. Arlington, VA: Information Resources Press, 1991.

128. Knight. *Managed Care: What It Is and How It Works*.

129. Knight. *Managed Care: What It Is and How It Works*, 99–100.

130. Knight. *Managed Care: What It Is and How It Works*, 235.

131. *2007 MCO Standards and Guidelines*. Washington, DC: National Committee for Quality Assurance, 2006.

132. Barton, Phoebe L. *Understanding the U.S. Health Services System*, 2nd ed., 2003. Chicago: Health Administration Press; 85.

133. *State Roles in Health,* 2nd ed., 11. Denver, CO: National Council of State Legislatures, 2005.

134. Coddington, Dean C., and Keith D. Moore. *Market-Driven Strategies in Healthcare,* 114–115. San Francisco: Jossey-Bass, 1987.

135. Johnsson, Julie. "Hospitals Dismantle Elaborate Corporate Restructurings." *Hospitals* 65 (July 5, 1991): 41–45.

136. Johnsson, Julie. "Hospitals Dismantle Elaborate Corporate Restructurings."

137. Leatt, Peggy, G. Ross Baker, and John R. Kimberly. "Organization Design." In *Healthcare Management: Organization Design and Behavior*, 5th ed, edited by Stephen M. Shortell and Arnold D. Kaluzny, 336–337. Clifton Park, NY: Thomson Delmar Learning, 2006.

138. National Roundtable on Healthcare Quality. *Statement on Quality of Care*, 11. Washington, DC: Institute of Medicine, 1998.

139. Ham, Chris, Ruth Kipping, and Hugh McLeod. "Redesigning Work Processes in Healthcare: Lessons from the National Health Service." *Milbank Quarterly* 81, 3 (September 2003): 415–439, p. 434.

140. From *The Role of the Healthcare Executive in a Change in Organizational Ownership or Control: Consolidations, Mergers, Acquisitions, Affiliations, Divestitures, or Closures*. Chicago: American College of Healthcare Executives, November 2005. Reprinted with permission of the American College of Healthcare Executives.

141. Institute of Medicine. *The Future of Public Health*. Washington, DC: National Academy Press, 1988.

142. Breslow, Lester, and Jonathan E. Fielding. "Public Health and Personal Health Services." In *Changing the U.S. Healthcare System*, 3rd ed, edited by Ronald M. Anderson, Thomas H. Rice, and Gerald F. Kominski, 591–608. San Francisco: Jossey-Bass, 2007.

143. From Orlikoff, James E., and Mary K. Totten. "Systems Thinking in Governance." *Trustee* 52 (January 1999 [workbook insert]): 4; reprinted by permission.

3

Healthcare Technology

The advancement and diffusion of technology are among the most complex and controversial aspects of health services. Technological innovations have given health services providers the means to diagnose and treat an increasing number of problems and illnesses. The same advances have been criticized, however, for their effect on the practice of medicine and on national healthcare expenditures. National healthcare expenditures are projected to be $2.4 trillion in 2008 and to grow to $4.1 trillion in 2016, or about 20.0% of GDP.[1]

Analyzing the effects of technology on health services and their costs is complex, especially in terms of costs.

> Some technologies increase costs. Some technologies decrease costs. And some technologies do both. Some raise costs in the short run, but save dollars over the full course of treatment; others lower costs by moving care to nonhospital settings, but increase costs overall because care is more accessible and used more often. How technology affects costs depends on the technology, where it is used, and—above all—on how the concepts of costs and benefits are defined. Indeed, that is the challenge.[2]

The dramatic rise in healthcare costs since 1950 is partly a function of proliferation of new technologies, increased use of existing tests and procedures (including attendant specialized staff), and paying for use of technological innovations. The cost of acquiring technology is significant, but its overall effect on national healthcare expenditures is minimal. Estimates of national expenditures to *purchase* healthcare technology, which ran the gamut from routine medical supplies to advanced diagnostic products and implantable devices to major capital equipment, ranged from 5.1% of healthcare spending in the mid-1990s[3] to 10% (about $200 billion spent) in 2004.[4]

That part of increased healthcare costs which is attributable to *application* of technology is uncertain. Estimates are as high as 70%.[5] There seems to be a consensus that approximately 50% of the rise in total healthcare expenditures results from the use of new technologies and the overuse of existing ones.[6] An analysis by the Health Care Financing Administration (HCFA), now the Centers for Medicare and Medicaid Services (CMS), showed, however, that from 1980 to 1990, new technologies contributed only 15% to the total increase in healthcare spending.[7] Recent analyses showed a range of 25%–33%. The wide variation is the result of using different definitions of *technology,* methods of cost estimation, measurement time frames, and types of expenditure analyzed.[8] Increases in the supply of technology tend to be related to higher utilization and spending for that service; greater availability of diagnostic imaging appears to be associated with incremental utilization rather than substitution for other services.[9] Suffice it to say, however, that the effect of technology on healthcare costs is significant.

Health economists conceptualize the issues in various ways. One theory examines the effect of technology on acute care hospital costs as measured by discrete units such as the labor and nonlabor inputs of using technology. A second theory analyzes the costs associated with specific acute care hospital-based technologies. A third theory examines the effect of technology on treating specific conditions and types of illnesses through time. A fourth theory measures the effect of technology on total healthcare expenditures. It is generally agreed that technology has increased how intensively resources are used to treat individual cases and that this has increased costs. Increased intensity has also resulted from the introduction of new technologies used on new diseases and categories of patients, in addition to the use of existing technologies in new ways. The exact contribution of the use of technology—new procedures, capabilities, and products—to healthcare costs cannot be determined; clearly it is a major contributor, however.

Medical technology is the procedures, equipment, and processes by which medical services are delivered, and is defined as "any discrete and identifiable regimen or modality used to diagnose and treat illness, prevent disease, maintain patient well-being, or facilitate the provision of health services."[10] This broad definition includes biologicals and pharmaceuticals; high technology such as positron emission tomography (PET) scanners and implantable defibrillators; low technology such as laboratory tests and nutrition services; facilities such as intensive care units; specific procedures such as endoscopy, laparoscopy, organ transplants, angioplasty, joint replacements, and coronary artery bypass; clinical and management information and control systems such as electronic medical records (EMRs) (or the broader concept of electronic health records [EHRs]), clinical and management decision support systems and telemedicine; and managerial and clinical technologies, including those that organize and provide care, such as home healthcare, and the use of physician extenders such as physician assistants and nurse practitioners.

A useful typology categorizing medical technologies by their characteristics is shown in Table 3.1. These technologies continue to be available predominantly in acute care hospitals. However, the increasing portability of technology allows it to be delivered in nonhospital and outpatient settings; the economic implications of this change for acute care hospitals are enormous. Portability does not necessarily lower *total* costs, however. On the contrary, home health services, once seen as lower-cost alternatives in delivery of services, have grown rapidly, which is further support for the assertion that demand for health services is virtually limitless—and, as here, only the location where it is provided changes.

Another way to describe medical technology is based on the charge for application. Laboratory tests, radiographs (x-rays), and other ancillary services that typically cost less than $100 are considered low-cost or "small-ticket" technologies compared with high-cost or "big-ticket" technologies such as magnetic resonance imaging (MRI) scans, with a cost of about $600, and organ transplantation, which costs from $30,000 to $200,000 or higher. The controversy over increasing costs focuses on high-cost technologies, but inexpensive technologies raise similar concerns because they are used in high volume

TABLE 3.1. TYPES OF MEDICAL TECHNOLOGIES

Type	Examples
Diagnostic	CT scanner
	Fetal monitor
	Computerized electrocardiography
	Automated clinical labs
	MRI
	Ambulatory blood pressure monitor
Survival (lifesaving)	Intensive care unit
	Cardiopulmonary resuscitation
	Liver transplant
	Autologous bone marrow transplant
Illness management	Renal dialysis
	Pacemaker
	PTCA (angioplasty)
	Stereotactic cingulotomy (psychosurgery)
Cure	Hip joint replacement
	Organ transplant
	Lithotripter
Prevention	Implantable automatic cardioverter-defibrillator
	Pediatric orthopedic repair
	Diet control for phenylketonuria
	Vaccines for immunization
System management	Medical information systems
	Telemedicine

From Rosenthal, Gerald. "Anticipating the Costs and Benefits of New Technology: A Typology for Policy." In *Medical Technology: The Culprit Behind Health Care Costs?* (Publication No. [PHS] 79-3216), 79. Washington, DC: Department of Health and Human Services, 1979, as updated.

and may be labor intensive. Data from the 1950s and 1960s show that the primary cost-raising changes were rapid increases in use of low-cost ancillary services, such as laboratories and x-rays. Data from the 1970s and 1980s, however, show that the use of small-ticket technologies hardly changed but that several new and expensive technologies came into common use, raising costs considerably.[11] In terms of costs, new technology may be a hybrid—its use reduces the costs of treatment or diagnosis, but the resulting higher volume increases total costs. Laparoscopic cholecystectomy is an example.[12]

Rather than classify technologies by cost, it is more useful to focus on the value obtained by their use, which can be done by emphasizing cost-effectiveness and clinical guidelines that reduce variation.[13] Despite differences in how technologies are described, the research, development, and application of technology will continue. It is useful to examine the factors behind this trend and its effects on the healthcare system and on individual health services organizations (HSOs) and health systems (HSs).

History and Background

The technology of modern allopathic (Western) medicine can be traced to the end of the 19th century and the advent of efficacious surgery. The most significant advances in diagnosing, treating, and managing disease, however, date from the 1950s, concomitant with the increasing prominence of the National Institutes of Health (NIH). Growth of the NIH was sparked by the renewed interest in curing disease, which was in turn prompted by new knowledge in the basic sciences. By the 1950s, immunizations to prevent infectious diseases such as polio and influenza, as well as drug therapies to treat noninfectious conditions such as pernicious anemia, diabetes, gout, and hyperthyroidism, were readily available. It was hoped that new technologies could be developed to cure or prevent chronic and life-threatening diseases such as heart disease, cancer, and stroke, which continue to be the leading causes of death by a significant margin.

Acute care hospitals are especially quick to add technology. No acute care hospital reported having MRI in 1984; by 1988, 10.6% had MRI.[14] The speed of generalizing this technology is astounding—in the late 1980s, an MRI unit cost $1.5 million to buy and $200,000 to install.[15] In 2004, the cost of MRI scanners varied by the weight and capacity of the magnet: a 3.0-tesla unit cost $2.5 million; a 1.5-tesla unit cost $1.5 million; a sub-1-tesla open MRI unit cost $1.4 million; and an extremity MRI unit cost $1.0 million.[16] To the cost of the machine must be added the costs of site preparation and installation. In the early 1990s, the ability to measure and map sources of electrical activity in the heart, the neuromuscular system, and especially the brain was substantially enhanced with the introduction of magnetic source imaging (MSI). Computerized tomography (CT) and MRI scans diagnose pathologies that leave lesions, but MSI provides important supplemental information. In the late 1990s, MSI units cost $2 million.[17] Proton beam therapy (PBT) is an advanced form of cancer radiation therapy technology that permits delivery of the maximum dose of radiation to a tumor site while reducing damage to normal tissue. PBT has distinct clinical advantages over other technology, was approved by the Food and Drug Administration (FDA) in 1988, and was approved for reimbursement by the CMS in 1997. Its use, however, has been limited by high cost— $100–$150 million depending on specific needs at the site of installation.[18]

Acute care hospitals are likely to make these technologies available to provide state-of-the-art care and remain competitive and because their physicians expect access to the new diagnostic information that MSI provides. In their residencies, physicians are trained using the most advanced technology for diagnosis and treatment; they will expect to have it available in the hospitals where they practice.

Diffusion of technology is also stimulated by the media and public perceptions that the procedures are safe, efficacious, available, and, in some instances, fashionable. Laparoscopic surgery had extraordinarily rapid diffusion—nearly 100% of hospitals and surgeons adopted it the first year that it was available.[19] Prominent examples early in the 21st century were open and laparoscopic bariatric surgery for the morbidly obese, and liposuction as an appearance-enhancing cosmetic procedure. Cosmetic surgery to correct various perceived or real natural defects in appearance is increasingly common and is being performed on children as young as 10.

Acute care hospitals are slow to abandon old (established) diagnostic technology when newer technology could replace it[20] or to substitute a newer, lower cost treatment for an older one, however.[21] Such inertia is explained largely by the practice patterns and preferences of physicians, as well as by other clinical treatment and support staff. Hence, acute care hospitals have a large financial investment in newly acquired equipment and in the high maintenance costs of established equipment that may be used less and less but cannot be abandoned. Physician expectations and competitive pressures are major reasons that acute care hospitals acquire technology.

Types of Technologies

DEFINITIVE (CURATIVE, PREVENTIVE) TECHNOLOGIES

Technologies are definitive when they cure or prevent a central disease agent or mechanism.[22] Some, such as vaccines and antibiotics, are relatively inexpensive, even considering the costs of research and development. Some, such as surgical intervention for acute appendicitis, are more expensive, but curative. Other definitive technologies, such as monitoring and screening programs, may or may not be expensive, depending on the cost of finding a true positive. Figure 3.1 shows the availability of clinical management and definitive technologies for several conditions. Progress in providing effective therapy differs widely for different conditions. For example, prevention, cure, and control have

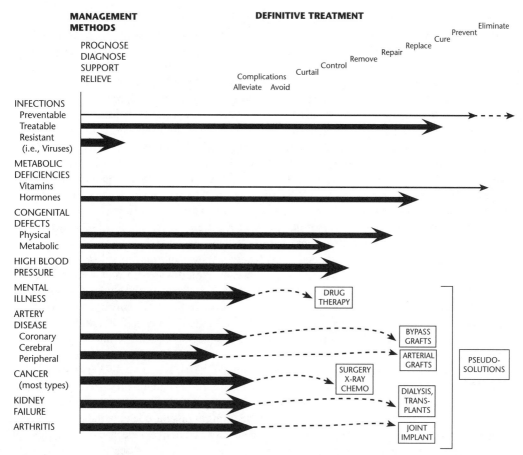

Figure 3.1. Advances in medical technology. From *Introduction to Health Services,* 3rd edition, edited by Stephen J. Williams (1989). Reprinted with permission of Delmar Learning, a division of Thomson Learning (www.thomsonrights.com). Fax 800-730-2215.

been attained for many infections. Many congenital malformations can be corrected by surgery, and high blood pressure can be effectively controlled with medications and weight loss. For conditions lacking definitive therapy, sophisticated technologies have been developed to replace or supplement the structure and function of affected organs, for example. These technical triumphs are pseudosolutions that assist current patients, but they have no effect on the underlying causes or the cures that must be developed if future generations are to benefit.

The development of two definitive technologies was stimulated by the risk of blood-borne diseases such as human immunodeficiency virus (HIV) and hepatitis B and C. One, a blood substitute to carry oxygen to tissues and carbon dioxide to the lungs, is expected to be available at a cost comparable to that of natural blood.[23] The other, a blood plasma–scrubbing technology that removes viruses, has received preliminary approval from FDA.[24] The benefits of avoiding blood-borne diseases are obvious.

HALFWAY (ADD-ON) TECHNOLOGIES

New medical technologies usually add to cost or generate new costs while achieving something not previously possible. Overwhelmingly, they are "halfway" or "add-on" technologies that can range from inexpensive interventions, such as feeding tubes, to treatments costing several hundred thousand dollars, an example of which is the iron lung that was used in the 1940s and 1950s to treat polio victims. Each halfway technology improves the clinician's ability to diagnose and/or treat an abnormality, and the technologies are used in addition to, not instead of, others.

Research in heart disease, cancer, and stroke has yielded primarily halfway technologies to diagnose and manage disease rather than prevent or cure it. New treatments produced by the "war" on cancer dating from the early 1970s have been disappointing; lower mortality reflects primarily the effects of changing incidence or early detection.[25] The historic trend line suggests that cancer incidence rates will increase because of improved screening, earlier detection, and effective treatment, all of which should lead to lower mortality rates, however.[26] A new efficacious technology to treat malignant tumors is PBT, which, as noted, delivers high doses of radiation to a tumor with minimal damage to normal tissue. The precision of PBT results from three-dimensional visualization of the malignancy and targeting the exact treatment point, thus minimizing side effects.[27]

Transplants are halfway technologies that improve the health status of a few but add considerably to overall healthcare costs. In 2006, there were 17,090 kidney, 6,650 liver, 2,192 heart, 463 pancreas, 1,405 lung, 31 heart/lung,[28] and about 40,000 cornea transplants performed.[29]

Halfway technologies have improved the diagnosis of brain disease. CT and MRI scans show the brain's structure. Brain electrical activity mapping (BEAM) enhances the study of brain waves. Blood circulation, energy consumption, and chemical neurotransmitter systems are measured with single photon emission computerized tomography (SPECT), PET scans, and functional magnetic resonance imaging (fMRI).[30] An example of applying neuroimaging is its use to understand the neuropsychiatric side effects of interferon in hepatitis C.[31] Other halfway technologies are transesophageal echocardiography (TEE), deep brain stimulation (DBS), and vagus nerve stimulation (VNS). TEE uses an ultrasound transducer mounted on a gastroscope to obtain images of the heart. It is recommended that acute care hospitals with cardiac surgery services have TEE and, perhaps, establish a dedicated ultrasound system to use it.[32] DBS requires placing a lead in the brain and connecting it to a neurostimulator or implantable pulse generator that delivers electric pulses to disrupt abnormal neurosignals associated with conditions such as Parkinson's disease. Similarly, VNS delivers intermittent electrical impulses from an implantable generator to the brain via the vagus nerve to treat patients suffering from epilepsy and chronic depression.[33]

DEFERRAL TECHNOLOGIES

Some technologies slow the progression of disease and may even dramatically improve a patient's condition. Nevertheless, the improvement is of short duration, and repeat treatments are usually required. Surgical treatment of coronary artery disease is an example. Coronary artery bypass grafting (CABG) is an expensive surgical procedure that must be repeated for many patients every 5–7 years. Development of percutaneous transluminal coronary angioplasty (PTCA) provided a simple, less invasive procedure that costs far less than bypass surgery. These attributes caused its use to grow rapidly. The data, however, showed no decline in bypass surgery. It is thought that after repeat angioplasties, bypass surgery is needed anyway. Thus, angioplasty defers the need for bypass surgery but does not eliminate it, while adding considerable costs.[34] Even after a technology is in wide use, its safety may be called into question, as happened with drug-coated carotid artery stenting.[35]

COMPETING TECHNOLOGIES

Technologies that compete may have similar results but very different costs. One example is the classic study involving the thrombolytic (blood clot–dissolving) agents streptokinase and tissue plasminogen activator (t-PA [Genentech's Activase]). In the mid-1990s, streptokinase cost $320 per dose; t-PA cost $2,750. The average cost-effectiveness of t-PA was $40,140 per life-year saved. Analysis showed that compared with the pattern of thrombolytic agent choice observed, targeting t-PA to the half of patients *most likely to benefit* could save 247 lives and $174 million nationally per year. It is difficult for clinicians to determine which thrombolic agent to administer, however. Some patients fare much better with streptokinase than t-PA, and others may actually be harmed by t-PA.[36]

As noted, CABG and PTCA are competing technologies to treat the same condition. Since the late 1990s, the number of CABG surgical procedures has declined, while the number of PTCA procedures has increased. The cost difference may partially explain the changes. The average cost of CABG is $24,000; for PTCA it is $11,000.[37]

Technologies competing to treat stenosis (narrowing) of the carotid artery are carotid endarterectomy (CEA) and carotid artery stenting (CAS). Costs are comparable, but CEA is $2,000–3,000 more expensive than CAS (excluding physicians' fees), and the median length of hospital stay for CEA is about 2 days longer.[38] CAS with the use of an emboli protection device is not inferior to CEA in high-risk patients.[39]

COST-SAVING TECHNOLOGIES

Few new technologies prevent disease for either individuals or populations (as vaccines protect future generations). Nonetheless, many reduce costs, especially when compared with old technologies that are used to treat the same diseases. Examples include arthroscopy, implantable infusion pumps, laparoscopic and endoscopic procedures, and lasers. These technologies may be halfway or deferral therapies, but if they replace more costly treatments or those of lesser quality in terms of efficaciousness, the result will be lower costs and better outcomes for the patient and the healthcare system. Costs and benefits are defined broadly and include hospitalization, sick days avoided, early return to work, reduced pain and discomfort, and short- and long-term quality of life. Assessing a technology must include these dimensions.[40] A laparoscopic technology that increases quality while reducing total costs is the port access system that enables surgeons to perform heart surgery without "cracking" the patient's sternum (breastbone). Specially designed catheters, surgical instruments, and imaging equipment are used. Patients avoid the trauma and pain of having their chests opened and are hospitalized only 3–5 days, compared with 8–12 days using open-heart techniques; also, they can return to work within 2 weeks, compared with 8–12 weeks after open-heart surgery. In addition, the risk of infection and other complications is greatly reduced.[41] The potential savings in costs, pain, and discomfort, as well as the increase in quality, are obvious.

Improved diagnostic technologies can reduce the costs of diagnosis and improve the quality of care, but they may increase overall costs because of a higher rate of use. Elasticity imaging of breast tissue using ultrasound allows radiologists to distinguish benign from malignant breast tissue with almost 100% accuracy. Malignant tissue is harder than normal tissue. By gauging movement (elasticity) when tissue is pushed, radiologists can distinguish the two types. The technique greatly reduces the need for needle biopsies, thus minimizing patient pain, discomfort, and anxiety.[42]

▬ Effects of Technology on Health Status ▬▬▬▬▬▬▬

Halfway and deferral technologies improve diagnosis and management of many diseases. For example, a CT scan may prevent or shorten a hospital stay and save other resources, such as exploratory surgery. However, the effect of halfway and deferral technologies on health status is uncertain. The modest increase in life expectancy from 1965 (at enactment of Medicare and Medicaid) to 1999 of only 2.7 years at age 65 and 1.0 year at age 85 suggest that advances in medical technology to that point had had little effect on longevity. Projections of average life expectancy at 2080 are for an additional 23.6 years at age 65 and 9.6 years at age 85.[43] While not insignificant, these projected increases in life expectancy seem modest.

An important dimension of understanding life expectancy and the effect of technology on longevity is the concept of active life expectancy, defined as the period of time expected to be free of disability.[44] Projections to 2080 show that all but about 12%–15% of the increase in life expectancy at age 65 will be active life expectancy; at age 85, active life expectancy is much lower, with 25%–40% of the additional years of life expectancy projected to include disability.[45]

Since 1968, death rates from coronary artery disease have declined by 63%, and death rates from strokes, by 62%.[46] Such declines generally are attributed to technology. It is possible, however, that the true cause-and-effect relationships are only partly known.[47]

Trying to credit technology with changes in health status indicators such as morbidity and disability raises other problems. It is paradoxical that by saving a life or preventing disease, technology increases the likelihood of morbidity and disability. Similarly, health promotion such as smoking cessation may actually increase healthcare costs in the long term.[48] This means, of course, that the results of technology and prevention are a double-edged sword; the quality of life is improved by reducing morbidity and mortality, but costs for long-term debilitating disease may be increased. A new body of data is developing, however, indicating that people with lower health risks because of better health habits have less lifetime disability, as well as less disability at any given age.[49] This does not, however, eliminate the almost certain need for long-term, labor-intensive services because of debilitating physical and mental impairment.

▬ Forces Affecting Development and Diffusion of Technology ▬▬▬

MEDICAL EDUCATION AND MEDICAL PRACTICE

Among the most important factors encouraging development and diffusion of technology after World War II were changes in medical training and the practice of medicine. Biomedical research funded by the NIH stimulated medical schools to investigate specialized areas of medicine, which led to the growth of specialty departments within academic medical centers. Increasingly, medical school graduates went on to postgraduate training and then to practice in a medical specialty.

Historically, specializing meant that physicians were trained to use technology. Not surprisingly, they expected to use the same technologies in their practices. This desire to have state-of-the-art technology and to use it as necessary, despite its cost, is called the "technological imperative." The technological imperative is most apparent in acute care hospitals and helps explain the proliferation of highly specialized technology in them. Chapter 1 includes data on physicians in primary care and in specialties.

In 2005, the healthcare and social assistance sector spent $73.8 billion for capital expenditures, a 14.3% increase over 2004. Compared with a 5.6% increase from 2003 to 2004, the significant growth in 2005 shows a resurgence in capital projects. Of the $73.8 billion, 53% was spent on capital structure projects and 47% on capital equipment. Spending by general acute care hospitals increased 15.1% from 2004, to $41.8 billion in 2005. Outpatient care centers and other ambulatory healthcare services spent $4.6 billion in 2005, a 32.1% increase from the previous year.[50]

Acute care hospitals must have state-of-the-art physical plants and acquire leading-edge technology to remain competitive. In addition, decreasing the number of staffed beds and increasing average patient acuity by means of earlier discharge has the result of a higher ratio of plant assets per bed. This results in hospitals that are increasingly expensive to operate and maintain.

The almost universal presence of technology should not suggest that it is applied similarly nationwide. There is wide geographic variation in treating patients with the same diagnoses.[51] These variations range from hospitalization rates and lengths of stay once admitted to treatment regimens, such as treatment of patients with coronary artery disease with risk factor modification (diet, exercise) and medication to reduce the frequency and severity of angina (chest pain) versus intervention with either PTCA or CABG.[52]

The cost implications of choosing different treatment regimens are significant and increase the controversy. A 1983 NIH study found that CABG was a commonly overused surgical procedure; it was estimated that 25,000 of the 200,000 (12.5%) CABG surgeries performed annually could be eliminated without jeopardizing patient care.[53] Later evaluation of CABG surgeries concluded that "surgical therapy improves prognosis in high-risk patients, but the advantage over medical therapy declines with longer follow up."[54] More recent evaluation concluded that 10% of CABG surgeries are inappropriate, with as many as 14% inappropriate in some states.[55] These findings of inappropriate CABG are virtually identical with those of 20 years earlier.

In 1991, the Department of Health and Human Services (DHHS) contracted with four acute care hospitals to provide CABG to Medicare patients on a fixed-fee (global payment) basis that included physician and hospital costs. Rates paid were 5%–30% lower, depending on the site.[56] With savings exceeding $35 million, the pilot CABG program was considered successful and was expanded to include more sites and other cardiac procedures, as well as hip and knee replacement. Although pilot hospitals' volumes did not increase, their financial margins did, probably because of greater efficiency.[57] Such efforts will increase as CMS seeks further reductions in Medicare spending. More recent analysis casts doubt on the potential cost savings of regionalizing CABG, however, with a 10% higher volume resulting in only a 2.8% reduction in average costs and a cost savings estimated to be only 3.5%. The potential savings may not justify the risks of reducing access to needed services.[58]

Interestingly, the reputation of coronary artery bypass surgeons among peers may be less closely associated with the quality of their work than with the number of procedures done (patient volume).[59] The relationship between the number of procedures and the quality of outcomes is shown by studies of other physicians and applies to hospitals as well.[60] Another form of variation in the application of technology is that physicians who have practiced longer than 15 years have significantly more inappropriate hospital admissions.[61] Beyond the application of technology is the question of treatment outcomes. Data show significant variation in mortality rates for some diagnoses by geographic region.[62]

Wide variation in practice patterns raises doubts about medicine's scientific certainty and whether low-technology, less interventionist, and less expensive treatment might not be as effective as high-technology, more interventionist, and more costly treatment. Understanding physician practice patterns and variation, as well as determining efficacy, will enable HSOs/HSs to deliver effective medical services more efficiently.

THIRD-PARTY REIMBURSEMENT OF SERVICES

Central to the diffusion of technological advances into medical practice and the existence of the technological imperative has been availability of third-party reimbursement. In traditional fee-for-service medical practice, decisions to use new technologies usually are made by individual physicians based on findings that the technology yields benefit with low probability of harm. Unlike other industries, innovations in medical technology have been judged, not primarily on the basis of performing some function better or more efficiently, but rather on whether they will yield a benefit to individual patients. Similarly, decisions to reimburse for new technologies have been based on the acceptance and use of those technologies by physicians. Manufacturers' prices for new technologies, particularly medications and devices, tend to be high in order to recover research and development costs. Provider charges are high to compensate for the skill and expertise that are involved in learning and offering a technology, as well as to recover the capital costs of acquiring it. Historically, once established in the reimbursement system, these charges have tended to remain high even after initial costs have been recovered.[63]

Assurance of payment for tests and procedures under cost-based reimbursement allowed HSOs to acquire technology, knowing that the costs of capital investment and operation would be met. Historically, there were few incentives to evaluate the cost-effectiveness of new technologies, and acquisition of technology was, and continues to be, stimulated by the need for HSOs/HSs to attract both physicians and patients. Changes in government funding of healthcare and growth of managed care suggest, however, that proper and timely reimbursement for new technology is no longer ensured.[64]

Like federal programs, payers such as health plans control costs through disease management programs and utilization review of high-cost diagnoses and treatments. For example, utilization management resulted in a 40% reduction in unneeded imaging by primary care physicians.[65] One study found that enrollees of not-for-profit health plans and health maintenance organizations (HMOs) had less access to three laser technologies than was available in for-profit and indemnity plans.[66] If true for access to technology generally, such findings have major implications for diffusion of technology as well as costs of health services.

DIAGNOSIS-RELATED GROUPS

In late 1983, the payment for Medicare patients in acute care hospitals was changed from cost-based reimbursement to a prospective payment system based on diagnosis-related groups (DRGs), which are discussed in Chapter 1. As noted, the incentive for hospitals under this payment method is to do less, not more, which is opposite of retrospective, cost-based reimbursement. Reimbursement is calculated using average cost per case for each DRG. This formula should create an incentive to carefully evaluate technology, use it more efficiently, and select cost-saving technologies when possible.

When DRGs were implemented, it was thought that acute care hospitals providing a service infrequently would be unable to compete with those providing it frequently. In theory, the latter group has lower average unit costs. It was also thought that because the costs of using technology were not reimbursed separately, acute care hospitals would have few incentives to adopt new technology that increases per-case cost by adding new operating expenses. It appears, however, that acquisition and use of technology by acute care hospitals not only is unchanged but may have accelerated. It may be that only when Medicare payments are reduced further will the full effect of DRGs on technology be felt.

Congress continues to try to reduce Medicare costs, primarily by reducing DRG payments. It appears that those who feared that the DRG system would stifle diffusion of new technology and adversely affect patient care were wrong; those who predicted that the need for acute care hospitals to be competitive and maintain admissions levels would necessitate acquiring technology were correct. Regardless, the long-term influence of DRGs on acute care hospitals and their use of technology remains to be seen. The real effect of DRGs may not comport with that intended.[67]

CENTERS FOR MEDICARE AND MEDICAID SERVICES

In the late 1980s, the HCFA, now CMS, began applying more uniform and stringent standards to judge appropriate use of technology. In early 1989, the HCFA issued proposed regulations to define for the first time the criteria *reasonable* and *necessary*. These words are used in Medicare to describe technology and procedures for which it will pay.[68] In defining *reasonable* and *necessary*, the final regulations rely heavily on FDA categorizations by requiring that technology and procedures be safe, effective, and noninvestigatory.[69]

Typically, states underfund Medicaid; this makes it noteworthy that considerable resources are devoted to transplants. The federal Early and Periodic Screening, Diagnosis, and Treatment Program requires that participating states provide "medically necessary" services that are interpreted to mean bone marrow, liver, heart, and lung transplants to people younger than 21 years of age. Historically, services available in Medicaid programs have been very comprehensive. Most provided bone marrow, liver, and heart transplants to adults; almost half provided lung transplants. Some states have put monetary limits on each type of transplant covered.[70]

THE PUBLIC

A third force influencing the diffusion of technology has been the public. The practice of highly technical and specialty-oriented medicine, coupled with widely publicized advances in medical care, fostered consumers' expectations that a technology is available to diagnose and treat every medical problem and that quality medical care necessarily involves extensive use of technology. Historically, Americans have expressed a willingness to pay the costs of health services and to spend what is needed to improve and protect their health.[71] More recently, however, the rapid increases in costs that have been reflected in health insurance premiums, copays, and deductibles have given the public pause and may result in reconsideration of their open-ended willingness to pay for whatever services are needed. People less economically protected by third-party reimbursement will likely be less willing to share their physicians' expectations that all possible technologies should be available. Payment systems that limit the use of technology threaten the traditional autonomy of patients and providers, an issue very near the surface in managed care and implicit in government-sponsored universal health services proposals.

COMPETITIVE ENVIRONMENT

Competition is an increasingly important fourth force in diffusion of technology. There is competition among HSOs/HSs, between physicians and HSOs/HSs, among physician specialties, and between physicians and nonphysician licensed independent practitioners (LIPs). One way acute care hospitals, and to a lesser extent other types of HSOs, compete is to acquire and offer advanced technology and shift services to outpatient settings, which have lower costs and offer greater convenience to users.

Historically, hospitals were the repository of medical technology because they had the capital, staff, and medical backup to support technology. Increasingly, medical technology is portable, which allows it to be applied outside acute care hospitals in nontraditional HSOs. Portability is creating a "medical arms race" between hospitals and physicians, as physicians deliver technically advanced services in their own specialty hospitals, freestanding ambulatory surgery centers, and their offices.[72] Finally, technological innovations disrupt the traditional demarcations among medical specialties, causing them to compete.

Technologies that enable health services to be safely moved from inpatient to outpatient settings include improved anesthesia that allows quicker return to consciousness with few aftereffects; better analgesics for pain relief; and minimally invasive procedures such as laser surgery, endoscopy, and laparoscopy.[73] In 1987, the number of outpatient visits surpassed the number of inpatient days.[74] Of the 50 million combined total outpatient and inpatient surgical and nonsurgical procedures performed annually, 31% (15.5 million) were performed in freestanding ambulatory surgery centers (ASCs). The number of freestanding ASCs increased by almost 25% from 2001 to 2006.[75] The minimally invasive surgical techniques that are revolutionizing cardiovascular surgery enable surgeons to operate on a beating heart. In the future, they may allow outpatient cardiovascular surgery.[76] The major shift into home health services is well underway.

New technology, much of it more portable and less costly to buy (or lease) and operate, coupled with efforts to limit the use of specialists, is blurring the traditional fiefdoms of physician specialties and causing fierce competition among them, as well as with nonphysician LIPs. Prominent among the specialties that have become more interventional in undertaking treatment are gastroenterologists, cardiologists, and radiologists. Medical imaging is a prime example of the increasing use of ambulatory testing performed outside the hospital, much of which may be done by nonradiologists.[77] These developments have major implications for the specialties involved, as well as for HSOs/HSs and, if the volume of procedures increases, have the potential to increase overall costs to the system. Generally, physicians are unconstrained by regulations such as certificates of need (CONs), which means that establishing an imaging center, for example, is a matter of raising capital and finding a location. Abuses resulting from physician ownership of HSOs that provide diagnosis and treatment caused state and federal governments to regulate self-referrals, which are defined as physicians sending patients to HSOs in which they have an ownership interest. The controversy over physician-owned cardiac specialty hospitals is only the latest example of hospitals competing with their physicians.[78]

Responses to Diffusion and Use of Technology

As HSOs/HSs acquired technology, issues of cost, benefit, and safety emerged. It became clear that diffusion and use of technology were only partially based on cost–benefit or cost-effectiveness considerations. Existing technological capabilities were often ignored or discounted, despite their proven efficacy. In addition, the hazards associated with a technology were inadequately understood. These concerns were the focus of federal laws to improve premarket evaluation of medical devices (i.e., amendments to the Food, Drug, and Cosmetic Act) and to influence acquisition and use of technologies, especially in acute care hospitals (i.e., professional standards review organizations [PSROs] were followed by peer review organizations [PROs], quality improvement organizations [QIOs], and CON). Another result was establishment of the congressional Office of Technology Assessment (OTA) and DHHS's National Center for Health Care Technology (NCHCT), both of which were later defunded.

Table 3.2 shows several of the public and private organizations that ensure the safety and efficacy of technology. Amendments to the federal Food, Drug, and Cosmetic Act in 1976 and 1990 gave the FDA a greatly expanded role in monitoring manufacturers and investigating devices linked to patient death or serious injury or illness.[79] State authorities are concerned with staff and patient safety—one of the traditional police powers of the state, described in Chapter 1—and may require the licensure of practitioners who use the equipment, approval of types of equipment by a national testing laboratory, and regular inspections, especially of radiation sources such as x-ray equipment. Private organizations have been important in producing consensus standards. Among them are the National Fire Protection Association, which has developed standards on design and use of facilities and some biomedical equipment, and The Joint Commission on Accreditation of Healthcare Organizations (The Joint Commission), whose standards govern equipment management and maintenance. Some standards affecting technology in HSOs have been stimulated by court decisions.

TABLE 3.2.   BIOMEDICAL EQUIPMENT REGULATION

Authority	Federal	State	Profession
	Food and Drug Adminstration (FDA)	Department of public safety/public health	JCAHO, NFPA, etc.[a]
Objectives	Manufacturer quality	Personal safety	Hospital quality
Standards	FDA specifications	National testing laboratory	JCAHO accreditation manual, NFPA codes, etc.

[a]From JCAHO, Joint Commission on Accreditation of Healthcare Organizations; NFPA, National Fire Protection Association.

PUBLIC SECTOR ACTIVITIES

Food and Drug Administration

Although FDA has been involved in premarket approval of drugs since 1962, evidence of the safety and efficacy of other medical technologies was not required. The Medical Device Amendments of 1976[80] to the Food, Drug, and Cosmetic Act extended FDA's premarket approval process to medical devices, divided into three classes. The most stringent regulation is for Class III—devices that support or sustain human life, are of substantial importance in preventing impairment of human health, or present a potential and unreasonable risk of illness or injury. Manufacturers must obtain approval from FDA before such devices may be marketed, a procedure that requires evidence of safety and efficacy.[81] FDA control of marketing new drugs and devices has been criticized as unnecessarily impeding introduction of technological innovations, because of the time and money that are required to conduct clinical trials and obtain approval. In the late 1980s, pressure on FDA from those wanting rapid access to new drugs to treat acquired immunodeficiency syndrome (AIDS) caused reconsideration of its review processes, especially those applying to drugs that were potentially beneficial in treating fatal illnesses.

Legal liability for HSOs/HSs increased when the Safe Medical Device Act of 1990[82] codified the need to report device-related serious injuries and death to the manufacturer and, in the case of death, to FDA. FDA defines *medical device* broadly; there are significant penalties for failing to report. A checklist form is recommended to guide incident investigation.[83] Medical devices range from simple tongue depressors and bedpans to complex programmable pacemakers with microchip technology and laser surgical devices. The lengthy official definition distinguishes between a medical device and other FDA-regulated products such as drugs. If the primary intended use of the product is achieved through chemical action or by being metabolized by the body, the product is usually considered a drug.[84]

Following FDA approval of the medical device, the organization developing the medical device must continue to evaluate and periodically report on the safety, effectiveness, and reliability of the device for its intended use. In addition, the organization must maintain records specified in the regulation.[85] FDA does not license technicians.[86] Absent licensure, voluntary certification programs such as those of the International Certification Commission and the Association for the Advancement of Medical Instrumentation ensure technicians' competence.[87]

PSROs, PROs, and QIOs

A general history of PSROs and how they were replaced by PROs beginning in 1984 is included in Chapter 1. In terms of medical technology, PSROs were established in 1972 as part of federal and state efforts to control healthcare costs by regulating the acquisition of new technology and reducing its use through review of utilization. PSROs sought to ensure that Medicare (and later Medicaid) services were "medically necessary, met professional standards of care, and were provided in the most economical setting possible consistent with quality care."[88] Initially, review focused on appropriateness of acute care hospital admission and length of stay. Later, services provided were also reviewed.

PSRO effectiveness was hampered by Medicare's interpretation of "reasonable and necessary." This concept meant that a procedure that is no longer experimental and that is accepted by the local community is deemed reasonable and may be necessary. PSROs determined indications for use.[89]

PROs replaced PSROs and had a similar role regarding technology. They reviewed validity of diagnostic and procedural information provided by hospitals; completeness, adequacy, and quality of care provided; and appropriateness of admissions patterns, discharges, lengths of stay, transfers, and services furnished in outlier cases.[90] Decisions of the PRO were usually binding as to reimbursement.

As Chapter 1 noted, PROs were officially renamed QIOs in 2001. QIOs are charged with quality improvement initiatives in numerous clinical areas and across healthcare settings. By evaluating the quality of outcomes, QIOs will effect more appropriate application of technology, as did PROs.[91] The effect will be indirect, however, and realized only over the long term.

Certificate of Need

States enacted CON and Section 1122 laws pursuant to the National Health Planning and Resources Development Act of 1974 (PL 93-641),[92] which required that acquisition of technology (and construction) by acute care hospitals be approved. Amendments in 1981 and regulations in 1984 increased dollar limits. In the 1980s, a philosophical shift at the federal level toward increased competition greatly reduced support for regulatory efforts such as CONs. Diminished federal support reduced state interest. As Chapter 1 noted, 35 states and the District of Columbia had CON laws in 2007.

CON and health planning legislation assumed that the availability of technology invites use and potential abuse and that its cost is paid by all healthcare system users. CT scanners became controversial because of wide availability and alleged overuse. In the 1990s, MRI and caesarean sections became a focus. These examples illustrate the problem inherent in one of the primary assumptions underlying CON legislation, that quality healthcare can be provided without the extensive use of technology. This assumption conflicted with societal expectations that appropriate technology would be available and used, as needed.

The CON laws were criticized because they

1. Gave no attention to low-cost technologies, whose high-volume use can significantly affect costs (e.g., electronic fetal monitoring, which is a widely used, low-cost technology whose capital cost excluded it from CON review)[93]
2. Did not consider the operating costs that are associated with installing and using technology, which typically exceed capital costs in a few years
3. Decreased competition by regulating acute care hospital services and types of technology, which eliminated a major incentive to compete
4. Focused on acute care hospitals, while increasingly portable technology allowed freestanding HSOs to become ubiquitous
5. Did not consider the role of professional staff in acquiring and using technology, as well as its importance in attracting and retaining physicians

Underutilization of high technology can be avoided by requiring that certain levels of use must be met before the regulatory process will approve new units.[94] The number of MRIs and their use varies considerably by country. Worldwide, Japan and the United States had the highest number of MRI scanners per million population, at 35.3 and 27.0, respectively, in 2004; Canada had 5.5. Compared with Canada, the United States performed more than three times the number of MRI exams, with 83.2 per 1,000 population in 2004–2005, compared with 25.5 in Canada. These data suggest, however, that Canada uses its MRI resources more efficiently.[95]

Tort Law

Concomitant with greater regulation of medical technology has been the application of more demanding liability standards. Strict liability has been applied to HSOs, and they may be liable for defects in devices that are unknown to the manufacturer. HSOs may be responsible for going beyond the maintenance recommendations of the manufacturer, if necessary. As noted above, they must inform FDA about experience contrary to that reported by the manufacturer. This area of the law will evolve, almost certainly toward more demanding and costly standards for HSOs.

PRIVATE SECTOR ACTIVITIES

The Joint Commission

Various private organizations have voluntary standards that guide HSOs/HSs in managing biomedical equipment. Among the most important is The Joint Commission. Standards applicable to biomedical equipment in hospitals are found in the "environment of care" section of the *Comprehensive Accreditation Manual for Hospitals (CAMH)*[96] and include 1) the hospital manages medical equipment risks and 2) medical equipment is maintained, tested, and inspected. These standards are emblematic of those applied to nonhospital HSOs and are addressed in detail below. As Chapter 1 noted, some acute care hospitals have abandoned Joint Commission accreditation in favor of complying with the federal "conditions of participation" that are applied without cost.

ISO 9000

The International Organization for Standardization has created a set of standards, known as ISO 9000, that organizations may voluntarily adopt to help them meet or exceed their customers' needs and expectations. Distilled to their essence, the principles of ISO 9000 are that high-quality service results only from a well-planned, well-documented, and well-executed quality management system. ISO 9000 is not quality control but quality assurance that embraces planning and implementing systems designed to ensure that quality requirements are met.[97] The history of ISO is discussed in Chapter 1; application of ISO standards is addressed in Chapter 7. Increased use of ISO 9000 standards in HSOs will diminish the importance and predominance of The Joint Commission in accreditation of HSOs.

▦ Healthcare Technology Assessment ▦

Healthcare technology assessment (HTA) evaluates the safety, efficacy, cost, and cost-effectiveness of technology and identifies ethical and legal implications, both in absolute terms and by comparison with competing technologies.[98] The Institute of Medicine of the National Academy of Sciences estimated that in 1983 only 2.9% of national health expenditures were for HTA.[99] Relative expenditures for HTA were declining, and it was estimated that in 1988 the budgets of the most prominent HTA programs, added to related activities of industry and exclusive of clinical trials, totaled only approximately $50 million.[100] In the late 1990s, the United States had 53 HTA programs and activities, most of them in the private sector.[101] Private and public organizations involved in HTA assessment include private insurers, managed care organizations (MCOs), professional and specialty societies, provider associations, group purchasing organizations, technology industry groups, disease-specific interest groups, private research groups (including academic medical centers, universities, and not-for-profit and for-profit research organizations), and various units of state and federal government.[102] This list suggests how decentralized HTA is in the United States. Decentralizing HTA and related activities widens the expertise available to the process, broadens perspectives, and diminishes or balances potential conflicts of interest. In all, these benefits add credibility to HTA processes and findings, and they lessen charges that assessments reflect narrow or self-serving interests of particular agencies or organizations.[103]

Figure 3.2 uses an input-process-outcome sequence to show the typical flow of HTA. These general methods include randomized clinical trials, evaluating diagnostic technologies, series of

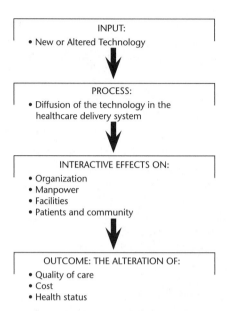

Figure 3.2. Technology assessment methods measure the impact on healthcare in an input-process-outcome sequence. (From Glasser, Jay H., and Richard S. Chrzanowski, "Medical Technology Assessment: Adequate Questions, Appropriate Methods, Valuable Answers," *Health Policy, 9,* 267–276 [1988], with permission from Elsevier Science.)

consecutive cases, case studies, registers and databases, sample surveys, epidemiological methods, surveillance, quantitative synthesis methods (meta-analysis), group judgment methods,[104] cost-effectiveness and cost–benefit analyses, and mathematical modeling. Important, too, are the social and ethical issues of HTA.[105]

PUBLIC SECTOR ACTIVITIES

In the 1990s, public sector HTA efforts included seven federal agencies (including the congressional OTA) and three state agencies (in Minnesota, New York, and Oregon). From 1974 to late 1995, OTA helped Congress understand and plan for the policy implications of applying technology by studying the efficacy of specific medical procedures, uses of health education, and quality of medical care.[106] OTA was abolished in late 1995, primarily as a cost-cutting measure.[107]

Concern about the proliferation of medical technology and its benefits, costs, and risks caused Congress to enact the Health Services Research, Health Statistics, and Health Care Technology Act of 1978 (PL 95-623).[108] NCHCT was established in the Public Health Service of DHHS as a clearinghouse for information on medical technology, the safety and efficacy of new technologies, and their cost-effectiveness. NCHCT was to advise HCFA as to cost-effectiveness, appropriateness, and medical validity of various technologies that might be reimbursed by Medicare and Medicaid.[109] NCHCT was defunded in 1981, however, and its role was transferred to the Office of Health Technology Assessment (later called the Center for Health Care Technology) of the National Center for Health Services Research,[110] which was reauthorized in 1987 as the National Center for Health Services Research and Health Care Technology Assessment (NCHSRHCTA).[111]

In 1989, the Agency for Health Care Policy and Research (AHCPR) was established in the Public Health Service to replace NCHSRHCTA. In 1999, AHCPR was reauthorized as the Agency for Healthcare Research and Quality (AHRQ) and became the lead federal agency on quality research and the primary source of government-sponsored HTA. AHRQ's Center for Practice and Technology Assessment conducts HTA internally or through contract and collaboration with its 13 evidence-based practice centers (EPCs).[112] Most of the EPCs are in academic health centers and other institutions, including three in Canada. They prepare "evidence reports" and HTA in support of clinical guidelines, coverage policies, and other practices and policies.[113]

AHRQ's highest priority is to support research that improves the quality of care. Its strategic goals are

- *Safety/quality*—Improving healthcare safety and quality for Americans through evidence-based research and translation
- *Efficiency*—Developing strategies to improve access, foster appropriate use, and reduce unnecessary expenditures
- *Effectiveness*—Translating, disseminating, and implementing research findings that improve healthcare outcomes
- *Organizational Excellence*—Developing efficient and responsive business processes[114]

Projects sponsored by AHRQ include research on bioterrorism, data development, chronic care management, socioeconomics of healthcare, informatics, long-term care, pharmaceutical outcomes, prevention, training, quality/safety of patient care, and organizational support.[115]

AHRQ's efforts to develop clinical practice guidelines in the mid-1990s failed because physicians saw them as a threat.[116] AHRQ collaborated with the American Medical Association and the American Association of Health Plans (now America's Health Insurance Plans) to establish a National Guideline Clearinghouse (NGC) that provides guidance for clinical management of specific conditions. The Internet site established by NGC became operational in 1998 and provides access to guidelines from public and private organizations.[117]

This brief description of public sector HTA efforts shows that, except for a few states and federal agencies, government plays a secondary role. The lack of comprehensive federal activities in HTA leads to the conclusion that "the United States is thus out-of-step with much of the developed world where government-linked agencies have been established with responsibility for providing advice to policy-makers at the national or regional level."[118] This observation continues to be true.

PRIVATE SECTOR ACTIVITIES

The majority of the 53 HTA programs and activities in existence in the late 1990s were private initiatives. They included 12 academic/not-for-profit organizations (often affiliated with major teaching hospitals), 11 health insurance companies (including managed care entities), 8 health professional societies, 5 hospitals or hospital chains, 4 consulting firms, and 3 medical industry manufacturers. In addition, there was an unknown number of private sector efforts that assessed technology or aided potential users and purchasers in decision making.[119] The HTA undertaken in the private sector will likely be available to a limited audience, or it may be available only for a fee. Thus, while private assessments avoid the pitfalls of publicly sponsored efforts, limited availability of results will slow dissemination of knowledge about technology.

SUMMARY

It is clear that both the private and public sectors are equivocal about giving HTA a high priority. This is difficult to understand, given that hundreds of billions of dollars are spent annually in a health services system driven to a significant extent by technology. The efforts described above cannot develop the information needed to assist HSOs/HSs to make decisions about acquiring technology and using it effectively and efficiently. In addition, information available about a technology may be difficult to find. Lack of a technology information clearinghouse and the absence of assistance in understanding and assessing technology must be decried. Developing a generic prototype for HTA by communities and HSOs/HSs should be a national priority.

HSO/HS Technology Decision Making

Assessment of technology at the operating level is very different from that done by national public or private groups. Among the most important differences is that, when machine- and chemical-based technologies become generally available to HSOs/HSs, questions of safety and efficacy have been answered by FDA. At the operating level, the safety and efficacy of new surgical techniques or innovative uses of already approved machine- and chemical-based technologies are reviewed almost exclusively by individual HSOs or HSs. It is less than reassuring to find that even well into the new millennium, many hospitals have no formal HTA program.[120]

Criteria that should be used by the HSO or HS to assess technology include appropriateness for the patient population; financial feasibility, cost-effectiveness, useful life, and operating costs; availability of trained technical personnel to staff it, expert physicians, and support services; availability of backup technologies, such as open-heart surgery if angioplasty fails; and adequacy of reimbursement.[121] Nonexotic technologies and replacement equipment should be scrutinized in the same manner, however. Furthermore, it is important to evaluate new technology 6–12 months after introduction, to determine its performance level and effect on the quality of patient care.[122] Generally, physicians are regarded as technically qualified to decide about acquiring technology, and HSOs/HSs give them great deference in decision making. Furthermore, it is believed that a high level of technology is essential to attract and retain the best physicians.

REVIEW AND PLANNING

Cost-containment pressures, increased legal liability, and competition have caused HSOs/HSs to reassess how they make decisions to acquire and use technology and to ensure safe operation and maintenance. One approach establishes annual review and financial planning processes for medical technologies that are separate from other capital expenditure decision making. This is crucial for financial planning, because many major technologies become obsolete before the end of the useful life estimated for depreciation purposes. As a result, depreciation and replacement allowances rarely meet the costs of newer technology. If the rate of technological innovation and diffusion increases, this problem will become more pressing. One example is the CT scanner, which sold for approximately $300,000 in 1973 with an estimated life of 5 years. Improved scanners costing more than $700,000 were available in 4 years.[123] In 1990, prices for CT scanners ranged from $195,000 to $1.6 million.[124] By 2007, the price was $0.5–$2.7 million, depending on capability.[125] Similarly, the cost of fluoroscopes with image intensifiers rose from $40,000 in 1965 to $200,000 in 1977.[126] In 1990, fluoroscopic units for cardiac catheterization cost as much as $600,000.[127] By 1998, their cost ranged from $600,000 to $2.3 million.[128] Despite the recent, significant investment in the technology for cardiac catheterization, an invasive procedure, it is rapidly being replaced by coronary imaging, which is even more effective and is noninvasive. This technology costs about $1.4–$3.0 million, depending on the specific imaging equipment utilized.[129] The transition to noninvasive diagnosis of the heart is a prime example of changing and improved treatment options that will increase the quality (and cost) of healthcare as HSOs make capital investments in the new technology.

HSOs/HSs should develop strategic technology plans to guide their technology acquisition, professional staff development, and market strategies. The plans should assess emerging medical technology in near-term and longer term time frames and identify niches where the HSOs/HSs should focus staff development and market strategies.[130]

FINANCING TECHNOLOGY

Acute care hospitals have the most capital- and technology-intensive physical plants of any type of HSO. Historically, acute care hospitals have had an annual capital equipment budget of several million dollars; technology had been financed out of internal funds and gifts because most capital equipment purchases were relatively small.[131]

In the new era of diminished reimbursement, successful healthcare executives must be creative to meet the costs of technology. Technology may be financed from current revenue, reserves, or charitable donations or by borrowing, through joint ventures, or using venture capital. Other strategies have been suggested: 1) merge interests with physicians and other HSOs, and develop complementary plans to minimize duplication of high-cost technology; 2) obtain manufacturer support for development, training, and maintenance of technology; 3) become a demonstration site for manufacturers; and 4) become a service center for other providers.[132]

EVALUATING AND ACQUIRING TECHNOLOGY — TEAM

A methodology to improve decision making about technology was developed by the American Hospital Association (AHA) and the Center for Health Services Research at the University of California, Los Angeles, in the late 1970s. The Technology Evaluation and Acquisition Methods (TEAM) assessment organized a review process, determined participation, and developed criteria. It addressed four common problems that acute care hospitals faced in evaluating and acquiring technology: 1) treating requests for medical technology in the same way as requests for other capital expenditures, 2) absence of multidisciplinary staff participation in planning and evaluation of technology requests, 3) sporadic and unorganized physician participation in acquisition decisions, and 4) reliance on the staff members who requested technology to also assess its need and feasibility.[133]

In TEAM, the governing body and chief executive officer (CEO) established a policy to ensure that requests for technology were compatible with the organization's mission and strategic plan. TEAM used an interdisciplinary standing committee to conduct miniassessments and make recommendations for each proposed technology regarding need and use; effect on staffing, space, and supply; effect on patient care; vendor and product evaluation; and financial impact.[134] Despite its potential, TEAM was not developed further by AHA.

NEWER ALTERNATIVES TO TEAM

Chief Technology Officer

Another approach to managing technology is to appoint a chief technology officer (CTO) to administer the organization's technology base and translate vision and planning into programs.[135] To accomplish this goal, the "line managers of technology," such as the chiefs of clinical pharmacy, clinical engineering, and information systems, should report directly to the CTO.[136] In practice, appointing a CTO, like TEAM, has had limited acceptance, perhaps because both affect or disrupt well-established responsibilities of senior managers, and technical support information flows up the organization only when solicited. An additional difficulty of appointing a CTO is finding someone who has suitable qualifications.

Technical Support Committee

An alternative to TEAM and a CTO that has less effect on recognized modi operandi is to establish a standing technical support committee that provides technical recommendations to senior management and resolves day-to-day technical problems.[137] The committee's strength lies in making decisions about acquiring technology, which requires answering questions about the costs of acquisition, maintenance, and replacement. The committee is chaired by a senior manager, and membership includes managers of plant operations, biomedical engineering, medical physics, information systems, and risk management and safety. The committee

1. Coordinates and maintains strategic technology planning compatible with the strategic plan
2. Coordinates Joint Commission–mandated "environment of care" plans and programs
3. Provides technical recommendations for HTA and equipment acquisition
4. Ensures equipment effectiveness
5. Identifies and secures funding for purchase, and monitors problem reporting and correction

Notably, and by design, the committee has no clinical members. Its recommendations present technologically acceptable options. As users, clinicians choose equipment from these options. Finally, such a committee goes far to maintain continuity of purpose and improve communication about biomedical equipment at the implementation level.

Multidisciplinary HTA Committee

The multidisciplinary technology assessment committee (M-TAC) approach is the broadest of those discussed in this section. The M-TAC draws on the organization's strengths and has three phases.[138] In Phase I, the capital planning process is modified to include the essential elements of HTA. The committee established in Phase I is multidisciplinary, emphasizes physician participation, and applies assessment criteria to technology within the context of the organization's mission, vision, and strategic plan. Phase II includes a technology inventory and postacquisition evaluation of technology. In Phase III, the M-TAC develops a strategic technology plan that includes identifying new technologies that meet service area and competitive needs. In all three phases, the committee can function as decision maker or advisory body. If the technology meets the predetermined criteria, the committee performs an in-depth analysis and asks questions such as Does it work? Is it safe? Is it an improvement over existing technology? Will it have organization-wide impact? What is its cost? Is it cost-effective? What are its potential effects on patient and community? Are there risk management and legal liability issues? Are there regulatory requirements? Will it assist in a managed care environment? What are its potential social, ethical, and political effects? Is it needed urgently?[139] The flow diagram in Figure 3.3 shows the capital planning and HTA process.

SUMMARY

Despite limited assistance, HSOs/HSs must make decisions about acquiring technology. In addition to the literature and government sources, there are private, for-profit technology assessment services, and various not-for-profit private groups that can provide information about technology. Generally, HSs have more resources for HTA. The generic process used to assess new technologies is to identify and set priorities; determine clinical efficacy, safety, and costs; synthesize information that is developed; disseminate assessments to users and make recommendations; initiate acquisition; and monitor after-purchase performance to assess the technology's benefits.[140]

Managing Biomedical Equipment in HSOs/HSs

Equipment used in delivering health services is commonly called biomedical equipment. Table 3.3 suggests how biomedical equipment diagnoses, treats, monitors, and supports patients. Although some equipment, such as an MRI scanner, is very expensive, most biomedical equipment is small, portable, and relatively low cost. In total, biomedical equipment is a major economic asset of the HSO and has significant potential to consume resources in terms of acquisition and operating costs,

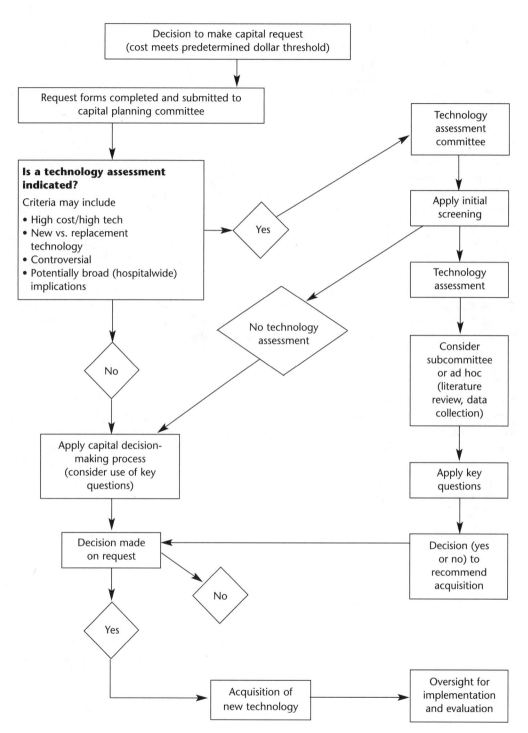

Figure 3.3. Flowchart for capital planning and technology assessment. (From Uphoff, Mary Ellen, Thomas Ratko, and Karl Matuszweski. "Making Technology Assessment Count." *Health Measures* 2 [March 1997]: 22; reprinted by permission.)

TABLE 3.3.   BIOMEDICAL EQUIPMENT CATEGORIES WITH EXAMPLES

Diagnostic	Therapeutic	Monitoring	Support
Body potentials	Resuscitation	Patient	Communication
Blood flow	Prosthetic and orthotic	Environment	Management
Chemical composition	Surgical support		Maintenance and testing
Radiant energy	Special treatment		Teaching
	Radiant energy		Records and statistics

training for users, and maintenance. Acute care hospitals carry an inventory of between 5,000 and 15,000 pieces of equipment.[141]

The staggering growth in the amount and complexity of biomedical equipment, coupled with increased legal liability for defects and malfunctions, necessitate considering biomedical equipment as one element in a complicated system that includes staff, internal environment, technology, organization, and external relations.[142] The categories of equipment shown in Table 3.3 are likely to affect one another. For instance, certain equipment supports a surgical process, even as the surgical process requires the equipment. Effective biomedical equipment use depends on internal factors such as the availability of trained staff, standard operating procedures, staff credentialing, and staff's willingness to accept and use new technology. Equipment use is also a function of external factors such as availability and receptiveness of patients, certification of staff by professional societies, and governmental regulation that governs the technology's safety and efficacy.

SYSTEMS ENGINEERING

Important to selecting biomedical equipment is whether the equipment under consideration can be integrated with the existing equipment, people, processes, and environment to provide a safe and effective system under both normal and contingency conditions. Figure 3.4 suggests these relationships. This integration requires technical expertise, especially when it involves multiple units of programmable equipment from several manufacturers or when facility modifications are necessary. This "systems engineering" may be completed by HSO staff with appropriate skills, by consultants from the HS or elsewhere, or by equipment manufacturers.

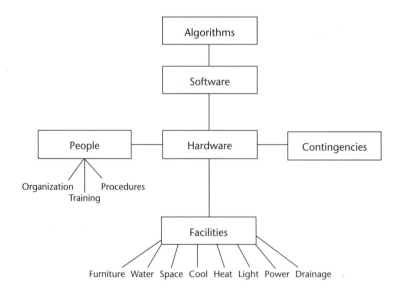

Figure 3.4.   Systems engineering components.

Managing computerized biomedical equipment is much more complex because it is likely to be part of the HSO's/HS's information system. As a result, more elements of the organization are affected; among the most important are clinicians, managers, and the governing body. Other areas that may be affected are fiscal affairs, plant maintenance and operations, biomedical engineering, risk management and safety, quality assessment and improvement, materials management, and information systems.

ORGANIZATION

External Standards

HSOs accredited by The Joint Commission must safely and effectively manage biomedical equipment. As noted, standards for hospitals in the *CAMH* are paradigmatic of those affecting other types of HSOs. Each applicable standard is stated below, followed by a summary of its elements.[143]

Standard EC. 6.10—The hospital manages medical equipment risks.

1. Develops and maintains a written plan to manage effective, safe, reliable operation of medical equipment
2. Identifies and implements one or more processes to select and acquire medical equipment
3. Uses risk criteria to identify, evaluate, and create an inventory of equipment in a medical equipment management plan before use
4. Identifies inspection and maintenance strategies for all equipment
5. Defines intervals for inspection, testing, and maintenance of equipment
6. Identifies and implements processes to monitor and act on equipment hazard notices and recalls
7. Identifies and implements processes to monitor and report incidents involving medical equipment
8. Identifies and implements a process for emergency procedures

Standard EC. 6.20—Medical equipment is maintained, tested, and inspected.

1. Has an inventory of all medical equipment
2. Documents performance and safety testing
3. Documents inspection and maintenance of equipment used in life support
4. Documents inspection and maintenance of non–life support equipment
5. Documents performance testing of all sterilizers
6. Documents chemical and biological testing of water used in renal dialysis and other applicable tests

The Joint Commission surveys determine if equipment management processes are appropriate and followed.

Maintaining and Servicing Biomedical Equipment

HSOs/HSs have four basic options for maintaining and servicing biomedical equipment: 1) having a facility-based biomedical engineering and management information system (MIS) support and service department; 2) having a combination of facility-based service and subcontracted service from equipment manufacturers or independent service companies; 3) expanding facility-based biomedical and MIS service departments to provide service to other HSOs/HSs to achieve economies of scale; and 4) outsourcing of maintenance, repair, and technical support.[144] It is common for large HSOs, and especially acute care hospitals, to have biomedical or clinical engineering departments with biomedical equipment technicians to perform equipment maintenance and management functions within staffing limitations. Historically, biomedical engineering included equipment research and develop-

TABLE 3.4.   CLINICAL ENGINEERING FUNCTIONS

1. Development and integration of new systems Planning System concept and design Facility, equipment, and interface diagrams Manufacturing and test specifications Cost estimates Operational and maintenance procedures Purchasing Sales literature files Sales quotations Buying decisions New installation Contractor liaison On-site installation and checkout support Training Scheduled nurse/technician training courses Educational seminars Evaluation System performance Statistics Cost-effectiveness	2. Operation, maintenance, and calibration Alignment and calibration Pre-operation preparation and checkout Routine performance/safety checks Equipment operation Failure repairs Incoming quality control inspection and test Spare parts inventories Schematic, instruction book, and reference library Operational improvements 3. Medical research and development support Proposal development New equipment design and construction Model shop operation Evaluation testing

From Shaffer, Michael J., Joseph J. Carr, and Marian Gordon. "Clinical Engineering—an Enigma in Health Care Facilities." *Hospital & Health Services Administration* 24 (Summer 1979): 81. © 1979, Foundation of the American College of Healthcare Executives. Used with permission from Health Administration Press.

ment, maintenance, and management support. As equipment proliferated and manufacturers became more active in research and development, however, biomedical engineering became the umbrella term for three subspecialties—bioengineering for research, medical engineering for development, and clinical engineering for integrating and servicing equipment. Nevertheless, many HSOs/HSs have kept the umbrella title *biomedical engineering* for their clinical engineering departments.

In larger HSOs/HSs with substantial equipment inventories, biomedical engineers may be added to provide systems engineering and a higher level of equipment management. The scope of a biomedical engineering department's functions is depicted in Table 3.4. Responsibility for some biomedical equipment may be vested in other departments, however. For instance, central supply may inspect and repair under contract some devices that are used throughout the HSO—intravenous pumps and suction equipment are in this category. Similarly, clinical departments such as anesthesiology, respiratory therapy, or radiology may prefer to manage their own equipment because of its specialized nature.

Organizationally, biomedical engineering normally reports to an assistant administrator or to the director of plant operations or materials management. This chain can create a communication gap between the department and equipment users. Rarely, however, does biomedical engineering report to upper management or the professional staff organization.

Figure 3.5 shows an organizational model in which the clinical departments perform setup and checkout and use their own biomedical equipment, and the administrative departments undertake management, inspections, and repairs. A critical care technician group is shown. Its purpose is to store, provide, and check out biomedical equipment that is used by several clinical departments in order to conserve equipment, ensure procedural consistency, and bridge the gap between clinical departments and biomedical engineering. Arterial pressure and cardiac output monitors and aortic balloon pumps used in special care units are examples of equipment for which critical care technicians are responsible.

Fiscal constraints and increasing cost pressures from managed care have forced many HSOs to downsize their biomedical engineering departments or to use external sources such as independent or

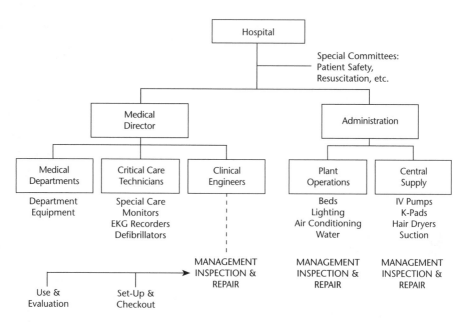

Figure 3.5. Organization of biomedical equipment. (From Shaffer, Michael J. "Managing Hospital Biomedical Equipment." In *Hospital Organization and Management,* 4th ed., edited by Kurt Darr and Jonathon S. Rakich, 283. Baltimore: AUPHA/National Health Publishing, 1989; reprinted by permission.)

manufacturer service organizations. Outsourced biomedical equipment maintenance and repair is often cheaper than repair by the manufacturer, the contractor may provide an on-site biomedical engineer, and there are fewer external organizations with which to deal.[145] Acute care hospital CEOs may be outsourcing as much as two thirds of biomedical engineering services, with very high levels of satisfaction.[146] In addition, service providers are moving from basic reactive repair and maintenance to value-added services such as consultation and customized, project-oriented services. This change has given rise to multivendor servicing (MVS), in which one company is responsible for servicing equipment from other manufacturers. This consolidates contracts, reduces costs, and provides one source of accountability.[147] General Electric provides a prime example of MVS, because it selects and services its biomedical equipment and that of other manufacturers, thus making it both advisor and vendor.[148]

In addition, service workloads have been reduced by improved equipment reliability, troubleshooting by substituting circuit boards, and eliminating preventive maintenance that has little effect on failure rates.[149] In many cases, it may be impossible to materially change mean time between failures. Such equipment is replaced before failure.[150] These factors, in conjunction with manufacturer offerings, such as corrective maintenance contracts that range from complete to partial after-sales support, built-in diagnostics, and manufacturer-provided remote online failure diagnosis, enable HSOs/HSs to employ less-skilled technician and engineering staff. As a result, more experienced technician and engineer staff believe that their future opportunities lie in consulting, manufacturing, and independent service organizations.[151] This may make them a vanishing resource in HSOs. Indeed, there has been a change from data dominance, which provides information for reasoning and calculation, to knowledge dominance that is based on practical experience and learning. These clinical information systems may increase the need for systems engineering in the HSO/HS. Shaffer has argued that the survival of biomedical engineering in hospitals will depend primarily on how well it supports clinical information systems and only secondarily on its ability to support the equipment-management interface for administration.[152]

Another approach is to broaden biomedical engineering to become directly involved in patient care activities. Part of this expanded role is to proactively provide HSO management and clinical staff with comprehensive information about potential equipment purchases through an ongoing process of HTA.[153]

Health Information Technology

Historically, most information technology applications in health services have been business related, with finance and administration foremost among them. Clinical applications have become much more common with the growth of computing power and storage capability. As with other technical areas, healthcare executives need not be expert in information technology, but they will need help from someone who is. Information technology assists in four areas:[154]

1. *Process management*—Redesigning processes to make them seamless and more efficient
2. *Care management*—Expert systems and other ways to assist clinicians, some of which are described below
3. *Demand management*—Especially useful in integrated systems to attract physicians, employers, health plans, and enrollees, as well as to direct patients to the least intensive setting able to meet their needs
4. *Health management*—Essential to store and retrieve risk assessment information, genetic profiles, family health histories, and similar data that predict and prevent disease, a use especially important in a capitated payment system

Of all information technology applications in HSOs/HSs, the subset used for clinical purposes is the focus here. Information technology applications in HSOs receive further attention in Chapter 10. Electronic applications in health (clinical) information have developed at the national, regional (community), and enterprise levels. This discussion addresses the latter two, which have the most direct effect on HSOs/HSs. Enterprise information networks, or corporate intranets, emphasize the internal applications of the electronic health record (EHR) but also link delivery sites in an HS. The following discussion uses the EHR as a generic concept to describe information technology as applied to someone's interactions with various healthcare providers that cover a gamut from acute care to prevention and wellness care and holistic medicine. The literature may use *EHR*. It is common, however, to see *electronic medical record, personal health record,* or *patient record,* which tend to reflect a narrower, episodic, and more acute care focus.

Health information networks date from the 1960s, when the National Library of Medicine initiated an online bibliography, academic medical centers experimented with telemedicine, and the first internal patient information networks were established. Later developments included computerized links among pharmaceutical manufacturers, wholesalers, retail stores, and payers; hospitals and suppliers; and hospitals and fiscal intermediaries who processed Medicare claims.[155]

In the late 1990s, it was estimated that there were 10,000 medical-based web sites; in addition, the Internet is used widely to connect service providers for clinical information interchange.[156]

A subset of information technology applications in health services is health information technology (HIT), defined as the application of information processing involving both computer hardware and software that deals with the storage, retrieval, sharing, and use of healthcare information, data, and knowledge for communication and decision making.[157] National expenditures for HIT were estimated at $11–$15 billion in 1997, with an increase to $17–$42 billion in 2004. Hospitals accounted for about 60% of these expenditures. The projection is that investment in HIT will increase 5%–18% per year. Despite these increasingly sizable expenditures, there continue to be significant deficiencies and inadequacies that technology could help remedy, and it is estimated that healthcare lags behind other industries in adopting information technology (IT) by at least 5–7, or as many as 10–15 years.[158] Wide application of HIT holds great promise with the expectation that it can improve patient safety, reduce hospital lengths of stay, increase appropriate medication use, facilitate chronic disease management, and reduce healthcare costs, generally. It is estimated that only about 20%–25% of hospitals and 15%–20% of physicians' offices have an HIT system; small hospitals are even less likely to have HIT.[159] In 2005, it was estimated that the 10-year costs of software, hardware, licenses, interfaces, training, implementation, maintenance, and opportunity costs to implement a national HIT system were $275 billion, with annual costs of $16.5 billion thereafter.[160]

REGIONAL HEALTH INFORMATION ORGANIZATIONS

From the late 1980s to the early 1990s, community health information networks (CHINs) were established to share health information among patients, providers, and the community for the mutual benefit of all involved, but especially the patient. The few CHINs that have survived into the new millennium are more focused on reimbursement transactions than sharing clinical information.[161] The successors to CHINs are regional health information organizations (RHIOs), with the ultimate goal of forming a national health information network. RHIOs are composed of hospitals, physicians, government agencies, insurers, laboratories, employers, and consumers. Other important stakeholders include schools, community agencies, and patients. By 2007, over 100 RHIOs had been formed. Although many are still in the formative stage, 20 were exchanging information. The federal government has encouraged development of RHIOs but has provided little funding.[162] Figure 3.6 shows healthcare data links similar to those in a RHIO.

Some RHIOs are informal collaborations among participating healthcare entities in a region;

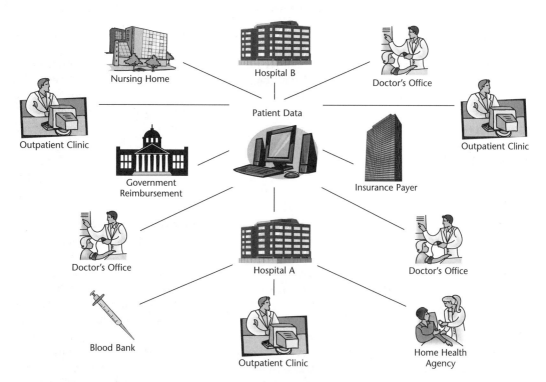

Figure 3.6. Example of healthcare data links. (From Sheldon I. Dorenfest & Associates, Ltd.; reprinted by permission.)

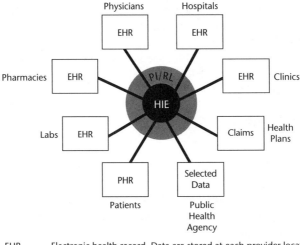

EHR	Electronic health record. Data are stored at each provider location, not in a central location.
PHR	Personal health record. Enables individuals to access their health records.
PI/RL	"Patient Index" and "Record Locator" software. These tools guide data requests through the network to the relevant information about the correct patient.
HIE	Health information exchange network. Information technology structure that enables health data transfer.

Figure 3.7. Regional health information organization: Federated system example. (From "A State Approach: Promoting Health Information Technology in California," February 2007. Retrieved August 10, 2007, from http://www.lao.ca.gov/2007/health_info_tech/health_info_tech_021307.aspx)

others are formally organized as for-profit or not-for-profit corporations. The means of sharing information vary, but there are four general types that connect participating entities in a RHIO: point-to-point systems (patient information is shared as needed); federated systems (each entity [doctor's office, hospital, etc.] stores patient information electronically and is linked to others through a wide area network [WAN]); centralized systems (all patient information is stored in a central database); and hybrid systems (elements of federated and centralized systems are combined).[163] Figure 3.7 shows a RHIO that uses a federated system.

RHIOs—CASE EXAMPLES

California. The California Regional Health Information Organization (CalRHIO) is a statewide collaborative whose focus is improving the safety, quality, and efficiency of healthcare through the use of information technology and the secure exchange of health information. CalRHIO intends to incrementally build a statewide information exchange for California; implement projects that build systems for data exchange, and demonstrate their feasibility and utility; ensure participation by safety net providers and underserved populations in data exchange and IT investment; build financial and business case models for health information exchange; facilitate creation of common governance, process, technology, and other elements needed for regional and statewide data exchange organizations; identify legislation and regulation necessary for statewide data sharing; and ensure that California's data exchange projects are consistent with national technology platforms and networks. Over 40 organizations ranging from hospitals and insurers to county government agencies have participated in CalRHIO through working groups and committees.[164]

Indiana. The Indiana Health Information Exchange (IHIE) is a not-for-profit corporation begun in 2004 with the collaboration of 13 healthcare organizations, including hospitals and other providers, public health organizations, and researchers. The first service available through IHIE was a messaging system that allowed physicians to obtain patients' test results electronically. Organizations such as laboratories that perform tests pay a fee to send the results electronically at about half the cost of sending results using hard copy. In addition, IHIE operates an EHR system that links 18 hospitals in Indianapolis. The EHR system allows emergency department (ED) physicians to gain immediate electronic access to the medical records of persons who present for treatment. Finally, since 1997, IHIE's HealthBridge has linked 18 hospitals that, in turn, connect thousands of physicians, nursing homes, independent laboratories, and imaging centers. HealthBridge provides clinical messaging services for laboratory, radiology, transcription, and health information, including some hospital inpatient records.[165]

PROBLEMS OF IMPLEMENTING RHIOs

In seeking to maximize health in their regions, RHIOs go well beyond the financial aspects of healthcare and use information for clinical, educational, research, and management purposes. Health information networks have long faced formidable barriers because they are complex and costly, are believed to threaten privacy, and have been resisted by professional groups and institutions.

Further impeding progress of RHIOs is that the health information community has not developed standards, such as those for data definitions, computer coding, and interfaces. These impediments greatly diminish the ability of RHIOs to have interoperable systems that facilitate data exchange.[166]

Sharing information is largely incompatible with a competitive environment, and HSOs/HSs may not want to share information with competitors.[167] There is often fragmentation of information about encounters and episodes of illness because patients receive care in different parts of a healthcare system at various times, and each entity has some of the information.[168] Unless all providers participate, the value of interoperability in a RHIO is diminished.

RHIOs may encounter some of the same issues of regulation and licensure as telemedicine. Avoiding them will require that a RHIO limit itself to one state, whereas the natural boundaries of a region may cross one or more state boundaries. The resulting legal issues are, for example, likely to compromise the ability of a physician in one state to provide consultation and coordination of care to a patient in another state. Legal issues of telemedicine are addressed in Chapter 4.

Regardless of the many impediments and difficulties RHIOs will encounter, there is reason to believe that RHIOs will increase in number and importance. Service boundaries of HSOs/HSs are ambiguous and constantly changing, but all of them must communicate if healthcare is to be comprehensive and effective. The market is likely to favor enterprise information networks that offer wider connections (including services on the Internet), and absent monopolistic control, the broader networks will prevail.[169]

ENTERPRISE-LEVEL EHRs

Despite several decades of effort and tens of billions of dollars spent by hospitals and other HSOs/HSs, the availability of a comprehensive, enterprise-wide EHR remains an elusive goal for most providers. The promise is enormous, however.

For example, the electronic medical (health) record system at the Mayo Clinic in Rochester, MN, was initiated in the mid-1990s. In 2007, this massive system included 16,000 active users, 360 million nurse documentation items, 200 million laboratory and procedure results, 44 million radiology reports, 19.2 million clinical notes, and 1.4 million inpatient orders. The system covers the continuum of inpatient and outpatient services, beginning with admission or patient appointment and continuing through examination and consultation, test results, consultation and diagnosis, and treatment (including surgery and postoperative treatment) and on to discharge. Authorized users may call up needed information from locations throughout the organization. The goals of the Mayo Integrated Clinical Systems are to improve patient safety and quality; improve clinical processes for patient care; enhance the ability to comply with regulations and accreditation; improve operational efficiency and reduce costs; enhance revenue recognition; and provide data for reporting, analysis, and research. The fully implemented paperless electronic medical record system improved operational efficiency and reduced costs by eliminating 200 full-time equivalent employees.[170]

A contemporary extension of the information explosion is medical informatics, a generic term for the application of computing and communication technology in health services. *Medical informatics* may be defined as the "systematic study, or science of the identification, collection, storage, communication, retrieval, and analysis of data about medical care services to improve decisions made by physicians and managers of healthcare organizations."[171] This definition is broad enough to incorporate management and health network applications such as WANs and RHIOs.

Despite significant applications of HIT, much remains to be done. Development of electronic health information systems in hospitals faces problems including standardization to achieve systems' interoperability, obtaining necessary funding, excessive regulation, privacy and information security issues, and a uniform approach to matching patients to their records.[172]

ADVANTAGES OF EHRs

There are numerous advantages to maintaining medical information in an electronic format. EHRs greatly facilitate using the medical and health information that is contained. Internally, the need to create, file, move, and store paper records is eliminated, and information is readily available anywhere in the HSO. Externally, the delivery of services at multiple sites is facilitated because all providers have access to the same medical and health information, something virtually impossible with paper records. A second advantage of EHRs is reduced offline storage and retrieval costs. Paper records require significant space and are costly to store. Third, EHRs improve the quality and coherence of the care process. For example, the logistics problems of paper records—loss or unavailability when needed, difficulty of finding information in them, illegibility—are largely solved.[173] A fourth advantage is that clinical guidelines can be automated to positively affect physician behavior and care processes. Computer-assisted decision support program reminders using local clinician-derived clinical guidelines can, for example, improve antibiotic use, reduce associated costs, and stabilize emergence of antibiotic-resistant pathogens.[174] Fifth, EHRs support research and quality improvement. Both are data driven, and ready access to medical and health information greatly facilitates them. Integrated EHR systems could be used to reduce variation in clinical processes and outcomes, thus lowering costs.[175] A sixth benefit of EHRs is that readily available data ease reporting of all types.

DISADVANTAGES OF EHRs

A major problem making EHRs operational is that the typical HSO has scores of electronic data sources—most complex are those in acute care hospitals. The number of such sources grew considerably with the ready availability of personal computers and increasingly powerful, inexpensive memory chips. Internal clinical information systems such as those in laboratories, pharmacies, EDs, and radiology are often different and cannot "talk" to one another, nor can they interface with administrative and support areas such as admission and discharge, patient billing, scheduling, risk management, and medical transcription. External systems such as those in physicians' offices, commercial pharmacies, freestanding affiliated outpatient units and surgical centers, home health agencies, and RHIOs store information that would facilitate the effective and efficient delivery of services were it available when needed. Both internal and external systems are rife with duplicate information, all of which is obtained and stored at significant cost to the HSO/HS and with inconvenience and frustration to the consumer.

Obtaining an interface among these various clinical systems, especially those internal to the HSO/HS, is key to realizing many of the advantages of an EHR. The interface problems are solvable with interface standards available. "Standards provide the bridges to the many islands of electronic patient data so that the data can be inexpensively combined into an electronic (health) record."[176] A remaining problem is to obtain physician information inexpensively in a coded or structured format compatible with electronic storage. Use of electronic documentation (dictation) into the EHR reduces the time a physician needs for dictation, as well as the time needed to access medical information, because most dictation occurs within the patient's medical (health) record. Also, electronic documentation requires fewer transcriptionists in the medical records department, an additional saving to the HSO.[177]

Confidentiality, privacy, and consent raise significant issues regarding EHRs. Confidentiality concerns may cause HSOs/HSs to control patient information so tightly that some or all of the advantages of EHRs are lost. For example, administration may determine that only the ordering physician can have access to test results. This will cause problems when nurses or on-call colleagues need test results, or in an emergency.[178] "Family charts" are produced by combining the health records of family members. This makes family practice more efficacious but raises issues of privacy and consent.[179]

For most patients, electronically linking internal health record information is unlikely to raise confidentiality concerns. Paper records are subject to the same issues of misuse as are electronic records. In fact, paper records are potentially more subject to inappropriate use than are EHRs, for which access codes and audit trails can be established. For some patients, however, the mysteries of electronic formats may create a greater psychological issue than do paper records.

The efficiencies achieved by linking external data sources benefit providers and insurers, but they ultimately accrue to the advantage of consumers. Consumers are much more likely to be concerned, however, about confidentiality and privacy issues as health information and data sets from external sources are linked. Beyond the reality is the psychological discomfort of knowing that comprehensive data banks contain personal, even embarrassing, information and that the potential for misuse exists. Confidentiality and privacy concerns, as well as the legal issues of consent and wrongful release of information, may cause so many restrictions on the use of information in EHRs that many of their advantages will be lost.[180] In addition to using dedicated electronic or hardwired links, providers can communicate over the Internet, which has sufficient security tools to alleviate confidentiality concerns.[181]

The efficiencies that will be realized with EHRs are unlikely to come from reductions in support staff. Implementing an electronic medical record in family practice residency programs did not decrease the need for support staff.[182] This finding is consistent with results from other clinical and nonclinical applications of HIT.

Gauging patient reaction to increased computer use by physicians must be done within the context that computers are ubiquitous. Concerns that patients may have less confidence in physicians who use computers to enter and retrieve patient-specific clinical information, provide access to decision support or an expert system, or search for reference information regarding diagnosis and treatment during a consultation are probably unfounded.[183] Similarly, patients do not seem to believe that physicians who use computers are paying inadequate attention to them; apparently, patients support physicians' use of computers.[184] In fact, it is likely that patients will increasingly interpret failure to use computers in consultations and treatment as practicing something less than state-of-the-art medicine.

SUMMARY

Paper medical records continue to be common but less and less the norm. Progress toward EHRs will continue slowly and at great economic cost. Electronic physician order entry as a means of reducing medication errors has become almost universal in HSOs. The ultimate EHR promises to retrieve whatever patient data are needed to perform tasks such as outcomes analysis, utilization review, profiling, and costing, abilities that are of special interest to CEOs in hospitals and MCOs.[185] Integrating the EHR with information retrieval systems to support diagnosis and treatment is a highly desirable, perhaps essential extension of the medical record in an electronic format.

Telemedicine

Telemedicine may be defined as the use of medical information exchanged from one site to another via electronic communications to improve patients' health status. Examples include videoconferencing, transmitting still images, e-health (including patient portals), remote monitoring of vital signs, continuing medical education, and nursing call centers. In 2007, there were approximately 200 telemedicine networks connecting nearly 2,000 medical institutions, half of which use telemedicine on a daily basis.[186] Clinical applications include radiology, dermatology, ophthalmology, cardiology, psychiatry, emergency medicine, pathology, obstetrics and gynecology, and orthopedics. Table 3.5 shows various types of telemedicine interactions.

The prototype of telemedicine was the telephone consultation between physicians; use of facsimile machines to transmit electrocardiograms and medical records is common. Newer technologies include interactive television. For example, physicians use digital cameras in their offices to obtain images of a patient's retinas and transmit them to an image-reading center for diagnosis of retinal disorders.[187] Using telemedicine in radiology—teleradiology—provides hospitals and patients in underserved communities access to consultations at a tertiary care hospital and broadens radiology residents' experience treating a wider variety of cases.[188]

In addition to clinical consultation, telemedicine has significant uses for administrative support and education. Many applications do not, however, require two-way, full-motion video. Still images are used for radiology and pathology, in which "store and forward" technologies transmit static images or video clips to remote storage devices for later retrieval, review, and consultation.[189] Telemedicine can be used when physical barriers prevent ready transfer of medical management information between patients and providers.[190] Monitoring patients at home is an example.

MCOs were early users of telemedicine, but as the technology becomes ubiquitous, its advantages as a means of marketplace differentiation will diminish. Military hospitals have been at the forefront of using telemedicine to serve personnel in remote locations where it is impossible to provide advanced technology, physician specialists, and other highly trained clinical staff.[191] Telemedicine offers opportunities for providers in the United States to consult and assist in providing healthcare to patients worldwide.

Five issues are unresolved in telemedicine:[192]

1. *Clinical expectations and medical effectiveness*—Much of the information about the clinical effectiveness of telemedicine is anecdotal.
2. *Matching technology to medical needs*—Inconvenience of interactive technology is a major obstacle to widespread use. Rural practitioners may lack the support technologies to apply it.
3. *Economics of telemedicine*—Acquiring and maintaining telemedicine equipment is very costly. Health plans may not pay for telemedicine. Medicare reimburses telemedicine. The Medicaid law does not recognize telemedicine as a distinct service, and CMS has not for-

TABLE 3.5. THE SPECTRUM OF CLINICAL TELEMEDICINE INTERACTIONS[a]

Purpose	Mode of interaction	Types of information transferred	Minimum bandwidth requirements[b]	Typical applications
Diagnostic or therapeutic consultation	Real-time, one-way or two-way interactive motion video	Voice, sound, motion video images, text, and documents	Moderate to high	Telepsychiatry and mental health applications, remote surgery, interactive examinations
	Still images or video clips with real-time telephone voice interaction	Voice, sound, still video images or short video clips, text	Low to moderate	Multiple medical applications, including dermatology, cardiology, otolaryngology, orthopedics
	Still images or video clips with text information; "store-and-forward," with data acquired and transmitted for review at a later date	Sound, still video images or short video clips, text	Low	Multiple medical applications, including dermatology, cardiology, otolaryngology, orthopedics
Medical education	One-way or two-way real-time or delayed video	Voice, sound, motion video images, text, and documents	Moderate to high	Distance education and training
Case management or documentation	Transfer of electronic text, image, or other data	Text, images, documents, and related data	Low to high	Community health information networks, medical record management

From Perednia, Douglas A., and Ace Allen. "Telemedicine Technology and Clinical Applications." *Journal of the American Medical Association 273* (February 8, 1995): 484; reprinted by permission.

[a] Omits telemedicine consultations performed using the telephone alone.

[b] Bandwidth is the transmission capacity of a telecommunication link. Conventional telephone lines have relatively little carrying capacity (low bandwidth). High-capacity lines are required to transmit large amounts of information (e.g., images) rapidly.

mally defined it. States may choose to provide the service, however; about half do.[193] The cost-effectiveness of telemedicine has been questioned.[194]

4. *Legal and social issues*—Remote licensure and liability must be addressed, as must the social and political issues relating to access to telemedicine. (Chapter 4 discusses the legal aspects of telemedicine.)
5. *Organizational factors*—Organizations must address issues surrounding telemedicine prospectively and specifically.

Telemedicine continues to be an essential element in health services delivery in the 21st century, and significant growth is certain. Managers must enable their HSOs/HSs to participate in it fully.

Future Developments

BIOMEDICAL EQUIPMENT

Some see cost containment as slowing biomedical equipment development, manufacture, and use. Conversely, some predict that competition among healthcare networks will encourage the purchase of advanced equipment and availability of new procedures. Decentralized facilities are likely to contain state-of-the-art biomedical equipment, but with little standby equipment and few spare parts. This necessitates increased reliability and speed of repair to minimize downtime.

These developments suggest that attitudes will change from

1. Performing maintenance because it is required to performing maintenance because it saves money
2. Purchasing based on price to purchasing based on life-cycle cost
3. Biomedical service as a part of maintenance to managing technology as part of managing healthcare
4. A focus on technology to a focus on information[195]

As technology continues to advance, HSO/HS managers must ensure that biomedical equipment is appropriate, complies with regulations, performs correctly, and is used properly. A major challenge will be achieving an interface among all the elements. Only if various types of technology can "talk" to one another will maximum benefit be realized. In addition, organizations will expect to get more from their equipment; this means that portability and a good fit with the environment will be important.[196]

CLINICAL SUPPORT AND INFORMATION SYSTEMS

Computer and communication technologies have supported the development of artificial intelligence; microprocessor and computer- and robot-assisted diagnosis and treatment; general applications of expert systems to integrate computers and machines; the Internet and intranets; and local area networks (LANs), WANs, and RHIOs, all of which give healthcare providers direct access to knowledge and information. In addition to the NGC noted earlier, current operational and experimental uses of the Internet include online patient registration, interactive question-and-answer services for disease management, dissemination of HMO guidelines to member physicians, and e-mail. In the late 1990s, it was reported that 176 sites on the Internet contained information on subjects such as consumer health information, support groups, physician specialties, disease tracking and reporting, physician recruitment, and long-term care facilities.[197]

Increasingly, physicians will use computerized scoring systems to determine the statistical effectiveness of treatments for critical care patients. One method uses a point system for age, seven morbid conditions that affect short-term mortality, and 16 physiologic variables that reflect values for vital signs, laboratory tests, and neurologic status.[198] Another expert system determines the optimum location of an HSO by using demographic surveys and factors such as anticipated financial, operational, and clinical performance; competing institutions; access roads; and ambulance support.[199] Most important, standards have been developed to transfer medical images and patient information, which brings medicine closer to the ultimate goal of a universal paperless electronic patient record.[200]

The Internet offers tremendous potential to centralize medical information in a patient-managed web site with controlled access, including read-only protection. Providers could view and download information in the record, as needed; entries would be made following treatment. Giving all providers access to the same database could greatly improve efficiency and efficaciousness, to the great benefit of the patient.

Technology and the Future of Medicine

Developments in tissue and genetic engineering, gene therapy, artificial organs and tissues, implantable computer chips and "smart" wafers, nanotechnology (microscopic machines and molecular-level tools), robotic "caterpillars" to deliver medication and treat internal organs, and minimally invasive, keyhole, and bloodless surgery have only begun to affect medicine in what is likely to become a cascade of change. Surgeons are increasingly using the body's natural openings—the nose, mouth, rectum, and vagina—to pass deep into the body the slender instruments that can be guided to perform surgery and other treatment. As with laparoscopic surgery, the procedure is much less traumatic, and recovery time is greatly reduced.

Advances in pharmaceutical research, including use of robochemistry—the science of applying computerization on a large scale to drug molecule research—will speed the basic research and development of medications.[201] Increasingly, allopathic (traditional Western medical) practice will be supplemented by holistic and nontraditional medicine. Complementary and alternative medicine includes chiropractic, homeopathy, naturopathy, and osteopathy; aroma, music, and massage therapies; biofeedback and visualization techniques; therapeutic touch; and Eastern medical theories, prominent among which are acupuncture, Chinese herbal remedies, and ayurvedic medicine. The sum of these technologies—as well as those yet to be developed— promises to revolutionize health and medicine, including the site at which the "technology" is available. The aggregate financial effect of wholesale use of an increasingly broad array of technologies is that private and governmental spending for "healthcare" will increase, perhaps dramatically. HSOs and HSs must be able to identify, acquire, and manage the technology needed. Effective managers are boundary scanners; medical technology is a critical aspect of this activity. There is no substitute for managers possessing basic knowledge about technology of all types.

Societally, we are experiencing an epidemic of diagnoses. One aspect of this epidemic is the medicalization of everyday life—the physical or emotional sensations that in the past were just a normal part of life are now seen as symptoms of disease. Thus, they require a diagnosis and, more important for the health services system, treatment. The other aspect of this epidemic is the drive to find disease early—to diagnose illness in people who have no symptoms, those with so-called pre-disease or those "at risk." The problem with this epidemic of diagnoses is that it leads to an epidemic of treatment. For the severely ill, the potential for harm from treatment pales in comparison with the potential for benefit. For others, it is important to remember that not all treatments have important benefits but that almost all can have harms, some of which may only be apparent years into the future.[202] Because they raise important considerations of ethics and costs, the implications of overdiagnosing and overtreatment lie well within the purview of managers.

▧ DISCUSSION QUESTIONS ▧▧▧▧▧▧▧▧▧▧▧▧▧▧▧▧▧▧▧▧▧▧▧▧▧▧

1. Describe the effect of medical technology on HSOs/HSs and the costs of health services. Link the theories of distribution of scarce lifesaving technology described in Chapter 1 (and in more detail in Chapter 4) with the problems that HSOs/HSs experience in managing medical technology.
2. Identify the effects of various types of payment mechanisms on the development of new medical technology. What are the likely effects on use? What are the implications for patient care?
3. The increasing portability of technology makes it available in settings other than traditional HSOs. As traditional settings for medical technology, acute care hospitals are greatly affected by portability. Identify the advantages and disadvantages from the standpoint of the HSO *and* the patient.
4. Trends suggest significant consumer interest in alternatives to traditional medicine. These include the low- or no-technology treatment found in holistic medicine, wellness care, and disease prevention. Identify the implications for society *and* traditional HSOs, such as hospitals.
5. The control of development and generalization of medical technology is fragmented. Identify control points, and suggest ways to improve them. Distinguish the private and public sectors.
6. Technology is present in HSOs/HSs because physicians ask for it and patients expect it. Describe changes in the external environment that affect availability and application of technology. Describe management's role in assessing technology.
7. The electronic health record promises to revolutionize the delivery of health services. Identify the advantages and disadvantages for the patient *and* for providers.
8. The internal management of biomedical equipment poses several problems for managers. How do managers involve clinical staff to solve these problems? Identify the types of equipment that managers can purchase without involving clinical staff.
9. Competition is a major force in health services, and marketing is critical to HSO/HS success. What are the relationships between marketing and acquisition and application of medical technology? Give examples from your experience or the literature.
10. Usually, little attention is paid to nonclinical technology such as financial or management data systems. Such technology can dramatically affect HSO/HS costs and effectiveness, however. Identify the types of nonclinical equipment and their effects on managing HSOs/HSs. What links are there between clinical and nonclinical technologies?

▧ Case Study 1: The Feasibility of BEAM

Brain electrical activity mapping (BEAM) is a technology for imaging the brain. It significantly improves the physician's ability to localize an abnormality. In response to increased demands for this procedure from staff radiologists and local neurologists and reports in the literature of the usefulness of BEAM testing, Metropolitan Hospital has decided to investigate the possibility of acquiring access to BEAM testing. Two options are to lease and to purchase. A third option is to ask nearby County Hospital to share its recently acquired BEAM machine.

A major unknown is uncertainty about the future of reimbursement. It is likely that Medicare DRG payments will be reduced. In addition, other third-party payers are requiring more stringent review of new technologies.

Because of the reimbursement issues and major expenditures involved, the governing body chair asked the CEO to form a committee and evaluate each option, including foregoing access to BEAM testing. The assessment will permit a final decision between BEAM and a proposed addition to the intensive care unit, a project that is supported strongly by the surgical staff and that has already been delayed twice.

The governing body would prefer to delay this decision until reimbursement is better understood, but several attending physicians think that BEAM testing is critical to their practices and have stated that, although they prefer the nursing staff at Metropolitan, quality of care considerations will force them to admit certain patients to County so they can have access to BEAM. Recently, you were told about a rumor that several prominent physicians want to develop a consortium to purchase and operate BEAM and other diagnostic equipment in a professional office complex that is under construction.

QUESTIONS

1. Propose the membership of a committee to assess the need for BEAM and, if it is to be made available at Metropolitan, to recommend whether to buy, lease, or use County's BEAM.
2. What types of information should be presented to the governing body in the committee's final report?
3. What political and economic complications are likely to be present in the decision-making process?
4. How should the political and economic complications be addressed? Be specific in identifying the sequence of steps.

Case Study 2: "Who Does What?"

When she purchased, installed, and staffed the single photon emission computerized tomography (SPECT) camera at a cost of more than $500,000, Andrea Berson thought it was one of the most difficult things she had done as chief operating officer at Sinai Hospital. Looking back, however, it could pale in comparison with the problem looming on the horizon. The SPECT camera's three-dimensional visualization of the heart makes it an exquisite diagnostic tool. Cardiologists commonly perform biplanar (two-dimensional) nuclear cardiology studies in their offices, but SPECT's high cost virtually precludes its use in physicians' offices.

Sinai has an exclusive contract with a radiology group to perform all inpatient radiology services. Four members of the group are board certified in nuclear medicine and credentialed for SPECT. Several cardiologists who refer patients to Sinai have expressed grave concerns about the quality of the readings of SPECT scans done by two of these four radiologists. When SPECT scans are done on their patients, these cardiologists want privileges to read the scans at Sinai. They threaten to refer patients for SPECT scans and other diagnostic radiology workups to a competing hospital if their request is denied.

The radiologists learned of the cardiologists' request and sent Berson a letter stating that they expect her to meet the terms of their exclusive contract. The letter stated that the radiologists who are board certified in nuclear medicine do high-quality work and have the training, experience, and proven ability to read SPECT scans. The letter emphasized that the change being contemplated would adversely affect the quality of patient care because the technologies involved in two- and three-dimensional scans are very different, and reading SPECT scans requires unique skills. In addition, granting these privileges to cardiologists would violate established relationships and cause other, unspecified disruptions. Berson suspected there just might be an economic reason as well.

The problem in radiology reminded Berson of the turf war between interventional radiologists and surgeons about using lasers and the turf war over which specialties should perform laparoscopic surgery. As she reread the letter, Berson mused about the course of modern medicine. It had reached the point at which many conditions could be diagnosed and treated without a scalpel. She thought briefly about Dr. McCoy, the *Star Trek* physician who had only to pass a small, handheld device over someone to make a diagnosis. Is that where we're headed? she wondered.

"But, enough of science fiction," she said to herself. "How do I solve yet another turf battle without too many casualties, not the least of whom could be me?"

QUESTIONS

1. Identify the quality-of-care issues. How are they similar to, and how are they different from, the economic issues?
2. What information should Berson possess to understand the facts and issues? To whom should Berson turn for advice?
3. Develop three options that Berson could use. Identify and justify your choice of the best.
4. Identify three other quality/economic controversies that occur among institutional or personal health services providers.

Case Study 3: "Let's 'Do' a Joint Venture"

In 1990, a consortium of churches established Arcadia Continuing Care Community as a not-for-profit, tax-exempt corporation. Located in the tidewater region of eastern Virginia near a major naval base, Arcadia had 200 apartments for independent and assisted living and a 30-bed skilled nursing facility. Arcadia featured indoor and outdoor recreational activities and emphasized maximum independence for residents in a supportive, caring environment.

By 2000, poor management had brought Arcadia to the brink of bankruptcy. It was rescued by a large loan from the consortium and put under professional management. Arcadia was soon on firm financial footing, and the board of directors determined that its services should be diversified. Arcadia developed a respite care program to provide weekend and day services for dependent older adults and give relief to family members. It also established a home hospice program.

The board hired a consultant to assist in strategic planning. Based on market analyses and community assessments, the consultant suggested several new programs. First on the list was a rehabilitation center. The consultant noted the absence of outpatient rehabilitation services in the area, that rehabilitation logically extended existing services (including respite care and residential services), and that reimbursement was adequate. Start-up costs, including leasing space and equipping and staffing a rehabilitation center, were estimated at $500,000. The board was enthusiastic, but it had less than $100,000 for a new venture. Arcadia was leveraged (mortgaged) to the maximum, and there was no ready source of new capital.

As the board grappled with this question, the consultant suggested a joint venture with a physiatry group located 35 miles away. The consultant proposed that they pool their capital and establish a for-profit subsidiary to offer rehabilitation services. A telephone call to the physiatrists showed that they were interested.

QUESTIONS

1. Critique what Arcadia is doing in terms of the technology that it has considered and is considering. Include both the positive and negative aspects.
2. Identify additional compatible activities that Arcadia could undertake. Be specific as to how they fit with its current activities and implied mission.
3. Identify the benefits and risks of forming a joint venture with the physiatry group.
4. What is the role of Arcadia's managers, especially the CEO, in these activities?

■ Case Study 4: Worst Case Scenario—The Nightmare

Randy Means dreams infrequently, but when she awoke this morning, she vividly recalled that she had had a nightmare. Means dreamt that it was past midnight when she was called by the night supervisor at the small acute care hospital at which Means is the CEO. The supervisor was quite aggravated and had trouble speaking. It took a few seconds for the message of the nightmare to become clear. The "worst case scenario" that sometimes crossed Means's waking mind had occurred. The four-bed intensive care unit (ICU) was full, and an emergency case had been stabilized in the ED after a car accident. The accident victim's injuries were severe, and transferring her to another facility would almost certainly cause her death. She had to get into the ICU in less than 2 hours. Only the ICU had the technology needed, such as a respirator and cardiac and other vital sign monitors, and the expert staff to keep her alive.

Almost pleading, Means asked the night supervisor if one of the ICU patients could be transferred elsewhere. Just as the nightmare ended, the night supervisor brusquely assured Means that physicians would not keep patients in the ICU unless they needed that level of care.

Means was shaken by the nightmare. There were no funds to add ICU beds, but Means was determined that the hospital had to plan for the worst case scenario—a full ICU.

QUESTIONS

1. Outline the steps Means should take in the planning process.
2. Identify by title the members of the hospital staff who should participate in the process.
3. Outline the contingency plan.
4. Identify external resources to be inventoried and involved in this type of contingency planning.

Notes

1. Centers for Medicare and Medicaid Services. "National Health Expenditure Projections 2006–2016." *http://www.cms.hhs.gov/NationalHealthExpendData/downloads/proj2006.pdf,* retrieved July 23, 2007.
2. Samuel, Frank E., Jr. "Technology and Costs: Complex Relationship." *Hospitals* 62 (December 5, 1988): 72.
3. Littell, Candace L., and Robin J. Strongin. "The Truth About Technology and Health Care Costs." *IEEE Technology and Society Magazine* 15 (Fall 1996): 11.
4. Beever, Charles, Heather Burns, and Melanie Karbe. "U.S. Health Care's Technology Cost Crisis." March 31, 2004. Booze Allen Hamilton, Inc., strategy+business enews. *http://www.strategy-business .com/press/enewsarticle/enews033104,* retrieved August 20, 2007.
5. Stevens, William K. "High Medical Costs Under Attack as Drain on the Nation's Economy." *The New York Times,* March 28, 1982, 50.
6. Newhouse, John P. "An Iconoclastic View of Health Cost Containment." *Health Affairs 1993* (12, Suppl.): 152; Bucy, Bill. "'Star Trek' Medical Devices Not So Far Out in the Future." *The Business Journal* 13 (January 29, 1996): 23.
7. Littell and Strongin, "The Truth About Technology," 12.
8. Cohen, Alan B., and Ruth S. Hanft. *Technology in American Health Care: Policy Directions for Effective Evaluation and Management,* 18–20. Ann Arbor, MI: The University of Michigan Press, 2004.
9. Baker, Laurence, Howard Birnbaum, Jeffrey Geppert, David Mishol, and Erick Moyneur. "The Relationship Between Technology Availability and Health Care Spending." Health Affairs Web Exclusive, November 5, 2003. *http://content.healthaffairs.org/cgi/reprint/hlthaff.w3.537v1?maxtoshow=&HITS =10&hits=10&RESULTFORMAT=&fulltext=imaging+technology&andorexactfulltext=and&searchid =1&FIRSTINDEX=0&resourcetype=HWCIT,* retrieved August 3, 2007.

10. Perry, Seymour, and M. Eliastam. "The National Center for Health Care Technology." *Journal of the American Medical Association* 245 (June 26, 1981): 2,510–2,511.

11. Scitovsky, Anne A. "Changes in the Costs of Treatment of Selected Illnesses, 1971–1981." *Medical Care* 23 (December 1985): 1345–1357; Showstack, Jonathan A., Mary Hughes Stone, and Steven A. Schroeder. "The Role of Changing Clinical Practices in the Rising Costs of Hospital Care." *New England Journal of Medicine* 313 (November 7, 1985): 1,201–1,207.

12. Chernew, Michael, A. Mark Fendrick, and Richard A. Hirth. "Managed Care and Medical Technology: Implications for Cost Growth." *Health Affairs* 16 (March/April 1997): 196–206.

13. Shine, Kenneth I. "Low-Cost Technologies and Public Policy." *International Journal of Technology Assessment in Health Care* 13 (1997): 562–571.

14. Souhrada, Laura. "Biotechnology, Cost Concerns Dominate in 1989." *Hospitals* 63 (December 20, 1989): 32.

15. Russell, Louise B., and Jane E. Sisk. "Medical Technology in the United States: The Last Decade." *International Journal of Technology Assessment in Health Care* 4 (1988): 275. By way of context, the most rapid generalization of new technology is almost certainly the diagnostic x-ray (radiograph). Discovered by German physicist Wilhelm Roentgen in 1895, it was only months before radiographs were in general use. Such rapid generalization was possible because scientists worldwide had similar apparatuses and made them available to clinicians. The chest x-ray continues to be the most common radiological procedure. (Lentle, Brian, and John Aldrich. "Radiological Science, Past and Present." *Lancet* 350 [July 26, 1997]: 280–285.)

16. Health Care Advisory Board. Annual Health Care Innovation Summit. "Future of Diagnostic Imaging: Charting a Course for Profitable Growth." *http://www.advisory.com/members/default.asp?contentID =41316&collectionID=1021&program=14&filename=41316_48_14_11-25-2003_1.pdf,* retrieved July 30, 2007.

17. Personal communication, Biomagnetic Technologies, Inc., San Diego, July 22, 1998.

18. The Edge. "T3 Compendium: Top Technology Trends from Sg2 - 2006," Sg2, Skokie, IL, 2007, p. 98–99. *http://www.sg2.com/ProductsServices/Publications/focusreports/Detail.aspx?Id=1761,* retrieved July 31, 2007.

19. Chernew, Fendrick, and Hirth. "Managed Care and Medical Technology."

20. Eisenberg, John M., J. Sanford Schwartz, F. Catherine McCaslin, Rachel Kaufman, Henry Glick, and Eugene Kroch. "Substituting Diagnostic Services: New Tests Only Partly Replace Older Ones." *Journal of the American Medical Association* 262 (September 1, 1989): 1,196–1,200.

21. Shine, Kenneth I. "Low-Cost Technologies and Public Policy." *International Journal of Technology Assessment in Health Care* 13 (1997): 563–564.

22. Kennedy, Donald. "Health Care Costs and Technologies." *Western Journal of Medicine* 161 (October 1994): 424–425.

23. Ross, Philip E. "Brewing Blood." *Forbes* 160 (November 17, 1997): 168.

24. Gillis, Judith. "Technology Cleans Donated Blood." *The Washington Post,* April 25, 1998, D1.

25. Bailar, John C., III, and Heather L. Gornik. "Cancer Undefeated." *New England Journal of Medicine* 336 (May 29, 1997): 1,569. From 1990 to 1995, the annual number (incidence rate) of new cancer cases fell slightly but steadily. This suggests an ebbing of the disease, not because of improved treatments but because of changing lifestyles, earlier detection, and more aggressive treatment of precancerous conditions. (Brown, David. "New Cancer Cases Decline in U.S." *The Washington Post,* March 13, 1998, A1.)

26. Sg2. "Cancer Fundamentals." *http://www.sg2.com/sg2_docs/fundamentals/Sg2U_Fundamentals_Cancer _Workbook.pdf,* retrieved August 13, 2007.

27. The Edge. "T3 Compendium: Top Technology Trends from Sg2 - 2006." Sg2, Skokie, IL, 2007, p. 98. *http://www.sg2.com/ProductsServices/Publications/focusreports/Detail.aspx?Id=1761,* retrieved July 31, 2007.

28. United Network for Organ Sharing. The Organ Procurement and Transplantation Network. "Transplants in the U.S. by Recipient Gender, U.S. Transplants Performed: January 1, 1988–April 30, 2007." *http://www.optn.org/latestData/rptData.asp,* retrieved July 30, 2007.

29. Mayo Foundation for Medical Education and Research. "Cornea Transplants: Restoring Sight with Donor Tissue." *http://www.mayoclinic.com/print/cornea-transplant/EY00004/METHOD=print,* retrieved July 30, 2007.

30. "Schizophrenia Update—Part I." *Harvard Mental Health Letter* 12 (June, 1995). Because fMRI allows imaging of soft tissue and concentrations of substances, scientists have been able to track human thought and emotion. ("Mapping Thought Patterns." *Biomedical Instrumentation & Technology* 31 [March/April 1997]: 111–112.)

31. Matthews, Scott C., Martin P. Paulus, and Joel E. Dimsdale. "Contribution of Functional Neuroimaging to Understanding Neuropsychiatric Side Effects of Interferon in Hepatitis C." *Psychosomatics* 45 (July/August 2004): 4.

32. "ECRI White Paper Makes Predictions on Equipment and Device Purchases." *Health Industry Today* 58 (May 1995): 6–7.

33. The Edge. "T3 Compendium: Top Technology Trends from Sg2 - 2006." Sg2, Skokie, IL, 2007, pp. 39–44. *http://www.sg2.com/ProductsServices/Publications/focusreports/Detail.aspx?Id=1761,* retrieved July 31, 2007.

34. Kennedy, Donald. "Health Care Costs."

35. Edelson, Ed. "Death Rate High in Drug-Coated Stent Trial." washingtonpost.com. July 10, 2007. *http://www.washingtonpost.com/wp-dyn/content/article/2007/07/10/AR2007071000740_p,* retrieved July 31, 2007.

36. Kent, David M., Sandeep Vijan, Rodney A. Hayward, John L. Griffith, Joni R. Beshansky, and Harry P. Selker. "Tissue Plasminogen Activator Was Cost-Effective Compared to Streptokinase in Only Selected Patients with Acute Myocardial Infarction." *Journal of Clinical Epidemiology* 57 (2004): 843–52.

37. Ho, Vivian, and Laura A. Petersen. "Estimating Cost Savings from Regionalizing Cardiac Procedures Using Hospital Discharge Data." Cost Effectiveness and Resource Allocation (2007) 5:7. *http://www.resource-allocation.com/content/5/1/7,* retrieved July 30, 2007.

38. Boston Scientific. "Treating Carotid Stenosis: Understanding Hosital Costs: Stenting and Carotid Endarterectomy Have Comparable Costs." November 2006. *http://www.carotid.com/pdf/treating carotidstenosisFAQ.pdf,* retrieved August 13, 2007.

39. Yadav, Jay S., et al. "Protected Carotid-Artery Stenting Versus Endarterectomy in High-Risk Patients." *New England Journal of Medicine* 351, 15 (October 7, 2004): 1,493–1,501.

40. A continuing useful discussion of the technology assessment process is found in Glasser, Jay H., and Richard S. Chrzanowski. "Medical Technology Assessment: Adequate Questions, Appropriate Methods, Valuable Answers." *Health Policy* 9 (1988): 267–276.

41. Ramage, Michelle. "New Devices Emphasize Less Trauma to Body and Billfold." *The Business Journal* 41 (January 20, 1997): 59.

42. "Elasticity Imaging Identifies Cancers and Reduces Breast Biopsies." *Medical News Today,* December 3, 2006. *http://www.medicalnewstoda.com/printerfriendlynews.php?newsid=57839,* retrieved February 22, 2007.

43. Manton, Kenneth G., XiLiang Gu, and Vicki L. Lamb. "Long-Term Trends in Life Expectancy and Active Life Expectancy in the United States." *Population and Development Review* 32, 1 (March 2006): 94.

44. "Instrumental activities of daily living (IADL) include heavy and light housework, laundry, cooking, grocery shopping, getting about outside, traveling, managing money, taking medication, and using a telephone. Activities of daily living (ADL) include eating, transferring in and out of bed or chair, getting around inside, dressing, bathing, and toileting. The absence of any chronic IADL or ADL impairment places individuals in the 'active' or nondisabled population." Manton, Kenneth G., XiLiang Gu, and Vicki L. Lamb. "Long-Term Trends in Life Expectancy and Active Life Expectancy in the United States." *Population and Development Review* 32, 1 (March 2006): 92.

45. Manton, Kenneth G., et al. "Long-Term Trends in Life Expectancy and Active Life Expectancy in the United States," 94.

46. Moore, Thomas J. "Look at the Mortality Rates; the 'War on Cancer' Has Been a Bust." *The Washington Post,* July 23, 1997, A23.

47. The significant decline of atherosclerosis (deposition of plaque on artery walls, an important factor in coronary artery disease) since the 1960s has been attributed to use of broad-spectrum antibiotics, particularly tetracycline, to cure other bacterial infections. Bacteria such as *Chlamydia pneumoniae* and *Bacteroides gingivalis* have been linked to atherosclerosis, as have viruses such as cytomegalovirus, which

can be treated but cannot be cured. (Mason, Michael. "Could You Catch a Heart Attack from a Common Germ?" *Health* 11 [November 21, 1997]: 90, 92–94.)

48. Health care costs for smokers at a given age are as much as 40% higher than those of nonsmokers. In a population in which no one smoked, the (health care) costs would be 7% higher for men and 4% higher for women. If all smokers quit, health care costs would be lower at first, but after 15 years, they would be higher. Over the long term, complete smoking cessation would cause a net increase in health care costs. (Barendregt, Jan J., Luc Bonneux, and Paul J. van der Maas. "The Health Care Costs of Smoking." *New England Journal of Medicine* 337 [October 9, 1997]: 1,052–1,057.)

49. Vita, Anthony J., Richard B. Terry, Helen B. Hubert, and James F. Fries. "Aging, Health Risks, and Cumulative Disability." *New England Journal of Medicine* 338 (April 9, 1998): 1,035–1,041.

50. U.S. Census Bureau. "Annual Capital Expenditures 2005." *http://www.census.gov/csd/ace/xls/2005/ace-05.pdf,* retrieved July 31, 2007.

51. Skinner, Jonathan, James N. Weinstein, Scott M. Sporer, and John E. Wennberg. "Racial, Ethnic, and Geographic Disparities in Rates of Knee Arthroplasty Among Medicare Patients." *New England Journal of Medicine* 349 (2003):1,350–1,359.

52. The Center for Evaluative Clinical Services, Dartmouth Medical School. *The Dartmouth Atlas of Health Care in the United States,* 115. Chicago: American Hospital Publishing, 1998.

53. Cohn, Victor. "Study Says Some Coronary Bypasses Are Unneeded." *The Washington Post,* October 27, 1983, A5.

54. Killip, Thomas. "Twenty Years of Coronary Bypass Surgery." *New England Journal of Medicine* 319 (August 11, 1988): 368.

55. Schneider, Eric C., Lucian L. Leape, Joel S. Weissman, Robert N. Plana, Constantine Gatsonis, and Arnold M. Epstein. "Racial Differences in Cardiac Revascularization Rates: Does 'Overuse' Explain Higher Rates Among White Patients?" *Annals of Internal Medicine* 135, 5 (September 4, 2001): 328–337.

56. "Medicare CABG Centers Chosen." *Health Policy Week* 20 (February 4, 1991): 1–2.

57. Weissenstein, Eric. "HCFA to Expand CABG Project, Add Others." *Modern Healthcare* 26 (February 5, 1996): 18–19.

58. Ho, Vivian, and Laura A. Peterson. "Estimating Cost Savings from Regionalizing Cardiac Procedures Using Hospital Discharge Data." *BioMed Central* 5 (2007): 7. *http://www.resource-allocation.com/content/5/1/7,* retrieved July 30, 2007.

59. Hartz, Arthur J., Jose S. Pulido, and Evelyn M. Kuhn. "Are the Best Coronary Artery Bypass Surgeons Identified by Physician Surveys?" *American Journal of Public Health* 87 (October 1997): 1,645–1,648.

60. Squires, Sally. "In Angioplasty, Experience Counts: Study Finds Higher Rate of Complications Among Doctors Who Perform Few of These Procedures." *The Washington Post,* November 19, 1996, Health, 11.

61. Agency for Health Care Policy and Research. "Longer-Practicing Physicians May Hospitalize More Patients Unnecessarily." *Research Activities* 136 (December 1990): 3.

62. Goodwin, James S., Jean L. Freeman, Daniel Freeman, and Ann B. Nattinger. "Geographic Variations in Breast Cancer Mortality: Do Higher Rates Imply Elevated Incidence or Poorer Survival?" *American Journal of Public Health* 88 (March 1998): 458–460.

63. Bunker, John P., Jinnet Fowles, and Ralph Schaffarzick. "Evaluation of Medical Technology Strategies: Effects of Coverage and Reimbursement." *New England Journal of Medicine* 306 (March 11, 1982): 622–623.

64. Kaden, Raymond J. "Ensuring Adequate Payment for New Technology." *Health Care Financial Management* 52 (February 1998): 46–50, 52.

65. Appleby, Chuck. "MRI's Second Chance." *Hospitals* 69 (April 20, 1995): 40–42.

66. Steiner, Claudia A., Neil R. Powe, Gerard F. Anderson, and Abhik Das. "Technology Coverage Decisions by Health Care Plans and Considerations by Medical Directors." *Medical Care* 35 (1997): 472. A contrasting view of technology availability in fee-for-service insurance compared with HMOs is found in Ramsey, Scott D., and Mark V. Pauly. "Structural Incentives and Adoption of Medical Technologies in HMO and Fee-for-Service Health Insurance Plans." *Inquiry* 34 (Fall 1997): 228–236.

67. Russell, Louise B., and Jane E. Sisk. "Medical Technology in the United States: The Last Decade." *International Journal of Technology Assessment in Health Care* 4 (1988): 280–282.

68. "Medicare Program: Criteria and Procedures for Making Medical Services Coverage Decisions that Relate to Health Care Technology. Proposed Rule. 42 CFR Parts 400 and 405." *Federal Register* 54 (January 30, 1989): 4,302–4,318.

69. "Section 405.201(a) (1). Subpart B—Medical Services Coverage Decisions that Relate to Health Care Technology." *Code of Federal Regulations,* pt. 42, ch. IV, 42. Washington, DC: Office of the Federal Register, October 1997.

70. Medicaid Organ Transplant and Experimental/Investigational Services Survey. Helena, MT: Montana Department of Public Health & Human Services, 1997.

71. Newhouse, John P. "An Iconoclastic View of Health Cost Containment." *Health Affairs 1993* (12, Suppl.): 164–165. A 1982 survey found that 51% of respondents were unwilling "to limit the opportunities for people to use expensive modern technology"; another 14% were uncertain. Most respondents were willing, however, to consider a change in the health care system that might reduce costs, such as having routine illnesses treated by a nurse or a physician assistant rather than by a doctor, and going to a clinic that assigned a patient to any available doctor rather than the patient's own private doctor. (Reinhold, Robert. "Majority in Survey on Health Care Are Open to Changes to Cut Costs." *The New York Times,* March 29, 1982, A2, D11.)

72. "Report Says Physicians, Hospitals Locked in 'Medical Arms Race.'" *Hospitals & Health Networks* 81, 1 (January 2007): 71–72.

73. Kozak, Lola Jean, Margaret Jean Hall, Robert Pokras, and Linda Lawrence. "Ambulatory Surgery in the United States, 1994." *Advance Data* 283 (March 14, 1997): 3. National Center for Health Statistics, Centers for Disease Control and Prevention, U.S. Department of Health and Human Services.

74. Robinson, Michele L. "Turf Battle Rocks Radiology." *Hospitals* 63 (November 5, 1989): 47.

75. Marcus, Mary Brophy. "The Spotlight Grows on Outpatient Surgery." *USA Today,* July 31, 2007. *http:www.usatoday.com/news/health/2007-07-29-outpatient-surgery_N.htm,* retrieved July 31, 2007.

76. Carrington, Catherine. "Finding a Gentler Way to Mend the Heart." *Health Measures* 2 (March 1997): 35–36, 41.

77. Robinson, Michele L. "Turf Battle Rocks Radiology," 47. A 1988 study by the American College of Radiology found that 60% of imaging studies were done outside the acute care hospital by nonradiologists.

78. Darr, Kurt. "Physician Entrepreneurs and General Acute-Care Hospitals - Part I." *Hospital Topics* 83, 3 (Summer 2005): 33–35; Darr, Kurt. "Physician Entrepreneurs and General Acute-Care Hospitals - Part II." *Hospital Topics* 83, 4 (Fall 2005): 29–31.

79. Medical Device Amendments of 1976, PL 94-295, 90 Stat. 539 (1976); Safe Medical Device Act of 1990, PL 101-629, 104 Stat. 4511 (1990).

80. *Medical Device Amendments of 1976.* Centers for Disease Control and Prevention. *http://wwwn.cdc.gov/cliac/pdf/Addenda/cliac0204/Addendum%20B_Post-market%20Activities_FDA.pdf,* retrieved February 5, 2008.

81. U.S. Department of Health and Human Services, Food and Drug Administration. Device Classes. *http://www.fda.gov/cdrh/devadvice/3123.html#class_3,* retrieved July 31, 2007.

82. *FORM FDA 2438g (12/03).* Food and Drug Administration. *http://www.fda.gov/cdrh/comp/guidance/7382.845.p1.pdf,* retrieved February 5, 2008.

83. Sloane, Elliot B. "Subacute: New Equipment, New Maintenance Concerns." *Nursing Homes* 44 (October 1995): 27.

84. U.S. Department of Health and Human Services, Food and Drug Administration. "Is the Product a Medical Device?" *http://www.fda.gov/cdrh/devadvice/312.html,* retrieved August 20, 2007.

85. U.S. Department of Health and Human Services, Food and Drug Administration. *http://www.accessdata.fda.gov/scripts/cdrh/cfdocs/cfcfr/CFRSearch.cfm,* retrieved July 31, 2007; U.S. Department of Health and Human Services, Food and Drug Administration. Title 21—Food and Drugs. [Code of Federal Regulations] [Title 21, Volume 8] [Revised as of April 1, 2006] [Cite: 21CFR814.82] *http://www.accessdata.fda.gov/scripts.cdrh/cfdocs/cfcfr/CFRSearch.cfm?fr=814.82,* retrieved July 31, 2007.

86. U.S. Department of Health and Human Services, Food and Drug Administration. *http://www.accessdata.fda.gov/scripts/cdrh/cfdocs/cfcfr/CFRSearch.cfm,* retrieved July 31, 2007.

87. Association for the Advancement of Medical Instrumentation. "Certification Leadership: The International Certification Commission (ICC)." *http://www.aami.org/certification/leadership.html,* retrieved

July 31, 2007; Association for the Advancement of Medical Instrumentation. "About AAMI." *http://www.aami.org/about/index.html,* retrieved July 31, 2007.

88. Lashof, Joyce C. "Government Approaches to the Management of Medical Technology." *Bulletin of the New York Academy of Medicine* 57 (January/February 1981): 40–41.

89. Lashof, "Government Approaches," 41.

90. Committee on Ways and Means, U.S. House of Representatives. *1998 Green Book Appendix D. Medicare Reimbursement to Hospitals.* Washington, DC: U.S. House of Representatives, 1998.

91. Bradley, Elizabeth H. "From Adversary to Partner: Have Quality Improvement Organizations Made the Transition?" LookSmart, Health Services Research. April 2005, p. 2. *http://findarticles.com/p/articles/mi_m4149/is_2_40/ai_n13720101/print,* retrieved July 16, 2007.

92. National Health Planning and Resources Development Act of 1974, PL 93-641, 88 Stat. 2225 (1974).

93. Cohen, Alan B., and Donald R. Cohodes. "Certificate of Need and Low Capital-Cost Medical Technology." *Milbank Memorial Fund Quarterly* 60 (Spring 1982): 307–328.

94. Brice, Cindy L., and Kathryn Ellen Cline. "The Supply and Use of Selected Medical Technologies." *Health Affairs* 17 (January/February 1998): 17. An example is Pennsylvania, where MRIs more than doubled between 1988 and 1993, to a total of 187 machines. Many were underused; now MRIs must operate at 85% of capacity before additional units are approved.

95. Canadian Institute for Health Information. "MRI Scanners in Canada Used More Intensively than Those in the United States and England." *http://www.cihi.ca/cihiweb/dispPage.jsp?cw_page=media_08feb2006_e,* retrieved August 1, 2007.

96. *Comprehensive Accreditation Manual for Hospitals (CAMH).* The Joint Commission. *http://www.jointcommission.org/AccreditationPrograms/Hospitals/Standards/FAQs/default.htm,* retrieved February 5, 2008.

97. Kantner, Rob. "ISO 9000—Quality Standards." *Global Opportunity* (1995): 62–66. (ISO is a nickname [a variant of *isos,* a Greek word meaning equal] and is not an acronym for the International Organization for Standardization.)

98. Perry, Seymour. "Technology Assessment in Health Care: The U.S. Perspective." *Health Policy* 9 (1988): 318.

99. Institute of Medicine, Committee for Evaluating Medical Technologies in Clinical Use. *Assessing Medical Technologies,* 9, 37. Washington, DC: National Academy Press, 1985.

100. Perry, Seymour, and Barbara Pillar. "A National Policy for Health Care Technology Assessment." *Medical Care Review* 47 (Winter 1990): 408.

101. Perry, Seymour, and Mae Thamer. "Health Technology Assessment: Decentralized and Fragmented in the U.S. Compared to Other Countries." *Health Policy* 40 (1997): 181.

102. Cohen, Alan B., and Ruth S. Hanft. *Technology in American Health Care: Policy Directions for Effective Evaluation and Management,* 220. Ann Arbor, MI: The University of Michigan Press, 2004.

103. U.S. National Institutes of Health. National Library of Medicine, National Information Center on Health Services Research and Health Care Technology. "HTA 101: Selected Issues in HTA." June 6, 2007. *http://www.nlm.nih.gov/nichsr/hta101/ta101012.html#Heading50,* retrieved August 1, 2007.

104. A concise discussion of consensus development conferences is found in Jacoby, Itzhak. "Update on Assessment Activities: United States Perspective." *International Journal of Technology Assessment in Health Care* 4 (1988): 100–101.

105. Institute of Medicine, Committee for Evaluating Medical Technologies in Clinical Use. *Assessing Medical Technologies,* 9, 70–175. Washington, DC: National Academy Press, 1985.

106. Office of Technology Assessment, U.S. Congress. *The OTA Health Program.* Washington, DC: Office of Technology Assessment, 1989.

107. Bimber, Bruce. *The Politics of Expertise in Congress,* 69. Albany, NY: State University of New York Press, 1996.

108. Health Services Research, Health Statistics, and Health Care Technology Act of 1978, PL 95-623, 92 Stat. 334 (1978).

109. Perry, "Technology Assessment," 320.

110. Perry and Thamer, "Health Technology Assessment," 194.

111. National Center for Health Services Research and Health Care Technology Assessment. *Program Pro-*

file: Office of Technology Assessment, 2. Washington, DC: U.S. Department of Health and Human Services, 1988.

112. Department of Health and Human Services, Agency for Healthcare Research and Quality. "AHRQ Plays an Important Role in Health Technology Assessment." *Research Activities* 264 (August 2002). *http://www.ahrq.gov/research/aug02/,* retrieved August 1, 2007.

113. U.S. National Institutes of Health. National Library of Medicine. National Information Center on Health Services Research and Health Care Technology. "HTA 101: Selected Issues in HTA." *http://www.nlm .nih.gov/nichsr/hta01/ta101012.html#Heading50,* retrieved August 1, 2007.

114. Department of Health and Human Services, Agency for Healthcare Research and Quality. "Final Fiscal Year 2005 GPRA Annual Performance Plan." *http://www.ahrq.gov/about/gpra2005/,* retrieved August 1, 2007.

115. Department of Health and Human Services, Agency for Healthcare Research and Quality. "Final Fiscal Year 2005 GPRA Annual Performance Plan."

116. Greene, Jan. "An Agency for Change." *Hospitals & Health Networks* 71 (October 20, 1997): 68, 70.

117. Department of Health and Human Services, Agency for Health Care Policy and Research. "AHCPR to Collaborate with AMA and AAHP to Develop a National Guideline Clearinghouse." *Research Activities* 205 (June 1997): 16. The National Guideline Clearinghouse is a public resource that can be accessed at www.guideline.gov.

118. Perry and Thamer, "Health Technology Assessment," 196.

119. Perry and Thamer, "Health Technology Assessment," 181.

120. Rogers, T. Lynn, Jr. "Hospital Based Technology Assessment." *Journal of Clinical Engineering* 27, 4 (Fall 2002): 277.

121. Perry, "Technology Assessment," 323.

122. Carrington, Catherine. "Community Hospitals Balance Progress and Costs." *Health Measures* 2 (March 1997): 9.

123. Sanders, Charles A. "Taming the Technological Tiger." *Trustee* 31 (March 1978): 24.

124. *Health Devices Sourcebook—The Hospital Purchasing Guide,* B 457. Plymouth Meeting, PA: ECRI, 1990.

125. Healthcare Advisory Board Company. "Technology Assessment Compendium 2007: Reference Guide to Emerging Clinical Innovations." *http://www.advisory.com/members/default.asp?contentid=67312 &collectionid=932&program=14,* retrieved August 1, 2007.

126. Sanders, "Taming the Technological Tiger."

127. *Health Devices Sourcebook,* B 407.

128. *Health Devices Sourcebook,* 1998, B 456.

129. Sg2. "Cardiovascular Services: Care Delivery Innovations Briefing 2004." *http://www.sg2.com/sg2 _docs/briefings/Edge_Briefing_Cardiovascular_Services_CDI_01002004.pdf,* retrieved August 1, 2007.

130. Coile, Russell C., Jr. "The 'Racer's Edge' in Hospital Competition: Strategic Technology Plan." *Healthcare Executive* 5 (January/February 1990): 22.

131. Anderson, Howard J. "Survey Identifies Technology Trends." *Medical Staff Leader* (October 1990): 30–33.

132. Miccio, Joseph A. "The Migration of Medical Technology." *Healthcare Forum Journal* (September/ October 1989): 24.

133. McKee, Michael, and L. Rita Fritz. "Team Up for Technology Assessment." *Hospitals* 53 (June 1, 1979): 119–122.

134. American Hospital Association. "Trustee Development Program: The Board's Role in the Planning and Acquisition of Clinical Technology." *Trustee* 32 (June 1979): 47–55.

135. Lodge, Denver A. "Someone Must Guide Technology Acquisition." *Modern Healthcare* 22 (December 7, 1992): 21.

136. Heller, Ori. "The New Role of Chief Technology Officer in U.S. Hospitals." *International Journal of Technology Management* 7 (Special Issue on the Strategic Management of Information and Telecommunications Technology, 1992): 455–461.

137. Shaffer, Michael D., and Michael J. Shaffer. "Technical Support for Biomedical Equipment and Decision Making." *Hospital Topics* 73 (Spring 1995): 35–41.

138. Uphoff, Mary Ellen, Thomas Ratko, and Karl Matuszewski, "Making Technology Assessment Count." *Health Measures* 2 (March 1997): 22.

139. Uphoff, Ratko, and Matuszewski, "Making Technology Assessment Count," 24.

140. Rogers, T. Lynn. "Hospital Based Technology Assessment." *Journal of Clinical Engineering* 27, 4 (Fall 2002): 278–279.

141. Blumberg, Donald F. "Evaluating Technology Service Options: Technology Services for Healthcare Organizations." *Healthcare Financial Management* 51 (May 1997): 72.

142. Heller, "The New Role of Chief Technology Officer."

143. *Comprehensive Accreditation Manual for Hospitals, Refreshed Core, EC 20-21.* Oakbrook Terrace, IL: Joint Commission on Accreditation of Healthcare Organizations, January 2007.

144. Blumberg, "Evaluating Technology Service Options," 72–74, 76, 78–79.

145. DeVivo, L., P. Derrico, D. Tomaiuolo, C. Capussotto, and A. Reali. "Evaluating Alternative Service Contracts for Medical Equipment." In *Proceedings of the 26th Annual International Conference of the IEEE EMBS.* San Francisco, September 1–5, 2004. *http://ieeexplore.ieee.org/iel5/9639/30463/01403978 .pdf?arnumber=1403978,* retrieved August 3, 2007.

146. Solovy, Alden. "No, You Do It." *Hospitals & Health Networks* 70 (October 20, 1996): 40–46.

147. Kasti, Mohamad S. "The Future of Clinical Engineering Practice: ACCE's Vision 2000." *Biomedical Instrumentation and Technology* 30 (November/December 1996): 490–495.

148. Spears, Jack. "Justice vs. GE: Two Sides to Every Story." *Healthcare Technology Management* 7 (October 1996): 5.

149. Keil, Ode R. "Accreditation and Clinical Engineering." *Journal of Clinical Engineering* (July/August 1996): 258–260.

150. Keil, Ode R. "Is Preventive Maintenance Still a Core Element of Clinical Engineering?" *Biomedical Instrumentation & Technology* 29 (July/August 1997): 408–409.

151. Ridgeway, Malcolm. "Changes in Industry Bring Opportunity." *Health Technology Management* 7 (October 1996): 48.

152. Shaffer, Michael J. "The Reengineering of Clinical Engineering." *Biomedical Instrumentation & Technology* 31 (March/April 1997): 178.

153. Rogers, T. Lynn. "Hospital Based Technology Assessment," 279.

154. Lando, MaryAnn. "Information Technology 101: What Every CEO Needs To Know." *Healthcare Executive* 13 (May/June 1998): 16–20.

155. Starr, Paul. "Smart Technology, Stunted Policy: Developing Health Information Networks." *Health Affairs* 16 (May/June 1997): 94.

156. Menduno, Michael. "Prognosis: Wired." *Hospitals & Health Networks* 72 (November 5, 1998): 2–30, 32–35.

157. U.S. Department of Health and Human Services and the Lewin Group. "Health Information Technology Leadership Panel Final Report." March 2005, p. 2. *http://www.hhs.gov/healthit/HITFinalReport.pdf,* retrieved July 30, 2007.

158. U.S. Department of Health and Human Services and the Lewin Group. "Health Information Technology Leadership Panel Final Report," 26.

159. Rand Health. "Health Information Technology: Can HIT Lower Costs and Improve Quality?" *2005. http://www.rand.org/pubs/research_briefs/RB9136/RAND_RB9136.pdf,* retrieved July 30, 2007.

160. U.S. Department of Health and Human Services and the Lewin Group. "Health Information Technology Leadership Panel: Final Report," 29.

161. Cohen, Michael R., and Margret Amatayakul. "Noble Concept." Advance Online Editions for Health Information Executives. *http://health-care-it.advanceweb.com/Common/editorial/editorial.aspx?CC =52106,* retrieved August 10, 2007.

162. Ferris, Nancy. "Regional Health Information Networks Gain Traction." June 9, 2005. *http://govhealth it.com/article89134-06-09-05-Web,* retrieved August 10, 2007.

163. "A State Policy Approach: Promoting Health Information Technology in California." February 2007. *http://www.lao.ca.gov/2007/health_info_tech/health_info_tech_021307.aspx,* retrieved August 10, 2007.

164. California Regional Health Information Organization. "About Us." *http://www.calrhio.org/?cridx=2,* retrieved August 10, 2007.

165. "A State Policy Approach: Promoting Health Information Technology in California." February 2007. *http://www.lao.ca.gov/2007/health_info_tech/health_info_tech_021307.aspx,* retrieved August 10, 2007.

166. Ferris, Nancy. "Regional Health Information Networks Gain Traction."

167. Muldoon, Jeannine D., and Joseph L. Sardinas, Jr. "Confidentiality, Privacy, and Restrictions for Computer-Based Patient Records." *Hospital Topics* 74 (Summer 1996): 32.

168. Kleinke, J.D. "Release 0.0: Clinical Information Technology in the Real World." *Health Affairs* 17 (November/December 1998): 29.

169. Starr, Paul. "Smart Technology, Stunted Policy: Developing Health Information Networks." *Health Affairs* 16 (May/June 1997): 102–103.

170. Mohr, David. "The Mayo Clinic EMR: What, When, How, Why?" PowerPoint presentation at the 2007 MN e-Health Summit: Lessons Learned Breakout Session. June 28, 2007.

171. Plex On-Line Resources. "Managed Care Glossary of Terms: Medical Informatics." *http://www.plexis web.com/glossary/words/m2.html,* retrieved August 10, 2007.

172. Umbdenstock, Rich. "Health IT Poses Major Challenges, but the Reward Is Worth Hospitals' Effort." *AHA News* 43, 13 (June 25, 2007): 4. An article discussing the problems of implementing an electronic medical record in a department of family and preventive medicine is Cacy, Jim, Frank Lawler, Nancy Viviani, and Donna Wells. "The Sixth Level of Electronic Health Records: A Look Beyond the Screen." *M.D. Computing* 14 (January/February 1997): 46–49.

173. McDonald, Clement J. "The Barriers to Electronic Medical Record Systems and How to Overcome Them." *Journal of the American Medical Informatics Association* 4 (May/June 1997): 213–221.

174. Pestotnik, Stanley L., David C. Classen, R. Scott Evans, and John P. Burke. "Implementing Antibiotic Practice Guidelines Through Computer-Assisted Decision Support: Clinical and Financial Outcomes." *Annals of Internal Medicine* 124 (May 15, 1996): 884–890.

175. Tierney, William M., J. Marc Overhage, and Clement J. McDonald. "Demonstrating the Effects of an IAIMS on Health Care Quality and Cost." *Journal of the American Medical Informatics Association* 4 (March/April 1997 [Suppl.]): S41–S46.

176. McDonald, Clement J. "The Barriers to Electronic Medical Record Systems and How to Overcome Them," 218.

177. Sangster, William M., and Robert H. Hodge. "Electronic Documentation vs. Dictation: How Do They Compare?" *Physician Executive* (March/April 2003). *http://findarticles.com/p/articles/mi_m0843/is _2_29/ai_99129944,* retrieved August 10, 2007.

178. Potts, Jerry F. "Electronic Medical Records: More Information but Less Access?" *Postgraduate Medicine* 101 (February 1997): 31–32.

179. Potts, "Electronic Medical Records," 35.

180. Potts, "Electronic Medical Records," 36.

181. McDonald, Clement J. "The Barriers to Electronic Medical Record Systems and How to Overcome Them," 218.

182. Swanson, Todd, Julie Dostal, Brad Eichhorst, Clarence Jernigan, Mark Knox, and Kevin Roper. "Recent Implementations of Electronic Medical Records in Four Family Practice Residency Programs." *Academic Medicine* 72 (July 1997): 611.

183. Gardner, Martin. "Information Retrieval for Patient Care." *British Medical Journal* 314 (March 29, 1997): 350–353.

184. Swanson, Dostal, Eichhorst, Jernigan, Knox, and Roper, "Recent Implementations."

185. McDonald, "The Barriers to Electronic," 219.

186. McMenamin, Joseph P. "Telemedicine: Technology and the Law." *For the Defense* 39 (July 1997): 13.

187. American Telemedicine Association. "ATA Defining Telemedicine." *http://www.atmeda.org/news/ definition.html,* retrieved August 10, 2007.

188. Elabd, Sonia. "Long-Distance Diagnosis—A Closer Look at Teleradiology." *Radiology Today. http:// www.radiologytoday.net/archive/rt_051004p20.shtml,* retrieved August 10, 2007.

189. Campbell, Sandy. "Will Telemedicine Become as Common as the Stethoscope?" *Health Care Strategic Management* 15 (April 1997): 1, 20–23.

190. Perednia, Douglas A., and Ace Allen. "Telemedicine Technology and Clinical Applications." *Journal of the American Medical Association* 273 (February 8, 1995): 483.

191. "Balancing Hospital Productivity, Health Care Utilization and Medical Expenditures." *Health Care Strategic Management* 15 (March 1997): 12.
192. Perednia and Allen. "Telemedicine Technology," 483–488.
193. Gray, Gayle A., H. Hudnall Stamm, Sarah Toevs, Uwe Reischl, and Diane Yarrington. "Study of Participating and Nonparticipating States' Telemedicine Medicaid Reimbursement Status: Its Impact on Idaho's Policymaking Process." *Telemedicine and e-Health* 12, 6 (2006): 681–690.
194. Whitten, Pamela S., Frances S. Mair, Alan Haycox, Carl R. May, Tracy I. Williams, and Seth Hellmich. "Systematic Review of Cost Effectiveness Studies of Telemedicine Interventions." *British Medical Journal* 324 (June 15, 2002): 1,434–1,437.
195. Zambuto, Raymond P. "Current Health Care Trends and Their Impact on Clinical Engineering." *Biomedical Instrumentation & Technology* 31 (May/June 1997): 233–234.
196. Sandrick, Karen. "Interview with John E. Abele." *Hospitals & Health Networks* 70 (January 5, 1996): 28–30.
197. Jaklevik, Mary C. "Internet Technology Moves to Patient Care Front Lines." *Modern Healthcare* 26 (March 11, 1996): 47–50.
198. Higgins, Thomas L. "Severity of Illness Indices and Outcome Prediction: Development and Evaluation." In *Textbook of Critical Care,* 4th ed., edited by Ake Grenvik, Stephen M. Ayres, Peter R. Holbrook, and William C. Shoemaker, 2,069–2,083. Philadelphia: W.B. Saunders, 2000.
199. "Inforum" brochure, Nashville, TN, 1994.
200. Steven, Peter. "All Roads Lead to the Electronic Patient Record." *Healthcare Technology Management* 7 (December 1996): 33–35.
201. Moukheiber, Zina. "A Hail of Silver Bullets." *Forbes* 161 (January 26, 1998): 76–81.
202. Welch, H. Gilbert, Lisa Schwartz, and Steven Woloshin. "What's Making Us Sick Is an Epidemic of Diagnoses." *The New York Times,* January 2, 2007, F1.

4

Ethical and Legal Environment

This chapter considers the ethical and legal environment of health services management. The relationships between ethics and the law are numerous, varied, and often dynamic.

The value system (moral framework) of a society is the context from which both ethics and law arise. Ethics is also the study of standards of conduct and moral judgment. In this respect, ethics is both a source for the law and a function of the law. With respect to a profession, ethics are the group's principles or code. Law is a system of principles and rules for human conduct that arises from a society's value system, is prescribed or recognized by society, and is enforced by public authority. This definition applies to both criminal and civil law.

Criminal law has a moral underpinning in that it reflects society's value system in terms of right and wrong—its moral code, or ethics. This also is true for civil law, which governs organizational and individual relationships such as contracts and malfeasance, including medical malpractice. Here, however, the underlying moral principles are more obscure.

Society and the Law

Some societies have regarded the law as a gift from the gods; Plato's Greece is an example. Plato considered written law an oversimplification that could not account for nuances, conditions, and differences among people and situations in a dispute. He believed that the best method of resolving a dispute was one in which a philosopher applied an unwritten law. His own experiences proved this impossible in practice, however, and Plato later accepted a written form of law in which the authorities become servants of the law and administer it without regard to the parties in dispute.[1] This principle of "a rule of law, not of men" is reflected in the Anglo-American legal system.

Beyond the written law, which reflects the most significant concerns of society, are other considerations. There are times when orderliness and continuity must yield to justice or fairness. Aristotle recognized the importance of unwritten law that incorporates concepts of justice too elusive or varied in their application to be readily codified.[2] Known as chancery, this concept of justice was established in England. American legal practice uses a similar concept, called equity, in which courts seek to do justice to parties in a dispute that is unique and unlikely to recur. Such a principle of law permits the right (fair) result to occur in a case in which blindly following the law would provide no remedy or one that is unsatisfactory.

Bodenheimer, a scholar of jurisprudence, divides sources of law into two major categories, formal and nonformal.

> By formal sources, we mean sources which are available in an articulated textual formulation embodied in an authoritative legal document. The chief examples of such formal sources are constitutions and statutes, executive orders, administrative regulations, ordinances, charters and bylaws of autonomous or semiautonomous bodies, treaties and certain other agreements, and judicial precedents. By nonformal sources we mean legally significant materials and considerations which have not received an authoritative or at least articulated formulation and embodiment in a formalized legal document. Without necessarily claiming exhaustive completeness for this enumeration, we have subdivided the nonformal sources into standards of justice, principles of reason and consideration of the nature of things *(natura rerum),* individual equity, public policies, moral convictions, social trends, and customary law.[3]

Health services organizations (HSOs) and health systems (HSs) use charters and bylaws of autonomous or semiautonomous bodies as formal sources of law. Courts look to these documents to determine the rights and obligations of those who are affected. State governments issue charters that establish corporations and create other types of organizations sanctioned by the law.

Bodenheimer's definition of *formal sources of law* includes the codes of ethics adopted by professional associations. Written codes with interpretations that guide application and decision making have the virtues of consistency and predictability. Commonly, professional codes of ethics set a higher standard than does the law. They state the profession's mission and philosophy, its goals and strivings, and minimally acceptable behavior. Formal sources of law supersede nonformal sources, except when the former lack comprehensiveness or require interpretation. All types of formal law—even treaties between the United States and foreign countries—may affect HSOs/HSs and their managers. Processes that produce the law are described in Chapter 1. Law is the basic grounding for society. Artistotle stated it well over two millennia ago when he wrote "for law is order, and good law is good order."[4]

▬ Relationship of Law to Ethics ▬

As a general rule, democratically derived laws reflect the majority's views of justice and fairness. Some in society may consider a law unjust or immoral and risk or invite punishment by breaking it. Classic contemporary examples are the widespread recreational use of marijuana and engaging in civil disobedience to protest government or private actions that are deemed morally wrong.

It is not necessarily true that what is lawful is ethical and what is unlawful is unethical. The law is the minimum performance expected in society. Professions demand that their members obey the law but simultaneously hold them to a higher standard. Thus, a profession's code of ethics requires members to act in ways different from members of society.

Henderson's models identify relationships of law and ethics.[5] Figure 4.1 shows the succession of events that results in public scrutiny of corporate decisions and a determination as to whether they are legal, ethical, or both. This judgment is retrospective, despite management's efforts to predict the effects of actions. The model suggests the difficulty of knowing whether those (e.g., law enforcement officials) who will eventually judge the decision will consider it legal and whether those (e.g., a profession or the public) who will eventually judge the decision will consider it ethical. This adds

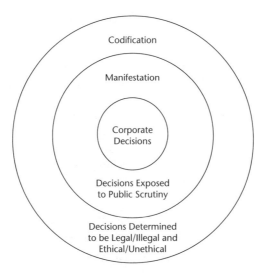

Figure 4.1. The relationship between law and ethics. (Reprinted from Henderson, Verne E. "The Ethical Side of Enterprise." *MIT Sloan Management Review* 23 [Spring 1982]: 37–47. By permission of publisher. Copyright © 1982 by Massachusetts Institute of Technology. All rights reserved.)

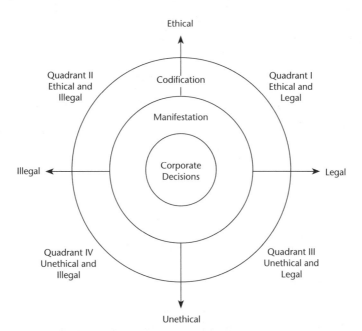

Figure 4.2. A matrix of possible outcomes concerning the ethics and legality of corporate decisions. (Reprinted from Henderson, Verne E. "The Ethical Side of Enterprise." *MIT Sloan Management Review* 23 [Spring 1982]: 37–47. By permission of publisher. Copyright © 1982 by Massachusetts Institute of Technology. All rights reserved.)

uncertainty to HSO/HS decision making. Predicting an action's legality is often easier than predicting whether it will be judged ethical.

Figure 4.2 shows the combinations of legal, illegal, ethical, and unethical factors that are involved in corporate decision making. Decisions made in Quadrant I are ethical and legal and easily identified: managers who obey the law are acting ethically and legally. Quadrant II includes decisions that are ethical but illegal. The American College of Healthcare Executives (ACHE) code of ethics states that obeying the law is minimal ethical conduct. This blanket prohibition means that only compelling moral justification exculpates an illegal act by a health services manager. An example is to disregard a law because obeying it will cause a significant injustice for a patient.

Quadrant III includes decisions that are unethical but legal. This quadrant is often reflected in a profession's code of ethics that requires performance more demanding than the law. Examples include failing to take all reasonable steps to protect patients from medical malpractice and managerial self-aggrandizement to the detriment of patients.

Quadrant IV includes activities that are both illegal and unethical. Examples are easy. Codes of ethics require that the law be obeyed; actions that break the law are both illegal and unethical. Failing to meet fire safety regulations, embezzlement, or knowingly filing a false Medicare report lie in this quadrant.

■ Ethics Framework

Ethical issues arise in all HSOs and HSs. Until recently, applications of medical technology in acute care hospitals were the sources of most significant ethical issues. In the 21st century, however, changes in the locus of care have meant that other types of HSOs increasingly confront ethical issues. The complexity and unique role of HSOs and HSs mean that ethical issues have legal dimensions and that legal issues have ethical aspects. Capable managers see both.

The dynamic relationship between ethics and law is sometimes synergistic, sometimes antagonistic. Each affects and is affected by the other. The law is the basic framework of society and is the context for application of ethics in health services.

MORAL PHILOSOPHIES

Teleology, deontology, and natural law have found extensive application in Western societies. Two other moral philosophies, casuistry and virtue ethics, have experienced a revival and are considered as well. These five moral philosophies provide a basis to study morals (ethics), provide a framework for a personal ethic and an organizational philosophy, and help determine the moral rightness or wrongness of an action.

Teleology

Teleology is derived from *telos*, Greek for *end*. The most prominent moral philosophy using this concept is utility theory; its followers are utilitarians. The underlying premise is that the moral rightness or wrongness of an act or decision is judged by whether it brings into being more good (utility) or ungood (disutility) than alternative decisions. Classical utilitarianism's most prominent proponent was the English philosopher John Stuart Mill (1806–1873). Utilitarians have no independent right or wrong to guide them. They look at the consequences of an act—the "good" is independent of the "right." Utilitarians are sometimes called consequentialists because they judge actions by their consequences.

Utilitarianism is divided into act utility and rule utility. Act utility assesses each decision and determines its consequences when judging moral rightness or wrongness. Act utilitarians judge each action independently, without reference to preestablished guidelines (rules). They measure the amount of good, or (nonmoral) value, brought into being and the amount of evil, or (nonmoral) disvalue, brought into being or avoided by acting on a particular choice. Each person affected is counted equally. This suggests a strong sense of objectivity. Act utilitarianism receives no further attention here because it is episodic and incompatible with developing and deriving the ethical principles needed for codes of ethics and a personal ethic.

Rule utility is more formal. It assesses courses of action (or nonaction) and measures their consequences—the amount of (nonmoral) good or ungood that is produced. The morally superior course of action must be taken, even though it may not produce the most good (or least ungood) in a specific application. Utility theory is the basis for cost–benefit analysis. A crude summary statement describing utilitarianism is "the end justifies the means."

Deontology

Deontology is based on the presence of an independent right or wrong. It does not consider consequences. *Deontology* is derived from *deon*, Greek for *duty*. The best-known proponent of a duty-based moral philosophy was the German philosopher Immanuel Kant (1724–1804). Briefly, Kantian deontology asserts that the end (result) is unimportant because human beings have duties to one another as moral agents, and these duties take precedence over consequences. For Kant, an act is moral if it arises from good will and if, therefore, one acts from a sense of duty. The Kantian test of morality is whether the act can meet the categorical imperative, which requires that we act in accordance with what we wish to become a universal law. The universal law is that what is right or wrong for one person is right or wrong for everyone, in all places and at all times. According to Kant, an action is right only if it can be universalized without violating the equality of human beings. For example, Kantians see it as logically inconsistent to argue that a terminally ill person should be euthanized (actively caused to die), because this is saying that life can be improved by ending it. Deontology may be summarized as never treating human beings simply as a means, but rather always as an end.[6] Another summary of deontology is to practice the Golden Rule, "do unto others as you would have them do unto you."

The work of a contemporary American philosopher, John Rawls (1921–2005), extended Kantian deontology. In *A Theory of Justice*, Rawls used elaborate philosophical constructs to develop the elements of a social contract among free, equal, self-interested, and rational persons. He reasoned that such persons would reject utilitarianism and select instead the concepts of right and justice as necessary to the good.[7]

Natural Law

Natural law states that ethics (morality) must be grounded in a concern for human good and is, therefore, teleological (consequential). Natural law is based on Aristotelian thought as interpreted and synthesized with Christian dogma by St. Thomas Aquinas (1225–1274).[8] It assumes a natural order in relationships and a predisposition among rational persons to do, or refrain from doing, certain things. Because human beings are rational, we are able to discover what we should do, and in that attempt we are guided by a partial notion of the eternal law that is linked to our capacity for rational thought. Because natural law guides what rational persons do, it is the basis for positive law, some of which is reflected in statutes. Natural law contends that the good cannot be defined only in terms of subjective inclinations; rather, there is a good for human beings that is objectively desirable, although not reducible to desire.[9] A summary statement of the basic precepts of natural law is that we should "do good and avoid evil."

Casuistry

Many historical definitions of casuistry are disparaging. Critics argue that it uses evasive reasoning and encourages rationalizations for desired ethical results. Regardless, contemporary advocates see casuistry as a pragmatic way to understand and solve ethical problems. Casuistry is case-based reasoning in historical context. It avoids excessive reliance on principles and rules, which may provide only partial answers and may not guide decision makers comprehensively. Casuistry allows problem solvers to use the concrete circumstances of actual cases and the specific maxims that people invoke in facing actual moral dilemmas.[10]

At base, casuistry is similar to the law, where court cases and the precedents they establish guide decision makers. "Cases in ethics are similar: Normative judgments emerge through majoritarian consensus in society and in institutions because careful attention has been paid to the details of particular problem cases. That consensus then becomes authoritative and is extended to relevantly similar cases."[11] HSOs use casuistry, for example, as ethics committees develop a body of experience with various ethical issues.

Both clinical medicine and management education rely on cases. This makes it natural to use them in health services, in which traditional ethics problem solving has applied moral principles to cases—from the general to the specific, or deductive reasoning. Modern casuists can profitably copy the classical casuists's reliance on paradigm cases, reference to broad consensus, and acceptance of probable certitude—assent to a proposition, but acknowledging that its opposite might be true.[12] Greater numbers of cases in HSOs/HSs and a body of experience will lead to consensus and more certainty in charting moral direction.

Virtue Ethics

Western thought about the importance of virtue can be partially traced to Aristotle. Similar to natural law, virtue is based on theological ethics but without a primary focus on obligations or duties. Like casuistry, it has received more attention, some of which results from a perception that traditional rules, or principle-based moral philosophies, deal inadequately with the realities of ethical decision making. This is to say that rules are of limited help in solving ethical problems. When there are competing ethical rules or situations to which no rules apply, something more than a coin toss is needed. Here, virtue ethicists claim to have a superior moral philosophy.

Contemporary authors argue that virtue ethics has three levels. The first two are observing laws and observing moral rights and fulfilling moral duties that go beyond the law. The third and highest level is the practice of virtue.[13]

> Virtue implies a character trait, an internal disposition habitually to seek moral perfection, to live one's life in accord with a moral law, and to attain a balance between noble intention and just action. . . . In almost any view the virtuous person is someone we can trust to act habitually in a good way—courageously, honestly, justly, wisely, and temperately.[14]

In this view, virtuous physicians (or managers) are disposed to the right and good intrinsic to the practice of their profession and will work for the good of the patient.

Some virtue ethicists argue that, as with any skill or expertise, practice and constant striving to achieve virtuous traits (good works) improve one's ability to be virtuous. Others argue that accepting in one's heart the forgiveness and reconciliation offered by God (faith) "would lead to a new disposition toward God (trust) and the neighbor (love), much as a physician or patient might be judged to be a different (and better) person following changed dispositions toward those persons with whom . . . [they] are involved."[15]

All people should live virtuous lives, but those in the professions have a special obligation to do so. Virtuous managers and physicians are not just virtuous people practicing a profession; they are expected to work for the patient's good even at the expense of personal sacrifice and legitimate self-interest.[16] Virtuous physicians place the good of their patients above their own and seek that good, unless pursuing it imposes an injustice on them or their families or violates their conscience.[17] Similarly, virtuous managers put the good of the patient above their own.

LINKING THEORY AND ACTION[18]

Figure 4.3 shows that principles, rules, and specific judgments and actions rely on or are based on ethical theories. Ethical theories do not necessarily conflict; diverse moral philosophies may

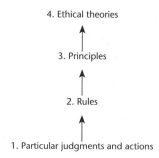

Figure 4.3. Hierarchy of relationships. (From Beauchamp, T.L., and James F. Childress. *Principles of Biomedical Ethics,* 4th ed., 6. New York: Oxford University Press, 1994; reprinted by permission of Oxford University Press, Inc.)

reach the same conclusion about an action, albeit through different reasoning or use of varying constructs.

Ethical theories and derivative principles guide development of rules that produce specific judgments and actions. Four principles should guide health services managers: respect for persons, beneficence, nonmaleficence, and justice. These principles should be reflected in the organization's philosophy, as well as in the manager's personal ethic.

Respect for Persons

The principle of respect for persons has four elements. The first, autonomy, requires that persons act toward others in a way that enables them to be self-governing. To choose and pursue a course of action, people must be rational and uncoerced (unconstrained). Sometimes physical or mental conditions cause people to become nonautonomous. They are owed respect, nonetheless, even though special means are needed to allow them to express their autonomy. Autonomy underlies the need to obtain consent for treatment, as well as the general way HSOs view and interact with patients and staff.

Autonomy is in dynamic tension with paternalism. The Hippocratic oath is antecedent to paternalism in the patient–physician relationship and suggests that physicians should act in their patients' best interests—as physicians judge those interests. Giving autonomy primacy limits paternalism to specific circumstances.

The second element of respect for persons is truth telling, which requires managers to be honest in all they do. At its absolute, truth telling eliminates "white lies," even if knowing the truth causes harm to the person learning it.

Confidentiality, the third element of respect for persons, requires managers and clinicians to keep secret what they learn about patients and others in the course of their work. Legal requirements necessitate morally justified exceptions to confidentiality.

The fourth element is fidelity, defined as doing one's duty or keeping one's word. Sometimes called promise keeping, fidelity, like the other three elements of respect, requires managers to be respectful of persons, whether they are patients, staff, or others.

Beneficence

The second principle, beneficence, is rooted in Hippocratic tradition and is defined as acting with charity and kindness. Contemporary health services applications of beneficence are broader, including a positive duty. Generally, beneficence anchors one end of a continuum, at the opposite end of which is the principle of nonmaleficence, defined as refraining from actions that aggravate a problem or cause other negative results.

Beneficence comprises conferring benefits and balancing benefits and harms. The former is well established in medicine; failing to provide benefits when one can violates an ethical obligation of clinicians. Modified in a way that is consistent with their role, beneficence applies to managers, too. The positive duty suggested by beneficence requires HSOs to do all that they can for patients. There is a lesser duty to aid those who are potential rather than actual patients. Application of this distinction varies with the HSO's values, mission, and vision and with the population served.

The second dimension of beneficence is balancing the benefits and harms of an action. This is the principle of utility, the philosophical basis for cost–benefit and risk–benefit analyses. Utility is but one of several considerations in health services decision making. Its more limited application results from a positive duty to act in the patient's best interests because one cannot act with kindness and charity if risks outweigh benefits. Regardless, utility cannot morally justify overriding patients' interests and sacrificing them to the greater good.

Nonmaleficence

The third principle applicable to managing HSOs is nonmaleficence. It, too, has deep historical roots in medicine. Nonmaleficence can be defined as *primum non nocere*—first, do no harm. This dictum to guide physicians applies to health services managers, too. Nonmaleficence gives rise to specific moral rules, but neither the principle nor any derivative rule is absolute. For example, it may be appropriate (with the patient's consent) to inflict harm (e.g., administer cancer chemotherapy) to avoid worse harm (e.g., a surgical procedure), and it may be appropriate to compromise truth telling if telling the truth would result in significant mental or physical harm.

Nonmaleficence most commonly applies to HSO relationships with patients. It also suggests that managers have duties to staff. Putting staff at unnecessary or extraordinary risk to their health and safety violates a manager's duty to them, even if the result meets the principle of beneficence to patients. Balancing benefits and harms also suggests application of the concept of utility.

Justice

The fourth principle, justice, is important in managerial decision making such as allocating the HSO's resources or developing and applying human resources policies. What is justice, and how does one know when it is achieved? Justice has various definitions. Some definitions require that all persons get their just desserts—what they are due. Rawls defined justice as fairness. But how are just desserts and fairness defined? Aristotle defined justice as equals being treated equally, and unequals unequally—a concept common to public policy analysis. Equal treatment of equals is reflected in liberty rights such as freedom of speech for all. Unequal treatment of people unequally situated is used to justify redistribution of wealth through the tax code. Aristotle's concept of justice is expressed in health services when greater resources are expended on those more ill and with greater needs. These concepts of justice are helpful, but they do not solve problems of definition and opinion that are so troublesome for managers. At a minimum, clinicians and managers act justly if they consistently apply clear and prospectively determined criteria in decision making.

SUMMARY

Moral philosophies and derivative principles provide a framework to hone and apply a personal ethic to analyze and solve ethical problems. Like philosophers, managers are unlikely to adopt one moral philosophy. Most will be eclectic in developing or reconsidering a personal ethic. In general, the principles of respect for persons, beneficence, nonmaleficence, and justice are useful in defining relationships among patients, managers, and organizations. The principles may carry different weights and take precedence over one another, depending on the issue. Justice requires, however, that they be consistently ordered and weighted as similar ethical issues are considered.

Personal Ethic and Professional Codes

The many written and unwritten codes of conduct that guide human behavior arise from family, religious training, professional affiliations and allegiances, and an often ill-defined personal code of moral conduct—an amalgam of intellect, reasoning, experience, education, and relationships. Guidelines may be vague or contradictory. Those solving ethical problems will find many difficult questions and choices but few easy answers. Such situations highlight the necessity of a well-developed, internalized personal ethic.

A personal ethic is a moral framework for decision making that allows persons to refine guidelines, judgments, and actions. Membership in a professional association with a code of ethics and employment in an HSO with an organizational philosophy reflected in values, mission, and vision statements are not substitutes for a coherent, consistent, and comprehensive personal ethic. Each of us is a moral agent whose actions, inactions, and misactions have moral consequences for which responsibility is borne. Morally, one's conduct cannot be excused by claims such as "I was following orders" or "that's not my area of responsibility." Demands from lawfully constituted public authorities pose special problems. Moral agents who judge such orders to be unjust disregard them at their peril and must bear the sanctions that are imposed. Ethical (moral) implications of acts must be considered independently of the acts.

One hallmark of a profession is a code of ethics that distinguishes acceptable from unacceptable behavior. Codes are common in health services, but general language and vague performance standards limit enforceability. It is best to see professional codes of ethics as guides for those seeking to do the right thing but in need of help to determine what that is. Those at the moral fringe of a profession are rarely dissuaded from questionable actions by a code of ethics.

Conflicts may arise between the HSO's ethic, as expressed in its values statement, and a manager's personal ethic. The concept of moral agency should cause managers to think carefully about the implications of acquiescing in specific expressions of an HSO's philosophy. It may seem easier to "go along to get along" than to risk one's position and economic association by speaking out. Failure to speak out when one should, however, violates the duty of moral agency.

State and federal "conscience clause" laws may support individual and institutional values on decisions not to provide certain types of treatment. The presence of such laws is a compelling reason to have fully articulated positions on value-laden medical treatment. For example, 46 states permit individual providers to refuse to participate in abortions; 43 allow religious, private, or in some states, all institutions to refuse to provide abortions.[19] The conscience clause reflected in federal law offers protection to HSOs and their staffs when religious beliefs or moral convictions prohibit performing sterilizations or abortions.[20]

Health Services Codes of Ethics

MANAGERS

American College of Healthcare Executives. The ACHE adopted its first code of ethics in 1939, 6 years after its founding. In its several iterations, the code has become more specific. In 2007, the code had five sections that detail the healthcare executive's responsibilities to the profession, to patients or others served, to the organization, to employees, and to the community and society. The final section charges affiliates with a positive duty to communicate the facts to the committee on ethics when they have reasonable grounds to believe that another affiliate has violated the code.[21] Biomedical ethical issues receive little attention. A major revision in 1987 recognized the concept of moral agent (since changed to *moral advocate*) and recognized a positive duty for affiliates to report violations.

The ACHE publishes ethical policy statements to guide affiliates on issues such as medical records confidentiality, decisions at the end of life, and professional impairment. The committee on ethics investigates allegations and makes recommendations regarding breaches of the code. Expulsion is the maximum disciplinary action.

American College of Health Care Administrators. This code of ethics guides managers of long-term care facilities, usually called nursing facilities. At this writing, the four "expectations" for managers are divided into prescriptions and proscriptions: 1) the welfare of those receiving care is paramount; 2) maintain professional competence; 3) maintain professional posture, holding paramount the interests of facility and residents; and 4) meet responsibilities to public, profession, and colleagues. Specific areas include quality of services; confidentiality of patient information; continuing education; conflicts of interest; and fostering increased knowledge, supporting research, and sharing expertise. Affiliates are expected to provide information to the standards and ethics committee of actual or potential code violations. No enforcement or appeals process is described.[22]

CLINICIANS

Physicians. The American Medical Association (AMA) is the preeminent professional association for allopathic physicians. The AMA's first "Principles of Medical Ethics" was adopted at its founding in 1847 and was based on the code of medical ethics developed by the English physician and philosopher Sir Thomas Percival (1740–1804) in 1803.[23] After several iterations, the 2001 principles emphasize providing competent medical care, honesty in all professional interactions, and safeguarding patient confidences. Members "shall . . . strive to report physicians deficient in character or competence, or engaging in fraud or deception, to appropriate entities."[24] Opinions of the AMA's Council on Ethical and Judicial Affairs assist in interpreting the principles. The 2001 principles continue the trend of recognizing responsibilities and rights that began in 1980. The 1980 iteration was "the opening to an ethics based on notions of rights and responsibilities rather than benefits and harms. It is the first document in the history of professional medical ethics in which a group of physicians is willing to use the language of responsibilities and rights."[25]

Nurses. The "Code for Nurses" was first adopted by the American Nurses Association (ANA) in 1950. The 2001 iteration has nine provisions including various expectations: principles to guide practice, primary commitment to patients' interests, advocating for patients, individual accountability, duties to self and others, improving healthcare, advancing the profession, collaboration, and obligations to the profession. An interpretive statement follows each. Like the ACHE, the American College of Health Care Administrators (ACHCA), and AMA, the ANA code obliges nurses to counter or expose problematic practice: "The nurse promotes, advocates for, and strives to protect the health, safety, and rights of the patient."[26]

INSTITUTIONAL TRADE ASSOCIATIONS

The American Hospital Association (AHA) is the leading trade association for hospitals. The AHA's "Patient Care Partnership" includes high-quality hospital care, a clear and safe environment, involvement in the patient's care, protection of the patient's privacy, help when the patient is leaving the hospital, and help with billing claims.[27]

The American Health Care Association (AHCA) includes for-profit and not-for-profit long-term facilities. The AHCA's code of ethics guides the organization and is a model for state affiliates and their members. Provisions include moral responsibility, good business practice, making difficult choices, acting responsibly, providing quality services, dealing with conflicting values, use of information, responsible advocacy, conflicts of interest, respect for others, and fair competition.[28]

America's Health Insurance Plans's statement of commitment guides member health plans. The three sections are commitments to improve quality, to give all Americans access through public and private coverage and through support for the public health infrastructure, and to improve affordability.[29]

BILLS OF RIGHTS

Patient bills of rights provide guidance about the relationship between health services consumers and HSOs. Organizations that have patient bills of rights include the AHA, The Joint Commission on Accreditation of Healthcare Organizations (The Joint Commisson), the U.S. Department of Veterans Affairs, and the American Civil Liberties Union.[30] They reflect the law regarding confidentiality and consent, and they meet Bodenheimer's definition of a formal source of law, but they have no legal effect. Rather, they set an ethical tone for the HSO's relationships with those it serves. Bills of rights are only as effective as the organization's willingness to make them known and develop processes that encourage and monitor their use.

Ethical Issues Affecting Governance and Management

FIDUCIARY DUTY

The concept of fiduciary arose in Roman jurisprudence. Today, the concept means that in certain relationships, a person in a position of superior knowledge and authority and in whom trust is reposed has obligations and duties toward others. This person is a fiduciary. Ethically (and legally), fiduciary duties arise in many relationships including physician–patient, priest–penitent, attorney–client, and professor–student. Fidelity, an element of respect for persons, beneficence, and nonmaleficence underpin the ethical aspects of fiduciary duty, as well.

Governing body members of for-profit and not-for-profit corporations are fiduciaries and have special obligations.[31] Fiduciaries have primary duties of loyalty and responsibility:

> Loyalty means that the individuals must put the interest of the corporation above all self-interest, a principle based on the biblical doctrine that no man can serve two masters. Specifically no trustee is permitted to gain any secret profits personally, to accept bribes, or to compete with the corporation.[32]

The fiduciary duty of responsibility means that in every governance activity, governing body members must exercise reasonable care, skill, and diligence in proportion to the circumstances. Governing body members can be held personally liable for gross negligence, which can be by acts of commission or omission.[33]

Trustees are fiduciaries responsible for assets held in trust. The law holds them to a very high standard. Trustees may not use their position for personal gain and must act only in the best interests of the beneficiary of the trust. Many governing body members of not-for-profit HSOs/HSs use the title *trustee*, even when they are not true trustees. Unless they are fiduciaries of a trust, the technically correct legal term is *director* or *corporate director*.

One of few federal court cases involving the fiduciary duties of not-for-profit HSO governing body members is *Stern et al. v. Lucy Webb Hayes National Training School of Deaconesses and Missionaries et al.**[34] In ruling on allegations of mismanaging, nonmanaging, self-dealing, and con-

---

*The full legal name of the hospital is The Lucy Webb Hayes National Training School for Deaconesses and Missionaries Conduct Sibley Memorial Hospital.

spiring among themselves and with various financial institutions, the court found no evidence of a conspiracy and determined that Sibley "trustees" were not true trustees and should be held to the lesser, corporate standard of care.[35]

CONFLICTS OF INTEREST

General Considerations

Interests with the potential for conflicts of interest occur in HSOs/HSs in several ways. The self-dealing in the Sibley Hospital case is one type. A conflict of interest occurs, too, when someone has multiple obligations that demand loyalty, and decisions based on these loyalties are different or in conflict. The element of fidelity (promise keeping) assists in ethical analysis of conflicts of interest. The principles of beneficence and nonmaleficence also provide an ethical framework to analyze conflicts of interest.

The ACHE code of ethics states only that the healthcare executive shall "avoid financial and other conflicts of interest," an admonition that provides scant guidance. "Matter of degree" provides useful guidance in determining when a duality of interests has devolved into a presumptive conflict of interest. It is unlikely that a conflict of interest arises when a vendor buys an inexpensive lunch for a manager. An expense-paid, two-week vacation presumptively indicates the presence of a conflict of interest. Large gifts are presumed to encourage or reward certain behavior. Extravagant gifts from vendors and self-dealing by executives are easily identified as causing conflicts of interest. Many are more subtle, however.

Is it ethical for a manager to use a position of influence or power to gain personal aggrandizement of titles and position at the expense of patient care? Is it ethical for a manager to be lax in implementing an effective patient-consent process? Is it ethical for a manager to keep negative information about performance from the governing body? Is it ethical for a manager who believes there are quality-of-care problems in a clinical department to ignore them? Is it ethical for managers who have concerns about their personal ability to meet the demands of their position to remain in it? The conflicts of interest suggested by questions such as these can be understood by continued questioning and self-analysis.

Managed Care

The duality of interests in managed care has an inherent potential for conflicts of interest because the goals, purposes, and objectives—the interests—of managed care organizations (MCOs) often differ from those of their members. Both the MCO and its members want a financially strong, well-functioning organization that meets member needs in a timely and effective manner. Beyond this congruence, there is significant divergence.

Marketing and Operations. The tension among the MCO and its members and potential members occurs as early as initial marketing when benefit packages and market segments are identified. For example, is marketing that focuses on healthy, low-risk people ethical?[36] Perhaps, but only if the MCO ignores high-risk groups because it has a greater duty to current than to potential members.

As a bureaucracy, MCO managers, physicians, and staff seek to maximize position, power, income, and other rewards with least disruption of homeostasis. Achieving these goals, especially maximizing income, may minimize service whether or not this is consistent with mission or contract provisions. The bureaucratic response may even be at variance with long-term survival. The member has a primary interest in retaining or regaining health and paying the least to do so. Members also want to maximize access to services to meet perceived needs. The goals of the MCO and members are congruent when members stay well with minimal costs and use existing services appropriately. It is rarely that simple, however.

MCO marketing must decide if it should "keep its light under a bushel basket." An MCO known as a leader in treating a certain medical condition may be overwhelmed by adverse selection if large numbers of people with, or at risk of, that medical condition enroll. The members of an MCO straining against adverse selection may experience diminished quality, restricted benefits, and increased premiums.

Utilization.   Using services has the greatest potential for conflicts of interest. In this regard, members may be divided into appropriate users and overusers, whether purposefully or not. The MCO's interests and those of appropriate users are congruent. To be competitive, however, overusers must be controlled. Even appropriate users are a potential financial threat to a MCO in a competitive environment. To trim costs, the MCO may seek to make members underusers. This sharpened duality of interests may result is a conflict of interest.

Physician Incentives and Disincentives.   Members will be concerned about subtle and potentially serious constraints that affect MCO-affiliated physicians. There are numerous dual interests among MCOs, members, and physicians. The Hippocratic tradition directs physicians to act in patients' best interests, a paternalistic ethic suggestive of safeguards. Physician treatment decisions are facilitated or inhibited by the MCO. Employment is the clearest example of a self-selection bias— physicians unable to accept the MCO's rules will work elsewhere. Independent physicians in an MCO network or MCO-sponsored independent practice association are less directly controlled, but they are subject to similar constraints. Independent physicians may choose to avoid an inhospitable MCO. The growing percentage of Americans enrolled in managed care may give them little choice but to participate.

MCO-affiliated physicians face numerous behavior-modifying guidelines: limits on referrals (especially out of plan) and hospitalization, financial disincentives (and incentives), quotas on numbers of patients seen (used in staff-model health maintenance organizations [HMOs]), and peer review. Undesirable physician practice patterns may result in various MCO actions. In order of increasing severity, they are data-based peer pressure, letters of warning or admonition, economic incentives or disincentives, nonrenewal, and dismissal. Constraints are positive when they encourage judicious but appropriate use of medical resources, which partly explains why MCOs use fewer ancillary services and hospital days.

The MCO may forgo purchase of high-technology diagnostic and treatment equipment, or it may contract with physicians or hospitals without such technology, strategies that reduce costs. Lower costs that enhance financial integrity and support availability of services make organizational and member interests congruent. This strategy has no advantage for those who might have benefited from an unavailable technology; to them it suggests a conflict of interest. When are constraints excessive and members deprived of needed services? When do constraints infringe on the principles of nonmaleficence and beneficence? Such questions defy simple answers. Constraints are a function of an MCO's willingness, prompted by the manager acting as a moral agent, to institute safeguards that balance competitiveness and financial viability with members' needs.

Minimizing Conflicts of Interest in Managed Care.   How are conflicts of interest prevented or minimized? An indispensable first step is acknowledging the many dual interests present in the relationships among MCOs, members, and physicians. Awareness permits avoiding or minimizing them. In addition, verification is needed. An ombudsman or consumer relations specialist can assist members to receive services they need. There should be readily accessible procedures to review members' concerns. Audits of utilization data and comparisons with other MCOs allow management to determine whether use was appropriate. Awareness of how and where conflicts of interest arise will help prevent them or minimize their effect.[37] These types of activities are essential if managers are to meet their ethical obligations to patients. Federally qualified HMOs must have an effective grievance procedure for members. All such efforts offer protection. They require, however, that members question the adequacy of care, something they may be unable to do.

Confidential Information

HSOs/HSs are rife with confidential information about patients, staff, and the organization. Managers are ethically and legally bound to use this information properly. Conflicts of interest occur if confidential information is used to benefit a manager or other people with whom the manager is associated or related, or to harass or injure.

Misuse of confidential information includes disclosing governing body decisions so that advantageous sales or purchases can be made by the insider's associates, selling or giving patient medical information to the media or attorneys, and providing the HSO's/HS's marketing strategies to competitors. An example that raises potential conflicts of interest and confidential information problems occurs when a manager serves on the governing body of a planning agency or potentially competing HSO/HS. Fidelity to one's own HSO/HS conflicts with the duty to objectively consider another HSO's certificate of need, for example. In addition, and more subtly, the manager becomes privy to information that is important to that manager's own HSO/HS. Duality of interests and antitrust law make cooperating with other HSOs/HSs difficult.

ETHICS AND MARKETING

HSOs/HSs are social enterprises with economic dimensions, not economic enterprises with social dimensions. Nevertheless, all HSOs/HSs market, and they did so long before marketing became acceptable. Marketing occurs in the physicians' hospital lounge, at health fairs, at new employee orientations, and in press releases. Applying the 4 *P*s of marketing—product, price, place, and promotion—to health services is easy; HSOs/HSs find that service, consideration, access, and promotion (SCAP) are more appropriate, however. Competition makes marketing a necessity.

Marketing and advertising raise questions as to how HSOs/HSs can meet their ethical obligations to serve those potentially in need while avoiding the creation of unnecessary demand. AHA guidance on advertising is instructive: "These guidelines are suggested to ensure that healthcare organizations implement their advertising with fairness, honesty, accuracy, and sensitivity to the special trust that exists between patients and healthcare providers."[38]

Responsible marketing is an important if elusive concept. HSOs/HSs whose focus is return on investment will view marketing and competition differently from those with other goals. To be responsible means tempering customers' desires and potential demand for a service with objective judgments of its value and usefulness. HSO/HS decision makers should determine if certain expenditures and goals are more worthy than others, a task consistent with mission statements and their expertise as providers. This approach has a significant element of paternalism.

▬ Biomedical Ethical Issues ▬▬▬▬▬▬▬▬▬▬▬▬▬▬▬▬▬▬▬

RESOURCE ALLOCATION

At both the macro and micro levels, resource allocation embodies the principle of justice. It necessitates making decisions—who gets what, when, and how. Value-laden criteria such as worth, usefulness, merit, and need are commonly used. Government involvement often brings political motives. Like governments, HSOs/HSs use macroallocation to determine what equipment to buy and whether to offer new programs. Microallocation includes a physician's willingness to refer, a patient's geographic access to services and technologies, and economic considerations. Often, micro-level decisions are guided (in a sense, predetermined) by policies and procedures of governments or HSOs/HSs. Often, the "greatest good" (utility) principle of utilitarianism is used for allocation decisions. It is at best a partial answer, because using principles of utility allows us to ignore considerations of need, fairness, and justice.

Numerous allocation theories have been proposed. At one end of a continuum is egalitarianism—the concept that persons are entitled to equal health services. Hyperegalitarianism holds that treatments not available to all should be available to none. At the other end of the continuum is a theory that health services are not a right guaranteed by society; rather, they are a privilege to be earned. This hyperindividualistic position holds that caregivers such as physicians have no obligation to render services but are free to choose to do so. Between these extremes is a view that society is obliged to encourage, develop, and perhaps even provide health services in certain situations. The macroallocation theory espoused by Charles Fried suggests that a "decent minimum" (routine services) should be available to all but that high-technology services are limited in several ways and should be available on a different basis.[39] Microallocation—allocation to persons—theories of exotic lifesaving services have been developed by James Childress and Nicholas Rescher. They consider the problem of how (by what criteria) decisions are to be made about who gets what. Both start by applying medical criteria to determine need and appropriateness for treatment. Then they diverge.[40] Rarely do HSOs/HSs address the ethical issues of resource allocation in an organized, prospective manner. Knowledge of the criteria used in decision making allows the public to know that the system of allocation is fair.

CONSENT

Background. Ethics and law treat consent similarly. The former is more demanding, however. Consent began at law as protecting the right to be free from nonconsensual touching. Ethicists greatly expanded the legal concept of consent, named it autonomy, included it in the principle of respect for persons (and self-determination), and found it reflected in the special relationship of trust and confidence (fiduciary relationship) between physician and patient. Consent reflects Kant's views of the equality of human beings. Ethically and legally, consent must be voluntary, competent, and informed. Ethically, HSOs should independently determine that these criteria are met.

Legal Aspects of Consent. The law recognizes that failing to obtain consent can lead to legal action for battery, an intentional tort. In addition, an action for negligence can be brought if physicians breach a duty to communicate information that the patient needs to make a decision.[41]

Questions of consent arise initially when a patient seeks treatment. Consent can be implied because the patient has sought treatment. Consent is implied, too, in life-threatening emergencies. Elective, routine treatment requires only general consent, as compared with the special consent needed for invasive, surgical, or experimental or unusual types of procedures. The law requires that consent be voluntary, competent, and informed.

Voluntary means that consent is given without duress that substantially influences the decision. Prisoners are a group whose incarceration greatly diminishes their independence; thus it is impossible for them to give voluntary consent to be part of a medical experiment, for example. Voluntariness is diminished if inducements to participate are so great that one becomes greedy, imprudent, and incautious. Similarly, there are circumstances when even small inducements reduce voluntariness; for example, starving people who are offered food may agree to take part in a risky medical experiment.

Beyond such obvious problems, the concept of voluntariness is elusive. Patients may be under duress to accept a physician's recommendations because they fear being seen as difficult and losing the physician's goodwill and cooperation. Patients are influenced by family and friends and may be persuaded (even coerced) by them to accept (or reject) treatment. It has been suggested that one's freedom to accept or reject medical treatment is reduced to only that of the right to veto unwanted procedures.[42]

Competent consent means that the patient knows the nature and consequences of what is contemplated or the decision to be made. The law presumes that an unemancipated minor is incompetent, as is an individual with a mental illness or a developmental disability.

The third element of consent is that it must be informed. Some discussions incorrectly refer to "informed consent" as if being informed were the only criterion, an assumption that ignores the other two elements. Historically, the legal standard for *informed consent* has required disclosure of the condition for which treatment was proposed, all significant facts about it, and an explanation of likely consequences and difficulties related to the proposed treatment. This standard was based on the amount of information that a reasonable physician would give in the same or similar circumstances. By comparison, ethical criteria suggest more active patient participation. Criteria developed by the President's Commission for the Study of Ethical Problems in Medicine and Biomedical and Behavioral Research state that patient sovereignty with complete participation in the process is preferred. The commission recognized that such participation is a goal not easily achieved, however.[43]

A number of courts have adopted a standard that is based on what a typical (reasonable) patient would want to know. A legal criterion that is oriented to patient sovereignty and used in a few jurisdictions asks What would *this* patient want to know? The latter legal standard is consistent with the President's Commission position and reflects the ethical view that a covenant (contract) between patient and physician should guide their relationship.

The consent procedures that HSOs use are covered later in this chapter. HSOs are likely to apply a legally oriented consent process whose primary purpose is self-protection. Typically, there is little emphasis on an ethical relationship with a higher standard of patient participation. This utilitarian approach is legally prudent but ignores the positive ethical obligation to the patient that is suggested by the principle of respect for persons.

End-of-Life Decisions

The historical definition of death as cessation of blood circulation and of circulation-dependent animal and vital functions such as respiration and pulsation (heartbeat) proved inadequate as technology advanced. A 1968 Harvard Medical School committee definition of irreversible coma was an important first step in redefining death.[44] The criteria were useful, but the President's Commission for the Study of Ethical Problems in Medicine and Biomedical and Behavioral Research noted several criticisms.[45] Since the mid-1990s, all states have recognized alternate criteria to determine death: irreversible cessation of circulatory and respiratory functions *or* irreversible cessation of all functions of the entire brain, including the brain stem (brain death). Most states have enacted the Uniform Determination of Death Act, which incorporates these criteria for determining death.[46]

LIFE-SUSTAINING TREATMENT

Decisions about life-sustaining treatment are a point of convergence for ethics and law. Hospitals and nursing facilities often face ethical issues regarding withholding or withdrawing life-sustaining treatment. Historically, risk of legal liability caused a reluctance to withdraw life support absent court intervention. The first case receiving national attention, *In re Quinlan*,[47] occurred in 1976 when the New Jersey Supreme Court permitted 21-year-old Karen Ann Quinlan's father to be appointed her guardian. He was authorized to withdraw extraordinary life-sustaining procedures if the family and physicians concurred that Quinlan had no reasonable possibility of emerging from a persistent vegetative state (PVS),[48] and if the hospital ethics committee confirmed the prognosis. This was an early recognition of a role for ethics committees in hospitals. Quinlan was weaned from the respirator and transferred to a nursing facility, where she died after 10 years in PVS.

In 1990, the U.S. Supreme Court first ruled on a case involving life-sustaining treatment,

Cruzan v. Director, Missouri Department of Health.[49] Nancy Cruzan had been in PVS since her 1983 automobile accident. She was a patient in a Missouri state hospital, where a gastrostomy tube had been inserted for nutrition and hydration. Cruzan's parents brought suit after the facility refused their request to remove the tube. The court held that the U.S. Constitution does not prevent Missouri from requiring "clear and convincing evidence" that an incompetent person in PVS would not wish to be kept alive artificially. The court distinguished the rights of competent people, who are assumed to have a constitutionally protected right to refuse life-sustaining hydration and nutrition, from the rights of incompetent people. Adopting a "clear and convincing evidence" standard recognized broad state latitude to protect and preserve human life in life continuation decisions. In late 1990, Cruzan's parents were granted a second hearing in state court, which the state of Missouri did not oppose. New evidence convinced a judge that Cruzan would not have wanted to live in PVS, and the feeding tube was removed. Cruzan died a few days later.

ADVANCE MEDICAL DIRECTIVES

Patient participation in and control of healthcare decisions were enhanced when the federal Patient Self Determination Act (PSDA) of 1989 (PL 101-508) took effect December 1, 1991. The PSDA requires that HSOs participating in Medicare and Medicaid give all patients written information about their rights under state law to accept or refuse treatment and to formulate advance medical directives (AMDs).[50] Medical records must document whether a patient has an AMD, and the HSO must educate staff and community about them. There is some evidence that the PSDA has increased the use of AMDs in nursing facility residents. Despite the PSDA and widespread state legislation, most patients do not have AMDs.[51]

Living Wills

Living wills have been available since the 1960s to allow persons to communicate their wishes regarding medical treatment when the time comes that they are not competent to do so. In theory, living wills allow someone to control treatment. Absent legislation or case law, however, living wills have no legal status; patients must rely on the willingness of caregivers to follow their directives.

Natural Death Act Statutes

Interest in living wills and public reaction to situations in which seemingly excessive treatment was provided led to state laws that codify the right of a competent adult to control treatment. This is another instance in which ethics (autonomy) and the law merge. Common titles for natural death act statutes are *living wills laws, natural death acts,* or *death with dignity laws.* All states have laws recognizing AMDs.[52] Each state's AMD form is available online.[53]

Natural death act statutes codify the competent person's right to direct caregivers as to how much and what types of treatment to render, including withholding or withdrawing life-sustaining treatment. Caregivers are legally bound to follow the directives if statutory requirements are met, and some states provide for penalties against caregivers who ignore AMDs. The laws may be drafted narrowly and apply only when a physician determines that the patient who signed the AMD is terminally ill with no prospect for recovery. States may require reaffirmation of the AMD when persons know they have a terminal illness. In addition to statutes, decisions of state appeals and supreme courts affect how AMD laws are interpreted. These decisions consider control (autonomy); roles of proxies, patients, and families; and to an extent, HSO and provider actions.

Problems with AMDs

Research into use of AMDs is not encouraging. Only 15–25% of patients complete AMDs; the majority do so only after a significant hospital event.[54] Only 15% of patients with AMDs are asked by their physicians or nurses about their preferences for end-of-life care.[55] Further diminishing their usefulness is that most AMDs are too vague to guide specific decisions about treatment.[56]

Furthermore, an AMD may be ignored because caregivers are unaware of it or disagree with it or because family members make other demands. Fragmented care complicates patients' use of AMDs and poses a special challenge to caregivers and managers. For example, an AMD in a nursing facility's medical record may be left behind if a patient is hospitalized. Other problems include establishing the presence of a terminal illness and determining patients' mental status and whether they comprehend the effect of what is being done. Ethical problems are more likely if statutory requirements for AMDs are unmet.

The HSO's challenge is to develop processes that promote AMD completion. Rates of completion can be improved by altering the time when they are distributed to patients.[57] Patients were far more likely to complete an AMD at a hospital when they received information several days before admission rather than on the day of admission. Patients were much more likely to read the information provided when it was available before hospitalization. The most common reason given for not completing an AMD was that it was not seen or was not read—a problem much more common in the hospital that did not provide information in advance.[58] Providing reminders, education, and feedback to attending physicians and a new documentation form used by physicians for AMDs can greatly increase the percentage of patients who have AMDs. After these changes, 87% of physician-attested directives agreed with the treatment preferences of patients interviewed, and physicians' attitudes and interest in AMDs improved.[59] Family physicians may be an underutilized resource in increasing the percentage of patients who complete AMDs.[60] Limitations in the extent and depth of the physician–patient relationship appear to be the most frequent impediments to writing do-not-resuscitate (DNR) orders.[61] Efforts to gain completion of AMDs are for naught, however, if physician orders that reflect patients' wishes are not available in medical records for staff to use.

Substituted Judgment

Surrogates make decisions for persons incompetent to make them because they are too young or have physical, intellectual, or mental disabilities. Before AMDs, a surrogate was appointed on petition to a court, which determined that a person was incompetent to make healthcare decisions. Statutes in many states have supplanted this cumbersome and expensive process. By 2004, 37 states and the District of Columbia had authorized surrogate decision making for persons without AMDs.[62]

Powers of attorney are another type of decision making by a surrogate. These delegations of authority are prepared before the fact, however, and may be general or limited. Powers of attorney are "durable" when the authority continues beyond the time the grantor becomes incompetent. Different names are used for these arrangements, but their effect is that healthcare agents and surrogate decision makers are granted durable powers of attorney for healthcare. These limited powers of attorney enable a surrogate to make legally binding decisions for the person who granted the power of attorney. By 2004, all states and the District of Columbia allowed appointment of healthcare agents.[63]

Do-Not-Resuscitate Orders

The DNR order is a type of AMD integral to delivery of services. Patients without a DNR order are presumed to want a "full code," or maximum cardiopulmonary resuscitation (CPR). Despite best efforts, CPR is very unlikely to be successful.[64]

Since most patients do not have AMDs, HSOs should implement policies regarding resuscitation of terminally ill patients and those for whom life-continuation decisions must be made, such as patients in PVS. This DNR policy should affirm the legal right of a patient or surrogate to direct caregivers and should identify specific chemical and mechanical technologies and their application.

Despite DNR orders, patients may require surgery and anesthesia management for palliative care, for relief of pain or distress, or to improve the quality of life—interventions that present unique ethical problems the HSO should address prospectively.[65] Key to appropriate DNR orders is whether patient wishes about CPR mesh with the physician's perception of what the patient wants.[66]

Prehospital DNR orders are a recent development that allow persons to refuse resuscitation in medical emergencies. They may be known as emergency medical services (EMS) do-not-resuscitate orders, EMS-DNRs, or durable DNRs. They make the patient's decisions about treatment legally binding in nonhospital settings. By 2003, 43 states and the District of Columbia authorized DNR orders outside hospitals, with special forms, wristbands, and registries used to document patient wishes.[67]

Summary

It has been suggested that widespread use of AMDs might encourage systematic rationing of healthcare, especially to the elderly. If a right to decline treatment becomes a duty to die, the living will and its progeny will have become a Frankenstein monster. Government attention to AMDs suggests a possible greater concern with economics than patient autonomy. HSO managers must consider the ethical issues of AMDs prospectively and implement policies that respect patients' wishes, consistent with organizational values.

EUTHANASIA

The Hippocratic tradition prohibited physicians from giving a deadly drug, and *euthanasia* (Greek for "good death" [*eu* and *thanatos*]) described care that made an inevitable death pain free. In contemporary use, however, *euthanasia* often describes mercy killing—active steps to cause death. It is important to understand the ethical distinctions between actively intervening to hasten death and providing palliative care that allows a pain-free, dignified death as a natural course of the disease. The latter is known as allowing natural death.

Ordinary versus Extraordinary Care

Hastening or causing death by increasing analgesics beyond those needed to control pain, for example, is euthanasia. As defined here, palliative care is ordinary care. Care that offers no hope of benefit is extraordinary. Normally provided hydration and nutrition are ordinary; those artificially provided are extraordinary, if they offer no hope of benefit.

> Ordinary means are all medicines, treatments, and operations which offer reasonable hope of benefit and which can be obtained and used without excessive expense, pain, or other inconvenience. Extraordinary means are all medicines, treatments, and operations which cannot be obtained or used without excessive expense, pain, or inconvenience, or which, if used, would not offer a reasonable hope of benefit.[68]

Ordinary and *extraordinary* do not mean usual and unusual, respectively. Instead, the measure is hope of benefit compared with excessiveness of expense, pain, or other inconvenience. Absent hope of benefit, any medicine, treatment, or operation is extraordinary. If there is hope of benefit, using the same medicine, treatment, or operation is not excessive and is ordinary treatment.

Comparing benefits and burdens is another way to judge treatment. Proportionality—*proportionate* and *disproportionate*—may be more descriptive than *ordinary* and *extraordinary*. Proportionate and disproportionate care are measured much as are ordinary and extraordinary care. The type of treatment and its complexity or risk, cost, and appropriateness are studied and compared with the results to be expected, taking into account the state of an individual's health and physical and moral resources.[69] Using this calculus, treatment is ethical if the benefit justifies the burden. These various comparisons of treatment are essentially qualitative. In sum, they ask Does the benefit justify the burden?

Types of Euthanasia

Euthanasia has four permutations: voluntary active (consenting person is killed), voluntary passive (person consents to allow natural death), involuntary active (nonconsenting person is killed), and involuntary passive (nonconsenting person is allowed a natural death). *Voluntary* means the person has consented freely. *Involuntary* means the person either has not consented freely or cannot consent freely but is presumed to want to die. *Active* means steps are taken to cause death, or killing. *Passive* means death is not hastened—the natural course of the disease causes death. Passive euthanasia always includes palliative care.

Rule of Double Effect

Like ordinary and extraordinary (proportionate and disproportionate) care, double effect is a subset of nonmaleficence. Classical formulations of the rule of double effect (RDE) require that four conditions or elements must be satisfied to justify an act with double effect. Each is necessary; in sum they form sufficient conditions of morally permissible action.

1. The nature of the act. The act must be good, or at least morally neutral (independent of its consequences).
2. The agent's intention. The agent intends only the good effect. The bad effect can be foreseen, tolerated, and permitted, but it must not be intended.
3. The distinction between means and effects. The bad effect must not be a means to the good effect. If the good effect were the direct causal result of the bad effect, the agent would intend the bad effect in pursuit of the good effect.
4. Proportionality between the good effect and the bad effect. The good effect must outweigh the bad effect. The bad effect is permissible only if a proportionate reason is present that compensates for permitting the foreseen bad effect.[70]

As an example, it is ethical under RDE to use increasing amounts of morphine to ease the pain of a dying patient, even though the morphine will hasten death.

PHYSICIAN-ASSISTED SUICIDE

Background. Also called "aid in dying," physician-assisted suicide (PAS) is not euthanasia. PAS has qualities of voluntary, active euthanasia, but it differs in a critical aspect. PAS occurs when a physician provides the means, medical advice, and (sometimes) assurance that death will result, but the person, not the physician, performs the act that causes death. Broadly defined, PAS is *eu thanatos* because it relieves suffering and is likely to be pain free. Physical disability prevents some from performing the final act to commit suicide. This means PAS is not an option for them; if they want to die, someone must cause their deaths—voluntary, active euthanasia. The Hippocratic tradition considered it unethical to deliberately cause death. Lacking further treatment, physicians were expected to "comfort always."

Dr. Death. The first widely publicized PAS occurred in 1990 when Janet Adkins, a 54-year-old with Alzheimer's disease, was aided in her suicide by Jack Kevorkian, a retired Michigan pathologist. Kevorkian, known to critics as Dr. Death, gained national prominence when he developed a device that enabled people wishing to commit suicide to self-administer chemicals, after initial help from a physician. Kevorkian's actions were criticized as procedurally flawed, and it was suggested that her Alzheimer's might have made Adkins incompetent to consent to PAS.[71] The case focused public attention on active, voluntary euthanasia and aid in dying.

Kevorkian's role varied in the more than 100 suicides he assisted. Kevorkian was criticized on professional and ethical grounds. He did not know his "patients," was unqualified to diagnose or understand illnesses because he was a pathologist, had a conflict of interest because he desired publicity for himself and (initially) his death machine, assisted people who were not terminally ill, and did not assess the mental competence of those receiving PAS. Kevorkian hoped to establish a clinic for terminally ill people—an obitorium—to assist in suicides.

In 1999, Kevorkian was convicted of second-degree murder in Michigan, where assisted suicide was made illegal after his "work" began.[72] He was sentenced to 10–25 years in prison. The Michigan parole board approved Kevorkian's release in 2007, after he served 8 years. He has promised not to assist more suicides.[73] By way of context, a substantial proportion of physicians receive requests for aid in dying. About 6% have complied at least once.[74]

Legal Aspects of PAS. Ballot initiatives in Washington (1991) and California (1992) to legalize PAS were rejected. After narrowly approving PAS in the so-called Death with Dignity Act in 1994[75] (52% to 48%), Oregon voters were asked by the legislature to repeal the law, a request they overwhelmingly rejected in November 1997 (60% to 40%). Thus, Oregon became the first state to legalize PAS.

Oregon's law permits physicians to prescribe, but not administer, fatal doses of oral drugs to competent, terminally ill adults with fewer than 6 months to live. The physician's minimal role of assisting in suicide distinguishes Oregon's law from Dr. Kevorkian's PAS. In Oregon, the physician's prescription allows access to medications necessary for self-administered *eu thanatos*, without the guarantee of death a physician's presence would provide. Absent this modest physician assistance and the legality conferred by the statute, such self-inflicted death would simply be a suicide.

Other requirements of the Oregon law are two oral requests separated by 15 days; a witnessed, written request to the doctor from the patient; consultations with other physicians; physician notification to pharmacists and state health authorities; and provision of information to the patient as to alternatives to assisted suicide.[76] Physicians who act in good faith are protected from professional discipline and legal liability.[77] The first suicide under the Oregon law was reported in March 1998.[78] The Blue Cross and Blue Shield plans of Oregon began covering PAS in early 1998.[79] In late 1998, the Oregon Health Plan (which covers Medicaid patients) added PAS to end-of-life palliative care and hospice.[80] Between 1998 and the end of 2006, a total of 292 Oregonians had been assisted in suicide.[81]

As of 2007, only Oregon had legalized PAS. In addition to Washington and California, unsuccessful attempts to pass PAS (or euthanasia) laws have been made in Michigan and Maine.[82] Similar legislation has been considered in more than a dozen other states.[83] PAS is illegal by specific statute or common law precedent in most states. Statutes in 39 states criminalize assisted suicide; in 6 states, the common law achieves the same purpose. Four states have neither statutory nor common law prohibitions against assisted suicide.[84] This legal context is inconsistent with polls cited below, showing that a large majority of Americans favor physician help in ending the lives of the terminally ill. In 1997, a unanimous U.S. Supreme Court ruled that states may ban PAS suicide without violating either the due process or equal protection clauses of the 14th Amendment to the U.S. Constitution. The court did not decide whether states could pass laws, as Oregon did, giving people the choice of assisted suicide.[85]

Physicians and PAS. Many physicians regard providing active assistance in dying as turning medicine on its head—those who traditionally guarded life are asked to end it. Organized medicine in the United States has condemned proposals that physicians provide aid in dying. Domestic survey findings suggest that this reaction is overstated.

Surveys show that a majority of physicians in Michigan (Kevorkian's home state) and Oregon favored legalizing assisted suicide, although a sizable minority in Oregon objected on moral grounds.[86] A national survey found that 6% of physicians responding who regularly care for the dying had either given lethal injections or written prescriptions so patients could kill themselves— at a time when physician assistance in suicide was illegal. The survey also found that one third of doctors would write prescriptions for deadly doses and that one fourth would give lethal injections, if they were legal. Opiates such as morphine were the drugs given most often to help patients die.[87] Aid in dying raises basic moral questions necessitating reexamination of the physician–patient relationship. In addition, there is ample evidence that physician participation in assisted suicide or euthanasia may have profound harmful effects on the physicians involved.[88]

Demedicalizing aid in dying reduces some ethical problems for physicians but raises others. German law, for example, makes it illegal for physicians to assist in suicide. Because suicide is not illegal and because assisting the suicide of people who are capable of exercising control over their actions and have freely made a responsible choice to commit suicide is not illegal, however, unique societal views about suicide and aid in dying have developed in Germany.[89]

International Comparisons. Assisted suicide has been available in parts of Switzerland since 1942; increasingly, it is a destination for "suicide tourists."[90] In 2002, Belgium legalized voluntary euthanasia and assisted suicide with a law similar to the one in the Netherlands.[91] In mid-2003, a year after passage of the original law, Belgian lawmakers proposed expanding euthanasia to children under 18.[92] PAS and euthanasia are being debated elsewhere in Europe, notably Spain and France. A 2002 survey in France showed that 88% favor or would tolerate euthanasia.[93]

Internationally, the vanguard of assisted dying is the Netherlands. Despite their illegality, euthanasia and PAS have been practiced there since the 1980s; 92% of the population supports euthanasia.[94] Before euthanasia and PAS were made legal in 1993, a 1990 government study found that about one third of patients whose lives were ended had not consented to assistance in dying.[95]

A 2002 revision of the 1993 law broadened use of euthanasia and assisted suicide, which are legally defined as medical treatments if performed in a medically appropriate manner.[96] The statute specifically allows euthanasia for legally incompetent patients. An individual of age 16 or older can make an advance written statement containing a request for euthanasia, which a physician may carry out. The statement can have been written years before and be based on views that have changed; regardless, the physician may administer euthanasia based on that prior written statement.[97]

In addition, the law allows other categories of persons to request and receive euthanasia or assisted suicide: Teenagers, with varying degrees of parents' or guardians' approval, depending on age, may request and receive euthanasia or assisted suicide. (Children as young as 16 may request termination of life in writing, which the physician can legally administer without parental or guardian approval, although they must be involved in the decision process.) Children as young as 12 may request and receive euthanasia or assisted suicide, with agreement of parents or guardians. Also, persons for whom the doctor "holds the conviction that the patient's suffering is lasting and unbearable" may be euthanized.[98]

The 2002 Dutch law requires that specific criteria must be met.

- *Voluntary*. The physician must be convinced that the patient has made a voluntary, persistent, and carefully considered request to die.
- *Suffering*. The physician must be convinced that the patient's suffering is unbearable and that there is no prospect of improvement of the patient's situation. (There is no requirement that the suffering must be physical or that the patient must be terminally ill).[99]
- *Informed*. The physician has informed the patient about his or her medical situation and medical prospects.

- *Alternatives.* The physician, together with the patient, must be convinced that there is no reasonable alternative.
- *Consultation.* The physician has consulted at least one other physician with an independent viewpoint who must have seen the patient and given a written opinion on the "due-care criteria."
- *Due care and attention.* The physician must have assisted the patient to die with due medical care and attention.[100]

The law does not prohibit physicians from administering euthanasia to a nonresident of the Netherlands.[101]

A stated hope is that the 2002 law will bring into the open euthanasia that has been hidden. Research published in 2004 showed that, although reporting has increased, about half of cases remain unreported.[102] Other concerns about "hidden euthanasia" surfaced only a year after the 2002 law went into effect. "Terminal sedation" occurs when physicians give patients in severe pain quantities of morphine large enough that death is hastened. Because euthanasia is defined as the active termination of life on request, such an overdose is not reportable—it is not clear that the death was intended. The death is considered a natural death.[103]

Legally sanctioning active euthanasia for various groups of "patients" (with varying degrees of consent from parents or guardians for some of them) is a significant change, and it moves euthanasia from the exceptional to an accepted way of dealing with medical conditions that are not serious or terminal illness. Palliative care in the Netherlands is one casualty of its history of physician-assisted deaths, and hospice care there lags behind other countries.[104]

Technically, PAS would seem to be simple. The Dutch data show, however, that a significant percent of cases have problems, even when a physician is present. Problems include medications not working as expected, technical difficulties, and unexpected side effects. In 16% of cases in which patients tried to kill themselves using doctor-prescribed drugs, the medication did not work as expected; 7% of the time, technical problems or unexpected side effects occurred. Physicians witnessing the attempted suicide felt compelled to intervene and ensure death in 18% of cases. Even when a doctor directly performed euthanasia, researchers found complications 3% of the time. In another 6%, patients took longer to die than expected, or they went into a drug-induced coma that was supposed to be fatal, but from which they awoke.[105] Thus, it appears that assisted suicide and euthanasia do not necessarily result in the easy, peaceful death—*eu thanatos*—that they promise and that, frequently, they add to the patient's misery and suffering. The data from the Netherlands are in stark contrast to Oregon data that show very few complications from PAS under the Death with Dignity Act.

That Dutch law has neither a requirement that suffering must be physical nor one that the patient must be terminally ill suggests a significant new use for active euthanasia and assisted suicide—by persons simply tired of living. In addition, persons in various states of aging or disability or in other ways unhealthy may now have to justify their existence. Given that Dutch physicians are willing to actively euthanize almost anyone, persons at risk fear that their lives will be ended without their consent.[106] This fear has caused many of the most vulnerable—the disabled or elderly—to carry cards specifying their desire to continue to live.[107]

Expansion of euthanasia in the Netherlands continues. In September 2005, the Dutch health ministry formulated guidelines know as the Groningen protocol (of the Groningen University Medical Center) that would allow euthanasia of children (including newborns) when "a child is terminally ill with no prospect of recovery and suffering great pain, when two sets of doctors agree the situation is hopeless, and when parents give their consent."[108] The Groningen protocol has been roundly criticized by disability rights groups.[109]

That a Western European democracy so willingly accepts active (voluntary *and* involuntary) euthanasia raises important ethical questions. The Dutch experience shows that active euthanasia, which seemingly began as a way to enhance individual self-determination, is not limited to those who request it. The continuing and troubling scenario of large numbers of persons involuntarily, actively euthanized highlights the slippery slope, defined by philosophers as one exception leading to other, more easily accepted exceptions.

HSOs/HSs and Ethical Issues. None of Kevorkian's "work" occurred in an HSO. Similarly, the Oregon statute has no role for HSOs. Nevertheless, HSOs often face the ethical issues present at the end of life and may be asked to provide aid in dying. A nursing facility, for example, may have a resident in PVS or a terminally ill resident too sick to transfer. The "conscience clause" found in state and federal laws protects caregivers and HSOs who refuse to participate in activities that compromise their ethics. MCOs and other insurers must decide if they will include aid in dying as a benefit. The organizational philosophy of all HSOs should prospectively address both voluntary and involuntary active euthanasia.

New forms of payment and organizational arrangements will change economic incentives, even as HSOs become less able to meet costs of services. Hospitals have already experienced a form of capitation in DRGs, which have the incentive to limit services. The increasing difficulty of cost shifting means HSOs/HSs must reduce costs through better quality, through greater productivity, or by changing the content of care. When physicians were less affected by cost reduction, they were a force to counterbalance organizational efforts to limit services. Traditional relationships are changing, however, and economically linking physician and HSO raises myriad ethical issues.

FUTILE TREATMENT

Background. In many ways, futility theory is old wine in new bottles. Its origins lie in the distinction between ordinary and extraordinary care, which are distinguished by "hope of benefit" and "excessive expense, pain, or other inconvenience." These distinctions make it ethical to withhold any medicine, treatment, or operation that offers no reasonable hope of benefit or that cannot be obtained or used without excessive expense, pain, or inconvenience.

Futility theory has quantitative and qualitative aspects. The *quantitative* is concerned with what the *probability of success* would be if a treatment were continued or attempted. *Probability of success* means the likelihood that the treatment can be successfully performed and achieve its intended purpose. So, for example, tube feeding will maintain the life of a PVS patient, but it will not restore cognition. This highlights the importance of viewing care as a continuum, not an isolated event.

Qualitative assumes a successful treatment that achieves its intended purpose, but it asks whether the result is such that the treatment *ought* to be undertaken. The quantitative determination is made by clinical experts. The qualitative determination (judgment) can be made only by the patient or, as necessary, the patient's surrogate. The concept of futility limits the qualitative decision.

Three basic variations of circumstances raise questions of futile treatment. The first is that patients demand services that offer no hope of benefit. Absent supporting data, these situations may be urban myth or misperception. Generally, AMDs limit medical intervention, although they may demand services clinicians deem futile.

A second type of futile treatment occurs when organizations insist on providing treatment that surrogates and physicians have determined offer no hope of benefit and should end. Karen Ann Quinlan and Nancy Cruzan are examples of such an organization policy, which for Cruzan was complicated by the fact that continued treatment was required by state law. The Quinlan and Cruzan cases suggest that questions of futility are better directed at legislators, HSOs, and staff than at patients and families.

The third type occurs when treatment is continued because surrogate decision makers demand it. An example is the case of Helga Wanglie, the Minneapolis woman in PVS whose husband demanded all efforts to keep her alive, despite a prognosis that doing so offered no hope of benefit. Another example was the treatment of Baby K, an anencephalic (missing a major part of the brain and skull) infant whose mother refused to authorize a DNR order and insisted that all treatment continue.

Futile-treatment Guidelines. Increasingly, acute care hospitals have futile-treatment guidelines or policies. Their use has been stimulated by perceptions that patients and/or surrogates demand treatment that clinicians deem to have little, if any, likelihood of benefiting the patient. Consent and autonomy drive the initial phases of decision making for patients able to participate. They should be given the information to make an informed choice about treatment or nontreatment options. Patients bear the brunt of continued, futile treatment, a fact that likely makes them more willing than surrogate decision makers to limit what will be done. Sometimes patients and surrogates have unrealistic goals or expectations of medical science. When patients' decisions (or demands) will not result in efficacious medical treatment or will only prolong suffering and the dying process, clinicians have a moral obligation to withhold or withdraw treatment. Guidelines for withholding or withdrawing life-sustaining treatment usually require agreement of attending and consulting physicians that treatment is futile.

The decisions about appropriateness of continued medical treatment are made within the context of the purposes of medical care. "There is . . . general agreement that the goals of standard medical treatment are to cure, restore, improve, or maintain some level of a person's ability to think, feel, and interact with others and the environment. Medical interventions that have little likelihood of achieving any of these treatment goals can be considered futile."[110]

The futility guidelines for Trinity Health, a nationwide, faith-based healthcare system, begin by positing the religious context for the guidelines, describing the role of the patient in decision making, the importance of professional integrity of caregivers, and the need for stewardship of resources. The guidelines continue by defining medically futile treatment and providing examples.[111] Medically futile treatment is defined as any treatment that, within a reasonable degree of medical probability, has little likelihood of having a positive physiological effect on the patient's condition; reversing the patient's imminent decline; or restoring the patient's cognitive, affective, and interactive functions.[112]

Several aspects of these futility guidelines are notable: 1) the criteria are stated in the alternative, (e.g., if reversing a patient's imminent dying is likely by applying a treatment, that treatment is not futile); 2) there is no consideration of "quality of life," as judged by either the patient or another; and 3) there is no specific attention to the economic dimensions of the treatment.

Examples of futile treatment in the guidelines include continued ventilator (breathing) support for a patient who meets brain death criteria, CPR for a patient with metastatic end-stage cancer or a patient with multiple organ failure, and aggressive therapies for a PVS-state or permanently comatose patient. The guidelines outline a process for making decisions about medical futility.[113]

The guidelines end by outlining a process for situations in which physicians and caregivers disagree regarding potentially futile treatments. Here, the ethics committee has a significant role. Throughout, dialogue with patients or surrogates is emphasized. Using a neutral third party to mediate allows important, positive opportunities to resolve disagreement on a course of action.

Futile-treatment guidelines or policies should emphasize that physicians have no moral (or legal) obligation to provide treatment that they judge inappropriate. Physicians' professional integrity is compromised and they fail to meet their duty to their patients if they provide treatment that has neither benefit nor hope of benefit. Physicians fail, too, in their ethical obligation to use resources parsimoniously if futilely ill patients consume them. Laws in almost all states give physicians and hospitals latitude in refusing to provide end-of-life treatment that is futile.

Some states have passed laws regarding futile treatment. For example, California's noncompliance provision for physicians and hospitals applies if a requested treatment "requires medically ineffective healthcare or healthcare contrary to generally accepted healthcare standards applicable to the healthcare provider or institution."[114] Despite such laws, however, it seems doubtful that either physicians or hospitals will refuse to provide treatment that they deem to be futile, except after considerable continued treatment and when the prognosis is beyond reasonable challenge. The potential for accusations from the public and media that passive, involuntary euthanasia is occurring or that patients are being treated cruelly or killed is too great. Reactions to highly publicized futile treatment cases show significant ignorance among the public. In such a milieu, strictly enforcing futile-treatment guidelines will cause a public relations nightmare. HSOs must have guidelines or a policy on futile treatment, nonetheless.

The presence of guidelines will encourage physicians to address the futility of a patient's treatment. Thus encouraged, their frank discussions with patients or surrogates may allow futile treatment to be withheld or withdrawn. By informing patients or surrogates of their moral objection to continuing medically inappropriate and harmful treatment, physicians may gain assent without invoking the HSO's guidelines. The "transfer out" option is unlikely to be viable but is useful to convince patients or surrogates how seriously physicians view the problem. In practical terms, patients may be too ill to transfer; more likely, no facility will accept them. Transfer becomes virtually impossible if all hospitals in a region agree to a common set of futile-treatment guidelines as, for example, in Knoxville and Houston. Thus, after a reasonable time in which no alternative source of treatment is found, the facility and its physicians must withhold or withdraw futile treatment. The concept of futile treatment is not without critics.[115]

Implications. Futility theory goes well beyond the contemporary concept of patient autonomy, which is a negative right. Autonomy, expressed as the need to consent, is the right to be free from unwanted treatment—the right to say "No, thank you." Futility theory limits exercise of what is *asserted* to be a positive right—the "right" to demand treatment after a determination that no medical benefit will accrue from receiving it. No such positive right exists at law or in ethics.

Futility theory is a proactive approach to circumstances of extraordinary, disproportionate, and burdensome treatment. Managers must address several issues when developing a futile-treatment policy. The first is determining the extent of the problem in the HSO. Other efforts, such as making education on AMDs more effective and increasing the likelihood that such directives are in the medical record, are appropriate as well, and should be taken in tandem with developing a futile-treatment policy. Effectively communicating to the patient (or surrogate) the gravity of the medical situation will reduce resistance to withholding or withdrawing treatment. The discussion of APACHE in Chapter 10 is germane here. Most important, a futile-treatment policy must provide guidelines and support for physicians, who will benefit from a definition of futile treatment. In turn, the policy may convince patients and surrogates that treatment without hope of benefit should be avoided or ended.

The most compelling ethical issue raised when considering futile treatment is that the right to die may become a duty to die. Do futile-treatment policies put HSOs and healthcare providers on a slippery slope? Will the policies become broader and more focused on the quality of life that clinicians decide would be (or should be) acceptable to the patient? These questions can be answered only in retrospect, in itself not a cheery prospect.

Organizational Responses to Ethical Problems

How do HSOs/HSs organize to solve administrative and biomedical ethical problems? The starting point is the organizational philosophy, which reflects the values of the HSO/HS and establishes moral direction and a framework for the vision and mission. As leaders, managers' personal ethics influence the organizational philosophy and are influenced by it. Ethical problem solving occurs in the context of the organizational philosophy, but it is affected by the manager's personal ethic, which is likely to be more specific and comprehensive. This dynamic reinforces the importance of the personal ethic. The organization's philosophy is subject to the external constraints of civil and criminal laws and derivative regulations that establish a minimum standard. External constraints, such as the "conscience clause" discussed above, support the values of HSOs and their staffs. Federal guidelines that protect human research subjects are the starting point for an HSO's relationship with patients who participate in research.

MEANS TO RESOLVE ETHICS ISSUES

The manager organizes the HSO to solve ethical problems. Since the 1970s, HSOs/HSs have developed various means to solve ethical problems; most prominent are institutional ethics committees (IECs), institutional review boards (IRBs), and infant care review committees (ICRCs). IECs provide a broad range of assistance on administrative and biomedical ethical issues. IRBs are specialized IECs that focus on preventing and solving ethical issues in research. ICRCs, too, are specialized IECs that prevent and solve ethical issues that arise in caring for infants with profound impairment.

Institutional Ethics Committees

Background. Progenitors to IECs were abortion selection committees that determined, prior to *Roe v. Wade*, whether a woman's health or life was at sufficient risk to justify an abortion. Similarly, medical morals committees in Roman Catholic hospitals reviewed certain treatment decisions in light of church teachings.[116] In the 1960s, ethics committees selected recipients of renal dialysis at a time when medically suitable patients greatly exceeded the capacity of treatment programs.

In 1976, the court decision regarding Karen Ann Quinlan directed establishment of an ethics committee to review her clinical prognosis to determine whether life support should be continued. Prognosis committees were known as "God squads" because they determined if treatment that sustained life should be withdrawn. Contemporary IECs have a much broader role. An early source of information about IECs was a national survey by the President's Commission for the Study of Ethical Problems in Medicine and Biomedical and Behavioral Research published in 1983.[117] The study estimated that there were fewer than 100 IECs in U.S. hospitals. The Quinlan decision encouraged hospitals to establish IECs. In New Jersey, where they were most common, 71% were formed because of the Quinlan case.

Studies in the mid-1980s showed rapid growth of IECs—from 26% of hospitals responding to 59%. Increase in the number of new IECs slowed in the late 1980s.[118] Lack of growth is confirmed by more recent estimates that nationally about 60% of hospitals have IECs; state and regional ethics networks suggest 65%–85%.[119] Largely because of The Joint Commission's 1992 mandate, it is likely that all hospitals have at least one IEC.[120] The IECs in hospitals are sufficiently mature that their role and mission should be reassessed. IECs should be involved in reviewing macroallocation decisions, considering the availability and use of AMDs, developing and monitoring a futile-care policy, reviewing relationships among various healthcare providers, addressing issues of diversity and cultural competence in service delivery, and educating patients and staff about ethical issues. Autonomy affects several aspects of care; special attention should be given to microallocation decisions that affect consent and decisions at the bedside.

Postacute care services and alternative delivery sites are increasingly important, and this means the growth in need and use of IECs will be greatest in sites such as nursing facilities, HMOs, and HSs. The American Association of Homes and Services for the Aging found that the percentage of IECs among members increased from 29% in 1990 to 45% in 1995; many others were planned.

These IECs perform case consultation, make and review proposed policies, and educate and advise staff and administration.[121] IECs in nonacute HSOs will develop consistent with their unique activities and roles. Compared with hospitals, physicians on nursing facility IECs will likely have a lesser role, while administrative staff will be more important.

Organizing IECs. Complex HSOs/HSs will benefit from establishing an IEC with subcommittees for administrative and biomedical ethical issues. An alternative is to have one ethics committee for administrative ethical issues, another for biomedical ethical issues. Specialization is necessary because a committee prepared to address administrative ethics issues may not be prepared for clinical ethics issues. More specialized committees, such as ICRCs, may be needed within the broad categories of administrative and biomedical ethics. Committee proliferation or overlap must be avoided, but solving unique ethics problems with specialized committees will improve results.

Purpose and Role of IECs. Since their early, focused beginnings, the purposes of IECs have evolved into two roles of general importance. One role is assisting to develop or reconsider the statement of organizational philosophy and derivative vision and mission statements. Here, the experience and range of interdisciplinary membership will produce more reasoned and thoroughly considered recommendations. Education is a second role—members' experiences make the IEC a reservoir of expertise. Using the resources of a well-prepared IEC will improve clinical and administrative decision making.

Before beginning its work, the IEC must develop a statement of its ethic within the general framework of the organizational philosophy. This exercise facilitates effectiveness by identifying and minimizing differences in members' personal ethics. Only by understanding and enunciating its own ethic can an IEC appreciate how its values differ from a patient's if, for example, patient autonomy is to be respected. The IEC's ethic does not determine how ethical problems are solved. Rather, these general principles are a framework for deliberations and recommendations.

Both administrative and biomedical IECs undertake generic activities such as policy development, education, case consultation, and guidance for staff and patients on request. Sample activities for administrative IECs include developing consent procedures, considering the ethics of macroallocation of resources, and whistle-blowing. Biomedical IECs could develop DNR and patient consent policies and advise on withholding or withdrawing life-sustaining treatment.

Membership of IECs. IECs should be and typically are interdisciplinary. Physicians and nurses are the most common types on IECs. Others are community and board members, risk managers, attorneys, clergy, and administrators. More than half of IECs' members are women.[122]

Relationships of IECs. IECs should be proactive in developing and revising the organizational philosophy and considering the ethical implications of macroallocation decisions. Similarly, they should take the lead in reviewing and revising consent procedures. They are more likely to be passive and wait to be consulted about conflicts of interest and misuse of confidential information, in the case of administrative IECs, or about specific clinical matters, in the case of biomedical IECs.

Generally, biomedical IECs will be more effective if they wait to be consulted rather than interpose themselves. Consultation means making recommendations, not final decisions.[123] IEC participation in biomedical and administrative decision making may be optional or mandatory. Whether the IEC's advice must be followed could be optional or mandatory as well. Table 4.1 shows the combinations. Physicians are unlikely to accept mandatory involvement in IECs that give mandatory advice. Even physicians unwilling to share decision making with an IEC will benefit from its analysis and recommendations.

The administrative location of the IEC is important. It may be a standing committee of the governing body, professional staff organization, or administration. Physician dominance of a clinical IEC may be avoided by making it part of governance or administration.

TABLE 4.6. OPTIONAL VERSUS MANDATORY USE OF AN IEC

Involvement of committee in decision making	Acceptance and use of advice given by IEC
Optional	Optional
Optional	Mandatory
Mandatory	Optional
Mandatory	Mandatory

Summary. IECs are not without problems. Organizational interests, especially legal aspects and avoiding public embarrassment, may overwhelm patient goals.[124] At the extreme, it is suggested that IECs cannot be objective because they are part of the HSO. This may cause IECs to fail as patient advocates because, when a dispute arises, they will take management's side to avoid risk.[125] Management must ensure that IECs are not subverted in this manner.

Overall, effective use of IECs will improve clinical and administrative decisions. It should not be assumed that the mere presence of an IEC means that it is successful or useful. IECs must be evaluated to improve their performance.[126]

Institutional Review Boards

Background. Defined as attempting new means, methods, and techniques, medicine has always engaged in research. Without research, medical knowledge would stagnate. Protecting the rights and welfare of human subjects remains problematic, however.

To protect human subjects, HSOs conducting research should establish an IRB, which is an independent committee composed of scientific and nonscientific members that meets the requirements of federal law.[127] IRBs conduct initial and continued review of research involving human subjects. Committees with similar activities are considered IRBs.

The Department of Health and Human Services (DHHS) and the Food and Drug Administration (FDA) are the most important federal entities that require an IRB to review, approve, and maintain oversight of research studies. DHHS requirements for IRBs and protection of human subjects are applicable to research funded by any of 17 federal agencies and departments that have adopted the "common rule" or "federal policy" for the protection of human subjects (i.e., research supported or conducted by and regulated under a specific research statute).[128] Federal agencies that use DHHS requirements include the departments of Defense and Veterans Affairs and the Environmental Protection Agency, the National Science Foundation, and the Consumer Product Safety Commission.

Research involving human subjects that is funded wholly or partly by federal government must be reviewed by an IRB with a process that meets DHHS criteria. Although technically not required, research funding applications typically include assurances that the organization will comply with DHHS IRB requirements for human subjects (and other DHHS requirements for the protection of human subjects) for *all* its research, whether or not federally funded.[129] FDA regulates interstate sale of drugs, biologicals, and medical devices and has the same requirements as DHHS. Unlike DHHS, however, compliance with FDA guidelines, including use of IRBs, is necessary regardless of funding source. A few states, such as New York, regulate medical research, but the regulation of most health-related research is performed by the DHHS or FDA. FDA regulates neither surgical experimentation nor innovative clinical care, which is defined as *new* uses of existing treatments, drugs, biologicals (vaccines), and devices.

Membership and Purpose. Institutions may choose specific IRB members, but federal regulations (and perhaps state law) govern composition of membership, nature of the review conducted, and conflicts of interest of IRB members.[130] IRBs review research proposals for conformance with the law, standards of professional conduct and practice, and institutional commitment and regulations. IRBs acceptable to DHHS have a minimum of five members with varying backgrounds (at least one with professional interests that are scientific and one with interests that are nonscientific) and who are capable of reviewing research proposals and activities of the type commonly performed by the organization.[131]

IRBs acceptable to DHHS must apply specific requirements when reviewing research activities:[132]

- Risks to subjects are minimized.
- Risks to subjects are reasonable in relation to anticipated benefit, if any.
- Selection of research subjects is equitable.
- Informed consent is sought from each prospective subject or the subject's legally authorized representative.
- Informed consent is appropriately documented.
- When appropriate, the research plan has adequate provision for monitoring the data collected to ensure the safety of subjects.
- When appropriate, there are adequate provisions to protect the privacy of subjects and maintain the confidentiality of data.

Additional safeguards are required when some or all of the subjects are likely to be vulnerable to coercion or undue influence; examples include children, prisoners, pregnant women, persons with mental disabilities, or persons with economic or educational disadvantages. Several provisions identify the information needed for informed consent.

FDA uses the same basic elements of consent as DHHS but applies special provisions when the subject is in a life-threatening situation that necessitates use of the test article and when the subject cannot provide legally effective consent, when time is insufficient to obtain consent from the subject's legal representative, and when no alternative method of generally recognized therapy that provides an equal or greater likelihood of saving the subject's life is available.

Requirements. Regulations issued in 1981 eliminated the requirement that any DHHS funding to an organization *required* use of DHHS guidelines in *all* research, regardless of funding source. This marked a shift in federal government's role in protecting human subjects, and in research generally. This change increased the role of managers and researchers and put greater reliance on the HSO's policies and procedures and on managers' personal ethics.

As a practical matter, and as noted, organizations with multiple research funding sources, one of them federal, are likely to use the same DHHS-qualified IRB for all research protocols. It is easy to slip, however, and managers must be alert to potential ethical problems in formal research programs, as well as in isolated innovative therapy or surgical experimentation.

It has been forcefully argued that nondiagnostic and nontherapeutic (without therapeutic benefit to the subject) research on children and adults who are legally incompetent should be prohibited.[133] Nontherapeutic research on children is permitted, however. A risk–benefit analysis is applied, and no child can be placed in unnecessary jeopardy. Assent from the child and consent from parents or legally authorized representatives are required. The ethical, economic, political, legal, and scientific problems of research involving children are daunting, however, and researchers are reluctant to undertake it. Congress *has not* given the FDA authority to *require* extensive testing on children. Despite efforts by Congress and the FDA to encourage testing of pharmaceuticals and biologicals on children, little research involving them is done, and most prescribing for children is based on physician trial and error.[134] It is estimated that 50%–75% of drugs used in pediatric medicine have not been studied adequately to provide appropriate labeling information.[135]

Exempt Research and Research Warranting Expedited Review. Six categories of research are exempt from DHHS requirements. Examples are research conducted in established or normally accepted educational settings involving normal educational practices; research involving use of educational tests, survey and interview procedures, or observation of public behavior; and research involving the collection or study of existing data, documents, records, and pathological or diagnostic specimens. Limits are specified.[136]

DHHS regulations identify research warranting expedited review as a category to which different provisions apply. Expedited review allows special procedures for approval of certain types of research that pose no more than minimal risk to human subjects.[137] Examples of research categories appropriate to expedited review are clinical studies of drugs and medical devices; collection of blood samples; collection of biological specimens such as hair and nail clippings and deciduous teeth; and collection of data through noninvasive procedures.[138] Expedited review greatly facilitates several kinds of research.

Summary. Regulations such as those imposed by DHHS focus responsibility on the organization and its IRB. Regardless of legal requirements, HSO managers have independent ethical duties to protect research subjects under the principles of respect for persons, beneficence, nonmaleficence, and even justice—for example, fairly allocating support for research. The virtues of honesty, integrity, and trustworthiness are also applicable. Managers must establish and maintain systems and procedures to prevent unauthorized research and to provide the necessary extra protection when innovative treatment or surgical research are proposed or undertaken. Most important are staff awareness about the parameters of acceptable practice and the courage to act.

Infant Care Review Committees

ICRCs are another type of specialized IEC. Their focus is biomedical ethical problems of infants with life-threatening conditions. The Child Abuse Amendments of 1984 directed DHHS to encourage establishment of ICRCs in health facilities, especially those with tertiary-level neonatal units. DHHS guidelines for ICRCs include 1) educate hospital personnel and families of disabled infants with life-threatening conditions, 2) recommend institutional policies and guidelines concerning the withholding of medically indicated treatment from infants with life-threatening conditions, and 3) offer counsel and review in cases involving infants with life-threatening conditions.[139]

The guidelines make it clear that DHHS considers it prudent to establish an ICRC but that HSOs decide whether to do so. Aspects of the ICRC's membership and administration recommended in the guidelines are notable. Members should include persons from varied disciplines and perspectives, because a multidisciplinary approach provides the expertise to supply and evaluate pertinent information. The committee should be large enough to include diverse viewpoints but not so large that effectiveness is hindered. Recommended membership includes a practicing physician (e.g., pediatrician, neonatologist, pediatric surgeon), practicing nurse, hospital administrator, social worker, representative of a disability group, lay community member, and a member of the facility's medical staff, who is the chairperson.[140]

DHHS suggested that the ICRC have staff support, including legal counsel; that the ICRC recommend procedures to ensure that hospital personnel and families know of its existence, functions, and 24-hour availability; that the ICRC self-educate about legal requirements and procedures, including state law requiring reports of known or suspected medical neglect; and that the ICRC maintain records of deliberations and summary descriptions of cases considered, and their disposition.[141]

Specialized Assistance

Analogues to IECs and specialized committees such as IRBs and ICRCs that can assist managers to identify and solve ethical problems are not well developed but may fit in some organizations.

Ethics Consultation Service (ECS). An ECS is one way HSOs can provide specialized personnel to advise and assist in solving biomedical ethics problems. Doing so is similar to establishing a clinical service. The ECS is staffed by ethicists with graduate degrees in philosophy, often at the doctoral level, and by clinical personnel who may be physicians or other caregivers. The clinicians have a special interest and/or preparation in ethics and provide a bridge between the ethicist and clinical staff attending the patient. They are also a resource for the ethicists. In this model, an ethicist is on call, and a clinical member of the ECS is involved as needed. The ECS reports to the hospital IEC, which develops and recommends policy to the governing body. The IEC also serves as a sounding board for problems that develop during ethics consultation. A variant model uses a primary consultant who is assisted by other members of the ECS. The primary consultants and those assisting them have varying backgrounds, but all have intensive and specialized training in ethics, and all participate in case reviews, ethics instruction, and regular meetings of ECS staff.[142]

Ethicists. A less formal approach than an ECS is common in larger hospitals and HSs, but it need not be limited to them. Such organizations may employ full- or part-time ethicists. Like ECSs, ethicists are often doctorally qualified. They may be university or medical school faculty who consult on biomedical ethical issues.

Organizations needing the assistance of an ethicist can look beyond universities and medical schools and consider anyone with specialized preparation in ethics and its application in health services. Here, as with the ECS, an ethicist is the clinically oriented, problem-solving extension of an IEC.

Dispute Resolution. Treatment options and decisions regarding them often cause disputes among stakeholders, such as clinicians, patient, and family. The various types of ethics committees—IECs, IRBs, and ICRCs—may be able to resolve disputes, but their connection to the HSO may raise concerns among some stakeholders as to their objectivity. Arbitration and mediation should be considered to resolve such disputes. Arbitration involves a neutral (person) to whom the parties in the dispute have given the authority to make a decision that all have agreed to accept. Mediators are neutrals who work with the parties to reach a result that is acceptable to them. Unlike arbitrators, mediators have no authority to impose a decision. Competent neutrals can minimize the power imbalances present in health services settings, especially when nonclinicians are involved in the dispute.[143] One objective of improved dispute resolution is to weld a multidisciplinary group into a cohesive, mutually supportive team so they can resolve their differences and improve patient care. Formal dispute resolution can also assist the various types of ethics committees, because it is overly optimistic to think that the act of establishing an interdisciplinary ethics committee means that it will be successful.

Ethics Officer. Appointing an ethics officer allows an HSO/HS to focus on internal ethics issues. An ethics officer can manage internal reporting systems, assess ethics risk areas, develop and distribute ethics policies and publications, investigate alleged violations, and design training programs. This senior-level executive can manage corporate compliance programs.[144]

Managers and the Law

Almost everything done in the delivery of health services is affected by statute, regulations, and court decisions. As with ethics, health services managers who have a basic understanding of the law and its effects on the HSO/HS will not only avoid problems, but be more effective.

CONTRACTS

A contract is an agreement between two or more parties that identifies rights and obligations. The parties agree to do or not do certain things. The definition of formal law in Chapter 1 includes understandings (contracts) between private parties or between private parties and government.

Decision makers in contract disputes first look to the generally applicable law and then interpret the private agreement within this context.

Elements of a Contract

A valid contract has several elements: (1) It is an agreement that is reached after an offer and an acceptance for which (2) there is consideration (something of value) that is (3) reached by parties who have the legal capacity to contract and (4) the objective of which is lawful. This seems simple enough, but applying the elements of contracts has resulted in a vast body of statutes, regulations, and case law.

Even small HSOs have scores of contracts for goods and services. Examples are collective bargaining agreements and contracts to buy supplies, equipment, and consulting services; sell maintenance, laundry, or clinical services; and employ staff. Many transactions are not and need not be in writing; for example, a food service manager asks a produce market to supply vegetables, with payment on delivery. Oral contracts are treated differently from written contracts, however; oral contracts may not be legally binding if they exceed a certain dollar amount or if their duration exceeds a certain length of time. Managerial control of contracting is maintained by using purchase orders that, when sent to the seller, constitute an *offer* to buy or, if sent in response to a previous offer to sell, constitute the *acceptance*. Increasingly, HSOs/HSs sell services. Hospitals sell laboratory services to physicians or contract with HMOs to provide hospital care to members. Visiting nurse agencies sell therapists' services to nursing facilities. Services are usually offered at predetermined prices, although cost-plus contracts may be used.

Breach of Contract

When compared with the total number of contracts that HSOs/HSs execute annually, breaches of contract are rare. A breach of contract occurs when one of the parties fails to perform as promised. There are defenses when a breach of contract occurs. The contract may be impossible to perform because of destruction or unavailability of the subject matter, death or illness, or legal prohibition. Three types of remedies are available when "impossibility" is not an issue and there is simply a breach of contract: rescission for a material breach, specific performance, or damages. *Rescission* means that the contract is null and void, and the parties are put into their original positions relative to each other, as far as possible. Specific performance requires the party who is in breach to do what was agreed in the contract. If neither rescission nor specific performance is the appropriate remedy, the aggrieved party may seek money damages.

Breaches of contract usually involve lawyers, legal fees, and often a trial, even if one party is clearly right and the other is clearly wrong. As a consequence, breaches should be avoided. An excellent preventive measure is to involve competent legal counsel in negotiating and drafting contracts. Binding arbitration is a common, low-cost means to resolve disputes. It is standard in commercial contracts and should be included in other types, as well.

TORTS

Breach of Contract and Tort Distinguished

A principle of Anglo-American legal tradition is that people are responsible for the harm they cause, whether they act intentionally or unintentionally (negligently). Such responsibility falls into the domains of both contract and tort obligations. *Tort* is derived from the Latin *tortus*, or *twisted*. As its use in standard English faded, *tortus* acquired a technical meaning in the law.[145]

A tort is a civil wrong, other than a breach of contract, for which courts provide a remedy in the form of an action for damages.[146] To be successful, the action must include certain elements: there must be a duty, a breach of that duty, and resulting harm that is causally linked to the defendant.

Defendants may be liable for punitive damages in addition to actual damages, depending on their intent and the circumstances.

Contract liability is distinguished from tort liability primarily by what is protected:

> The distinction between tort and contract liability, as between parties to a contract, has become an increasingly difficult distinction to make. It would not be possible to reconcile the results of all cases. The availability of both kinds of liability for precisely the same kind of harm has brought about confusion and unnecessary complexity. . . .Tort obligations are in general obligations that are imposed by law—apart from and independent of promises made and therefore apart from the manifested intention of the parties—to avoid injury to others. By injury here is meant simply the interference with the individual's interest or an interest of some other legal entity that is deemed worthy of legal protection. . . . Contract obligations are created to enforce promises which are manifestations not only of a present intention to do or not to do something, but also a commitment to the future. They are, therefore, obligations based on the manifested intention of the parties to a bargaining transaction.[147]

This statement suggests that breach of contract and tort are more easily distinguished in theory than application. This is especially true in the breach of an implied warranty, a hybrid of contract and tort. In general, there is an implied warranty that goods are fit (merchantable) for their usual and customarily intended purposes.

> The doctrine of (strict) liability imposes liability on those responsible for defective goods which pose an unreasonable risk of injury and which do in fact result in injury, regardless of how much care was taken to prevent the dangerous defect. An important distinction has been made between products and services, and the doctrine does not normally apply to the latter. For example, in attempts to hold hospitals strictly liable for injuries caused by blood transfusions, courts generally have held that hospitals are providing a service and not in the business of selling blood; therefore strict liability does not apply.[148]

The legal concept of implied warranty is widely applied to medical products and devices. Clearly, the legal distinction between products and services is important to health services providers.

Intentional Torts

Some torts result from intentional rather than negligent conduct. The actor's intent need not be hostile or result from a desire to harm; rather, there is an intent to "bring about a result which will invade the interests of another in a way that the law will not sanction."[149] The intentional torts most likely to affect HSOs include battery, defamation, false imprisonment, invasion of privacy, tortious interference in contractual obligations, wrongful discharge of an employee, and wrongful disclosure of confidential information. Assault is often linked to battery in criminal proceedings, but rarely in civil law. Assault must raise a reasonable apprehension of harmful or offensive contact and can occur without the physical touching necessary for battery. As noted, to be ethical, consent must be informed, voluntary, and competent. Legal requirements are similar. Consent is discussed here in the context of intentional torts, but a legal action regarding consent can arise in negligence, as well.

Written consent is rarely obtained for routine outpatient visits if no invasive or potentially dangerous medical treatment is rendered. Consent is presumed when treatment is sought; this is sufficient for routine care. Because of the likelihood of significant medical treatment, hospital staff obtain written general consent for routine services when patients are admitted.

Nonroutine diagnostic, surgical, or other invasive procedures require special consent. Usually, an HSO's role in special consent is secondary and limited to obtaining the patient's signature on a form that authorizes it to participate in treatment ordered or rendered by physicians. For example, before admitting a patient to the hospital for surgery, the attending physician provides information the patient needs to give informed consent. This consent is recorded in the physician's office. After admission but before treatment, the hospital determines that the medical record includes the special consent signed by the patient that verifies the patient received an explanation of the treatment and gave consent. HSOs concerned with the ethics of consent independently determine that patients whose treatment requires special consent understand the treatment's nature and consequences. This may be ethically appropriate, but doing so exceeds the legal standard of care.

Important to informed consent are how much the patient must be told and the judgment made by the physician as to the patient's understanding. States apply three different legal standards to how much information the patient should be given: 1) that given by a reasonable physician, 2) that given to a reasonable patient, and 3) as a minority view, what this patient wants. The legal concept of therapeutic privilege allows physicians to withhold information if they judge that the patient might be harmed by, or engage in harmful behavior due to, having it.

In future, the consent process may oblige physicians to divulge their mental and physical health status, clinical experience and competence, outcomes for the procedure being contemplated, and whether they have been sued for malpractice or disciplined for poor clinical work. It is difficult to argue that such information is unimportant to informed decision making. The law is evolving in that direction. At the forefront of a duty to disclose are *Behringer v. The Medical Center at Princeton* and *Doe v. Noe,*[150] which held that HIV-positive physicians have a duty to disclose that fact to their patients.

The earlier discussion of the ethical issues of consent suggested that myriad factors, including education, intellect, emotional status, and general physical and psychological conditions, make it difficult or even impossible for patients to give truly informed consent. Many patients put themselves in their physicians' hands and accept their recommendations, thus minimizing the burden of consent for both.

Negligence

Background. Negligence is defined as not doing something that a reasonable person who is guided by reasonable considerations that ordinarily regulate human affairs would do, or doing something that a reasonable and prudent person would not do.[151] The test in health services is the actions or nonactions of a reasonable and prudent physician, nurse, manager, or governing body. As with the law of contracts, this seems straightforward, but volumes have been written to define and apply the concept of "reasonable person." What the reasonable person would do is called the "standard of care." The standard of care is used to measure performance of the acts (actions) in question—the alleged negligence. If the plaintiff—the party who brought the lawsuit and must prove the allegations (bears the burden of proof)—convinces the finder of fact (a jury or judge) by a preponderance of the evidence that the acts (actions) deviated from the standard of care, the finder of fact will find for the plaintiff. *Preponderance of the evidence* refers to evidence that produces the stronger effect or impression, has a greater weight, and is more convincing as to its truth—its effect is greater. If the burden of proof is not met by a preponderance of the evidence, the finder of fact must find for the defendant.

The person who commits a tort is always liable for damages. Commonly, however, HSOs/HSs are named as defendants because of legal theories discussed below. To be successful, a lawsuit for negligent medical conduct must meet four elements:

1. The caregiver(s)—physician(s) or other care provider(s)—must have had a duty to provide care of a certain quality (standard of care).
2. There must have been a breach of that duty—the care provided must have been less than the established standard for a reasonable provider of that type of care.

3.   The breach of duty must have been a substantial factor in causing the harm (proximate cause).
4.   The patient must have been injured.

Should any of the elements be absent, the plaintiff cannot recover damages on a theory of negligence.

Duty. With few exceptions, laws in the United States place no positive duty on one person to aid another. This is true for physicians and other caregivers, as well. Once a duty is established, however, care may be discontinued only if alternate provisions have been made and the patient is protected from harm. Abandonment is an intentional tort that supports a lawsuit.

Standard of Care. How is the standard that providers have a duty to provide services of a certain quality determined? The standard of care has evolved, from a locality rule that used the provider's geographic location, to a broader standard using the practice in communities of similar size and medical resources, to the current expectation that providers must meet a national standard. In general, providers are held to the standard of care appropriate under similar circumstances for that type of practitioner, delivered with the same reasonable and ordinary care, skill, and diligence as those in good standing would ordinarily exercise in like cases. This is the "average standard of the profession test,"[152] which is a national standard. Because providers are of different types, using various theories about disease causation and cure, practitioners must meet the standards for their types of practice.

Breach. The breach of the standard of care is shown by testimony from persons able to testify as to what is normally expected of that type of practitioner delivering care with ordinary and reasonable care, skill, and diligence. This is done through expert witnesses. In addition, breach of the standard of care may be established by citing the treating physician's own statements, calling that physician as a hostile or adverse witness, using standard medical textbooks or similar sources, or invoking a doctrine known as *res ipsa loquitur* (the thing speaks for itself), which is a legal theory limited to specific circumstances. Sometimes the negligence is a matter of common knowledge, and expert testimony is not needed.

Proximate Cause. The third element necessary for negligent medical conduct—causation—has several aspects:

> In addition to proving that a physician was negligent, that is, failed to meet the standard of care, and that the patient was injured, a malpractice plaintiff must also prove that the injury resulted from the negligence. Although this element of proof is called "causation," the term has a different sense from that used in medical circles. The law considers an injury to be caused by a negligent act if the injury would not have occurred but for the defendant's act, or if the injury was a foreseeable result of the negligent conduct. The legal cause of an injury is often termed the proximate cause. Note that the plaintiff need not prove that the negligent act caused the result, but only the strong likelihood that it did. Also, the negligence need not be the sole cause, but only a significant factor in the injury. It must be remembered that the purpose of a malpractice trial is not to convict the defendants of malpractice, but to decide whether the loss caused by the injury should be allocated to the defendants. The standards of proof are thus lower than for a criminal trial, for example.[153]

To solve questions of liability when two causes act together to bring about an event and either one of them alone would have brought the same result, some courts use the concept of substantial factor. Was the defendant's conduct a substantial factor in bringing about the injury? An example of substantial factor occurs when two physicians treat a patient essentially simultaneously in an emergency situation and both are negligent, so either could have caused the injury. This concept was applied by the California Supreme Court in *Landeros v. Flood,* a medical malpractice case in which the defendant negligently failed to diagnose and report battered child syndrome to authorities. The plaintiff child was returned to the same environment, where continued battering caused further injuries. The court ruled that actors may be liable if their negligence is a substantial factor in causing injury and that they are not relieved of liability because of the intervening act of a third person if such act was reasonably foreseeable at the time of their negligent conduct.[154]

Injury. The finder of fact must determine that the plaintiff was injured, the extent to which the injuries diminish quality of life or economic opportunities, and the costs the plaintiff will incur to meet the special needs that resulted from the injuries. Damages awarded to the plaintiff can be nominal, actual, and/or punitive. Nominal damages are paid when the plaintiff proves the case but cannot prove the extent of damages. Actual damages are awarded for past and future medical expenses and loss of income, as well as for physical pain and mental suffering. Plaintiffs are awarded punitive damages when the finder of fact determines that the defendant should be punished. Punitive damages may be called exemplary damages. They are similar to a fine levied against a defendant in a criminal case. Punitive damages are appropriate when conduct has been reckless, willful, malicious, or grossly negligent.

Torts and HSOs/HSs

The previous discussion about torts emphasized the roles of persons who commit the civil wrong, intentionally or unintentionally (negligently). This section identifies and analyzes legal theories used to find liability against HSOs/HSs when there is an employment relationship or when physicians or other licensed independent practitioners (LIPs) are independent contractors. Two legal doctrines result in liability for HSOs/HSs: agency, and the general concept that organizations owe a duty to patients and others. The legal risk for HSOs/HSs has expanded greatly since the 1960s.

Historically, the legal doctrines of governmental immunity and charitable immunity allowed HSOs to avoid liability for employees' negligent acts. Governmental immunity derived from the sovereign power of a monarch to be free from civil actions. The doctrine of charitable immunity arose from the concept that assets of a charitable HSO were unacceptably threatened if actions for medical malpractice could be brought against them. Court decisions and statutes such as the Federal Tort Claims Act[155] have eroded the doctrines of charitable and governmental immunity; in some jurisdictions or circumstances, they have disappeared completely.

AGENCY AND CORPORATE LIABILITY

Agency. The master's responsibility for a servant's negligence was established in English common law. It is the basis for the law of agency and is embodied in the Latin phrase *respondeat superior,* let the master answer. Though not masters per se, principals are responsible for their agents' acts. The negligence of a servant or agent is imputed (by vicarious liability) to the person best able to exercise control—the master or principal. An important pragmatic consideration underlying *respondeat superior* is that courts sometimes search for a "deep pocket," and employers usually have one. This doctrine applies to HSO/HS employees' acting within the scope of their employment. It has limited applicability to caregivers who are independent contractors, because they exercise control over the means and methods of performing their tasks, rather than being controlled by the HSO/HS. Therefore, the legal theory of agency cannot be used to hold the HSO/HS liable for the negligent acts of independent contractors. Physicians are the most common type of independent contractor in

HSOs. The legal doctrine of apparent or ostensible agency is applied when a patient is wittingly or unwittingly led to believe that the HSO is an employer of a caregiver who would otherwise be defined as an independent contractor. A reasonable person standard is used.

Corporate Liability. The other legal basis for liability of HSOs/HSs is the general theory that the HSO/HS owes a duty to patients (as well as to others, such as visitors) to protect them from harm. This is known as corporate liability, an area of tort law that expanded rapidly in the last third of the 20th century. In the past, this legal doctrine allowed recovery by patients and visitors who were injured because the HSO failed to keep buildings, grounds, and equipment in a safe condition. Further, the HSO/HS has a duty to take reasonable steps in selecting and retaining those who provide services as independent contractors. HMOs, for example, may be found liable for the negligence of their independent contractor physicians, using legal theories such as nondelegable duties by contract or by statute, joint venture, agency, or apparent or ostensible agency.[156] MCOs face similar risks.

Merged Concepts. Southwick has concluded that the two concepts of organization liability for malpractice found in agency and corporate liability have virtually merged into one:

> It should . . . be acknowledged that in the hospital setting there is no longer a viable distinction between the rules of respondeat superior, on one hand, and corporate or independent negligence, on the other. Essentially, the two theories have become one. . . . In the delivery of healthcare services in an institutional setting it is increasingly difficult to determine factually who is in control of whom. As allied healthcare professionals proliferate and are accorded a greater degree of independence from the direct supervision and control of the attending physician, the matter of the right to control another's actions becomes a very difficult question both as a matter of fact and of law. It therefore becomes necessary to place either sole or joint liability upon the institution which, in the final analysis, is ultimately responsible for arranging, providing, and coordinating the activities of a host of professional individuals, all of whom must work together in the care of patients.[157]

This evolution of legal doctrine has major consequences for HSOs/HSs. They are not yet guarantors of the results of medical treatment, but the field is moving toward unequivocal accountability for activities that fall below the standard of care. HSOs use quality assessment, continuous quality improvement, and risk management to establish and maintain quality, concepts that are considered in Chapter 7.

ENTERPRISE LIABILITY

The concept of enterprise liability includes elements of strict liability and corporate liability, which were discussed previously, and no-fault, which is discussed below. The failed Clinton health proposal of 1993 included tort reform, a prominent part of which was enterprise liability. Also known as organizational liability, enterprise liability changes the locus of liability for patient injuries without other significant alterations to the rules of proof and damages.[158] Channeling liability to HSOs is justified on several grounds:

> First, insurers would have an improved ability to price insurance, since difficulties in pricing for individual physicians in high-risk specialties would be eliminated; in most other areas of tort law, from environmental to products risk, business enterprises bear the cost of insuring against liability. Second, by eliminating the insurance problems inherent in the fragmented malpractice market, specialties such as obstetrics would no longer face onerous burdens, nor will physicians have to face premiums that fluctuate excessively from year to year. Third, physicians would be freed from the psychological stress inflicted by being named defendants in malpractice suits. Fourth, admin-

istrative and litigation costs would be reduced by having only one defendant, rather than the multiplicity of providers named in the typical malpractice suit. Fifth, and most important, patterns of poor medical practice would be deterred by placing liability on institutions rather than individuals, since organizations have superior data collection abilities and management tools for managing risks.[159]

Proponents argue that a compensation system that rewards more claimants, especially small ones, in a more evenhanded and rapid fashion than does the current tort system will be an improvement, even if it is not cheaper.[160] Opponents of enterprise liability argue that persons rather than HSOs should be accountable for medical care, excessive power will accrue to HSOs, and physicians will be pitted against HSOs.[161] Enterprise liability is a logical extension of the evolution of vicarious liability and corporate negligence, which have moved the locus of much medical liability from independent contractor physicians to HSOs. It may well be effectively adopted by court decisions even absent legislative enactment.

▬ Reforms of the Malpractice System ▬

The direct costs of the medical malpractice system, $28 billion per year, do not consider the costs of defensive medicine, defined as ordering procedures and tests not clinically indicated.[162] Early state efforts at tort reform included limiting noneconomic damages, primarily recovery for pain and suffering; capping plaintiffs' legal fees; and allowing juries to learn how much money plaintiffs received from other sources (modifying the collateral source rule). Some state supreme courts have found such limitations constitutional.[163] Other legislative proposals include modifying the joint liability doctrine, allowing defendants to pay in installments, establishing malpractice screening panels, establishing patient compensation funds, granting immunity, and implementing a no-fault scheme.[164] It is argued that such reforms do not address the root of malpractice because the basic system is unchanged. Caps on damages and attorneys' fees reduce insurance premiums, but "patients with the most serious injuries are the ones who pay the price for the strategy."[165] Tort reform has had mixed results.[166] It is estimated that in the 28 states that limit malpractice payments, healthcare expenditures have been reduced 3%–4%.[167]

It is argued that reforms such as no-fault, which compensate injured persons without litigation or assigning liability, are key to reducing medical malpractice costs. Workers' compensation, which pays medical expenses and lost income to workers injured on the job, is an example of no-fault. No-fault malpractice systems in Virginia and Florida apply to newborns who suffer neurological damage caused by medical treatment during delivery. Both states allow recovery for medical and rehabilitation expenses, as well as compensation to replace lost future wages and noneconomic losses.[168] Because all those injured may file claims, no-fault may actually increase rather than decrease costs, however. There is mounting evidence that (primary care) physicians who communicate effectively with their patients are sued less often and that physicians who admit errors and apologize for them are less likely to be sued.[169]

NONJUDICIAL MEANS OF RESOLVING DISPUTES

Most lawsuits are settled before trial; some are settled after trial begins. Settlement occurs at the behest of counsel, or the parties perceive the advantages of avoiding a trial, such as uncertainty of outcome, desire to control the result, and avoiding a trial's negative publicity. State law may require settlement efforts; many courts have mandatory procedures to settle cases.

Resolving disputes in court is expensive and time-consuming. Since the mid-1980s, much attention has been given to alternative dispute resolution (ADR). ADR includes binding and nonbinding arbitration (which may be voluntary or nonvoluntary), mediation, minitrials, neutral fact finding, and variations of these techniques. ADR is private, inexpensive, and efficient—attributes especially useful for HSOs/HSs. Each type of ADR has attributes that make it the best choice for certain disputes. For example, mediation is most effective when the parties want a continuing relationship. In particular, professional staff should be aware of ADR's advantages; their bylaws should reflect its use. A number of private organizations provide mediators, arbitrators, and others who are expert in ADR.

Mediation is common in court-annexed programs. For example, the Superior Court of the District of Columbia requires mediation of all cases in its small claims division (for monetary compensation claims under $5,000). Judges may order mediation or case evaluation, which is similar to neutral fact finding, for cases in the civil division. Medical malpractice cases may be mediated in the civil division. In both divisions, cases that do not settle are scheduled for trial.[170]

Arbitration is common in managed care and health plans. In 2001, it was reported that the 30 health plans that enrolled 80% of the 23 million Californians in managed care required arbitration for some disputes.[171] Generally, courts dislike contracts of adhesion and may rule that provisions such as mandatory arbitration are unenforceable.[172] This general view is buttressed by strong constitutional safeguards of the right to a jury trial.[173] In future, more HSOs/HSs are likely to use mediation or voluntary binding arbitration to resolve malpractice claims. *Voluntary* here means that if the parties agree to arbitrate, the arbitrator's award is binding and judicial remedies are unavailable.

This discussion of ADR has focused on medical malpractice. Numerous other types of problems occur in HSOs/HSs, including professional staff appointment and credentialing issues, disputes regarding sales agreements and employment and construction contracts, debt collection, and zoning appeals. ADR is common outside health services, and it has significant potential for expanded application in HSOs/HSs.

Selected Legal Areas Affecting HSOs/HSs

PEER REVIEW

Historically, antitrust lawsuits against physicians and HSOs arose in hospitals in which members of the professional staff organization (PSO) conducted peer review of other physicians' clinical work. When peer decisions caused PSO members to lose or be denied clinical privileges, the actions were alleged to be anticompetitive because they were based on economics, not efforts to improve quality. In *Patrick v. Burget*, a physician alleged federal antitrust violations when a peer review action ended his clinic practice and caused suspension of his hospital privileges.[174]

The chilling effect of such lawsuits on peer review and other efforts to improve quality resulted in passage of the Health Care Quality Improvement Act (HCQIA) of 1986 (PL 99-660).[175] HCQIA grants limited immunity from paying damages in private lawsuits under federal or state law (except civil rights laws) for any "professional review action" (including peer review) if the professional review follows standards established in the law. Standards include a reasonable belief that the action was justified in furthering the quality of healthcare, there was a reasonable effort to obtain the facts, and the physician (or dentist) was given adequate notice and a fair hearing or such other procedures fair under the circumstances. *Austin v. McNamara* and *Egan v. Athol Memorial Hospital* show that HCQIA's peer review protections are achieving their purpose.[176]

EMERGENCY MEDICAL TREATMENT AND ACTIVE LABOR ACT

The Emergency Medical Treatment and Active Labor Act (EMTALA) (PL 99-272) was passed in 1985.[177] This unfunded mandate requires that hospitals participating in Medicare provide screening examinations to persons who seek treatment at their emergency departments, regardless of ability to pay. If an emergency condition exists, the hospital must treat and stabilize the patient unless the patient requests a transfer in writing with knowledge of the hospital's obligation under EMTALA or unless a physician certifies that the benefits to the patient of an unstabilized transfer outweigh the risks. The means of transportation used for transfer must meet statutory requirements as to adequacy of equipment and personnel, the receiving facility must agree to accept the transfer, and medical records must be provided to the receiving facility. In 1989, EMTALA was amended to apply to women in any stage of labor, rather than merely active labor.[178] Women in labor are in an emergency condition if transfer cannot occur before delivery or if transfer presents a health threat to the woman or unborn child.[179]

MEDICARE AND MEDICAID FRAUD AND ABUSE

Since Medicare and Medicaid were enacted in 1965, a large body of law has resulted from the amendments, regulations, and court decisions that followed. A special focus of Congress has been what is generically called fraud and abuse, defined broadly to include lying, stealing, providing too few or too many services, improperly coding services, bribes and kickbacks, and self-referrals.[180] Congress has been of some assistance to providers by identifying exceptions and by authorizing DHHS "to issue 'safe harbor' regulations delineating conduct that DHHS determined would not be subject to prosecution or exclusion under the anti-kickback statute."[181] Of the numerous actions defined by Medicare and Medicaid as fraud and abuse, only fraudulent billing and self-referral are addressed here.

Fraudulent Billing. In addition to the *qui tam* actions described below, there are civil and criminal penalties for false claims made to Medicare and Medicaid. Fraudulent billing is a common type of false claim. Some infractions are presumptively fraudulent; for example, a psychiatrist billed Medicaid for 4,800 hours in a year (40 hours/week = 2,080 hours/year). Other cases are less clear. A court upheld a $258,000 fine against anesthesiologists whose defense was that, at most, they were guilty of "unartfully" describing services rendered. The court found that the standard of care to be applied was exacting and that "unartful descriptions" were descriptions of services not rendered as claimed.[182]

Physician Self-Referral. A second example of fraud and abuse is physician self-referral. Amendments to Medicare in 1989 and 1993 to restrict self-referral are known as Stark I and Stark II, respectively, after the congressman instrumental in their passage. Stark I restricted referral of Medicare patients for clinical laboratory services by physicians who had financial relationships with the laboratory.[183] Stark II expanded restrictions on self-referral to services such as physical and occupational therapy; radiology services; radiation therapy; durable medical equipment and supplies; parenteral and enteral nutritional services; prosthetics, orthotics and prostheses; home health; outpatient prescription drugs; and inpatient and outpatient hospital services.[184] Penalties are substantial. Civil penalties of thousands of dollars *per item or service*, plus assessments of two or three times the amount claimed, can be imposed. Some infractions can result in criminal sanctions. Providers can be excluded from participating in Medicare and Medicaid, the penalty that might be the harshest of all.[185]

HEALTHCARE INTEGRITY AND PROTECTION DATA BANK

Section 221 of the Health Insurance Portability and Accountability Act of 1996 (PL 104-191)[186] created the Healthcare Integrity and Protection Data Bank (HIPDB), the purpose of which is to record adverse actions against healthcare providers, suppliers, or practitioners. Included are civil judgments against a provider, supplier, or practitioner related to delivery of healthcare; criminal convictions related to delivery of a healthcare item or service; adverse actions by federal or state agencies responsible for licensing and certification; exclusion of a provider, supplier, or practitioner from federal or state healthcare programs; and any other adjudicated actions or decisions that the secretary of DHHS establishes by regulations.[187] This well-intentioned legislation highlights the need for HSOs/HSs to have access to legal advice. HIPDB may well achieve far less than its intended results, and at considerable cost to providers.

QUI TAM ACTIONS

The vast amounts of money spent by federal programs cause significant potential for fraud, abuse, and waste. In 1986, Congress enacted the False Claims Act Amendments (PL 99-562) to strengthen Civil War–era legislation that protected whistle-blowers who report fraud, abuse, and waste in federally funded programs.[188] One provision allows whistle-blowers, whom the law calls relators, to sue in the name of the federal government, with the incentive that they may receive 15%–30% of triple damages and fines imposed. Such suits are known as *qui tam*, from the Latin for "who as well." Healthcare fraud is the leading type of federal *qui tam* lawsuit, accounting for 46% of cases and recoveries of $5 billion from 1987 to 2005. A 2005 federal law encourages states to pass their own *qui tam* statutes by increasing their share of Medicaid fraud recoveries.[189]

TAX-EXEMPT STATUS OF HSOs/HSs

Federal tax law has long recognized the special role of organizations performing charitable work. HSOs/HSs organized as not-for-profit corporations may apply to the Internal Revenue Service (IRS) to become tax-exempt organizations under Section 501(c)(3) of the Internal Revenue Code. If approved, the HSO/HS is exempt from federal income and excise taxes, and donors are allowed to deduct gifts to them in calculating federal income taxes. If local and state governments accept the IRS determination, the HSO avoids property, inventory, excise, sales, and other taxes typically levied on for-profit businesses. Being tax exempt provides significant economic benefits.

From 1956 to 1969, the IRS required a tax-exempt hospital to "be operated to the extent of its financial ability for those not able to pay for the services rendered and not exclusively for those who are able and expected to pay."[190] A 1969 IRS revenue ruling removed the requirement to render service to those unable to pay and stated that promoting health was a sufficient charitable purpose that benefited the community as a whole. By operating an emergency room open to all and providing care for community members unable to pay, a hospital was promoting the health of a class of people broad enough to benefit the community. The IRS position was upheld in the legal challenge that followed.[191] Thus, less emphasis on treating those unable to pay did not cause loss of tax-exempt status. The 1969 IRS revenue ruling criteria are reflected in the "community benefit" standard of Section 501(c)(3). The economics of community benefit include charity care (the total of uncompensated care, bad debt, and the differences between billings to Medicare and Medicaid and payments from them) and hospital spending such as that on health fairs.[192] Other indicators of charitable purpose and community benefit include a mission to provide community benefit: providing essential services, educating the public, and serving unmet human needs.[193]

Despite a consistent approach by the IRS, the issue is far from resolved at other levels of government. The stakes are high. The Congressional Budget Office (CBO) estimated that in 2002, the total value of hospitals' tax-exempt status was $12 billion.[194] Historically, state and local governments accepted the IRS determination. This has changed. Several state and local governments have successfully argued that hospitals provided too little public service and charity care to justify their tax-exempt status. Some tax-exempt hospitals paid voluntarily; others fought the challenge and won.[195] Seemingly politically motivated challenges to tax-exempt status occurred in Urbana, IL, when local authorities alleged that two hospitals were overly aggressive in collecting unpaid patient accounts, that some of their property was used in for-profit businesses, and that they did not provide charity care to all who needed it.[196]

Adding political impetus to review of tax-exempt status by state and local jurisdictions is that many hospitals and other HSOs are involved in service integration, diversification, reorganization, mergers, and joint ventures, all of which suggest for-profit businesses, not charitable, tax-exempt-worthy activities. Reports of highly compensated executives have also stirred political interest. Such developments diminish the public perception of "community benefit" that previously distinguished not-for-profit HSOs/HSs. A public that believes not-for-profit HSOs/HSs are just like any other business will not support tax-exempt status. Further clouding issues of tax-exempt status and charitable purpose are data from a CBO analysis that found that tax-exempt hospitals provided only slightly more uncompensated care as a percentage of operating expenses than did for-profit hospitals, which receive none of the tax benefits enjoyed by not-for-profit hospitals.[197]

A tax-exempt organization may participate in activities unrelated to its exempt purpose if they are insubstantial parts of operations. Beyond that proviso, Congress has imposed an unrelated business income tax to eliminate unfair competition from tax-exempt entities.[198] Overall, the trend is to narrow tax-exempt status, with Congress tying continued tax-exemption to minimum levels of charity care that are likely to be a percentage of the benefit of being tax exempt.

TELEMEDICINE

The law of contract, negligence, malpractice, and strict liability will apply to telemedicine, but like the technology, the law of telemedicine is evolving and is unlikely to achieve stability for decades. Several areas—confidentiality, data compression, artificial intelligence, licensure, and consent—are legally problematic.

Confidentiality. Electronic patient records with multiple users and distributed computer systems make information security problematic. Confidentiality issues include improper disclosure, such as leaving visible or easily retrievable data on a screen; unauthorized access, such as by hackers; aggregating data to identify individual patients; and data integrity and authenticity.[199] Providers' liability for failing to maintain the confidentiality of patient information is well established; largely undetermined is the duty of organizations providing telemedical support.[200]

Data Compression. The great amount of data in health services requires special handling so the system is not overwhelmed. Compressing files makes the data stream more manageable, but greater compression ratios increase the risk of image degradation. This means, for example, that teleradiology may be unable to achieve the reliability of in-person reading of x-rays.[201] Resulting faulty diagnoses or treatments will raise liability issues.

Artificial Intelligence. Telemedicine includes aids to decision making, one of which is artificial intelligence (AI). Expert systems are a type of AI that helps practitioners solve problems by asking questions, discarding irrelevant information, and producing an explained, reasoned conclusion.[202] An example of applying expert systems is the Acute Physiology and Chronic Health Evaluation (APACHE), which helps manage intensive care unit patients by monitoring various indicators and calculating the probability of death.[203] Studies comparing the conclusions of expert physicians with those of AI diagnostic systems found that the systems provided useful but potentially misleading information. In addition, AI could lead to claims of information overload distracting to the physician, or it may be used to unfairly question a physician's treatment when, in fact, it is the technology that is limited.[204] Such findings suggest that AI's contribution to health services may increase in the future, but it brings potential legal problems.

Licensure. States regulate physicians and other LIPs. An LIP unlicensed in the state in which a consultation occurs has engaged in unauthorized practice in that state. Concomitantly, if the LIP was not practicing in the state (e.g., because no physician–patient relationship had been established), reimbursement may be denied. Such barriers have limited the more widespread use of telemedicine. Several states are addressing aspects of telemedicine as they apply to Medicaid.[205] The AMA fully supports state-based licensure for physicians; the American College of Radiology recommends that physicians who interpret teleradiology images be licensed at both the transmitting and receiving sites; the College of American Pathologists takes the position that a physician must be licensed in the state where the patient is located.[206]

Although not necessarily affecting HSOs/HSs directly, at least in the near term, the availability of prescription drugs from web sites on the Internet raises complex legal and ethical issues and potentially disastrous health risks for "patients" who self-diagnose and self-prescribe. These web sites have little or no review by physicians, and remote prescribing raises issues of unlicensed practice.[207] Further, there are few, if any, controls or prospects of control by state or federal government.

Consent. The use of telemedicine makes the legal aspects of patient consent much more complex. Disclosing involvement of LIPs via telemedicine becomes legally more important as "direct" participation increases, as, for example, in robotic surgery. Prudence suggests that patients should be informed and asked to consent when their treatment is being directed by other than their attending physician.[208]

Summary. Each year, the environment for telemedicine improves. An important reason telemedicine has not expanded into routine care is the stringent regulation of Medicare reimbursement for such services. Some federal-level barriers were removed with passage of the 2000 Omnibus Budget Bill.[209] Telemedicine offers a cost-efficient means to improve access and the quality of medical services everywhere, but the barriers to wider application are significant.

Legal Process of a Civil Lawsuit

This discussion is on the legal process of a civil lawsuit based on a tort, not a breach of contract. A civil lawsuit begins when a plaintiff files a complaint in a court with jurisdiction to hear the case. This filing makes the complaint an official document and a matter of public record. It is served on (delivered to) a defendant by a process server, who is often a marshal or a sheriff's deputy. The defendant's response to the complaint is known as an answer, and it must be filed within a limited period of time. The answer may deny the allegations in the complaint in whole or in part, or it may assert specific affirmative defenses, such as that the complaint is barred by the statute of limitations and the suit may not be brought, the plaintiff assumed the risk, or the plaintiff was partly to blame for the injury (contributory negligence). The defendant may also make certain motions before the court—for example, a motion to dismiss because the complaint fails to state a cause of action or a motion to dismiss because the complaint was filed in a court that lacks jurisdiction. Few cases are dismissed at this stage. The next phase is discovery, which allows each party to learn about the opponent's case. The plaintiff seeks information to support the allegations of tortious conduct; the defendant seeks to determine the strength of the plaintiff's case, and vice versa.

During discovery, the plaintiff is likely to make motions that ask the court to require the defendant(s) to produce documents (production) needed to prepare its case. The defendant may ask the court to deny the motions for reasons such as statutory privilege, relevance, and reasonableness of demands. In addition, the parties obtain information through written interrogatories (questions) and by taking sworn depositions (statements) of the parties, other people with knowledge of the alleged injuries, or those who will testify as expert witnesses. With rare exceptions, all states protect the results of peer review by health services providers from discovery. The discovery phase may take months or years; statutes determine the time. Procedural maneuvering to prevent a party (usually the plaintiff) from obtaining documents and information adds time and expense.

Many cases are settled during the discovery phase or when it is complete, primarily because the parties have learned enough about the accuracy of the allegations and the strength of the case to make an informed decision. States have various requirements to determine the merits of a medical malpractice claim, as well as alternative means of settling cases.

If the case has merit but is not settled, a trial date is set. The trial begins with opening statements by counsel, in which they outline their cases and suggest what they will attempt to show. The plaintiff's case is presented first, and the elements of a tort must be proven by a preponderance of the evidence. This is done by introducing evidence consisting of documents and testimony by persons who may have observed the event or can offer other information, and by expert witnesses. If there is no direct evidence as to the cause of the tort, the plaintiff must use circumstantial evidence from which inferences can be drawn that convince the finder of fact (the jury, or judge sitting without a jury) as to causation. Both parties will object to introduction of evidence that may damage their cases. The judge rules on the admissibility of evidence and any motions that are made by counsel during the trial. If present, a jury hears and sees the evidence and makes findings of fact.

Witnesses are questioned in several steps. The party calling the witness asks questions first; this is called direct examination. After direct examination, opposing counsel asks questions to cross-examine the witness. Cross-examination permits counsel to impeach the witness by raising questions about the accuracy of the witness's memory, veracity, reputation, and the like. This tests the witness's testimony and allows the finder of fact to give it whatever weight is considered appropriate. After cross-examination, redirect examination allows counsel to rehabilitate the witness—to minimize undesirable impressions left by cross-examination. The last round of questions is called re-cross-examination. A major theory of the law is that truth will emerge from this adversarial process and that the finder of fact can determine the reliability of the witnesses.

The defendant's case is presented following the plaintiff's and uses the same steps. When the evidence has been heard (and seen), the jury is charged (given instructions) by the judge. This means that the judge instructs the jury in writing that if it determines certain facts are present, the law requires it to find in specific ways. Jury instructions are very important, and both sides submit proposed instructions from which the judge chooses. Proposed instructions are cast by each party in the light most favorable to its case. If there is no jury, the judge considers the evidence and renders a decision. In some jurisdictions, the decision to find for the plaintiff or defendant is separate from a decision on damages, if the finding is for the plaintiff.

At various times during the trial, the parties make motions for the judge to consider and make rulings on. For example, the defendant usually moves for a directed verdict after the plaintiff's case has been presented. This motion asks the judge to rule that the plaintiff has not presented enough evidence to support the claim—that it is not a prima facie case—and as a matter of law, the plaintiff is not entitled to damages. If the motion is granted, which is rare, the trial ends because the judge has found for the defendant. Both parties may move for a directed verdict after all the evidence has been presented. When the jury finds for one of the parties, the other may ask for a judgment notwithstanding the verdict or, alternatively, for a new trial. If the judge grants the former, which is rare, the jury verdict is overturned, and judgment is entered for the other party. If the latter is granted, a new trial is set. Motions are supported or opposed by briefs from the parties that cite legal precedents and arguments as to why their motions should be granted or their opponents' denied.

If the defendant loses and the jury awards damages that the defendant believes are excessive as a matter of law, the defendant can petition the court for *remittitur,* which allows the judge to decrease the award, if granted. Again, the defendant's brief will argue that the evidence and/or the law do not support the verdict. The plaintiff submits a brief in opposition. Similarly, the doctrine of *additur* allows the court to increase a jury award that the judge finds to be inadequate.

The losing party may appeal the verdict. Appeals are based on alleged errors made by the trial court and that represent misapplication of the law by the judge. These appeals are entered in the appeals court (the intermediate level) or, on further appeal, in the highest court of a state. Typical errors alleged by the losing party are admitting (or not admitting) evidence, granting (or not granting) a motion, content of jury instructions, and the judge's decision to qualify or refuse to qualify expert witnesses.

Trial and appeals court proceedings are very expensive. Discovery before trial requires paying fees for documents, deposing parties and witnesses, and paying the costs of expert witnesses. Usually, such costs must be paid as they are incurred. There are major costs to defendants who must answer interrogatories, produce documents, and cope with the disruption and other aspects of defending the suit. Trial appearances by attorneys command higher fees than are charged for other work. In addition, court costs must be paid. An appeal requires a transcript of the stenographic record of the trial. This record is several thousand pages long, even for a short trial, and costs thousands of dollars to prepare. High stakes, however, warrant such costs. Contingency fees for attorneys are suggested as a cause of the large number of medical malpractice suits. However, contingency fee arrangements allow injured patients to seek redress even if they cannot pay for an attorney to prepare and try the case.

Special Considerations for the Manager

Managers face a range of problems in effectively handling legal and quasilegal matters that arise regularly. These run the gamut, from patients with a grievance and who are potential litigants to instructing staff on the maintenance and confidentiality of medical records. It must be remembered that HSOs/HSs have an independent ethical obligation to the patient and community that is separate from and more demanding than that arising from their legal obligations.

RECORD KEEPING

Lacking adequate medical records, healthcare providers have great difficulty proving that their actions comport with the standard of care. Medical records hold no special legal magic. The information contained in medical records is admissible only under an exception to the hearsay rule of evidence. They are used to refresh the recollection of caregivers who participated in treatment and made entries in the record. In addition, the record is the basis for opinions by expert witnesses. The complexity and extent of events and treatment, the mobility of caregivers, and fading memories necessitate that medical records be complete, accurate, and legible.

Persons who fear that information in a medical record may lead to embarrassment, dismissal, or a law suit may alter the medical record. Doing so violates a basic ethical duty and breaks the law. Alterations are likely to be discovered, however, and not only make juries more willing to award damages, but may persuade a judge to punish the defendant by allowing award of punitive damages. Effective risk management requires that a responsible person obtain custody of the medical record at the first indication of a potentially compensable event. This control should be exercised continuously until the dispute has been resolved, including any appeal.

A common problem with paper medical records is that handwritten entries are hard to read or illegible. An electronic medical record (EMR) eliminates legibility issues. The transition to an EMR will be slow, however; in the meantime, the HSO's medical records committee or its equivalent must work to monitor and improve legibility of entries. It must also ensure that records are properly organized, authenticated, completed properly and in a timely fashion, and available when needed. Advantages and disadvantages of EMRs are discussed in Chapter 3.

EFFECTIVE USE OF RETAINER AND HOUSE COUNSEL

HSOs/HSs obtain legal advice in two basic ways. Often, smaller organizations pay a retainer to an attorney to guarantee consultation as needed. Considering the law's importance in managing HSOs/HSs and the need for ongoing advice and counsel, however, this may not be the most desirable option. Usually, larger HSOs/HSs employ in-house counsel. In this arrangement, the attorney is a staff assistant to management and the governing body. Access to either retainer counsel or in-house counsel is essential because HSOs/HSs can no longer rely on free advice from an attorney who is a member of the governing body, for example. Health services law is so specialized and frequently applied that casual or informal relationships are insufficient.

Effective use of legal counsel poses the same problems for management as does interacting with other technical staff. Specifics vary depending on whether in-house or retainer counsel is used. A major advantage of in-house counsel is that they are integrated into the systems that alert management to legal problems or prevent them from occurring, such as the risk management program. Furthermore, greater contact with in-house counsel enhances managers' knowledge of the law and potential legal problems, and they will be more likely to seek timely guidance. In-house counsel is committed to one organization and not distracted by other clients. Finally, in-house counsel will be expert in the HSO's/HS's unique characteristics and special problems. In sum, these considerations offer enhanced effectiveness. Legal expertise can be obtained in other ways, too. Law school graduates with dual degrees—with one in management or a clinical area—allow HSOs/HSs to hire managers and program directors with legal training, thus enhancing their ability to comply with the law.

Having in-house counsel does not entirely eliminate the need for outside counsel. Specialized areas of the law and litigation are referred to outside attorneys. Like medicine, the practice of law has become highly segmented. Appropriate skills will optimize the outcome.

TESTIFYING

During their careers, health services managers are likely to testify in legal proceedings. Common is testimony to provide information about how the HSO/HS is organized or how it functioned in a specific circumstance. Less common is providing information about an incident about which the manager has firsthand knowledge.

Written interrogatories ask managers and staff to answer questions about the organization, staffing, functions, and similar topics. The answers are prepared with assistance of legal counsel. Interrogatories aid counsel in requesting specific documents and information and often are the first step in the discovery process. Managers may be deposed by counsel for the opposing party. The deponent (manager) swears (or affirms) to answer questions truthfully. The HSO's/HS's attorney is present and may object to questions, but they are usually answered. A verbatim record is made. If the deposition is used in court, the judge rules on the objections that counsel made during the deposition. The finder of fact weighs the testimony of witnesses, who are expected to testify in an honest and forthright manner.

Expert witnesses are ubiquitous in legal proceedings involving HSOs/HSs. The experience and education of health services managers qualifies them to be expert witnesses regarding the organization and management of HSOs/HSs about which they are knowledgeable. Once qualified by the court, the expert renders an opinion as to whether the organization, management, and performance of an HSO/HS or its staff met the standard of care. Hypothetical questions may be used to establish the standard of care, but they are less common than in the past. Questions are as likely to be formulated in terms of whether performance conformed with the standard of care. Being an expert witness requires no special skills beyond a knowledge of one's field and a clear understanding of how it applies to the case.

▰ DISCUSSION QUESTIONS

1. Describe the relationship between law and ethics. Which is the more demanding standard? Why? Identify and be prepared to explain examples other than those described in the chapter.
2. Identify health services laws or regulations based on 1) a utilitarian philosophy, 2) a deontological philosophy, and 3) elements of both. How compatible are these philosophies when included in the same law or regulation?
3. What does a professional code of ethics reflect? How can enforcement be made meaningful? Must a profession "police" its standards? Why or why not?
4. Describe uses and limitations of codes of ethics that apply to HSOs/HSs. Should they be communicated to patients who are served by the organization? If so, how?
5. What is the HSO's/HS's role regarding patient rights? Are some duties or obligations surpassed by the organization's duty to patients? If so, give examples of where this occurs.
6. Define *fiduciary*. Give some examples in and out of health services. Are HSOs/HSs and their services unique in terms of this concept? If so, how?
7. Define *conflict of interest*. Give examples in HSOs or HSs. How can they be minimized? What is the manager's role?
8. What should be the role of managers in allocating resources at the micro and macro levels? What can be done to reduce the likelihood that ethical problems will arise?
9. What types of experimentation might occur in HSOs/HSs? Distinguish surgical experimentation from that involving drugs and devices, in terms of safeguards. How can patients be protected?
10. Identify the types of advance directives. What are their effects on HSOs? How do managers ensure that HSOs interact effectively with patients in terms of such directives?
11. What is euthanasia? What are the types of euthanasia? Distinguish euthanasia from physician-assisted suicide. Develop brief scenarios that highlight the differences between the various types of euthanasia and physician-assisted suicide.
12. Some research indicates that the majority of patients are willing and able to participate in end-of-life decisions by speaking about their preferences for care. Do such findings diminish hospitals' need to develop a futile care policy? Explain how futility theory is compatible with physician-assisted suicide.

▰ Case Study 1: "What's a Manager to Do?"[210]

S.L. Rine joined the managerial staff of a large health services provider after gaining several years of experience. Rine is an affiliate of the American College of Healthcare Executives (ACHE) and wants to build the best set of credentials in the shortest possible time. Rine wants to become a chief executive officer.

Rine is responsible for several support departments as well as some clinical areas. Rine realized quickly that the HSO is very political. Much of what happens at the senior level is the result of personal relationships.

One of Rine's departments, maintenance, is responsible for all grounds. Rine found that grounds crews were being sent to homes of senior members of the governing body to maintain their lawns, shrubs, and trees. Rine asked the maintenance director to explain and was told that the practice had a long history; he suggested that it would be best not to make any changes. When Rine asked the maintenance director for a cost estimate of the grounds work being done at the private homes, he refused to give it. He said he didn't want to incur the wrath of the governing body members who were benefiting. Rine pondered what to do.

Shortly after talking to the maintenance director, Rine had lunch with the laboratory director. Without discussing specifics, Rine described the problem in maintenance. The laboratory director exclaimed, "That's nothing!" and described how two governing body members were selling reagents, supplies, and equipment to the laboratory at what she thought were higher than market prices. Rine asked if she had done anything about it; she replied that her predecessor had tried to stop the practice and had been fired. Rine pondered what to do.

QUESTIONS

1. Identify the ethical problem(s) that face the governing body members and the managers. Do similar problems face those not directly involved?
2. Are the grounds maintenance and the sale of reagents, supplies, and equipment to the laboratory ethically different? State your reasons. Are the two likely to be distinguished in the "real world"?
3. What steps should managers like Rine take if they have the moral courage to risk their jobs to try to solve the problems? Short of risking their jobs, what steps could they take?
4. What sources of assistance are there for Rine outside the organization? How should they be involved?

■ Case Study 2: Bits and Pieces[211]

John Henry Williams was pleased with his new job in the radiology department of Affiliated Nursing Homes and Rehabilitation Center. He was appointed acting department head because his predecessor, Mary Beth Jacobson, had been granted 6 months maternity leave. John Henry would be responsible for the equivalent of two-and-a-half full-time technicians, an appointment clerk, and $250,000 in equipment. He would have authority to purchase supplies, including certain types of x-ray film. The annual value of these purchases was about $90,000. Most were obtained from three vendors, companies from which the center had bought for years.

During her orientation for John Henry, Mary Beth emphasized how much she liked the meetings with sales representatives from the three vendors. Over the years, one had become a personal friend. Most meetings were held at the nice restaurant near the center. Some were held in Mary Beth's office, and if so, the sales representative always brought along a "little something." When John Henry asked what she meant, Mary Beth gave some examples: perfume, a bottle of French brandy, and a pen set in a leather case. John Henry remembered thinking that his wife would like the perfume, but he was more interested in the lunches. It would be a chance to get away from the dreary cafeteria, as well as his boring sack lunches. Mary Beth described the lunches as nothing fancy. She estimated that the typical cost to the sales representatives was the same as for a small gift—in the $40–$50 range.

John Henry asked Mary Beth whether there was a policy about accepting gifts from vendors. Mary Beth was angered by the question because it implied something was wrong with what she was doing. She responded curtly that the center trusted its managers and allowed them discretion in such matters.

John Henry asked if her behavior might suggest to other staff that her decisions were influenced by the gratuities she received from the sales representatives. Mary Beth's anger flashed. "I know you think that this doesn't look right. That isn't fair! I work long hours as a manager and get paid very little extra. It takes more effort and time to order and maintain proper inventory. If things go wrong, I get the blame. These gifts make me feel better about my efforts. My work has been exemplary. I'd be happy to talk to anyone who thinks otherwise!!"

QUESTIONS

1. Develop arguments that support Mary Beth's position on the gratuities she has been receiving. List them in order of importance.
2. Describe the importance of business custom in the relationship Mary Beth has with the sales representatives. Should this influence the ethics of the situation?
3. Develop a policy regarding gratuities that Affiliated Nursing Homes and Rehabilitation Center could use. Identify the underlying ethical principles, and be prepared to defend the policy.
4. Describe incidents from your own experience that are similar to the issues in the case. Did they have detrimental effects on the organization? Were they resolved? If so, how?

Case Study 3: Understanding[212]

The department of public health of Alplex County offers a variety of health promotion and disease prevention services. Patients who require medical or surgical intervention are referred to hospital-affiliated clinics or physicians' offices, as appropriate. These provider sites have an arrangement with the health department and receive reimbursement on a sliding scale, according to a prearranged fee schedule.

Eighteen-year-old Shirley Brown was seen by a nurse practitioner (NP) at a health department clinic. She was referred to a private practice gynecologist, who diagnosed severe dysmenorrhea. Ms. Brown was treated with a regimen of medications. Several months later, she returned to the health department clinic complaining of the same problem. The NP explained that surgery might be necessary to correct her problem. Ms. Brown returned to the gynecologist, telling him that the NP had discussed the surgical option. The gynecologist told her that the surgical option was a last resort. She was so distressed by the severe dysmenorrhea that she told the gynecologist to do whatever was necessary to make her feel better.

Ms. Brown was admitted to the hospital and underwent a hysterectomy. Only after her recovery from the surgery did she grasp the meaning of the procedure and that, as a result, she was unable to bear children. The realization caused her to become extremely distraught. She went back to the NP, with whom she had developed good rapport, to complain about her lack of understanding of the implications of surgical treatment.

DISCUSSION QUESTIONS

1. Describe the role of each provider involved, including the hospital, regarding patient consent.
2. Describe how the roles are complementary. How are they different?
3. Identify how a patient's age is important in the consent process.
4. Outline a process by which situations like Ms. Brown's could have been prevented.

Case Study 4: Allocation[213]

You are the coordinator of disease prevention for the health department of Grant County, which is geographically large and ethnically diverse and has urban and suburban population centers totaling 600,000. A recent outbreak of mumps and the shortage of mumps vaccine prompted your boss, the commissioner of health for Grant County, to ask you to update the county's plan for allocating vaccines that might be in short supply. The commissioner's memorandum to you directs that the plan must take a comprehensive, countywide approach. It references the importance of considering both the vaccines and antiviral medications for high-risk, infectious diseases. The memo uses the example of avian (bird) flu as one to consider in developing the plan. You are aware that bird flu affecting human beings has rapid onset and a high case fatality rate and tends to be more deadly for persons 20–40 years of age than other age groups.

You spend the next several hours in front of your PC preparing an outline of the plan. You include all major health services providers in the county. Of special concern to you is the need to preface and support your plan with a clearly identifiable value system (ethical basis) by which vaccines and antivirals should be allocated.

QUESTIONS

1. Which HSOs in Grant County should be included in the plan? Why?
2. What value system do you recommend as the underlying philosophy(ies) to guide allocation of scarce vaccines?
3. Outline the steps to inform the HSOs and relevant government agencies about the plan and to involve them in the contingency planning for implementation. (Should law enforcement officials participate?)
4. Should the residents of Grant County be involved in the planning process? Justify your answer.

Notes

1. Bodenheimer, Edgar. *Jurisprudence: The Philosophy and Method of the Law,* 6. Cambridge, MA: Harvard University Press, 1974.
2. Bodenheimer, *Jurisprudence,* 6.
3. Bodenheimer, *Jurisprudence,* 325.
4. Aristotle. *Politics,* 287. Translated by Benjamin Jowett. New York: The Modern Library, 1943.
5. Henderson, Verne E. "The Ethical Side of Enterprise." *Sloan Management Review* 23 (Spring 1982): 41–42. "Can a Corporation Know the Difference Between Right and Wrong?" In *State v. Christy-Pontiac, GMC, Inc.* (354 N.W.2d 17), the Minnesota Supreme Court held that a corporation could form the specific intent necessary to commit theft and forgery and thus be subject to criminal fines. The irony of the case lies in the fact that corporate officers were found not guilty when tried separately on the same charges. (Simonett, John E. "A Corporation's Soul." *Minnesota Bench & Bar* (September 1997): 34–35.
6. Kant, Immanuel. "Fundamental Principles of the Metaphysics of Morals." Translated by Thomas K. Abbott. In *Knowledge and Value,* edited by Elmer Sprague and Paul W. Taylor, 535–558. New York: Harcourt, Brace, 1959.
7. Rawls, John. *A Theory of Justice,* 60. Cambridge, MA: Belknap Press, 1971.
8. Bodenheimer, *Jurisprudence,* 23.
9. Arras, John, and Nancy Rhoden. *Ethical Issues in Modern Medicine,* 3rd ed. Mountain View, CA: Mayfield Publishing, 1989.
10. Jonsen, Albert R., and Stephen Toulmin. *The Abuse of Casuistry: A History of Moral Reasoning,* 13. Berkeley, CA: University of California Press, 1988.
11. Beauchamp, Tom L., and LeRoy Walters. *Contemporary Issues in Bioethics,* 4th ed., 21. Belmont, CA: Wadsworth, 1994.
12. Jonsen, Albert R. "Casuistry and Clinical Ethics." *Theoretical Medicine* 7 (1986): 71.
13. Pellegrino, Edmund D., and David C. Thomasma. *For the Patient's Good: The Restoration of Beneficence in Health Care,* 121. New York: Oxford University Press, 1988.
14. Pellegrino and Thomasma, *For the Patient's Good,* 116.
15. Carney, Frederick S. "Theological Ethics." In *Encyclopedia of Bioethics,* vol. 1, edited by Warren T. Reich, 435–436. New York: The Free Press, 1978.
16. Pellegrino and Thomasma, *For the Patient's Good,* 121.

17. Pellegrino, Edmund D. "The Virtuous Physician and the Ethics of Medicine." In *Contemporary Issues in Bioethics,* 4th ed., edited by Tom L. Beauchamp and LeRoy Walters, 53. Belmont, CA: Wadsworth, 1994.

18. This section is adapted from Darr, Kurt. "Linking Theory and Action." In *Ethics in Health Services Management,* 4th ed., 25–29. Baltimore: Health Professions Press, 2005; used with permission.

19. State Policies in Brief. "Refusing to Provide Health Services." Washington, DC: Guttmacher Institute, March 1, 2007. (Photocopy.)

20. Also known as the Church Amendment, the federal conscience clause was enacted in 1973. It relieves from adverse consequences those HSOs whose religious beliefs or moral convictions prohibit performing sterilizations or abortions, and it similarly protects staff who refuse to participate in these activities even if organizational values permit them.

21. ACHE Code of Ethics. *http://www.ache.org/ABT_ACHE/code.cfm,* retrieved February 5, 2007.

22. American College of Health Care Administrators. Code of Ethics. *http://www.achca.org/achca.asp?DP =content&FN=code_of_ethics.asp,* retrieved February 5, 2007.

23. *Current Opinions of the Judicial Council,* vii. Chicago: American Medical Association, 1982.

24. American Medical Association. Principles of Medical Ethics. *http://www.ama-assn.org/ama/pub/category/ 2512.html,* retrieved February 1, 2007.

25. Veatch, Robert M. "Professional Ethics: New Principles for Physicians?" *Hastings Center Report* (June 1980): 17.

26. *Code of Ethics for Nurses.* Washington, DC: American Nurses Association, 2001.

27. American Hospital Association. "The Patient Care Partnership: Understanding Expectations, Rights, and Responsibilities." © 2003. *http://www.aha.org/aha/content/2003/pdf/pcp_english_030730.pdf,* retrieved April 24, 2007.

28. Code of Ethics for the American Health Care Association. *http://www.ahca.org/quality/qfi/code_of _ethics.pdf,* retrieved December 5, 2006.

29. "A Commitment to Improve Health Care Quality, Access, and Affordability." Board of Directors Statement. Washington, DC: America's Health Insurance Plans, 2004.

30. Annas, George J. *The Rights of Patients: The Basic ACLU Guide to Patient Rights,* 2nd ed. Totowa, NJ: Humana Press, 1992.

31. Bryant, L. Edward, Jr. "Ethical and Legal Duties for Healthcare Boards." *Healthcare Executive* 20, 4 (July/August 2005): 46, 48.

32. Showalter, J. Stuart. *The Law of Healthcare Administration,* 4th ed., 91. Chicago: Health Administration Press, 2004.

33. Showalter, *The Law of Healthcare,* 93.

34. Stern et al. v. Lucy Webb Hayes. The governing body was called a board of trustees, and its members were known as trustees even though no trust was involved and they functioned as corporate directors.

35. Stern v. Hayes, 381 *Federal Supplement* 1003 (1974).

36. A furor resulted from a report that some Medicare HMOs' advertising targeted healthy seniors. (Hilzenrath, David S. "Study: HMOs Target Healthiest Seniors." *The Washington Post,* July 14, 1998, C3.)

37. Some physicians are "gaming" MCO constraints—sometimes through fraud and deception—so that their patients can get medical treatment that is needed but that the MCO will not authorize. Such actions go well beyond the physician-as-advocate role and raise several ethical issues. (Hilzenrath, David S. "Healing vs. Honesty? For Doctors, Managed Care's Cost Controls Pose Moral Dilemma." *The Washington Post,* March 15, 1998, H1.)

38. American Hospital Association. "American Hospital Association Guidelines: Advertising by Health Care Facilities." *http://www.100tophospitals.com/exclusives/guidelines/,* retrieved January 4, 2007.

39. Harron, Frank, John Burnside, and Tom Beauchamp. *Health and Human Values: A Guide to Making Your Own Decisions,* 148. New Haven, CT: Yale University Press, 1983.

40. Childress rejects subjective criteria (utilitarianism) because these comparisons demean people and run counter to the inherent dignity of human beings. He argues that the only ethical system of allocation is one that views all people needing a specific treatment as equals. To properly recognize human beings, we should provide treatment on a first-come, first-served basis or, alternatively, through random selection, as by a lottery. (Childress, James F. "Who Shall Live When Not All Can Live?" *Soundings, An Interdisciplinary Journal* 53 [Winter 1970]: 339–355.)

Rescher uses a two-tiered approach. The first tier includes basic screening for factors such as constituency served (service area), progress of science (benefit of advancing science), and prospect of success by type of treatment or recipient, such as denying dialysis to the very young or very old. The second tier considers individual patients and judges biomedical factors, including relative likelihood of success for the patient and life expectancy, as well as social aspects, including family role, potential future contributions, and past services rendered. When all factors are equal for two people, Rescher uses random selection to make a final choice. (Rescher, Nicholas. "The Allocation of Exotic Medical Lifesaving Therapy." In *Unpopular Essays on Technological Progress,* 30–44. Pittsburgh: University of Pittsburgh Press, 1980.) Because they result from value judgments, the social aspects are the most difficult. Rescher considered it irrational, however, to base choice on chance (after meeting medical criteria), as Childress advocated.

Each of these microallocation theories has advantages (and disadvantages); the resulting decisions will not satisfy everyone. The decision frameworks address issues and problems in an organized fashion, however. The choices of which people will receive extraordinary lifesaving treatment may be unpredictable, in the case of random allocation (Childress), or rational and almost totally predictable (Rescher). It may be left to chance and, in that sense, be fair to all needing treatment (Childress). Or it may be a matter of primarily subjective criteria (Rescher). Kantian principles of respect for persons and not using people as means to ends are reflected in Childress's theory. Conversely, Rescher's criteria are predominantly utilitarian.

41. Contrast this view with a case in Japan, in which a physician told a patient that she had gallstones rather than frighten her by telling her that she actually had gallbladder cancer. She delayed surgery. The cancer spread and she died. Her family sued. The court said that the patient herself was to blame because she had not followed the physician's advice to have the surgery and that the physician had no obligation to inform her of the true condition. (Hiatt, Fred. "Japan Court Ruling Backs Doctors." *The Washington Post,* May 30, 1989, A9.)

42. Katz, Jay. "Informed Consent—A Fairy Tale." *University of Pittsburgh Law Review* 39 (Winter 1977): 137–174.

43. President's Commission for the Study of Ethical Problems in Medicine and Biomedical and Behavioral Research. *Making Health Care Decisions,* vol. 1. Washington, DC: President's Commission, 1982.

44. Harvard Medical School. "A Definition of Irreversible Coma." *Journal of the American Medical Association* 205 (August 5, 1968): 337–338.

45. President's Commission for the Study of Ethical Problems in Medicine and Biomedical and Behavioral Research. *Defining Death: Medical, Legal, and Ethical Issues in the Determination of Death,* 25. Washington, DC: President's Commission, 1981.

46. Capron, Alexander Morgan. "Brain Death—Well Settled Yet Still Unresolved." Editorial. *New England Journal of Medicine* 344, 16 (April 19, 2001): 1,244.

47. In re Quinlan, 70 N.J. 10 (1976).

48. *Permanent* is used instead of *persistent* after a vegetative state has continued longer than a year.

49. Cruzan v. Director, Missouri Department of Health, 110 S. Ct. 2841 (1990).

50. Patient Self Determination Act of 1989, PL 101-508, 104 Stat. 1388-27 (November 5, 1990).

51. Bradley, Elizabeth H., and John A. Rizzo. "Public Information and Private Search: Evaluating the Patient Self-Determination Act." *Journal of Health Politics, Policy and Law* 24 (April 1999): 239–273.

52. Commission on Legal Problems of the Elderly. "Health Care Power of Attorney and Combined Advance Directive Legislation." Chicago: American Bar Association, September 1, 2004. (Photocopy.)

53. States' AMDs are at *http://www.caringinfo.org/i4a/pages/Index.cfm?pageid=3425,* retrieved January 4, 2007.

54. Wissow, Lawrence S., Amy Belote, Wade Kramer, Amy Compton-Phillips, Robert Kritzler, and Jonathan P. Weiner. "Promoting Advance Directives Among Elderly Primary Care Patients." *Journal of General Internal Medicine* 19, 9 (September 2004): 944–951.

55. Hahn, Michael E. "Advance Directives and Patient–Physician Communication." *Journal of the American Medical Association* 289 (January 2003): 96.

56. Colburn, Don. "Patients' Directives on Dying Have Little Effect on Care." *The Washington Post,* April 15, 1997, Health, 5.

57. Brown, Jonathan Betz, Arne Beck, Myde Boles, and Paul Barrett. "Practical Methods to Increase Use of Advance Medical Directives." *Journal of General Internal Medicine* 14 (1999): 21–26. Mailing written

materials to older adults with a substantial baseline placement rate increased the placement of AMDs in the medical record.

58. Cugliari, Anna Maria, Tracy Miller, and Jeffery Sobal. "Factors Promoting Completion of Advance Directives in the Hospital." *Archives of Internal Medicine* 155 (September 25, 1995): 1,893–1,898.

59. Reilly, Brendan M., Michael Wagner, C. Richard Magnussen, James Ross, Louis Papa, and Jeffrey Ash. "Promoting Inpatient Directives About Life-Sustaining Treatments in a Community Hospital." *Archives of Internal Medicine* 155 (November 27, 1995): 2,317–2,323.

60. Crane, Monica K., Marsha Wittink, and David J. Doukas. "Respecting End-of-Life Treatment Preferences." *American Family Physician* 72, 7 (October 1, 2005): 1,263–1,268.

61. Eliasson, Arn H., Joseph M. Parker, Andrew F. Shorr, Katherine A. Babb, Roy Harris, Barry A. Aaronson, and Margaretta Diemer. "Impediments to Writing Do-Not-Resuscitate Orders." *Archives of Internal Medicine* 159, 18 (1999): 2,213–2,218.

62. "Surrogate Consent in the Absence of an Advance Directive." Chicago: American Bar Association, Commission on Law and Aging, July 1, 2004. (Photocopy.)

63. "Health Care Power of Attorney and Combined Advance Directive Legislation." Chicago: American Bar Association, Commission on Legal Problems of the Elderly, September 1, 2004. (Photocopy.)

64. Shmerling, Robert H. "CPR: Less Effective than You Might Think." *InteliHealth*. Last updated and revised on November 29, 2005. *http://www.intelihealth.com/IH/ihtIh/WSIHW000/35320/35323/372221 .html?d=dmtHMS,* retrieved March 30, 2007. The article cites success rates of CPR in several settings: 2% to 30% effectiveness when administered outside the hospital; 6% to 15% for hospitalized patients; and less than 5% for elderly patients with multiple medical problems.

65. Jacobson, Bonnie S. "Ethical Dilemmas of Do-Not-Resuscitate Orders in Surgery." *AORN Journal* 60 (September 1994): 449–452; "Proposed AORN Position Statement on Perioperative Care of Patients with Do-Not-Resuscitate (DNR) Orders." *AORN Journal* 60 (October 1994): 648, 650; "Statement of the American College of Surgeons on Advance Directives by Patients: 'Do Not Resuscitate' in the Operating Room." *ACS Bulletin* (September 1994): 29; Margolis, Judith O., Brian J. McGrath, Peter S. Kussin, and Debra A. Schwinn. "Do Not Resuscitate (DNR) Orders During Surgery: Ethical Foundations for Institutional Policies in the United States." *Anesthesia and Analgesia* 80 (1995): 806–809.

66. Teno, Joan M., Rosemarie B. Hakim, William A. Knaus, Neil S. Wenger, Russell S. Phillips, Albert W. Wu, Peter Layde, Alfred F. Connors, Neal V. Dawson, and Joanne Lynn, for the SUPPORT Investigators. "Preferences for Cardiopulmonary Resuscitation: Physician–Patient Agreement and Hospital Resource Use." *Journal of General Internal Medicine* 10 (April 1995): 179–186.

67. "Out-of-Hospital/EMS/Bedside Do-Not-Resuscitate Orders." *http://www.atthecloseofday.com/outof hospitalDNR.htm,* retrieved April 19, 2007.

68. Kelly, Gerald. "The Duty to Preserve Life." *Theological Studies* 12 (December 1951): 550.

69. "Declaration on Euthanasia." Rome: Vatican Congregation for the Doctrine of the Faith, June 26, 1980.

70. Beauchamp, Tom L., and James F. Childress. *Principles of Biomedical Ethics,* 4th ed., 207. New York: Oxford University Press, 1994.

71. Gibbs, Nancy. "Dr. Death's Suicide Machine." *Time,* June 18, 1990, 69–70.

72. Walsh, Edward. "Kevorkian Sentenced to Prison." *The Washington Post,* April 14, 1999, A2.

73. Gray, Kathleen. "Kevorkian Paroled: 'I'm Not Going to Do It Again.'" *Detroit Free Press,* December 14, 2006. *http://www.freep.com/apps/pbcs.dll/article?AID=/20061214NEWS06/612140349/1007/,* retrieved December 18, 2006.

74. Meier, Diane E., Carol-Ann Emmons, Sylvan Wallenstein, Timothy Quill, R. Sean Morrison, and Christine K. Cassel. "A National Survey of Physician-Assisted Suicide and Euthanasia in the United States." *New England Journal of Medicine* 338 (April 23, 1998): 1,193–1,201.

75. Death with Dignity Act (ORS 127.865 (2)). Oregon Department of Human Services. *http://www.oregon .gov/DHS/ph/pas/,* retrieved February 22, 2008.

76. State of Oregon, Department of Human Services, Office of Disease Prevention and Epidemiology. "Eighth Annual Report on Oregon's Death with Dignity Act," 7–8. (March 9, 2006) *http://www.oregon .gov/DHS/ph/pas/docs/year7.pdf,* retrieved August 15, 2006.

77. State of Oregon, Department of Human Services, Office of Disease Prevention and Epidemiology. "Eighth Annual Report on Oregon's Death with Dignity Act," 8.

78. Booth, William. "Woman Commits Doctor-Assisted Suicide." *The Washington Post,* March 26, 1998, A7. The Oregon Health Plan, which covers Medicaid patients, and the Blue Cross and Blue Shield plans of Oregon began covering physician-assisted suicide in early 1998. ("Oregon Health Plans Proceed with Caution on Suicide Coverage." *AHA News* 34 [March 16, 1998]: 5.)

79. "Oregon Health Plans Proceed with Caution on Suicide Coverage." *AHA News* 34, 10 (March 16, 1998): 5.

80. "Assisted-Suicide Coverage Could Be Expanded." *AHA News* 34, 43 (November 2, 1998): 6.

81. State of Oregon, Department of Human Services, Office of Disease Prevention and Epidemiology. "Ninth Annual Report on Oregon's Death with Dignity Act." (March 8, 2007). *http://www.oregon .gov/DHS/ph/pas/docs/yr9-tbl-2.pdf,* retrieved March 30, 2007.

82. Earll, Carrie Gordon. "Status of Physician-Assisted Suicide Law." CitizenLink Focus on Social Issues. February 27, 2001. *http://www.family.org/cforum/fosi/bioethics/euthanasia/a0028006.cfm,* retrieved November 4, 2003.

83. Lisko, Elaine A. "Oregon Task Force's Guidelines for Physician-Assisted Suicide Are Likely to Have Broad Impact." (March 5, 1998). *http://www.law.uh.edu/healthlawperspectives/Bioethics/980305Oregon .html,* retrieved November 4, 2003.

84. "Doctor-Assisted Suicide—A Guide to Web Sites and the Literature." (January 13, 2004) Longwood University. *http://www.longwood.edu/library/suic.htm,* retrieved February 2, 2006.

85. Washington v. Glucksberg, 521 U.S. 702; Vacco v. Quill, 521 U.S. 793. In *Lee v. Harcleroad,* 118 S. Ct. 328, *cert.* den., the Court declined to review a lower court ruling that a group of terminally ill people and their physicians had no standing to challenge the constitutionality of Oregon's physician-assisted suicide law because it posed no personal danger to them. (Biskupic, Joan. "Oregon's Assisted-Suicide Law Lives On." *The Washington Post,* October 15, 1997, A3.)

86. Bachman, Jerald G., Kirsten H. Alcser, David J. Doukas, Richard L. Lichtenstein, Amy D. Corning, and Howard Brody. "Attitudes of Michigan Physicians and the Public Toward Legalizing Physician-Assisted Suicide and Voluntary Euthanasia." *New England Journal of Medicine* 334 (February 1, 1996): 303–309; Lee, Melinda A., Heidi D. Nelson, Virginia P. Tilden, Linda Ganzini, Terri A. Schmidt, and Susan W. Tolle. "Legalizing Assisted Suicide—Views of Physicians in Oregon." *New England Journal of Medicine* 334 (February 1, 1996): 310–315.

87. Haney, Daniel Q. "6 Pct. of Physicians in Survey Say They Have Assisted Patient Suicides." *The Washington Post,* April 23, 1998, A9.

88. Stevens, Kenneth R., Jr. "Emotional and Psychological Effects of Physician-Assisted Suicide and Euthanasia on Participating Physicians." *Issues in Law & Medicine* 21, 3 (Spring 2006): 187–200.

89. Battin, Margaret P. "Assisted Suicide: Can We Learn from Germany?" *Hastings Center Report* 22 (March/April 1992): 44–51.

90. Langley, Alison. "'Suicide Tourists' Go to the Swiss for Help in Dying." *The New York Times,* February 4, 2003, A3.

91. Humphry, Derek. "A Twentieth Century Chronology of Voluntary Euthanasia and Physician-Assisted Suicide." (March 9, 2003). *ERGO. http://www.finalexit.org/chronframe.html,* retrieved January 1, 2004.

92. "Belgian Lawmakers Propose Euthanasia for Children." WorldNetDaily, June 21, 2003. *http://worldnet daily.com/news/article.asp?ARTICLE_ID=33199,* retrieved November 17, 2003.

93. Soulas, Delphine. "Euthanasia Debate Renewed: Mercy Killing of Frenchman Forces Society to Re-Examine Right to Die." *The Washington Times,* October 27, 2003, A14.

94. Truehart, Charles. "Holland Prepares Bill Legalizing Euthanasia." *The Washington Post,* August 15, 1999, A19.

95. Simons, Marlise. "Dutch Parliament Approves Law Permitting Euthanasia." *The New York Times,* February 10, 1993, A10.

96. Holland's Euthanasia Law. "International Task Force on Euthanasia and Assisted Suicide." (November 4, 2003). *http://www.internationaltaskforce.org/hollaw.htm,* retrieved December 5, 2003.

97. Holland's Euthanasia Law.

98. Holland's Euthanasia Law.

99. Holland's Euthanasia Law.

100. Vos, Joris, Ambassador, Embassy of the Netherlands. "The Netherlands' Euthanasia Law Explained." Letter to the Editor. *The Washington Times,* May 3, 2001, A18.

101. Vos, Joris. "The Netherlands' Euthanasia Law Explained."

102. Onwuteaka-Philipsen, Bregje D., Agnes van der Heide, Martien T. Muller, Mette Rurup, Judith A.C. Rietjens, Jean-Jacques Georges, Astrid M. Vrakking, Jacqueline M. Cuperus-Bosma, Gerrit van der Wal, and Paul J. Van der Maas. "Dutch Experience of Monitoring Euthanasia." *British Medical Journal* 331 (September 24, 2005): 691–692.

103. Richburg, Keith B. "Death with Dignity, or Door to Abuse?" *The Washington Post,* January 4, 2004, A1.

104. Hendin, Herbert, Chris Rutenfrans, and Zbigniew Zylicz. "Physician-Assisted Suicide and Euthanasia in the Netherlands." *Journal of the American Medical Association* 227 (June 4, 1997): 1,720–1,722.

105. "Assisted Suicide Takes a Hit." *The Washington Times,* February 24, 2000, A7.

106. Nolan, Jenny. "Dutch Legalize Euthanasia and Assisted Suicide." (2001). *http://www.nrlc.org/news/ 2001/NRL05/dutch.html,* retrieved November 14, 2003.

107. Allen, Anne. "Euthanasia Is Threat to Our Freedom." *The Express on Sunday,* Global News Wire, April 15, 2001, 1.

108. Sterling, Toby. "Dutch Target Terminally Ill Newborns." *The Washington Times,* September 30, 2005, A18.

109. Drake, Stephen. "Euthanasia Is Out of Control in the Netherlands." *The Hastings Center Report* 35, 3 (May/June 2005): 3.

110. "Q&A: Guidelines on Medically Futile Treatment." In *Trinity Health Guidelines on Medically Futile Treatment.* Novi, MI: Trinity Health, 2007.

111. *Trinity Health Guidelines on Medically Futile Treatment.* Novi, MI: Trinity Health, 2007.

112. *Trinity Health Guidelines on Medically Futile Treatment.* Novi, MI: Trinity Health, 2007.

113. *Trinity Health Guidelines on Medically Futile Treatment.* Novi, MI: Trinity Health, 2007. Steps include the following: 1) Judgment that a treatment is futile is made by agreement of the attending physician, medical consultants, and caregiving team. 2) The attending physician informs the competent patient or surrogate, as appropriate, that the treatment judged medically futile will not be started, or that it will be stopped if already underway. Assurance is given that comfort care will be provided. 3) If the competent patient or surrogate, as appropriate, agrees, then appropriate orders are written in the chart. 4) If there is disagreement, the ethics committee is consulted. The ethics committee will determine whether the guidelines' criteria have been met and will assist with communication and negotiation between the parties involved. 5) Judgments about futile treatment involving incompetent patients without a surrogate are to be reviewed by the ethics committee. If it concurs, the attending physician will document the process in the chart and write appropriate orders. 6) If the ethics committee concurs with the attending physician that a treatment is medically futile and a competent patient or surrogate, as appropriate, refuses to agree, then a mediator will be used to try to resolve the dispute. 7) If the patient or surrogate chooses to remain in the facility, or remains because no alternative facility can be found, one of three courses will be followed—the medically futile treatment will not be started, or it will be started or continued for a goal-specified or time-limited trial as the result of a formal mediation process, or (if started) it will be discontinued.

114. Foubister, Veda. "California Law Facilitates Advance Directives for End-of-Life Medical Care." *AMNews* (August 14, 2000). *http://www.ama-assn.org/amednews/2000/08/14/prsb0814.htm,* retrieved November 14, 2003.

115. Valko, Nancy. "Futility Policies and the Duty to Die." *Voices* (online edition) (2003). *www.wf-f.org/ 03-1-Futility.html.*

116. Ross, Judith Wilson, John W. Glaser, Dorothy Rasinski-Gregory, Joan McIver Gibson, and Corrine Bayley. *Health Care Ethics Committees: The Next Generation,* 1. Chicago: American Hospital Publishing, 1993.

117. President's Commission for the Study of Ethical Problems in Medicine and Biomedical and Behavioral Research. *Deciding to Forego Life-Sustaining Treatment: Ethical, Medical, and Legal Issues in Treatment Decisions,* 443. Washington, DC: President's Commission, 1983.

118. "Right-to-Die: An Executive Report." *Hospitals* 63 (November 20, 1989): 34.

119. Ross, Glaser, Rasinski-Gregory, Gibson, and Bayley, *Health Care Ethics Committees,* ix.

120. Bernt, Francis, Peter Clark, Josita Starrs, and Patricia Talone. "Ethics Committees in Catholic Hospitals." *Health Progress* 87, 2 (March/April 2006). *http://www.chausa.org/Pub/MainNav/News/HP/Archive/ 2006/03MarApril/Articles/Specia,* retrieved February 22, 2007.

121. *Summary Report: Survey on Ethics Involvement in Aging Services.* Washington, DC: American Association of Homes and Services for the Aging, 1995.

122. Bernt, Clark, Starrs, and Talone. "Ethics Committees in Catholic Hospitals."

123. Freedman, Benjamin. "One Philosopher's Experience on an Ethics Committee." *Hastings Center Report* 11 (April 1981): 20–22.

124. Mannisto, Marilyn M. "Orchestrating an Ethics Committee: Who Should Be on It, Where Does It Best Fit?" *Trustee* 38 (April 1985): 17–20.

125. Annas, George, and Amy Haddad. "Do Ethics Committees Work?" *Trustee* 47 (July 1994): 17.

126. Scheirton, Linda S. "Measuring Hospital Ethics Committee Success." *Cambridge Quarterly of Healthcare Ethics* 2 (1993): 495–504.

127. Section 46.107 - IRB Membership. *Code of Federal Regulations.* Title 45, Department of Health and Human Services, Part 46, Protection of Human Subjects, and Title 21, Part 56.

128. Barnes, Mark, and Sara Krauss. "Conflicts of Interest in Human Research: Risks and Pitfalls of 'Easy Money' in Research Funding." *BNA's Health Law Reporter* 9, 35 (August 31, 2000): 1,383.

129. Barnes and Krauss. "Conflicts of Interest."

130. Barnes and Krauss. "Conflicts of Interest."

131. Section 46.107 - IRB Membership. *Code of Federal Regulations,* Title 45, Department of Health and Human Services, Part 46, Protection of Human Subjects, effective December 13, 2001. *http://ohrp.osophs.dhhs.gov/humansubjects/guidance/45cfr46.htm,* retrieved August 17, 2003.

132. Section 46.111 - Criteria for IRB approval of research. *Code of Federal Regulations,* Title 45, Department of Health and Human Services, Part 46, Protection of Human Subjects, effective December 13, 2001. *http://ohrp.osophs.dhhs.gov/humansubjects/guidance/45cfr46.htm,* retrieved August 17, 2003.

133. Ramsey, Paul. "Research Involving Children or Incompetents." In *The Patient as Person,* 252. New Haven, CT: Yale University Press, 1970.

134. Budetti, Peter B. "Ensuring Safe and Effective Medications for Children." *Journal of the American Medical Association* 290, 7 (August 20, 2003): 950–951.

135. Roberts, Rosemary, William Rodriguez, Dianne Murphy, and Terie Crescenzi. "Pediatric Drug Labeling: Improving the Safety and Efficacy of Pediatric Therapies." *Journal of the American Medical Association* 290, 7 (August 20, 2003): 905–911.

136. Office for Protection from Research Risks. "Summary of Basic Protections for Human Subjects," 2. (December 23,1997). *http://ohrp.osophs.dhhs.gov/humansubjects/guidance/basics.htm,* retrieved August 17, 2003.

137. Section 46.110 - Expedited review procedures for certain kinds of research involving no more than minimal risk, and for minor changes in approved research. *Code of Federal Regulations,* Title 45, Department of Health and Human Services, Part 46, Protection of Human Subjects, effective December 13, 2001. *http://ohrp.osophs.dhhs.gov/humansubjects/guidance/45cfr46.htm,* retrieved August 17, 2003.

138. "Categories of Research that May Be Reviewed by the Institutional Review Board (IRB) Through an Expedited Review." (November 9, 1998). *http://ohrp.osophs.dhhs.gov/humansubjects/guidance/expedited98.htm,* retrieved August 17, 2003.

139. Department of Health and Human Services, Office of Human Development Services. (1985). Final Rule, Child Abuse and Neglect Prevention and Treatment Program, 45 *Code of Federal Regulations* §1340.

140. Department of Health and Human Services, Office of Human Development Services. (1985). "Services and Treatment for Disabled Infants; Model Guidelines for Health Care Providers to Establish Infant Care Review Committees." 50 *Federal Register* 14893.

141. Department of Health and Human Services, Office of Human Development Services. 50 *Federal Register* 14893.

142. Fletcher, John C., Margo L. White, and Philip J. Foubert. "Biomedical Ethics and an Ethics Consultation Service at the University of Virginia." *HEC Forum* 2, 2 (1990): 89–99.

143. Roscoe, Jerry P., and Deirdre McCarthy Gallagher. "Mediating Bioethical Disputes: Time to Check the Patient's Pulse?" *Dispute Resolution Magazine* 9, 3 (Spring 2003): 21–23.

144. Petry, Edward. "Appointing an Ethics Officer." *Healthcare Executive* 13 (November/December 1998): 35.

145. Keeton, W. Page, ed. *Prosser and Keeton on the Law of Torts,* 5th ed., 2. St. Paul, MN: West Publishing, 1984.

146. Keeton, *Prosser and Keeton,* 2.

147. Keeton, *Prosser and Keeton,* 655–656.

148. Southwick, Arthur F. *The Law of Hospital and Health Care Administration,* 2nd ed., 67–68. Ann Arbor, MI: Health Administration Press, 1988.

149. Prosser, William L. *Handbook of the Law of Torts,* 4th ed., 31. St. Paul, MN: West Publishing, 1971.

150. Behringer v. The Medical Center at Princeton, 249 N.J. Super. 597, 592 A.2d 1251 (1991); Doe v. Noe, Ill. App. Ct. December 26, 1997.

151. *Black's Law Dictionary,* 5th ed., 930. St. Paul, MN: West Publishing, 1979.

152. *American Jurisprudence,* 2nd ed., Cumulative Supplement, section 205, vol. 61. St. Paul, MN: West Publishing, 1997.

153. Southwick, *The Law of Hospital,* 69.

154. Landeros v. Flood, 17 Cal. 3d 399 (1976).

155. Federal Tort Claims Act of 1946, 60 Stat. 842 (August 2, 1946).

156. Baumberger, Charles H. "Vicarious Liability Claims Against HMOs." *Trial* 34 (May 1998): 30–33, 35

157. Southwick, *The Law of Hospital,* 580.

158. Furrow, Barry R., Thomas L. Greaney, Sandra H. Johnson, Timothy S. Jost, and Robert L. Schwartz. *Health Law: Cases Materials and Problems,* 3rd ed., 353. St. Paul, MN: West Publishing, 1997.

159. Furrow, Greaney, Johnson, Jost, and Schwartz, *Health Law,* 353.

160. Furrow, Greaney, Johnson, Jost, and Schwartz, *Health Law,* 354.

161. Thornhill, Michael C., and William H. Ginsburg. "Enterprise Liability: Cure or Curse." *Whittier Law Review* 16 (Spring 1995): 143–156.

162. Howard, Philip K. "Strong Medicine." *Wall Street Journal,* January 6, 2007, A6.

163. Goldstein, Avram. "Va. High Court Upholds Malpractice Cap." *The Washington Post,* January 9, 1999, B3. The unanimous opinion upheld the constitutionality of Virginia's $1 million cap on medical malpractice damage awards, including punitive damages, lost wages, future medical costs, and interest on unpaid judgments against doctors and hospitals. Supporters argue that the cap has stabilized the physicians' malpractice insurance market and eased their ability to get malpractice insurance.

164. Wencl, Annette, and Margaret Brizzolara. "Medical Negligence: Survey of the States." *Trial* 32 (May 1996): 21.

165. Grant, Ruth Ann. "Tinkering on Tort Reform Not Enough to Solve Problem: Experts." *AHA News* 27 (March 18, 1991): 2.

166. Grant, "Tinkering on Tort Reform," 5; *Health Care Statistics and the Effect of Caps on Noneconomic Damages,* 17–18. Washington, DC: Citizen Action, 1996; Best v. Taylor Machine Works 179 Ill.2d 367, 689 N.E.2d 1057 (1997); Smith, William C. "Prying Off Tort Reform Caps: States Striking Down Limits on Liability and Damages, and Statutes of Limitations." *ABA Journal* 85 (October 1999): 28–29.

167. Hellinger, Fred J., and William E. Encinosa. "The Impact of State Laws Limiting Malpractice Damage Awards on Health Care Expenditures." *American Journal of Public Health* 98, 6 (August 2006): 1,375–1,381.

168. Wencl, Annette, and David Strickland. "No-Fault Med Mal: No Gain for the Injured." *Trial* 33 (May 1997): 20.

169. Darr, Kurt. "Communication: The Key to Reducing Malpractice Claims." *Hospital Topics* 75 (Spring 1997): 4–6.

170. Superior Court of DC. Small Claims Mediation Program. *http://www.dccourts.gov/dccourts/superior/multi/small.jsp,* retrieved February 8, 2007; Superior Court of DC. "Civil Mediation and Case Evaluation Program." *http://www.dccourts.gov/dccourts/superior/multi/civil.jsp,* retrieved February 8, 2007.

171. Bravin, Jess. "Patient–Insurer Arbitrations Criticized." *The Wall Street Journal,* January 11, 2001, B-12. *http://proquest.umi.com/pqdweb?index=1&did=66545361&SrchMode=1&sid=4&Fmt=3...,* retrieved April 12, 2007.

172. "Arbitration Accepted as a Means for Resolution of Medical Malpractice Disputes." *American Journal of Orthodontics and Dentofacial Orthopedics* 3 (March 1997):349–351. This reference includes a form to contract for arbitration of medical malpractice disputes.

173. White, Jeffrey Robert. "Mandatory Arbitration: A Growing Threat." *Trial* 35 (July 1999): 32–34, 36.

174. Patrick v. Burget, 800 F.2d 1498 (9th Cir. 1986), reversed, 486 U.S. 94 (1988), rehearing denied 487 U.S.

1243 (1988). Dr. Patrick prevailed in the antitrust claims in the trial court. The court of appeals reversed the decision because the peer review activity that was established by Oregon was determined to be state action, which is exempt from federal law. The Supreme Court reversed the appeals court on a finding that the state judiciary did not supply active supervision and raised the question of whether state court review could constitute state action.

175. Health Care Quality Improvement Act of 1986, PL 99-660, 100 Stat. 3784.
176. Austin v. McNamara, 731 F.Supp. 934 (C.D. Cal. 1990), affirmed 979 (F.2d) 726 (9th Cir. 1992); Egan v. Athol Memorial Hospital, 971 F.Supp. 37 (D. Mass. 1997), affirmed *per curiam* 134 F.3d 361 (1st Cir. 1998), *certiorari* denied, 119 S.Ct. 409 (1998).
177. Emergency Medical Treatment and Active Labor Act of 1985, PL 99-272, 100 Stat. 174.
178. Furrow, Greaney, Johnson, Jost, and Schwartz, *Health Law,* 547.
179. Furrow, Greaney, Johnson, Jost, and Schwartz, *Health Law,* 539.
180. Furrow, Greaney, Johnson, Jost, and Schwartz, *Health Law,* 638.
181. Furrow, Greaney, Johnson, Jost, and Schwartz, *Health Law,* 648.
182. Furrow, Greaney, Johnson, Jost, and Schwartz, *Health Law,* 641–642.
183. Crane, Thomas S., Richard G. Cowart, Robert G. Homchick, Ellen P. Pesch, Sanford V. Teplitzky, and Harvey Yampolsky. "Stark II Proposed Regulations." *Health Law Digest* 26 (February 1998): 3–4.
184. "Spotlight on the Stark II Regulations." *Health Lawyers News* 2 (February 1998): 6.
185. Furrow, Greaney, Johnson, Jost, and Schwartz, *Health Law,* 643.
186. Health Insurance Portability and Accountability Act of 1996, PL 104-191, 110 Stat. 1936 (August 2, 1996).
187. "New Healthcare Integrity and Protection Data Bank Casts Wide Net." *Health Lawyers News* 2 (December 1998): 7.
188. False Claims Act Amendments of 1986, PL 99-562, 100 Stat. 3153 (October 17, 1986).
189. Gibeaut, John. "Seeking the Cure." *ABA Journal* 92 (October 2006): 46.
190. Havighurst, Clark C. *Health Care Law and Policy: Readings, Notes, and Questions,* 204. Westbury, NY: Foundation Press, 1988.
191. Havighurst, *Health Care Law,* 204–205.
192. Francis, Theo. "Lawmakers Question If Nonprofit Hospitals Help Poor Enough." *The Wall Street Journal,* July 30, 2007, A5.
193. Clarke, Richard L. "Consumerism: A Matter of Trust." *Trustee* 60, 6 (June 2007): 27.
194. Francis, Theo. "Lawmakers Question If Nonprofit Hospitals Help Poor Enough."
195. Fischer, Kevin B. "Tax Exemption and the Health Care Industry: Are the Challenges to Tax-Exempt Status Justified?" *Vanderbilt Law Review* 49 (January 1996): 163.
196. Monson, Mike. "Provena Facing Tax Bill of $1.1 Million." *The News-Gazette Online,* March 13, 2004. *http://www.news-gazette.com/story.cfm?Number=15615,* retrieved April 7, 2004. The opportunity for Urbana officials to review Provena's tax status occurred because in Illinois the new owner of a charitable organization must reapply for tax-exempt status. Provena was formed in 1997 by consolidation of the health activities of three religious orders of sisters, but reapplication for tax-exempt status did not occur until 2002. Lagnado, Lucette. "Hospital Found 'Not Charitable' Loses Its Status as Tax Exempt." *The Wall Street Journal,* February 19, 2004, B1.
197. Francis, Theo. "Lawmakers Question If Nonprofit Hospitals Help Poor Enough."
198. Stanley, J. Mark, and David R. Ward. "UBIT May Hit Common Transactions." *Tax Advisor* 25 (September 1994): 557.
199. McMenamin, Joseph P. "Telemedicine: Technology and the Law." *For the Defense* 39 (July 1997): 11.
200. McMenamin, "Telemedicine," 11.
201. McMenamin, "Telemedicine," 13.
202. McMenamin, "Telemedicine," 13.
203. McMenamin, "Telemedicine," 13.
204. McMenamin, "Telemedicine," 14.
205. Kelly, Beckie. "Telemedicine Begins to Make Progress." *Health Data Management* 10, 1 (January 2002): 73.
206. American Medical Association. "Physician Licensure: An Update of Trends," 6. (August 11, 2005). *http://www.ama-assn.org/ama/pub/category/print2378.html,* retrieved February 15, 2007.

207. Neergaard, Lauran. "Patients Bypass Doctors' Visits with On-Line Prescription Sales." *The Washington Times,* December 25, 1998, B11.

208. Daar, Judith R., and Spencer Koerner. "Telemedicine: Legal and Practical Implications." *Whittier Law Review* 19 (Winter 1997): 25.

209. Kelly, Beckie. "Telemedicine Begins to Make Progress." *Health Data Management* 10, 1 (January 2002): 72; Omnibus Budget Bill of 2000, PL 106-554, 114 Stat. 2763 (2000).

210. Adapted from Darr, Kurt. *Ethics in Health Services Management,* 4th ed., 147–148. Baltimore: Health Professions Press, 2005; used by permission.

211. Adapted from Darr, Kurt. *Ethics in Health Services Management,* 4th ed., 132–133. Baltimore: Health Professions Press, 2005; used by permission.

212. Written by Gary E. Crum, Ph.D., M.P.H., Executive Director, Graduate Medical Education Consortium, The University of Virginia at Wise, (Past Director, Northern Kentucky Health Department). Used with permission.

213. Written by Gary E. Crum, Ph.D., M.P.H., Executive Director, Graduate Medical Education Consortium, The University of Virginia at Wise, (Past Director, Northern Kentucky Health Department). Used with permission.

PART II

Managing Health Services Organizations and Systems

5

The Practice of Management in Health Services Organizations and Health Systems

It has been observed that leading HSOs/HSs "are demonstrating how to satisfy customers, improve quality of care, and meet cost goals simultaneously."[1] The leading organizations and systems are setting the standard for the practice of management in the 21st century, and they are accomplishing this to a great extent through the work of their managers.

Managers perform one of three distinct but interrelated types of work in HSOs/HSs.[2] Direct work performed in these settings entails some combination of patient care, research, education, and the production of products or services. A second type of work, support work, is a necessary and facilitative adjunct to the direct work. Support work involves such activities as fund-raising and development, provision of legal counsel, marketing, public relations, finance, and human resources. The third type of work, management, is the focus of the remainder of the book. It involves establishing an appropriate organizational mission and objectives in relation to the entity's external environment. Management work also involves assembling and effectively utilizing resources—including human resources, material/supplies, technology/equipment, information, capital resources, and patients/customers—so that direct work, aided by support work, can accomplish the objectives and fulfill the mission.

The people who perform management work in HSOs/HSs—those who occupy positions of managerial authority—face unprecedented challenges. These challenges result from many forces: remarkable scientific and technological advances in medicine (see Chapter 3), new organizational forms and relationships through which to provide health services (see Chapter 2), and new policies and programs for financing the provision of these services (see Chapters 1 and 4), to name some of the most important. It is fair to say that managers in these organizations and systems are accustomed to challenges. They routinely face the high expectations of consumers and patients, of clinicians, and of those who pay for health services. They are scrutinized for the costs and quality of the services they provide. Demands for greater efficiency in the delivery of services and for effectiveness in service delivery are familiar challenges to these managers.

As will be seen in this chapter, there are several ways to assess and study management work. The work of managers can be approached in terms of the *functions* managers perform, the *skills* they use in doing their work, the *roles* they play in performing their work, and the *competencies* they need to do the work well. Each of these approaches is considered in this chapter and used to illustrate important aspects of management work throughout the book. Overall, however, the remaining chapters in this book focus on the *process* of management, that is, on what managers actually do. The chapter concludes with the description of a comprehensive model of management in HSOs/HSs; this model forms a framework that puts the previous chapters in perspective for managers and guides the structure and content of the book's remaining chapters.

▬ Key Definitions ▬

The terms *health services, health services organizations,* and *health systems* have already been used in this book. To some extent, their meanings are intuitive. However, we want to give them explicit meanings as a preface to also defining the terms *managers* and *management*.

HEALTH SERVICES

As noted in Chapter 1, healthcare is the total societal effort, undertaken in the private and public sectors, focused on pursuing health. Within the larger domain of healthcare, health services are specific activities undertaken to maintain or improve health or to prevent decrements of health. These services can be preventive (e.g., blood pressure screening, mammography), acute (e.g., surgical procedures, antibiotics to fight an infection), chronic (e.g., control of diabetes or hypertension), restorative (e.g., physical rehabilitation of a stroke or trauma patient), or palliative (e.g., pain relief or comfort in terminal stages of disease).

In general, health services can be divided into two basic types. Public health services are activities that are conducted on a communitywide or populationwide basis, such as communicable disease control, sanitation, food and water safety, the collection and analysis of health statistics, and air pollution control. Personal health services, in contrast, are activities directed at individuals and include promotion of health, prevention of illness, diagnosis, treatment (sometimes leading to a cure), and rehabilitation. Thus, activities as diverse as the emergency department treatment of a child with acute asthma and the conduct of education programs about the practice of safe sex to prevent the spread of human immunodeficiency virus (HIV) are examples of health services.

HEALTH SERVICES ORGANIZATIONS (HSOs)

Health services are provided through a variety of organizational arrangements. HSOs are entities that provide the organizational structure within which the delivery of health services is made directly to consumers, whether the purpose of the services is preventive, acute, chronic, restorative, or palliative. Historically, HSOs were predominantly independent, freestanding organizations. In a movement beginning in the 1970s and gaining momentum through the 1980s and 1990s, however, many HSOs have joined together to form systems of organizations. More discussion of this shift can be found in Chapters 1 and 2.

One way to envision the diversity of HSOs is to consider a continuum of clinical health services that people might use during the course of their lives and to think of the organizational settings that provide them. Prebirth, the continuum could begin with HSOs that minimize negative environmental impact on human fetuses or that provide genetic counseling, family planning services, prenatal counseling, prenatal ambulatory care services, and birthing services. This would be followed early in life by pediatric ambulatory services; pediatric inpatient hospital services, including neonatal intensive care units (NICUs) and pediatric intensive care units (PICUs); and both ambulatory and inpatient psychiatric services for children.

For adults, the most relevant HSOs are those providing such services as ambulatory surgery centers and emergency and trauma services; adult inpatient hospital services, including routine medical, surgical, and obstetrical services, specialized cardiac care units (CCUs), medical intensive care units (MICUs), surgical intensive care units (SICUs), and monitored units; stand-alone cancer units with radiotherapy capability and short-stay recovery beds; ambulatory and inpatient rehabilitation services, including specific subprograms for orthopedic, neurological, cardiac, arthritis, speech, otological, and other services; ambulatory and inpatient psychiatric services, including specific subprograms for people with psychoses and day programs, counseling services, and detoxification; and home health services.

In their later years, people might add to the list of relevant HSOs those providing skilled and intermediate nursing services; adult day services; respite services for caregivers of homebound patients, including services such as meal provision, visiting nurses and home health aides, electronic emergency call capability, cleaning, and simple home maintenance; and hospice care and associated family services, including bereavement, legal, and financial counseling.

HEALTH SYSTEMS (HSs)

The continuum of health services outlined previously has been provided traditionally by autonomous or independent HSOs, often in an uncoordinated and disjointed manner. However, many HSOs have significantly changed how they relate to one another. Mergers, consolidations, acquisitions, and affiliations between and among previously independent HSOs are pervasive (see Figure 2.9). At the extreme end of this activity is vertical integration, in which HSOs join into unified organizational arrangements or systems of organizations.[3] This phenomenon of integration is likely to continue into the foreseeable future.[4] In fact, among the most important contemporary developments in the infrastructure of healthcare is the integration of HSOs into HSs. HSs are formally linked HSOs, possibly including financing arrangements, joined together to provide more coordinated and comprehensive health services. The development of vertically integrated HSs capable of providing a largely "seamless" continuum of health services, including primary, acute, rehabilitation, long-term, and hospice care, increasingly characterizes the organizational context of healthcare.

The most extensively integrated situations arise in the formation of integrated delivery systems, or IDSs (synonymous with organized delivery systems or integrated delivery networks). Whatever the name, the further development of these highly integrated HSs requires "significant investment in the components of system building (e.g., integrated information systems) that is essential for ensuring the coordination of care across the full spectrum of healthcare providers and services."[5]

Although the question of how far HSOs will integrate remains unanswered, it is a reality that more integration will characterize health services in the future. The implications of HSOs integrating into HSs are considered throughout this book. Whether autonomous or integrated, however, all HSOs and HSs must be managed. Thus, definitions of managers and of management are important; they form the substance and focus of this book.

MANAGERS

Managers are those who are formally appointed to positions of authority in organizations or systems and who enable others to do their direct or support work effectively, who have responsibility for resource utilization, and who are accountable for work results. In HSOs/HSs, this broad definition includes people with titles such as nurse team manager; maintenance director; dietary, surgery, or medical records director or supervisor; pharmacy, laboratory, outpatient clinic, social services, or business office director; medical director; chief medical officer (CMO); chief nursing officer (CNO); chief financial officer (CFO); chief information officer (CIO); vice president; or president or chief executive officer (CEO). The variety of managers in these settings can be identified, in part, by the level of the organization at which they work. Note that some of these are in support roles.

Classification schemes typically identify managers as senior-level, middle-level, and supervisory or first-level managers. Regardless of title or level, managers have several common attributes: 1) they are formally appointed to positions of authority, 2) they are charged with directing and enabling others to do their work effectively, 3) they are responsible for utilizing resources, and 4) they are accountable to superiors for results.

The primary differences among levels of managers are the degree of authority and scope of responsibility. For example, CEOs and other senior-level managers comprising the executive office have authority over and are responsible for entire HSOs/HSs—all staff, resources, and individual and organizational results—because governing bodies (GBs) grant authority to them and expect accountability in return. Reporting to senior-level managers are numerous middle-level managers, each of whom is responsible for smaller segments of the organization or system. Middle-level managers, such as department heads and heads of services, have authority over and are responsible for specific segments, in contrast to the HSO/HS as a whole. Finally, first-level managers, who generally report to middle-level managers, have authority over and are responsible for overseeing specific work and a particular group of workers. Managers at each of the various levels are responsible for different types of activities. However, all of these activities are important, and no HSO/HS can be successful unless the management work at each level is done well and unless the work is carefully coordinated and integrated within and across levels.

MANAGEMENT

No matter what their level, all managers perform management work by engaging in the process of management. Management is defined as the process, composed of interrelated social and technical functions and activities, occurring within a formal organizational setting for the purpose of accomplishing predetermined objectives through the use of human and other resources. Management at all levels has four main elements:

- It is a process—a set of interactive and interrelated ongoing functions and activities.
- It involves accomplishing organizational objectives.
- It involves achieving these objectives through people and the use of other resources.
- It occurs in a formal organizational setting, whether a single organization or a system, which invariably exists in the context of larger external environments.

By definition, managers focus on establishing and achieving organizational missions and objectives. The scope of managerial work includes providing the organizational context within which direct and support work can be performed effectively. Managerial work also includes preparing organizations and systems to deal with both the threats and opportunities from their external environments. Managers influence all work in the entities as they manage because they influence the context, framework, and premises of decisions about work and conditions under which it is done. In effect, managers help shape the culture and philosophy of the entities they manage in important ways; more than anyone, they determine the overall performance that is achieved by their organizations or systems.

▬ Management and Organizational Culture, Philosophy, and Performance ▬▬▬▬▬▬▬▬

This section discusses the vital relationships between management and the development and maintenance of appropriate organizational cultures and philosophies in HSOs/HSs and between management and organizational performance. Managers make unique contributions to cultures, philosophies, and performance.

MANAGEMENT AND ORGANIZATIONAL CULTURE AND PHILOSOPHY

All organizations have identifiable cultures. The organizational cultures of HSOs/HSs typically differ from those of business enterprises because they provide services that are unique in society and because they are humanitarian in nature. Their CEOs and other senior-level managers both help establish and maintain the culture and manage in the special context of that culture.

Organizational culture is the pattern of shared values and beliefs—along with associated behaviors, symbols, and rituals—that is acquired over time by members of the HSO/HS.[6] It is the historically developed sense of the institution's "legacy"—what it is and what it stands for—that permeates the entire organization or system and is known to all who work in it.[7] Examples of important values are duty, respect, trust, integrity, honesty, equity, and fairness. Examples of shared beliefs are the commitment to patients and to meeting their needs and respecting them as people, with the unshakable belief that they are the primary reason for the entity's existence. These values and beliefs shape organizational objectives and prescribe acceptable behavior for managers and other employees, as well as acceptable relationships between the organization and its external stakeholders. By adhering to these values and beliefs, HSOs/HSs retain their unique character and the privileges that society has accorded them.[8]

An HSO's/HS's philosophy is its explicit and implicit view of itself and what it is. Generally expressed in its mission statement, the philosophy is directly linked to and rooted in the cultural values and beliefs that drive and guide the organization or system.[9] The philosophy and culture must be compatible, and each must reflect the other. One important aspect of an organization's philosophy is that it depicts the desired nature of relationships with its stakeholders—that is, between the organization and the individuals, groups, or other organizations who are affected by the HSO/HS and who may seek to influence it.[10] A well-thought-out and implemented philosophy about stakeholders is prerequisite to strategic planning, resource allocation and utilization, customer service, and ability to cope with the external environment. An organization's stakeholders can be classified into three groups.[11] Internal stakeholders operate entirely within the HSO/HS and typically include management and professional and nonprofessional staff members. Interface stakeholders function both internally and externally and include members of the professional staff organization (PSO), the GB, and stockholders in for-profit situations. External stakeholders include suppliers, patients, third-party payers, competitors, interest groups, local communities, labor organizations, and regulatory and accrediting agencies.

HSO/HS managers must determine which stakeholders represent potential threats and which represent potential opportunities. Appropriate behavior toward stakeholders is based on these assessments, and it ranges from ignoring to negotiating to co-opting and cooperating. Careful assessments also can indicate which of the conflicting priorities, needs, demands, and pressures presented by stakeholders should be addressed. Balancing the demands of multiple stakeholders with different interests is a major challenge. Finally, the conduct of managers conveys to all stakeholders the HSO's/HS's values and beliefs (its culture) and its philosophy. Culture and philosophy are expressed through approaches to customer service, attitudes about staff, and attitudes about stakeholder relations in general.

A philosophy about staff, for example, is clearly rooted in an organization's values. It may include concepts such as respect for them as persons, whether they are viewed as the principal component in accomplishing organizational objectives, the extent of their involvement and participation in decision making about work and work systems design, and the way in which management oversees their work.[12]

MANAGEMENT AND ORGANIZATIONAL PERFORMANCE

Organizations and systems are formed for the purpose of accomplishing certain missions and objectives that participants could not achieve as well acting alone. From this fact arises the central purpose of management work and of all managers: to help achieve high performance in relation to organizational objectives. A higher-performing organization more completely fulfills its mission and meets more of its objectives than a lower-performing organization. Managers are judged by these contributions because they occupy positions that permit them to make unique contributions to organizational performance, and they are judged by the degree to which organizational missions are accomplished and objectives are successfully fulfilled.[13]

There is no universally accepted formula by which managers maximize their contributions to performance in their organizations or systems. However, the evidence of the contributions managers make to organizational performance is substantial. For example, studies conducted in a variety of HSOs/HSs have demonstrated that the way managers set goals, objectives, and standards;[14] coordinate and integrate various workgroups;[15] make decisions and involve others in decision making;[16] structure compensation systems;[17] and design their organizations[18] and professional staff organizations (PSOs)[19] affect organizational performance. Effective managers create work environments and conditions that are conducive to superior organization-level performance, as well as performance of individuals in the organization or system.

Measuring Performance

From a management perspective, performance measurement is requisite to managing and improving the level of performance at the organization and system levels, as well as the at the levels of their components, including the level of individual performance. Among the fundamentals of effective performance are measuring and tracking, and determining how this information is used. The most effective approaches to measuring organization-level or system-level performance utilize multiple dimensions of performance. Although the widespread use of multicriteria approaches to measuring organizational performance in HSOs/HSs is a recent development, the concept emerged much earlier. In seeking to answer the focused question of how best to measure quality of care, Avedis Donabedian established a lasting multicriteria paradigm for measuring clinical and nonclinical aspects of performance as well.[20] His answer to how best to measure quality of healthcare was to use three types of measures: *structural measures* (innate characteristics of those who provide services and of the settings in which they are provided); *process measures* (what service providers do to patients/customers); and *outcome measures* (what happens to the health of patients/customers as a result of services). This was the beginning of a multicriteria approach to measurement and is explained more fully in Chapter 10.

A popular model used in multidimensional performance measurement is the Balanced Scorecard (BSC),[21] started in the business sector and now well established in leading HSOs/HSs.[22] BSCs used in HSOs/HSs are selected to reflect the critical stakeholders and strategic plan and typically include such perspectives as patient satisfaction, human resources, clinical effectiveness, operational effectiveness, market share, and financial results. For each dimension of performance, a number of specific measurements are used. For example, performance in the financial dimension is assessed by return on assets, operating margins, and bond ratings. The quality dimension is assessed by measures such as case severity-adjusted mortality, patient satisfaction, and percentage of hip surgery patients walking 6 weeks postsurgery.

A variation of BSC is the Data Dashboard, a concept derived from airplane cockpits or automobile dashboards, where various types of information are conveniently displayed. The dashboard

TABLE 5.1.   THE NATIONAL HEALTH SERVICE (U.K.) PERFORMANCE ASSESSMENT FRAMEWORK

(1) *Health improvement*
- Deaths from all causes (ages 15–64)
- Death from all causes (ages 65–74)
- Deaths from cancer
- Deaths from all circulatory diseases
- Suicide rates
- Deaths from accidents
- Serious injury from accidents

(2) *Fair access*
- Inpatients waiting list
- Adult dental registrations
- Early detection of cancer
- Cancer waiting times
- Number of GPs
- GP practice availability
- Elective surgery rates
- Surgery rates—coronary heart disease

(3) *Effective delivery of appropriate healthcare*
- Childhood immunizations
- Inappropriately used surgery
- Acute care management
- Chronic care management
- Mental health in primary care
- Cost effective prescribing
- Returning home following treatment for a stroke
- Returning home following treatment for a fractured hip

(4) *Efficiency*
- Day case rate
- Length of stay
- Maternity unit costs
- Mental health unit costs
- Generic prescribing

(5) *Patient/carer experience of the NHS*
- Patients who wait less than two hours for emergency admission (through A&E)
- Cancelled operations
- Delayed discharge
- First outpatient appointments for which patients did not attend
- Outpatients seen within 13 weeks of GP referral
- Percentage of those on waiting lists waiting 18 months or more
- Patient satisfaction

(6) *Health outcomes of NHS healthcare*
- Conceptions below age 18
- Decayed, missing or filled teeth in five-year-old children
- Readmission to hospital following discharge
- Emergency admissions of older people
- Emergency psychiatric readmissions
- Stillbirths and infant deaths
- Breast cancer survival
- Cervical cancer survival
- Lung cancer survival
- Colon cancer survival
- Deaths in hospital following surgery (emergency admissions)
- Deaths in hospital following surgery (non-emergency admissions)
- Deaths in hospital following a heart attack (ages 35–74)
- Deaths in hospital following a fractured hip

Source: Data are from NHS Executive. *Quality and Performance in the NHS; NHS Performance Indicators.* London: The Stationary Office, 2000.

approach to measurement and display of information on organizational performance is based on the idea that "When data are presented in a clear and concise format, healthcare leaders, managers, and clinicians can monitor progress, identify needed improvements, and make rapid and better data-driven decisions."[23] Another variation of multicriteria performance measurement is the "report card."[24] When applied to HSOs/HSs, these report cards are so new that there is little agreement as to what should be reported and to whom. Even so, *Consumer Reports* lists four report cards currently in use nationally, and many more at the state level. The National Committee for Quality Assurance (NCQA) provides a Health Plan Report Card, which is available to consumers to help them choose among health plans.[25]

In the United Kingdom, performance of the organizations in the National Health Service (NHS) is assessed through the use of a BSC-like device called the Performance Assessment Framework (PAF). The PAF utilizes six dimensions of performance: health improvement, fair access, effective delivery of appropriate healthcare, efficiency, patient/carer (caregiver in the United States) experience, and health outcomes of NHS care.[26] The NHS says that the PAF "is based on the BSC approach. The use of the BSC allows organizations to get a more rounded view of performance by identifying different key elements of performance and understanding how changes in them may have implications for others."[27] Utilizing data from the NHS, Table 5.1 illustrates the measures used in the PAF, including the six dimensions of performance and the set of specific performance indicators used in this approach to performance measurement. [28]

Going forward, the use of multicriteria performance measurement—whether through balanced scorecards, report cards, or dashboards—will increase because these devices provide useful information in clear and concise formats. In the executive suites of HSOs/HSs, use of the devices permit monitoring and tracking of organizational performance across strategic, clinical, operational, and financial dimensions. GBs can use the information in these multicriteria performance measurement devices to track the fulfillment of their entities' obligations to various stakeholders. Consumers are likely to use such information increasingly to make decisions about providers and plans necessitated by the emergence of consumer-driven healthcare.

Management Functions, Skills, Roles, and Competencies

As noted earlier, there are several different possible approaches to considering management work. In this section, the most important ones—functions, skills, roles, and competencies—are considered and summarized in Table 5.2. No single approach provides a comprehensive framework for understanding management or the management work performed in HSOs/HSs. However, each contributes something, and all together they provide a comprehensive framework. The functions that are fulfilled in the management process are considered first.

MANAGEMENT FUNCTIONS

The set of social and technical functions inherent in the management process (see the definition of management presented earlier) includes planning, organizing, staffing, directing (motivating, leading, and communicating), and controlling. Decision making pervades each of these functions, and although some authorities list it as a separate function, it is best viewed as integral to each of the management functions.

These management functions are the result of logical grouping of generic management activities. All managers perform these functions to some degree regardless of hierarchical level. Figure 5.1 illustrates the interdependence among the management functions. In considering management in terms of its functions, it is convenient to separate them so that each can be discussed independently; but the process should not be seen as a series of separate functions. In practice, a manager performs these functions simultaneously, not sequentially, and as part of an interdependent mosaic of func-

TABLE 5.2. APPROACHES TO CONSIDERING MANAGEMENT WORK

Functions	Skills	Roles	Competencies
Planning	Technical	Interpersonal	Conceptual
Organizing	Human	Informational	Technical managerial/clinical
Staffing	Conceptual	Decisional	Interpersonal/collaborative
Directing (motivation, leading		——	Political
and communicating)			Commercial
Controlling		Designer	Governance
Decision making		Strategist	——
		Leader	Transformation
			Execution
			People

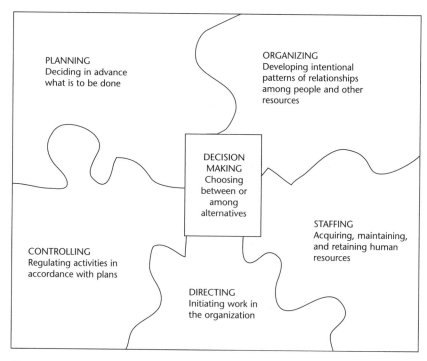

Figure 5.1.   The management functions are interrelated like the pieces of a puzzle.

tions, as shown in Figure 5.1. The separation of management functions is necessary for purposes of discussion, but it is an artificial treatment of the reality of managing.

Planning Function

Planning means deciding prospectively what to do—charting a course of action for the future. Planning establishes and devises the means to achieve organizational missions and objectives. Without planning, disjointed, even random, activities can prevail. Planning is a necessary precursor to other management functions; it lays the foundation for organizing. An organizational structure designed to carry out plans dictates the objectives and activities toward which managers lead other members of the organization. Part of the planning function, when managers carry out their controlling function, is establishing desired objectives and standards against which actual performance can be measured.

There are many reasons that planning is crucial to the successful operation of HSOs/HSs. None is more important than that planning focuses attention on objectives. Good planning yields appropriate organizational objectives and develops the means through which they can be met. In this way, planning contributes to integrating the actions of organizational participants toward common ends.

Another reason that planning is important is because it helps offset the pervasive uncertainty that HSOs/HSs face. Typically, the only certainty about the future is uncertainty. However, when managers think systematically about the future and plan for contingencies, they greatly reduce the chances of being unprepared. The profound changes occurring in delivering and financing health services require that HSOs/HSs be adaptable and flexible; planning is critical for both.

A third reason that planning is important is that it enhances efficiency and effectiveness. Health services are expensive, and whereas many aspects of their cost are beyond the control of managers, others can be minimized through planning for efficient operation. Planning substitutes integrated effort for random activity, controlled flow of work for uneven flow, and thoughtful decisions for snap judgments. As the delivery of health services becomes more dependent on costly technologies and more and more centered in complex organizations and systems, the managerial function of planning in these settings becomes increasingly important.

Finally, planning is important because it facilitates fulfillment of the management function of controlling. Controlling implies comparing actual results with predetermined desired results and correcting deviations when they occur. The planning function yields information that can be used to set standards against which actual results can be compared. As third parties, government (principally) and private employers have assumed a greater share of the financial burden of health services, and they have required significantly more accountability from service providers. This accountability goes beyond costs, to include both the quality of care and the manner in which it is delivered. The trend toward more accountability and the concurrent necessity for control that it implies will become increasingly important in HSOs/HSs in the years ahead. The effect of planning on managers' efforts to control the activities for which they are responsible is one of the most important values in effective planning.

Planning is done by all managers in HSOs/HSs, although the work varies by level. Senior-level managers typically are concerned with the planning function activities of external environment assessment and of formulating and reformulating missions and objectives for the entire organization or system. Objectives that are consistent with and support the mission and organizationwide objectives are set by middle-level and first-level managers for their areas of responsibility. Planning by these managers focuses on program and operations design, as well as on implementation procedures and work scheduling.

Organizing Function

Mission and supporting objectives are established by planning, but managers must design an organization that is capable of achieving them if they are to become reality. If the mission and objectives of HSOs/HSs are to be effectively pursued, their managers must develop intentional patterns of relationships among staff and other resources. The resulting structure is called the organization design, and the developmental efforts and activities are the organizing function of management.

The design of organizations begins with the establishment of individual positions, which typically are determined by how an HSO's/HS's work is divided and specialized. Conceptually, organization design proceeds from individual positions to clustering positions into workgroups such as departments and units, then further clustering workgroups into larger subdivisions of the organization, and eventually clustering these into an entire organization and, in some cases, into systems or networks of organizations.

Successful designs depend on appropriate distributions of responsibility and authority as the organization is built through successive rounds of clustering. Authority is the power that is derived from a person's position in an organization or system. Responsibility can be thought of as the obligation to execute work, whether it is direct, support, or management work. All staff have responsibilities as a result of their organizational positions. The source of responsibility is one's superior in the organization. By delegating responsibility and accountability to a subordinate, the superior creates a relationship based on obligation between superior and subordinate. When responsibility is delegated to individuals, they also must be given the authority to make commitments, use resources, and take the actions necessary to fulfill their responsibilities.

HSOs typically are departmentalized functionally. Effective interactions among the departments are essential, as are integration and coordination. One must recognize the relationship between the degree to which an organization's work is divided and specialized and subsequent requirements for integration and coordination of the work. The more work is differentiated and specialized, the more difficult integration becomes. Large hospitals and systems are among the most complex organizations in terms of differentiation of work and worker specialization. These organizations are characterized by detailed division of work into a number of different jobs. The work done is so specialized and performed by such a variety of workers that very significant problems involving integration and coordination of work often arise. Furthermore, in these organizations, the direct, support, and management work is highly interdependent. This functional interdependence makes integration and coordination of work an important aspect of successfully organizing.

Successful organization designs include features that ensure a high level of integration and coordination of work. The essential challenge of effectively integrating and coordinating the work in these settings stems from the fact that individuals often perceive objectives differently and may also favor various methods of accomplishing them. Effectively integrating and coordinating work often means managing conflicts that may arise between and among the subparts of an organization, such as between the PSO and senior-level management or between the nursing service and the pharmacy or laboratory. There also may be conflicts involving pairs of individuals or conflicts between individuals and the organization.

In HSs, relationships between and among component organizations have the potential for conflict. Not all conflict is bad, but even low-level conflict, such as "disliking" and "difficulty in getting along with," reduces organizational effectiveness. Integration and coordination are managerial activities concerned with preventing conflicts and misunderstandings. Organization designs that facilitate integration and coordination are very important to the success that managers achieve in carrying out the organizing function.

Staffing Function

Staffing HSOs/HSs with competent employees involves a wide range of centralized activities, programs, and policies related to acquisition, retention and maintenance, and separation of human resources. All managers play a part in and have some degree of responsibility for the staffing function, including selection, performance appraisal, promotion, training and development, discipline and corrective counseling, and compensation of their employees. However, the staffing function is centralized in and coordinated by a single human resources (HR) department—or in the case of a HS, a corporate office—that establishes organizationwide/systemwide policies and procedures and provides human resources acquisition, retention, and separation services for other departments/units. HR activities are detailed in Chapter 10.

The contemporary designation for the centralized staffing function is human resources management (HRM) or strategic human resources management (SHRM).[29] As Fottler has noted, "SHRM refers to the comprehensive set of managerial activities and tasks designed to develop and maintain a qualified workforce that contributes to organizational effectiveness as defined by the organization's strategic goals."[30] *HRM* is used here to refer to the set of centralized staffing activities, programs, and policies concerned with the acquisition, retention and maintenance, and separation of employees, as well as labor relations (i.e., union–management relationships). *Human resources department* refers to the organizational component responsible for staffing and labor relations activities, programs, and policies; *human resources managers* refers to people who manage these departments or offices.

The human resources department is responsible for bringing employees into the organization and placing them in the existing structure (acquisition); enhancing the competencies of existing employees and keeping those who are effective in the organization (retention and maintenance); facilitating the exit of those who leave (separation); and developing policies for employees in the organization (coordinating). Human resources departments assist other departments and managers with special expertise and programs. Because the HR department has a centralized role and because employees are the organization's most important resource, the human resources manager is typically a member of senior-level management who influences the formulation and implementation of human resources policies for the whole HSO/HS. More important, this manager integrates all HRM activities with the entity's strategic plans.[31]

Even though staffing activities are centralized in the human resources department, other managers must be familiar with them. First, HRM policies provide structure and define the interactions among managers, who are ultimately accountable for the quality and productivity of their operations and employees. Second, HRM policies reflect societal norms that are expressed in legislation and judicial decisions in areas such as nondiscriminatory hiring, discipline, promotion, and compensation. Better informed managers will be more effective in using human resources and less likely to act unethically or illegally.

Staffing Activities

The interconnected activities that comprise the staffing function are described more fully in Chapter 10 but include the following. *Acquisition* includes human resources planning, recruitment, selection, and orientation. *Retention and maintenance* include placement, performance appraisal, training and development, discipline and corrective counseling, compensation and benefits administration, employee assistance and career counseling, and safety and health. *Separation* occurs when employees leave HSOs/HSs for various reasons—better job opportunities, discharge, retirement, or death. Most human resources departments engage in activities to assist and monitor exit. Traditional activities include easing the individual's departure; collecting employer-provided equipment, keys, and records; completing personnel records; processing final pay; and collecting information through an exit interview. Other activities include preretirement planning and outplacement.

Human Resources Planning

Acquisition requires careful human resources planning to precede the recruitment, selection, and orientation of new employees. An HSO/HS determines staffing needs through human resources planning. The workforce must be considered in the context of a changing environment because organizations and systems are dynamic and needs change. Present staff must be evaluated and retained and new employees recruited to meet changing needs.[32]

Staff needs in HSOs/HSs are driven by organizational growth and employee turnover. Growth occurs through increased demand for services, facility expansion, the addition of new services, or intensification of services. Furthermore, staffing needs differ when services are eliminated or point of delivery changes. Each change may necessitate a different level of employees and mix of skills. Employee turnover through resignation, discharge, and retirement is the normal process of employee separation (exit). In addition to employee turnover and organizational growth, changes in technology drive the need for staff with different skills. The human resources manager must constantly monitor the need for new employees to ensure that current and future needs for adequate numbers of qualified employees are met. This makes human resources planning integral to HRM, and the HR plan must be supportive of the organization's strategic plans.

Directing Function

Directing is social-behavioral in nature and focuses on initiating action in the organization or system. Effectively directing others in organizations depends on ability of managers to lead, motivate, and communicate with those they direct. Leading others is important to successful directing at all levels of HSOs/HSs. First- and middle-level managers rely on their ability to lead those whom they directly manage. HSOs/HSs also require leadership at the organization or system level. Leadership at this level reflects the ability to develop and instill in HSO/HS members a common vision and to direct adherence to that vision.

Leading effectively means managers must inspire and influence others to contribute to the attainment of the HSO's/HS's mission and objectives. Leading requires interactions between managers and those they manage in a wide variety of organizational situations. A single pattern of leadership behavior will not fit the diversity of these situations. Thus, the successful manager cannot be locked into a particular leadership style but must choose the method that is most appropriate in a given situation.

Success in the directing function is influenced by how effectively managers motivate others and by how well they communicate with them. Following directions is caused behavior. Thus, skill at motivating people is crucial to effective directing. Similarly, managers who effectively articulate and communicate their visions and preferences are more likely to have them followed.

Controlling Function

The controlling function of management involves gathering information and monitoring activities and performance, comparing actual results with expected results, and when appropriate, intervening to take corrective action. That is, controlling is the regulation of activities and performance in accordance with the requirements of plans. By definition, the controlling function is directly linked to the planning function through measuring and correcting activities of people and things in an organization or system to ensure that the mission is pursued and that objectives developed in the planning function are accomplished. Controlling is a function of managers at all levels, and its basic purpose is to ensure that what is intended is done. Senior-level managers focus on controlling their organization or system's overall results, such as quality of care, expenditures compared with revenues, and resource utilization. First-level managers focus on control in their areas of responsibility—for example, number of laboratory tests performed per employee per day, number of meals served, or time between dictation and transcription of medical records. The control function monitors outputs and inputs, but it also must monitor processes, or how work is done. Improving performance requires that all processes be systematically monitored, evaluated, and changed if performance is to be maximized.

A Model of Controlling[33]

Control activities have the same basic elements regardless of whether people, quality of services, expenses, or morale are being controlled. Control, wherever it is applied, involves three steps: 1) monitoring performance, 2) comparing actual results with previously established desired results and standards, and 3) correcting deviations that are found. Figure 5.2 illustrates these three interrelated parts of controlling applied to controlling performance in the laboratory of a program intended to screen for HIV infection.

In this model, inputs and resources are used in processes to produce desired outputs, outcomes, and impact. Desired outputs, outcomes, and impact are the performance targets for this laboratory. Standards typically are those established by professions, regulators, and accrediting agencies. Together, the desired results and the standards become the criteria against which performance can be compared and judged.

Controlling is facilitated when the criteria against which performance will be assessed are expressed in objective, quantifiable terms. For example, a desired outcome of high employee morale may be more difficult to specify in objective terms than a desired outcome of not exceeding an established operating budget. However, ways of subjectively determining achievement of a desired outcome of improved morale can be devised and used.

The manager of this laboratory may find an information system (IS) useful in controlling the laboratory's work and results.[34] ISs can be designed so that information relevant to control can be collected, formatted, stored, and retrieved in a timely way to support the monitoring and comparing aspects of controlling. An IS can be relatively simple or very elaborate but should report deviations at critical points. Effective control requires attention to those factors that actually affect performance. A good IS will report deviations promptly and will contain elements of information that are understandable to those who use the system. Finally, a good IS will point to corrective action. A control system that detects deviations from accomplishment of desired results or from standards will be little more than an interesting exercise if it does not show the way to corrective action. A good IS will disclose where failures are occurring and what is responsible for them so that corrective action can be undertaken.

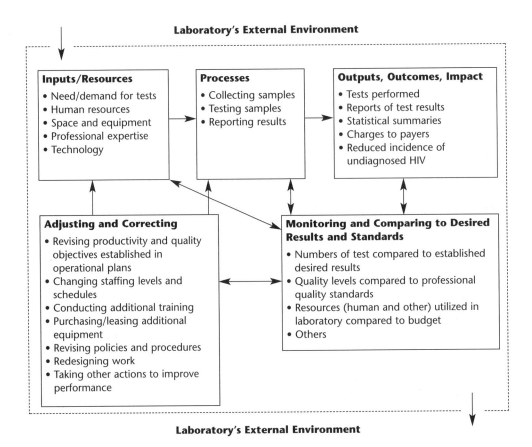

Figure 5.2.   Control of performance in an HIV-screening program's laboratory. Source: Beaufort B. Longest, Jr. *Managing Health Programs and Projects.* San Francisco: Jossey-Bass, 2004: 58. Reprinted with permission.

Monitoring and comparing will reveal deviations from the accomplishment of desired results or from adherence to chosen standards. When deviations occur, effective control requires adjustments or corrective actions to curb undesirable results and bring performance back into line, as shown in Figure 5.2.

Effective managers carefully analyze the situation, starting by comparing desired results and standards against monitored performance. After all, the desired results may have been poorly conceived; conditions may have changed, rendering them inappropriate; and standards undergo revision from time to time.

Only after a thorough analysis of a deviation should this laboratory's manager take effective corrective action that will secure improved results in the future. Such corrective action may consist of revising the definition of desired results, changing a process, redeploying resources, holding a simple discussion with employees about their work, changing technology employed, providing more training, providing better equipment, allowing more time, developing a new schedule, or any of a wide range of other means of rectifying the situation. Control receives further attention in Chapter 10.

The Pervasiveness of Decision Making

As noted earlier and shown in Figure 5.1, decision making is intertwined with each function of management. All managers are decision makers. They make decisions when they monitor and control work; when they plan, establish, or change organizational arrangements, work process, and content; when they acquire and assign personnel; and when they direct work activity. All managers make decisions, but their decisions vary in scope and nature, as well as in techniques used, depending on the manager's level in the organization or system. Senior-level managers make policy decisions that affect entire organizations or systems, and they make resource allocation decisions that affect the various parts of the organization; middle- and first-level managers make decisions about allocating and utilizing resources provided by senior-level management within their areas of authority and responsibility. Chapter 6 addresses decision making as a product of problem solving.

MANAGEMENT SKILLS

Consideration of the management functions of planning, organizing, staffing, directing, controlling, and decision making helps one understand management work. Strong evidence from empirical studies shows that much of what managers do can be categorized into one or more of these functions.[35] However, identifying management functions says very little about skills managers need to properly execute the functions. Thus, another way to consider management work is to examine the set of skills that people must possess and use in doing this work well.

As shown in Table 5.2, effective managers utilize three distinct types of skills.[36] Technical skills of managers include their abilities to use the methods, processes, and techniques of managing. It is easy to visualize the technical skills of a surgeon or a physical therapist, but counseling a subordinate or developing a departmental budget also require specific technical skills. Human, or interpersonal, skills are the abilities of managers to get along well with others, to understand them, and to motivate and lead them in the workplace. Conceptual skills reflect the mental abilities of managers to visualize the complex interrelationships in a workplace—relationships among people, among departments or units, among various organizations in a system, and even between an organization or system and its external environment. Conceptual skills permit managers to understand how the various factors in particular situations fit together and interact.

Not all managers use these skills to the same degree or in the same mix, although every manager must rely on all three types of skills in performing management work. For example, the management work that takes place in a hospital nursing service reflects different levels of management and requires different mixes of these technical, human, and conceptual skills. The vice president for nursing (a senior-level manager) is vitally concerned with how the nursing service fits into the hospital's operation. However, the vice president can rely on nursing service staff to accomplish the technical work. In contrast, a director of nursing (a middle-level manager), whose primary responsibility is to "troubleshoot" an entire nursing staff on one shift, may be constantly required to make decisions on the basis of technical knowledge of nursing while rarely having time to think about the relationship of the nursing service to other hospital departments. A nurse in charge of a nursing unit will use a considerable amount of technical skill because, in addition to being a manager, this individual also must practice nursing. Almost all this manager's work involves direct contact with people and, consequently, also requires human relations skills more than the work of either the vice president or director of nursing.

The extent to which each management skill is needed and utilized varies with the manager's position in the organizational hierarchy; degree of authority; scope of responsibility; and number, types, and skills of subordinates. Senior-level managers typically use disproportionately more conceptual skills in their jobs than middle- or first-level managers. Conceptual demands include recognizing and evaluating multiple, complex issues and understanding their relationships; engaging in planning and problem solving; and thinking globally about the organization or system and its environment. In contrast, first-level managers tend to use more job-related technical skills and skills that involve specialized knowledge than either middle- or senior-level managers. Figure 5.3 shows the

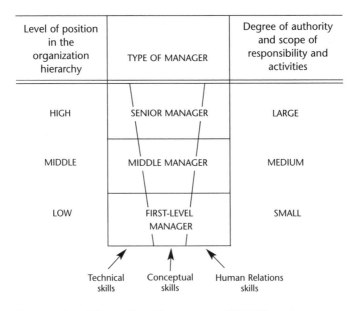

Figure 5.3.   Skills used by different types of HSO/HS managers.

relationship of these skills, degree of authority, and scope of responsibility and activities for each management level.

MANAGEMENT ROLES

All managers engage in management functions of planning, organizing, staffing, directing, and controlling; all managers utilize some mix of technical, conceptual, and human relations skills; and all managers constantly engage in decision making, although this does not capture all that managers do. For example, a hospital CEO or other senior-level manager may serve on an areawide mental health task force, an HMO president may testify before a legislative body, the administrator of a nursing facility may serve on a state licensing board, the vice president of nursing at an academic medical center may present a guest lecture in a nursing baccalaureate program, and a Department of Veterans Affairs senior official may provide testimony before Congress to justify budget increases. However, such activities are not fully encompassed in traditional descriptions of management functions or skills.

Mintzberg's Interpersonal, Informational, and Decisional Roles

In an important study of management work, Henry Mintzberg observed a sample of managers over a period of time, recording what they did. He concluded that management work can be described meaningfully in terms of roles that all managers play. Roles in organizations are the typical or customary sets of behaviors that accompany particular organizational positions. Mintzberg compared the roles of managers to those of actors on a stage and concluded that, just as actors play roles, managers, because they are managers, should adopt certain patterns of behavior when filling managerial positions. He viewed the work of managers as a series of three broad categories of roles—interpersonal, informational, and decisional—with each category comprising several distinct but interrelated roles.[37] Figure 5.4 summarizes Mintzberg's view of management roles. Thus, a third

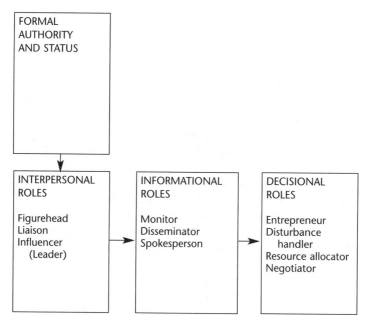

Figure 5.4.   The manager's roles. (Reprinted by permission of *Harvard Business Review* from Mintzberg, Henry. The manager's job: Folklore and fact. 53 [July–August 1975]. Copyright © 1975 by the Harvard Business School Publishing Corporation; all rights reserved.)

way to examine the work of managers is to consider the different roles that they play (see Table 5.2).

Interpersonal Roles

In Mintzberg's schema, all managers are granted formal authority over the organizations, systems, or organizational units they manage, and that leads to their interpersonal roles as figurehead, leader, and liaison. The figurehead role is played by managers, especially by senior-level managers, when engaging in ceremonial and symbolic activities such as presiding over the opening of an addition to their organization's physical plant or giving a speech about healthcare to a local civic club. Managers play an influencer, or leader, role when they seek to motivate, inspire, and set examples through their own behavior. The liaison role allows managers, in formal and informal contacts both inside their HSOs/HSs and with their external stakeholders, to establish relationships that will help them advance organizational performance and achieve organizational missions and objectives. Playing interpersonal roles provides managers with opportunities to gather and use information, which generates a second set of roles.

Informational Roles

The informational roles of managers include monitor, disseminator, and spokesperson. As monitors, managers gather information from their networks of contacts, including those established in their liaison roles; filter the information; evaluate it; and decide whether to act as a result of the information. The disseminator role grows out of managers' access to information and ability to choose what to do with that information. In dissemination, managers have many choices about who, inside and outside their organizations or systems, should receive information. The third informational role, spokesperson, is related to managers' figurehead role and involves their communicating the positions of their entities to internal and external stakeholders who affect their areas of responsibility.

Decisional Roles

Managers' decisional roles include entrepreneur, disturbance handler, resource allocator, and negotiator. The authority granted to them and supported by their interpersonal and informational roles permits managers to play decisional roles. As entrepreneurs, managers are initiators and designers of changes intended to improve performance in their organizational domains. When playing this role, managers act as change agents. In their disturbance handler role, managers decide how to handle a wide variety of problems or issues that arise as they carry out their daily work. For example, senior-level managers may face disturbances created by their PSOs, by regulatory agencies, or by the actions of competitors. First-level managers may face a variety of disturbances, ranging from a heavy snowfall that keeps necessary staff from their work, to conflict among subordinates, to budget cuts. The ability to make good decisions about handling disturbances is an important determinant of managerial success.

In their resource allocator role, managers must allocate human, physical, and technological resources among alternative uses. The decisions about resource allocation become more difficult, and more important, as resources are constrained. As negotiators, managers interact and bargain with employees, suppliers, regulators, customers and clients, and others. Negotiating includes deciding what objectives or outcomes to seek through negotiation and how to conduct the negotiations.

Integrating Mintzberg's Interpersonal, Informational, and Decisional Roles

The 10 managerial roles shown in Figure 5.4 cannot be neatly separated. In practice, they are intertwined into what psychologists term a *gestalt*, or an integrated whole. Management work is much more than the sum of these 10 roles. When the interconnected roles are each played well, the result is synergistic. Being a good negotiator makes a manager a better disturbance handler. Playing the informational roles effectively improves performance in the decisional roles because managers have better information with which to make decisions.

Obviously, each manager will use different combinations of these roles. In part, the manager's level in the organization will determine the optimum mix. Senior-level managers in HSOs/HSs engage in figurehead, entrepreneur, and spokesperson roles more frequently than do other managers. Middle-level managers, often heavily involved in disturbance handler and resource allocator roles, rely on their abilities to successfully play informational roles in their work. First-level managers may play leader, disturbance handler, and negotiator roles extensively in their daily work. The point is that all managers engage in these roles, but specific circumstances, work conditions, and their responsibilities will dictate the most appropriate mix of roles.

Designer, Strategist, and Leader Roles

Figure 5.5 illustrates another conceptualization of roles managers play, a trinity of roles: designer, strategist, and leader.[38] Like Mintzberg's model, this depiction of the roles of managers can apply in all types of organizational settings and to the management work that occurs at the various levels of organizations and systems. In this model as well, managers in differing circumstances must use varying mixes of the roles if they are to achieve optimal performance.

Designer Role

The designer role is fulfilled as managers establish intentional patterns of relationships among staff and other resources in their organizations or systems. Managers at all levels of organizations and systems play the designer role, although in different ways. First-level managers are more concerned with designating individual positions and aggregating them into the workgroups that they manage (teams, departments, units, and so forth). Middle-level managers cluster workgroups into the major

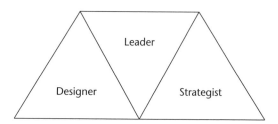

Figure 5.5. The trinity of managerial roles. (From Zuckerman, Howard S., and William L. Dowling. The managerial role. In *Essentials of Health Care Management,* edited by Stephen M. Shortell and Arnold D. Kaluzny, 47. Albany, NY: Delmar Publishers, 1997; reprinted by permission of Delmar Learning, a division of Thomson Learning (www.thomsonrights.com). Fax 800-730-2215.)

divisions of their organizations and determine how various workgroups and clusters of workgroups are integrated and coordinated. In their designer roles, senior-level managers are likely to focus on arranging the workgroups and clusters of workgroups into entire organizations, perhaps even into integrated HSs or alliances of organizations.

Strategist Role

The strategist role is played as managers participate with GBs to establish missions and then develop and implement suitable strategies capable of achieving their organizational objectives. When managers think strategically, they are thinking about how to adapt their organizational domains to the external challenges and opportunities presented by the environment.[39] HSOs/HSs are dynamic, open systems that exist within complex external environments where they engage in ongoing exchanges and are influenced, sometimes dramatically, by events. Managers who think strategically understand that each part within an organization or system has similar relationships with other parts or components.

Important to the strategist role is the ability of managers to discern essential information in their environments. They engage in situational analysis through which they see and assess pertinent information in their environments. At the macro level, managers must scan an enormous amount of biological, cultural, demographic, ecological, economic, ethical, legal, political, psychological, social, and technological information to assess its potential effect on their organizations. In addition, managers must analyze internal organizational conditions, decisions, and actions to ascertain their effects.

Good situational analysis, however, includes more than merely discerning important information. It also includes organizing information and evaluating it in order to chart the issues that are likely to have significant impact. In addition, it includes assessing the internal strengths and weaknesses of the organization or system and its mission and objectives, as well as the values held by those inside. Only after all of this information is considered can managers most effectively make strategic decisions about the objectives they wish to pursue and the means they wish to use in doing so.

Managers' strategist roles also involve them in acting on information garnered through situational analysis. They formulate objectives (the ends to be achieved) and decide on strategies (broad patterns of actions) necessary to achieve objectives. Senior-level managers, sometimes called strategic managers, are responsible, along with the GBs of their HSOs/HSs, for establishing the overall strategic directions of their organizations or systems. Middle- and first-level managers who implement organization-level strategies frequently provide valuable input to the formulation of these strategies. In addition, they must develop and implement objectives and the means to accomplish what they directly manage. Thus, all managers play strategist roles, although differently.

Leader Role

As discussed earlier, all organizations are dependent on the quality of leadership that is exercised by their managers. Only effective leadership will encourage and motivate staff to fulfill missions and accomplish organizational objectives. The leader role is not isolated from other roles that managers play. Leadership is affected directly by the context in which it takes place. How well managers play their designer and strategist roles will affect their leader roles. For example, leadership is facilitated where

- The existence of long-standing shared values and a commonly accepted philosophy help shape the HSO's/HS's mission and objectives and resolve conflicts among competing views about them
- A history of service helps legitimize claims for support from internal and external stakeholders
- The technical ability to plan strategically helps provide a sense of organizational purpose, stability, and self-control

Successfully playing the leader roles in all organizations is a challenge. This is especially true in HSOs/HSs for several reasons, but most important is that these institutions operate in such dynamic environments. "The most difficult leadership challenges arise when changes in the environment require transformation of organizational cultures, or reexamination of organizational goals."[40]

A second reason that the leader role is difficult in HSOs/HSs is that their managers must satisfy diverse constituencies. The communities served by these organizations and systems, as well as the wishes of the people who work, govern, or practice in the organizations and systems, must be considered. Only rarely are the preferences of these various groups in harmony.

A third cause of difficulty of leading in HSOs/HSs is that, unlike many other organizations, they often require extensive sharing of the leadership role. The managers certainly play leadership roles, but so do the members of their GBs and PSOs. The president plays a key organizational leadership role, but it would be very difficult to play this leadership role properly without support and validation provided by the GB. Furthermore, clinical leadership primarily resides with clinicians—including physicians and, increasingly, others with clinical responsibilities.[41] Consequently, the issue of who provides organizational leadership is often cloudy. What is clear, however, is that the challenge of leadership is made more complex by the ambiguities about who is responsible for it.

MANAGEMENT COMPETENCIES

The fourth way to consider management work is in terms of the competencies needed by managers if they are to perform well. This approach builds on and overarches the function, skill, and role approaches. Competencies are sets of skills and knowledge that managers need in order to do their management work. Two models of management competencies are presented below. The first, the Health Leadership Competency Model of the National Center for Healthcare Leadership (www.nchl.org), is summarized here. The full model can be applied to leadership by managers at first-, middle-, and senior-level. The second model presented below applies primarily to senior-level managers.

As has been noted, the "definitions and terminology surrounding the concept of competency are replete with imprecise and inconsistent meanings, resulting in a certain level of bewilderment among those seeking to identify the concept."[42] For our purposes, we will use the following definition of a competency: "a cluster of related skills, knowledge, and ability (sometimes referred to by the acronym SKA) that: 1) affect a major part of one's job (a role or responsibility), 2) correlate with performance on the job, 3) can be measured against well accepted standards, and 4) can be improved by training and development."[43]

Health Leadership Competency Model

The National Center for Healthcare Leadership (NCHL) is a not-for-profit organization seeking to ensure that competent leaders (managers) are available and can ensure the delivery of quality patient healthcare in the 21st century. "NCHL's goal is to improve health system performance and the health status of the entire country through effective healthcare management leadership."[44]

The competency model developed by NCHL contains 26 specific leadership competencies organized into three interrelated competency domains: transformation, execution, and people, as follows:[45]

TRANSFORMATION

Visioning, energizing, and stimulating a change process that coalesces communities, patients, and professionals around new models of healthcare and wellness. Competencies include:

Achievement Orientation: A concern for surpassing a standard of excellence. The standard may be one's own past performance (striving for improvement); an objective measure (results orientation); outperforming others (competitiveness); challenging goals, or something that has not been done previously (innovation).

Analytical Thinking: The ability to understand a situation, issue, or problem by breaking it into smaller pieces or tracing its implications in a step-by-step way. It includes organizing the parts of a situation, issue, or problem systematically; making systematic comparisons of different features or aspects; setting priorities on a rational basis; and identifying time sequences, causal relationships, or if-then relationships.

Community Orientation: The ability to align one's own and the organization's priorities with the needs and values of the community, including its cultural and ethnocentric values, and to move health forward in line with population-based wellness needs and national health agenda.

Financial Skills: The ability to understand and explain financial and accounting information, prepare and manage budgets, and make sound long-term investment decisions.

Information Seeking: An underlying curiosity and desire to know more about things, people, and issues, including the desire for knowledge and staying current with health, organizational, industry, and professional trends and developments.

Innovative Thinking: The ability to apply complex concepts, develop creative solutions, and adapt previous solutions in new ways for breakthrough thinking in the field.

Strategic Orientation: The ability to draw implications and conclusions in light of the business, economic, demographic, ethno-cultural, political, and regulatory trends and developments, and to use these insights to develop an evolving vision for the organization and the health industry that results in long-term success and viability.

EXECUTION

Translating vision and strategy into optimal organizational performance. Competencies include:

Accountability: The ability to hold people accountable to standards of performance or ensure compliance using the power of one's position or force of personality appropriately and effectively, with the long-term good of the organization in mind.

Change Leadership: The ability to energize stakeholders and sustain their commitment to changes in approaches, processes, and strategies.

Collaboration: The ability to work cooperatively with others as part of a team or group, including demonstrating positive attitudes about the team, its members, and its ability to get its mission accomplished.

Communication: The ability to speak and write in a clear, logical, and grammatical manner in formal and informal situations, to prepare cogent business presentations, and to facilitate a group.

Impact and Influence: The ability to persuade and convince others (individuals or groups) to support a point of view, position, or recommendation.

Information Technology Management: The ability to see the potential in and understand the use of administrative and clinical information technology and decision-support tools in process and performance improvement. Actively sponsors their utilization and the continuous upgrading of information management capabilities.

Initiative: The ability to anticipate obstacles, developments, and problems by looking ahead several months to over a year.

Organizational Awareness: The ability to understand and learn the formal and informal decision-making structures and power relationships in an organization or industry (e.g., stakeholders, suppliers). This includes the ability to identify who the real decision makers are and the individuals who can influence them, and to predict how new events will affect individuals and groups within the organization.

Performance Measurement: The ability to understand and use statistical and financial methods and metrics to set goals and measure clinical as well as organizational performances; commitment to and employment of evidence-based techniques.

Process Management and Organizational Design: The ability to analyze the design or improve an organizational process, including incorporating the principles of quality management as well as customer satisfaction.

Project Management: The ability to plan, execute, and oversee a multi-year, large-scale project involving significant resources, scope, and impact. Examples include the construction of a major building, implementation of an enterprise-wide system (patient tracking, SAP), or development of a new service line.

PEOPLE

Creating an organizational climate that values employees from all backgrounds and provides an energizing environment for them. Also includes the leader's responsibility to understand his or her impact on others and to improve his or her capabilities, as well as the capabilities of others. Competencies include:

Human Resources Management: The ability to implement staff development and other management practices that represent contemporary best practices, comply with legal and regulatory requirements, and optimize the performance of the workforce, including performance assessments, alternative compensation and benefit methods, and the alignment of human resource practices and processes to meet the strategic goals of the organization.

Interpersonal Understanding: The ability to accurately hear and understand the unspoken and partly expressed thoughts, feelings, and concerns of others.

Professionalism: The demonstration of ethics and professional practices, as well as stimulating social accountability and community stewardship. The desire to act in a way that is consistent with one's values and what one says is important.

Relationship Building: The ability to establish, build, and sustain professional contacts for the purpose of building networks of people with similar goals and that support similar interests.

Self-Confidence: A belief and conviction in one's own ability, success, and decisions or opinions when executing plans and addressing challenges.

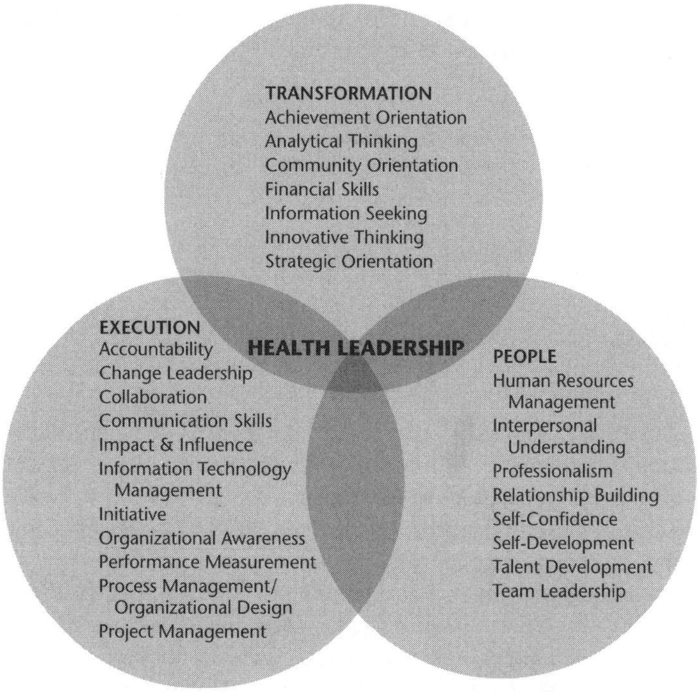

Figure 5.6. NCHL Health Leadership Competency Model. (National Center for Healthcare Leadership. *NCHL Health Leadership Competency Model,* Version 2.0. Chicago: National Center for Healthcare Leadership, 2004. Reprinted by permission.)

Self-Development: The ability to see an accurate view of one's own strengths and development needs, including one's impact on others. A willingness to address needs through reflective, self-directed learning and trying new leadership approaches.

Talent Development: The drive to build the breadth and depth of the organization's human capability, including supporting the top-performing people and taking a personal interest in coaching and mentoring high-potential leaders.

Team Leadership: The ability to see oneself as a leader of others, from forming a top team that possesses balanced capabilities to setting the mission, values, and norms, as well as holding the team members accountable individually and as a group for results.

Although the NCHL Health Leadership Competency Model will continue to evolve with use and new information about necessary competencies for managers in HSOs/HSs, Figure 5.6 depicts how the current competencies fit together to produce health leadership.

Competencies Needed by CEOs[46]

The NCHL model of managerial competencies is designed to apply to all levels of managers. Presented here is a model designed specifically for CEOs. With some overlap among them, six distinct competencies are required for successful CEOs. The clusters of knowledge and skills that make up these competencies are 1) conceptual, 2) technical managerial/clinical, 3) interpersonal/collaborative, 4) political, 5) commercial, and 6) governance. In part, this categorization of managerial competencies builds on Katz's model of the conceptual, technical, and interpersonal skills used by managers.[47] The set of competencies described here includes conceptual competence, albeit of a more expansive nature than that envisioned by Katz. The set also includes a technical managerial/clinical cluster of knowledge and skills as well as an interpersonal/collaborative cluster, each of which is an extension of elements in Katz's model. The political, commercial, and governance clusters represent important additional competencies that are increasingly required of CEOs.[48]

Conceptual Competence

In all organizational settings, possession of an adequate cluster of conceptual knowledge and skills is a competency that permits managers to envision the places and roles of their organizations or systems in the larger society. This competency also allows them to visualize the complex interrelationships within their organizations and systems—relationships among staff and other resources, among units of an HSO, and among the various organizations in an HS. In short, adequate conceptual competence allows CEOs to identify, understand, and interact with their organization's or system's myriad external and internal stakeholders. Conceptual competence also enhances CEOs' abilities to comprehend organizational cultures and historically developed values, beliefs, and norms and to visualize the futures of their organizations and systems.

HSOs/HSs are always works in progress. Typically, their structures and operations are changing continually, with each change expanding the notion of an adequate level of conceptual competence. Apart from organizational and operational complexities, CEOs face new or expanded conceptualizations of mission. When missions change, everything about organizations and systems, including their organizational cultures, also may change. The missions of HSs differ from those of their component HSOs, although the missions are interrelated. Furthermore, as HSOs join other organizations in HSs, CEOs face new and more complex conceptualizations of their own managerial roles as well as the roles of other managers with whom they work. In particular, they are more likely to share their leadership responsibilities with physicians. As noted elsewhere, "success in integrated healthcare absolutely requires physicians in leadership positions."[49]

In HSs, CEOs and other senior-level managers must shift their concepts of managerial success from advancing individual HSOs to attaining the more complex integration among sets of HSOs and perhaps other entities. The more extensive and demanding conceptual challenges of increasingly integrated health services significantly broaden the notion of conceptual competence for managers. To achieve success, CEOs working within HSs and other types of strategic alliances must be creative and able to synthesize ideas into new forms and patterns. They must be creative in adapting their domains to constantly evolving circumstances by relying on information, often from disparate sources, to build frameworks, concepts, and hypotheses about the future. These CEOs will be required to identify and evaluate options for solving ever more complex challenges and to select from among them.

Technical Managerial/Clinical Competence

The cluster of knowledge and associated skills that compose technical competence for CEOs covers a broad range of managerial activities: planning for a new service or facility, devising and operating an incentive-based compensation program, arranging the financing of long-term debt, and much more. Traditionally, CEOs in HSOs/HSs were required to know something of the clinical work to obtain the necessary resources, and they relied on the help of experts to ensure an acceptable level of quality. Knowledge and relevant skills in using or applying clinical knowledge are increasingly important. However, effective CEOs also rely on clinically *and* managerially based technical knowledge, and sometimes both simultaneously.

As with conceptual competence, the technical managerial/clinical competence that is required of CEOs in complex HSs is generally more extensive than what is needed for an independent HSO. All CEOs and senior-level managers in HSOs/HSs need to possess a significant degree of clinical and management expertise. However, this increases, especially at the clinical level of integrated situations in which HSs are formed among multiple entities involved in diverse aspects of clinical care.

In highly integrated HSs, for example, CEOs lead their systems in providing continua of health services. In doing so, CEOs face difficult work imperatives requiring new or expanded competencies as they assess health needs in populations they serve and measure performance as improvements in the health status of their client populations; as they use population-based data to determine appropriate system size and configuration in terms of primary and specialty providers, acute care and nursing facility beds, home health, hospice, and related components of the continuum of service; and, perhaps, as they assume financial risk for the provision of services.

Interpersonal/Collaborative Competence

An important ingredient in managerial success always has been the cluster of human interaction knowledge and related skills and relations by which managers direct or lead others in the pursuit of organizational objectives. A survey of executives conducted to determine management competencies that are most important to success in management performance in ambulatory health services settings found interpersonal skills rated most highly.[50]

Interpersonal competence incorporates knowledge and skills that are useful in effectively interacting with others, including the knowledge and related skills that permit a CEO to develop and instill a common vision and stimulate a determination in others to pursue the vision and fulfill objectives related to it. The essence of the interpersonal competence of managers is knowing how to motivate people, how to communicate their visions and preferences, how to handle negotiations, and how to manage conflicts.

The core elements of traditional interpersonal competence expand considerably when HSOs are involved in establishing and maintaining strategic alliances with other organizations, particularly in the formation and operation of HSs. This expansion results from the differences between interpersonal relationships that occur within organizations and those that occur among organizations in a system or strategic alliance. Achieving and managing integration and coordination with other organizations relies on knowledge and skills that facilitate synergistic interaction among the organizations involved.

Two sets of knowledge and skills form collaborative competence. The first element of collaborative competence is the ability to partner—to create and maintain multiparty organizational arrangements, negotiate complex agreements and contracts that sustain these arrangements, and produce mutually beneficial outcomes through such arrangements.[51] The second element, closely related to but distinct from partnering ability, is the ability to manage within the context of an HS. This context is different from an independent HSO and requires different decisions and actions by CEOs and other senior-level managers.

A partnering skill crucial to success in establishing and maintaining effective HSs is the ability of CEOs to develop a common culture. In this context, culture is the pattern of shared values and beliefs that become ingrained in HS participants over time and influence their collaborative behaviors and decisions. A senior manager in one HS noted, "Nothing is more important to the long-term success of integrated systems than developing a culture. We have to do it or we won't survive. Without it, we won't be able to stand the pressures and develop the team approach we need."[52]

Collaborative competence also may mean establishing not only new mission statements and associated organizational objectives, but also new types of missions and objectives that fit the HS's needs and toward which others can be led. In independent HSOs, organizational objectives typically pertain to success in meeting volume, revenue, market share, and narrowly specified quality targets. HSs' organizational objectives at the system level are added and can pertain to such objectives as enhancing the health status of a defined population and integrating functionally diverse organizations.

The core interpersonal/collaborative management challenge for CEOs and other senior managers is to convince CEOs and senior managers of the system's component organizations to avoid thinking of success in terms of "advancing individual organizational priorities and favorably positioning the organization within the wider system"[53] but to consider the system's broader vision, values, and objectives. They must suboptimize individual unit performance to optimize performance of the whole system. Managers at all levels of an HS's component HSOs are challenged to adjust their mind-sets regarding success and to help subordinates do the same by changing perceptions and ingrained habits acquired during years of pursuing narrower definitions of success.

In the context of independent HSOs, conflict management responsibilities primarily involve managers in resolving issues of intrapersonal conflict (within a person), interpersonal conflict (between or among individuals), intragroup conflict (within a group), or intergroup conflict (between or among groups). Increased levels of integration among HSOs as they form HSs, especially the larger and more complex HSs, mean that CEOs must add management of conflicts between and among the organizations participating in the system to this substantial list of traditional conflict management responsibilities.

As integration levels increase through formation of HSs or other types of interorganizational alliances, CEOs and other senior-level managers become involved in interorganizational conflict. Integration of providers at different points in the patient services continuum brings into proximity disparate organizations, particularly when HSs are linked with insurers or health plans such as managed care organizations. Conflicts are unavoidable, and the knowledge and skills that are useful in managing them effectively are imperative. Interpersonal/collaborative competence is required of CEOs and other senior-level managers in all HSOs, but it is even more complex and important in HSs.

Political Competence

Political competence, defined as the dual abilities to accurately assess the impact of public policies on the performance of the CEO's domain of responsibility and to influence public policy making at state and federal levels, is extraordinarily important for CEOs.[54] CEOs can utilize position-, reward-, and expertise-based sources of power to influence public policy making. Influence can be exerted in the entire policy-making process at all levels of government. This process includes policy formulation, which incorporates legislative agenda setting and the development of laws, and policy implementation, which incorporates rule making and policy operation.[55]

CEOs and other senior-level managers can influence the public policy environments of their HSOs/HSs at many levels. For example, they can help define problems that policies address; they can design solutions; or they can create the political circumstances necessary to advance solutions through the policy-making process.[56] Their central vantage points in the health industry enable CEOs to thoroughly understand healthcare and related problems, such as Medicare and Medicaid coverage and financing, that must be addressed through public policies. By permitting their organizations to serve as demonstration sites for assessing possible solutions, CEOs can identify feasible solutions to problems through mechanisms that can help shape the political circumstances surrounding a policy issue including interest groups, lobbying, and the courts.

Furthermore, individually and through interest groups, CEOs can participate in drafting legislative proposals, and they can testify at legislative and regulatory hearings. They also can influence the public policy-making process in the implementation phase by focusing on rule making. Procedurally, rule making typically precedes and guides the implementation of public policies and is designed to include input from those who will be affected by the regulations in the form of formal comments on proposed rules.

Political competence in the context of an HS requires successful interactions with more policy decisions, as well as policy makers, than is typical for an independent HSO. Contrast the numbers and variety of policy decisions that are relevant for a single, independent community hospital with those of relevance to a large, vertically integrated HS.

Commercial Competence

In any setting, commercial competence is the ability of managers to establish and operate value-creating situations in which economic exchanges between buyers and sellers occur. *Value* in health services has a specific meaning. It requires that buyers and sellers think about both quality and price. Value is quality divided by price.[57] Value in health services is created when services have more of the quality attributes desired by buyers than competitors offer. Value is also created when an HSO/HS sells a set of quality attributes desired by buyers at a lower price than its competitors. Of course, determining value in health services is not quite as straightforward as these relationships might suggest.

The quality of a single health service, such as the repair of a hernia, is difficult to assess. Creating value in health services more typically involves the quality of a large and diverse package of services, which is more difficult to assess than the value of a single service. Similarly, comparing price is difficult because packages of services are being purchased. True price comparisons are of the same benefits or services in the various packages, including any associated copayments or deductibles. Despite these difficulties, however, the commercial success of HSOs/HSs increasingly requires that they compete on value.

Commercial competence in any setting is based on knowledge and associated skills in identifying markets and positioning in markets, and in establishing product/service strategies that enhance the ability to compete effectively. Increasingly, commercial success for HSOs/HSs is determined by their ability to contract with health plans to provide a package of integrated services and, in some cases, to contract with employers to provide services directly to their employees. Indeed, the ability to enter into such contracts is one of the principal motives in forming many HSs.

Governance Competence

Each HSO/HS relies on its CEO and other senior-level managers and GB working in concert at its "strategic apex"[58] to establish a clear vision for the organization or system, to foster a culture that supports the realization of the vision, to assemble and effectively allocate the resources to realize the vision, to lead the organization through various challenges, and to ensure proper accountability to multiple stakeholders.[59] *Accountability,* in the context of governance, means "taking into account and responding to political, commercial, community, and clinical/patient interests and expectations."[60] Although the boundaries between management and governance are not always clear-cut, governance is perceived as the unique function in the organization that "holds management and the organization accountable for its actions and that helps provide management with overall strategic direction in guiding the organization's activities."[61]

The knowledge and associated skills incorporated in governance competence are important for CEOs and other senior-level managers for three reasons. First, CEOs often participate directly in the governance function as members of the GBs of their organizations or systems.[62] Chief executives of HSs are almost universally included. In HSs, other managers, such as CFOs and CMOs with specific expertise, also are typically added to GBs.

A second reason for CEOs and other senior-level managers to possess governance competence is that, at the strategic apex, it is difficult to separate what occurs under the rubric of governance from what occurs in the context of strategic management. Consequently, effective CEOs and other senior-level managers must be knowledgeable about management *and* governance. Governance competence enables CEOs and certain other managers to help the GBs fulfill five somewhat overlapping governance/management responsibilities.[63]

- Those who govern are responsible for establishing a vision for the organization or system from which a mission and associated objectives grow. Although GBs are responsible for final approval of vision, mission, and associated objectives, the CEOs and other senior-level managers who must achieve them can be instrumental in establishing these guideposts to action in an effective manner.

- GBs are responsible for ensuring suitable performance from CEOs and other senior managers. Steps in fulfilling this responsibility typically include selecting the CEO, specifying performance expectations, and periodically appraising the chief executive's actual performance.
- GBs and CEOs have overlapping governance/management responsibility for the quality of care in HSOs/HSs. The legal responsibility of governance in this area is well established and includes credentialing licensed independent practitioners on professional staffs; seeing that procedures for quality management, utilization management, and risk management issues are in place; and assessing both the processes and outcomes of care, increasingly at the level of populations.[64] HSOs/HSs face unprecedented opportunities for the application of algorithms, guidelines, or pathways to improve clinical outcomes, as well as new opportunities for improved service quality and improved levels of customer satisfaction among the populations served. The managers who implement GB-developed goals for quality can be very helpful in establishing them.
- GBs also bear responsibility for the finances and financial performance of their organizations or systems. This responsibility entails establishing appropriate financial objectives, maintaining adequate controls over financial matters, and ensuring that the organization's or system's financial obligations, including investments, are met.
- GBs have governance responsibility for self. That is, those who govern must do so effectively and efficiently. Fulfilling this responsibility includes establishing and maintaining appropriate bylaws to guide the governance process, selecting GB members who can and do serve well, and ensuring that processes function to evaluate board performance and develop members.

The third reason that CEOs and senior-level managers must possess governance competence is that such competence enables them to assist other GB members to do a better job. This includes providing development programs for members of their organization's or system's GB.

The degree to which CEOs and other senior-level managers possess these six competencies—conceptual, technical managerial/clinical, interpersonal/collaborative, political, commercial, and governance—will largely determine their contributions to the performance of their HSOs/HSs.

SUMMARY OF APPROACHES TO CONSIDERING MANAGEMENT WORK

The work of managers has been considered from four perspectives: the functions that managers perform, the skills that they use in carrying out these functions, the roles that managers fulfill in managing, and the set of management competencies that is needed to do the work well. These perspectives form a mosaic—a more complete picture than any one perspective—of management work. Building on and integrating these perspectives on management, a comprehensive model of management in HSOs/HSs is described in the next section.

A Management Model for HSOs/HSs

Earlier in this chapter, management was defined as the process, composed of interrelated social and technical functions and activities, occurring within a formal organizational setting for the purpose of accomplishing predetermined objectives through the use of human and other resources. It was noted

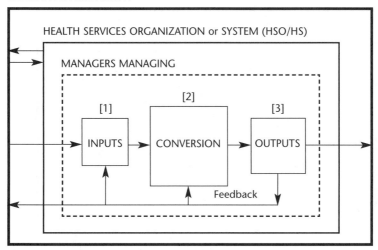

Figure 5.7.   Management as an input–conversion–output process.

and shown in Table 5.2 that all HSO/HS managers perform the management functions of planning, organizing, staffing, directing, and controlling, and that all managers engage in decision making as they perform these functions. These interrelated functions enable managers to establish and accomplish objectives through people and by using other resources in a formal organizational setting. In undertaking these functions, managers use conceptual, technical, and human relations skills; fulfill interrelated interpersonal, informational, and decisional roles, as well as managerial roles as strategists, organization designers, and leaders; and rely on extensive sets of management competencies, including conceptual, technical managerial/clinical, interpersonal/collaborative, political, commercial, and governance competencies; or as conceptualized in another competency model, transformation, execution, and people competencies.

As seen in the schematic model in Figure 5.7, management can be conceptualized as an input–conversion–output process, which is set within the larger environment. Healthcare organizations and systems are open systems (see Chapter 8) that are constantly interacting with their external environment. Within HSOs/HSs, inputs (human and physical resources and technology) are converted, under the catalytic influence of management, into desired outputs (accomplishment of organizational missions and objectives regarding services, products, markets, quality, and other parameters of organizational performance). Figure 5.7 depicts several important relationships.

- HSOs/HSs are formal organizational settings where outputs are produced (mission fulfilled and objectives accomplished) through use (conversion) of inputs (resources).
- Managers and the management work that they perform are the catalyst that converts inputs to outputs.
- HSOs/HSs (and their managers) interact with—are affected by and affect—their external environments; this makes them open systems because inputs are obtained from their external environment and outputs go into that environment.

The input–conversion–output model is expanded into the more comprehensive management model in Figure 5.8. The expanded model incorporates the input–conversion–output perspective but is significantly more detailed. (*Note:* The following discussion of the model references the major components of the model by numbers in brackets.)

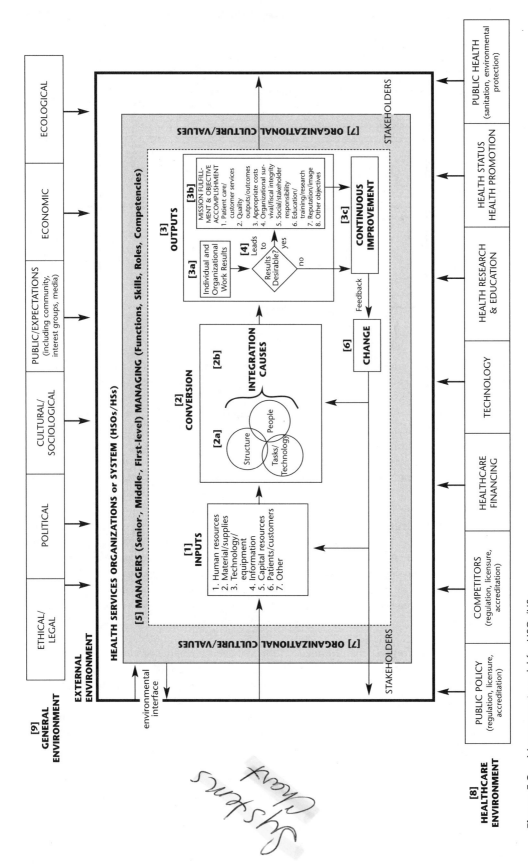

Figure 5.8. Management model for HSOs/HSs.

INPUTS (RESOURCES)

The "inputs" component [1] in Figure 5.8 shows that resources are acquired and used to generate "outputs" [3]. Inputs include human resources, material/supplies, technology/equipment, information, capital resources, and patients/customers. Examples of human resources in HSOs/HSs include managers, physicians, dentists, nurses, technologists, pharmacists, dietitians, social workers, and clerical and housekeeping staff. Material inputs (resources) are supplies of all types, such as medical forms, food, linens, drugs, and instruments. Technological resources include equipment, such as magnetic resonance imagers, heart catheterization equipment, and fetal monitors, as well as knowledge possessed by the staff. Internal information sources include diverse areas such as patient data, reports, schedules, and budgets. External information sources include public policy, stakeholder views and opinions, economic data and forecasts, and the more immediate environment—the healthcare system, which includes regulation, accreditation, competition, and third-party payers. Capital resources are physical plant and funds. Finally, patients or customers are an input resource in the healthcare context.

A great variety of inputs is necessary. Eliminating or restricting them may compromise the effectiveness of the whole organization or system. For example, a rapid rise in supply costs could affect an output, such as the cost of care or provision of a service, or high interest rates may prevent capital expansion. Obsolete equipment may detract from providing better care, or an inadequate supply of human resources may mean that some services are unavailable.

OUTPUTS (MISSIONS AND OBJECTIVES)

The "output" component [3] of the model in Figure 5.8 shows that individual and organizational work results [3a] are produced by the conversion [2] of inputs. Outputs for HSOs/HSs include both specific individual and overall organizational work results [3a]. When work results are appropriate and desirable [4], they lead to fulfilling missions and achieving objectives [3b]. Mission fulfillment and objective accomplishment [3b] in HSOs/HSs typically include patient care and customer services; quality of care; delivering care at appropriate costs; organizational survival and fiscal integrity; meeting responsibilities to stakeholders and society; participating in medical education, training, and research; and maintaining reputation and image.

Missions and organizational objectives vary by type of organization or system. For example, a home health agency seeks primarily to provide high-quality patient care services at appropriate costs to clients in their homes. By comparison, a nongovernmental acute care hospital seeks primarily to provide a range of diagnostic, restorative, and palliative services of different intensity to the community it serves in both inpatient and outpatient settings; it also may have the objective of training medical residents. A veterans medical center may have the primary mission of caring for veterans. A community health center provides care to an indigent population. A genetics counseling center provides counseling and appropriate referral services. A public health department seeks to improve general health through preventive measures in its community. An academic health center may have a complex mission and multiple objectives related to patient care; providing specialized treatment, which requires different inputs, combinations of sophisticated equipment, and medical specialists; training healthcare personnel; and research.

CONVERSION (INTEGRATION)

Conversion [2] of inputs to outputs occurs when managers [5] integrate [2b] structure, tasks/technology, and people [2a] in the context of the organizational culture [7] and in response to meeting the needs of internal, interface, and external stakeholders.

The "structure" element [2a] in Figure 5.8 conceptualizes formally designed organizational arrangements such as authority and responsibility, and superior and subordinate relationships; grouping work activities; and coordination, communication, information, and control mechanisms. The "tasks/technology" element [2a] represents work specialization: job design; work processes, methods, and procedures; and logistical and work flows. It also represents technological characteristics such as equipment, cybernetics, and to some degree, information and knowledge that are used by managers and others in performing their work. Work occurs only through the "people" element [2a]; the accomplishment of work requires that managers integrate [2b] structure, tasks/technology, and people within the context of the shared beliefs and values of the entity's culture [7].

MANAGERS MANAGING

As managers manage [5] by carrying out their functions—using appropriate skills and competencies and successfully fulfilling managerial roles—they determine the nature of the model's components and link and integrate them. Figure 5.8 shows this with the dotted boundary line that surrounds the inputs [1], conversion [2], outputs [3], continuous improvement [3c], and change [6] components. When managers plan, they determine the individual and organizational work that will lead to accomplishing objectives. Once determined, human and other input resources [1] can be identified, acquired, and allocated. When managers organize and staff, they shape the setting in which conversion [2] occurs—the structure, tasks/technology, and staff relationships. When managers direct, they initiate activity that is intended to accomplish appropriate and desirable individual and organizational work results [3a]. When managers control, they monitor individual and organizational work results [3a] and compare them with standards and expectations to determine whether missions and objectives [3b] are being fulfilled and achieved. If results are inconsistent with standards, expectations, or both [4], managers make changes [6] through a feedback loop. For example, if comparison with best clinical practices determines that care in an HSO/HS should be improved, then managers change the structure, tasks/technology, and people components, change input resources, or both. Even if missions are being fulfilled and objectives are being met [3b], the philosophy of continuous quality improvement (CQI) requires that assessment and improvement of HSO/HS activity be continuous [3c]. The essential implication of the CQI philosophy is that outcomes in all organizational performance dimensions can be improved by continuously evaluating, changing [6], and improving [3c] processes that are used in conversion [2] or the inputs used [1], or both.

EXTERNAL ENVIRONMENT (AN OPEN SYSTEMS PERSPECTIVE)

No organization or system is isolated from its external environment. Its managers receive and interpret information from the external environment and seek to help shape the environment. The outer black boundary in Figure 5.8 denotes the external environment and presents its two major components: the general environment [9] and the more proximate healthcare environment [8]. HSOs/HSs are affected by the external environment—their inputs come from it; they also affect the external environment—their outputs go into it.

Managers seek to understand, influence, modify, and change the external environment of their organization or system. This is denoted by the change loop arrow [6] in Figure 5.8 that extends to the environment. For example, advocacy and lobbying with the public policy component of the healthcare environment is a responsibility of senior-level managers,[65] who rely upon full political competence or the dual abilities to accurately assess the impact of public policies on the performance of the (manager's) domain of responsibility and to influence public policy making at state and federal levels to the benefit of their domains of responsibility.

Managers interact with the multiple components of the external environments of their organizations and systems in other ways as well. They might affect the flow of supplies by joining group purchasing cooperatives, for example. They might influence the supply of a particular human resource, such as nurses, by interactions with schools of nursing. They might seek to influence the numbers of potential patients for the services of their organizations and systems by participating in efforts to upgrade the economic conditions or other quality of life aspects of their communities.

Systems theory provides a framework within which to conceptualize the relationships between an HSO/HS and its external environment. A system is a set of interrelated and interdependent parts. A subsystem is part of a system; a suprasystem is a system of systems. An organization or health system may be viewed as a system composed of many subsystems, such as those for patient care, ancillary services, professional staff, financial services, and information, among others. An HSO/HS also may be viewed as a subsystem of the larger system of HSOs/HSs found in the healthcare environment [8], which is, in turn, part of the suprasystem called the general environment [9].

A suprasystem, its systems, and their subsystems are interrelated and interdependent, and they simultaneously affect one another at all levels. The general environment ([9] in Figure 5.8) is a suprasystem composed of many systems, including ethical/legal, political, cultural/sociological, public (i.e., external stakeholders such as the community at large, interest groups, and media), economic, and ecological systems and the systems that compose the healthcare environment [8].

More proximate to, and having a more direct effect on, the HSO is the healthcare environment. The forces and influences in the healthcare environment affecting HSOs/HSs, their managers, and how they manage are presented in Figure 5.8 [8]. A variety of external stakeholders such as patients, third-party payers, government, special interests, local communities, and licensure, regulatory, and accrediting agencies are important. Other forces in the healthcare system include competitors; numbers and skills of practitioners; public and private financing of healthcare; and resource entities for technology, equipment, and materials. A final, more remote group of healthcare environmental forces includes health research and education; health status, wellness, prevalence of disease, and health promotion and awareness; and the status of public health, general sanitation, and protection from hazardous substances and injurious working conditions.

The Challenges of Management

The management model presented in Figure 5.8 details the management process. The challenges facing HSOs/HSs and their managers—which must be met daily—are considerable. Managers must be

> Concerned with the overall health status of their communities while continuing to provide direct patient services. They should take a leadership role in enhancing public health and continuity of care in the community by communicating and working with other healthcare and social agencies to improve the availability and provision of health promotion, education, and patient care services.
>
> [They] are responsible for fair and effective use of available healthcare delivery resources to promote access to comprehensive and affordable healthcare services of high quality. This responsibility extends beyond the resources of the given [HSO/HS] to include efforts to coordinate with other healthcare organizations and professionals and to share in community solutions for providing care for the medically indigent and others in need of specific health services.
>
> All [HSOs/HSs] are responsible for meeting community service obligations which may include special initiatives for care for the poor and uninsured, provision of needed medical or social services, education, [and] various programs designed to meet the specific needs of their communities.[66]

Looking Forward

Building on the previous chapters, which have described the setting through which healthcare and services are provided, this chapter sets the stage for the remaining chapters, which focus on the process of managing in HSOs/HSs in the following order:

In Chapter 6, Managerial Problem Solving and Decision Making, the pervasive decision-making function is examined, particularly as it relates to the challenge of solving problems. A problem-solving model is used to structure the chapter.

Chapter 7, The Quality Imperative, focuses on continuous improvement of quality and productivity. The concepts of process improvement, as well as methods to improve productivity through better work methods, flows, job design, facilities layout, and scheduling, are discussed.

Chapter 8, Strategizing, details how managers determine the opportunities and threats emanating from the external environments of their organizations and systems, and how they respond to them effectively.

Chapter 9, Marketing, details how managers understand and relate to the markets they serve.

Chapter 10, Controlling and Allocating Resources, presents a general model of control and focuses on controlling individual and organizational work results through techniques such as management information systems, management and operations auditing, human resources management, and budgeting. Control of medical care quality through risk management and quality assessment and improvement is discussed. The chapter concludes with applications of quantitative techniques that are useful in resource allocation, such as volume analysis, capital budgeting, cost–benefit analysis, and simulation.

Chapter 11, Designing, provides conceptual background for understanding HSO/HS organizational structures. It contains information on general organization theory, including classical principles as well as contemporary concepts as they relate to organizations, systems, and alliances of organizations.

Chapter 12, Leading, differentiates transactional and transformational leadership and models and defines leadership. The extensive literature on leader behavior and situational theories of leadership is reviewed. Motivation is defined and modeled. The concept of motivation and its role in effectively leading other people and entire HSOs/HSs are discussed.

Chapter 13, Communication, describes a communication process model and applies it in communicating within organizations and systems and between them and their external stakeholders.

▬ DISCUSSION QUESTIONS ▬

1. What is the distinction between an HSO and an HS?
2. Define the term *manager*.
3. Define *management* and include the basic ingredients of the definition. Why is management a process?
4. How are managers at various levels in HSOs/HSs classified and differentiated?
5. Figure 5.4 shows various managerial roles. Relate these roles to the management functions and to management competencies.
6. What relationship do managers have to the input–conversion–output perspective?
7. Carefully examine Figure 5.8. Describe and discuss 1) its components and how they flow and link and 2) the way in which management functions, skills, roles, and competencies interrelate with the components.
8. Figure 5.8 shows that outputs are composed of individual and organizational work results that accomplish objectives. How do individual and organizational work results fulfill objectives? Choose an HSO or HS with which you are familiar (or find one's web site), and identify its organizational objectives.
9. Figure 5.8 shows two external environments and the forces that affect HSOs/HSs. How do these forces affect HSOs/HSs? Are there others?
10. Identify an organization or system and identify its internal and external stakeholders. For each group, indicate whether each stakeholder is 1) important, 2) influential, and/or 3) a positive influence or a threat.

▣ Case Study 1: The CEO's Day

Terry Blaze, the 45-year-old president and CEO of Midvale Community Hospital, rose early on Monday morning. A busy schedule of meetings and several major issues that would require full attention and careful decisions lay ahead. While getting dressed, Blaze thought about what to say to two county commissioners at a breakfast meeting in a local restaurant at 6:30 a.m. The county coroner had called Blaze the previous Wednesday, asking if Midvale Community Hospital would permit the coroner's office to use some of the hospital's facilities. As a 500-bed teaching hospital with more than 2,000 full-time employees and a medical staff of 450 physicians, Midvale was the largest of the four hospitals located in the metropolitan area, which had a population of about 400,000. Recent budget reductions for the coroner's office by the county commissioners had prompted the coroner's request; he was searching for ways to run his office on a reduced budget by drawing on the goodwill and resources of other community organizations.

Blaze had scheduled the meeting with the commissioners to see whether they were aware of the coroner's request. Blaze was relatively open-minded about the situation, wanted to maintain the existing good relations between the commissioners and the hospital, and wanted to respond to the needs of the community, provided that the hospital's basic objectives were not jeopardized or its resources inappropriately used. However, getting caught in the middle of the county's political problems could be disastrous.

At 7:30 a.m., Blaze attended a campaign fund-raiser breakfast for the state senator who represented the district in which Midvale was located. Blaze spoke to the senator about how the state's recently announced Medicaid payment reductions under their managed care program would affect Midvale and asked the senator to use his influence to try to have funding levels increased. After circulating among the other guests, Blaze went to the hospital. As soon as Blaze arrived at the office at 8:15 a.m., the executive secretary, Ms. Billings, mentioned that Dr. Smith wanted to see him. Dr. Smith, president of the PSO, composed of physicians, dentists, podiatrists, and clinical psychologists having privileges at Midvale, insisted on speaking privately with Blaze about a problem involving a staff physician before the scheduled 9:00 a.m. meeting of the PSO executive committee. Blaze immediately called Dr. Smith, and at the end of the conversation wondered whether it had been a correct decision to tell Dr. Smith to handle the problem as he thought appropriate. Relations between administration and the PSO are always delicate, but this time it seemed best to let Dr. Smith handle the situation and keep Blaze informed.

At 8:30 a.m., the vice president for operations arrived and accompanied Blaze to the hospital's conference room. All department heads were present. Because of a recent decision by Blaze and the board to establish a satellite facility in an adjacent county, most departments would be expanded, work loads would be increased, and coordination mechanisms between the hospital and satellite facility would need to be developed. Blaze explained the reasons for the decision, described the planning that had occurred before the decision was made, indicated how Midvale would work with the state planning agency in obtaining a certificate of need, and described how it would affect Midvale and its patients, as well as other area hospitals. Blaze asked the department heads to inform their subordinates before the official announcement was made to the press on Wednesday. A question-and-answer session followed.

Blaze arrived at the 9:00 a.m. PSO executive committee meeting 10 minutes late and found that it had been postponed until the next day. Because the next meeting on the day's schedule was not until 10:00 a.m., Blaze returned to the office and asked Billings to hold all calls. Blaze had given considerable thought over several months to the governing body's directive that options be evaluated for expanding the scope of the hospital's services, particularly in light of the government's attitude favoring competition among HSOs, the actions of other area hospitals, and the area's newly formed HMO. Mindful of the hospital's resource constraints, rising costs, and changing patient mix, as well as the continued tightening of Medicare and Medicaid reimbursement, Blaze was concerned about accomplishing the hospital's objectives during the next 5 years in this changing environment. Particularly worrisome was the restlessness of some members of the PSO, who wanted new services and an on-site medical office building.

Blaze recalled the discussions that had occurred at past governing body and management executive staff meetings. After weighing the options, Blaze realized that the hospital would need three feasibility studies to be performed by external consultants. Blaze dictated a memo to the vice president for operations and the assistant vice president for planning, instructing them to begin studies for expansion of the hospital's cardiac services and the addition of 34 psychiatric beds and a physicians' office building adjacent to the hospital. Blaze did not approve a study for a regional burn unit because this service, although desirable, would contribute less to the hospital's objectives than the others, and limited resources meant some projects could not be undertaken.

At 10:00 a.m., Blaze met with the chair of the department of psychiatry. Blaze informed him of the feasibility study, but the meeting also continued negotiations about making the psychiatry department chair a salaried position. This would be the first such position in the hospital and would set a precedent with long-term implications.

At 10:30 a.m., Blaze interviewed a finalist for the position of director of marketing. At 11:00 a.m., Dr. Loren, who had requested clinical privileges, arrived for a meeting. It was a long-standing policy for the president of the PSO and the CEO to interview all those seeking privileges.

At 11:30 a.m., Blaze returned telephone calls that required immediate attention. The first was to a governing body member whose husband was being admitted for minor surgery. The second was to a former patient with a complaint about his statement. Billings told Blaze that the former patient had already spoken to patient accounts but was still dissatisfied. Blaze spoke briefly with him and gave assurances that the matter would be rectified. The last telephone call was to the director of human resources. They decided that the human resources director should accept the mayor's invitation to serve on the health department's personnel evaluation task force. This would require approximately 8 hours per week for 6 months, but they agreed it would help the hospital and community.

As was customary, Blaze had lunch in the hospital cafeteria and circulated among the staff before and after eating. It was a simple yet effective way to stay in touch with them.

Two major meetings were scheduled in the afternoon. From 1:00 to 3:00 p.m., the budget committee reviewed next year's operations and capital expenditures budgets. The executive staff and controller had prepared options for review. Among those Blaze approved for presentation to the governing body were an increase in the number of nursing service employees, a reduction in the equipment budget, and the annual pay increase for nonprofessional personnel that had been discussed previously. Blaze had positive relations with the governing body and told the executive administrative staff that the recommendations would likely be approved. However, a source of displeasure was last month's adverse overtime budget variance and the cost overrun on supplies. Both were unacceptable because census and patient days were below expectations. Blaze firmly told the senior managers to monitor their areas closely and report variations weekly.

The second meeting that afternoon was with the governing body task force on diversification. Near the end of the meeting, Blaze told them about ordering the physicians' office building feasibility study and told them they should be thinking about incorporating a for-profit subsidiary to own and manage the office building. The major consideration was how reimbursement would be affected by allocating overhead to either the not-for-profit hospital or the for-profit subsidiary. The board task force asked Blaze to include these revenue–cost implications in the feasibility study.

On returning to the office at 4:00 p.m., Blaze approved the agenda for Friday's weekly senior management staff meeting, gave Billings several items for the agenda of the next governing body meeting, and returned phone calls. At 5:00 p.m., Blaze left the hospital to attend a 5:30 p.m. area hospital executives' council quarterly meeting. The meeting featured a presentation by the new dean of the medical school located in Midvale about how her plans would affect teaching hospitals and their medical education and residency programs. During the half-hour drive to and from the medical school, Blaze dictated several letters and memoranda and took a cell phone call. Blaze went to a restaurant at 7:00 p.m. for dinner and left at 8:00 p.m. to attend a United Way trustees board meeting. At 10:00 p.m., Blaze returned home and did paperwork for an hour before retiring.

QUESTIONS

1. Terry Blaze engaged in activities related to the functions of management and roles of managers. Identify which of Blaze's activities relate to the management functions and managerial roles presented in this chapter.
2. Use the environmental portion of the management model in Figure 5.8 to 1) identify internal, interface, and external stakeholders with whom Blaze interacted and 2) identify other environmental forces that affected Blaze, as well as Blaze's actions that affected the environment.

■ Case Study 2: Projection of Registered Nurse Shortage[67]

The chart below depicts projections of supply and demand for registered nurses (RNs). It appeared in the *Trendwatch Chartbook, 2007* published by the American Hospital Association and Avalere. The chart is based on analysis by the Health Resources and Services Administration, Bureau of Health Professions. Other projections exist, and some of them predict smaller shortages in future years. However, there is widespread agreement that the United States has a shortage and faces a continuing shortage of registered nurses. Examine the chart and think of some of the potential impacts and managerial implications in the case that these projections are realized.

TRENDWATCH CHARTBOOK 2007
Workforce

Chart 5.12: National Supply and Demand Projections for FTE RNs, 2000–2020

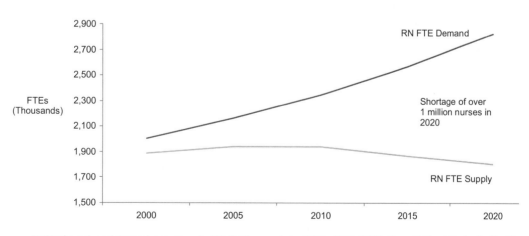

National supply and demand projections for FTE (fulltime equivalent) RNs, 2000–2020. (From National Center for Health Workforce Analysis, Bureau of Health Professions, Health Resources and Services Administration. *What Is Behind HRSA's Projected Supply, Demand, and Shortage of Registered Nurses?* September 2004. Available at www.aha.org/aha/trend watch/2006/cb2006chapter5.ppt. Reprinted by permission of the American Hospital Association.)

QUESTIONS

1. What effects does this trend have on HSOs/HSs?
2. What steps should a hospital CEO take to address this trend?
3. What should an HS's vice president for nursing do to manage this trend's impact on the HS.

Case Study 3: Very Brief History of Management Theories

Views on management have changed substantially over the past century—particularly in the past few decades. Some of the major theories follow.

Scientific Management Theory

At the turn of the 20th century, the most notable businesses were large manufacturing organizations that involved ongoing, routine tasks and manufacturing processes that yielded a variety of products. The United States highly prized scientific and technical matters, including careful measurement and specification of activities and results. Management tended to be the same. Frederick Winslow Taylor developed the scientific management theory, which espoused this careful specification and measurement of all organizational tasks. Tasks were standardized as much as possible. Workers were rewarded and punished. This approach appeared to work well for organizations with assembly lines and other mechanistic, routinized activities.

Bureaucratic Management Theory

Throughout the middle third of the 20th century, Max Weber embellished the scientific management theory with his bureaucratic theory. Weber focused on dividing organizations into hierarchies and establishing strong lines of authority and control. He suggested that organizations develop comprehensive and detailed standard operating procedures for all routinized tasks.

Human Relations Movement

Throughout the last third of the 20th and into the 21st century, unions and government regulators reacted to the rather dehumanizing effects of these earlier theories. More attention was given to individuals and their unique capabilities in organizations. Management alleged that organizations would prosper if their workers prospered as well. Human resource departments were added to organizations. The behavioral sciences played a strong role in helping to understand the needs of workers and how the needs of the organization and its workers could be better aligned. Various new theories were spawned, many based on the behavioral sciences.

QUESTIONS

1. Which of these approaches to managing would you prefer to practice? Why?
2. Why was each approach popular in its day?
3. Does the human relations approach fit well with contemporary HSOs/HSs?

Case Study 4: The Business Office

At 4:45 p.m. on Friday, Mary Hite, an employee in the business office, walked into the office of Henry Staffs, business office manager, and asked to talk with him privately. Hite told Staffs that she had been elected by the other employees of the business office to speak on their behalf about practices that they wished would be modified or eliminated. One practice concerned employee evaluations, which they thought were unfair, poorly executed, and used as an excuse for not paying higher salaries. A second practice not accepted well was the arbitrary way in which management determined employee vacation schedules. Hite said that one employee was given a 2-day notice before he had to take his first week of vacation and a 5-day notice before his second week. Staffs listened attentively and told Hite that, because it was so late in the day, he would consider these requests the first part of next week. During the following week, Hite noticed that Staffs was out of town and that no action was taken concerning her remarks. Her fellow employees tended to treat her like a heroine for representing them before Staffs.

When she picked up her check the next Friday afternoon, Hite was shocked to find a discharge notice and 2 weeks' severance pay in the envelope.

QUESTIONS

1. What should Staffs have done when Hite came to see him?
2. What messages did Staffs communicate to Hite and the other employees?
3. What will be the outcome of the action he took?
4. Is there any way that Staffs can improve communication in the business office?

Notes

1. Griffith, John R. "Can You Teach the Management Technology of Health Administration? A View of the 21st Century." The Andrew Pattullo Lecture, the Association of University Programs in Health Administration, Washington, DC, June 1998.
2. Charns, Martin P., and Jody Hoffer Gittell. "Work Design." In *Healthcare Management: Organization Design and Behavior,* 5th ed., edited by Stephen M. Shortell and Arnold D. Kaluzny, 212–236. Clifton Park, NY: Thomson Delmar Learning, 2006; Charns, Martin P., and Carol Ann Lockhart. "Work Design." In *Essentials of Healthcare Management,* edited by Stephen M. Shortell and Arnold D. Kaluzny, 198–219. Albany, NY: Delmar Publishers, 1997.
3. Shortell, Stephen M., Robin R. Gillies, David A. Anderson, Karen Morgan Erickson, and John B. Mitchell. *Remaking Healthcare in America: Building Organized Delivery Systems.* San Francisco: Jossey-Bass, 1996; Shortell, Stephen M., Robin R. Gillies, David A. Anderson, Karen Morgan Erickson, and John B. Mitchell. *Remaking Healthcare in America,* 2nd ed. San Francisco: Jossey-Bass, 2000.
4. Satinsky, Marjorie A. *The Foundations of Integrated Care: Facing the Challenges of Change.* Chicago: American Hospital Publishing, 1997.
5. Luke, Roice D., and James W. Begun. "Permeating Organizational Boundaries: The Challenge of Integration in Healthcare." *Frontiers of Health Services Management* 13 (Fall 1996): 46–49.
6. Conner, Daryl. "Corporate Culture: Healthcare's Change Master." *Healthcare Executive* 5 (March/April 1990): 28.
7. Deal, Terrence E. "Healthcare Executives as Symbolic Leaders." *Healthcare Executive* 5 (March/April 1990): 25.
8. Friedman, Emily. "Ethics and Corporate Culture: Finding a Fit." *Healthcare Executive* 5 (March/April 1990): 18.
9. Gibson, Kendrick C., David J. Newton, and Daniel S. Cochran. "An Empirical Investigation of Hospital Mission Statements." *Healthcare Management Review* 15 (Summer 1990): 35–36.
10. Blair, John D., and Myron D. Fottler. "Effective Stakeholder Management: Challenges, Opportunities and Strategies." In *Handbook of Healthcare Management,* edited by W. Jack Duncan, Peter M. Ginter, and Linda E. Swayne, 19–48. Malden, MA: Blackwell, 1998.
11. Fottler, Myron D., John D. Blair, Carlton J. Whitehead, Michael D. Laus, and Grant T. Savage. "Assessing Key Stakeholders: Who Matters to Hospitals and Why?" *Hospital & Health Services Administration* 34 (Winter 1989): 525–546.
12. Metzger, Norman. "The Changing Healthcare Workplace: A Challenge for Management Development." *Journal of Management Development* 10 (Special Issue on Healthcare, 1991): 55.
13. Flood, Ann B., Jacqueline S. Zinn, and W. Richard Scott. "Organizational Performance: Managing for Efficiency and Effectiveness." In *Healthcare Management: Organization Design and Behavior*, 5th ed.,

edited by Stephen M. Shortell and Arnold D. Kaluzny, 415–454. Clifton Park, NY: Thomson Delmar Learning, 2006.

14. Nauert, R.C. "The Quest for Value in Healthcare." *Journal of Healthcare Finance* 22, 3 (1996): 52–61; Shortell, Stephen M. "High Performing Healthcare Organizations: Guidelines for the Pursuit of Excellence." *Hospital & Health Services Administration* 30 (July/August 1985): 7–35.

15. Longest, Beaufort B., Jr. "Relationships Between Coordination, Efficiency, and Quality of Care in General Hospitals." *Hospital & Health Services Administration* 19 (Winter 1974): 65–86; Shortell, Stephen M., Selwyn W. Becker, and Duncan Neuhauser. "The Effects of Management Practices on Hospital Efficiency and Quality of Care." In *Organizational Research in Hospitals,* edited by Stephen M. Shortell and Montague Brown, 90–107. Chicago: Blue Cross Association, 1976; Alexander, Jeffrey A., and Thomas G. Rundall. "Public Hospitals Under Contract Management: An Assessment of Operating Performance." *Medical Care* 23 (1985): 209–219.

16. Payne, Beverley C., Thomas F. Lyons, and Evelyn Neuhaus. "Relationship of Physician Characteristics; to Performance Quality and Improvement." *Health Services Research* 19 (August 1984): 307–332; Shortell, Stephen M. "High Performing Healthcare Organizations: Guidelines for the Pursuit of Excellence." *Hospital & Health Services Administration* 30 (July/August 1985): 7–35; Kaluzny, Arnold D. "Revitalizing Decision-Making at the Middle Management Level." *Hospital & Health Services Administration* 34 (Spring 1989): 39–51.

17. Flood, Ann B., David M. Bott, and Elizabeth Goodrick. "The Promise and Pitfalls of Explicitly Rewarding Physicians Based on Patient Insurance." *Journal of Ambulatory Care Management* 23, 1 (2000): 55–70.

18. Mark, Barbara. "Task and Structural Correlates of Organizational Effectiveness in Private Psychiatric Hospitals." *Health Services Research* 20 (June 1985): 199–224; Morlock, Laura L., Charles Nathanson, Susan Horn, and David Schumacher. "Organizational Factors Associated with the Quality of Care in Seventeen General Acute Hospitals." Presented at the Annual Meeting of the Association of University Programs in Health Administration, 1979, Toronto; Flood, Ann B., and William R. Scott. *Hospital Structure and Performance.* Baltimore: Johns Hopkins Press, 1987.

19. Flood, Ann B. "The Impact of Organizational and Managerial Factors on the Quality of Care in Healthcare Organizations." *Medical Care Review* 51, 4 (1994): 381–428.

20. Donabedian, Avedis. *Explorations in Quality Assessment and Monitoring, Volume I: The Definition of Quality and Approaches to Its Assessment.* Chicago: Health Administration Press, 1980.

21. Kaplan, Robert S., and David P. Norton. *Alignment: Using the Balanced Scorecard to Create Corporate Synergies.* Boston: Harvard Business School Publishing, 2006; Kaplan, Robert S., and David P. Norton. *Balanced Scorecard: Translating Strategy into Action.* Boston: Harvard Business School Publishing, 1996.

22. Cartwright, Jonathon W., Steven C. Stolp-Smith, and Eric S. Edell. "Strategic Performance Management: Development of a Performance Measurement System at the Mayo Clinic." *Journal of Healthcare Management* 45, 1 (2000): 58–68; Chow, Chee W., Denise Ganulin, Kamal Haddad, and James Williamson. "The Balanced Scorecard: A Potent Tool for Energizing and Focusing Healthcare Organization Management." *Journal of Healthcare Management* 43, 3 (1998): 263–280; Oliveira, Jason. "The Balanced Scorecard: An Integrative Approach to Performance Evaluation." *Healthcare Financial Management* 55, 5 (2001): 42–46; Sioncke, Gratienne. "Implementation of a Balanced Scorecard in a Care Home for the Elderly: Useful or Not?" *Total Quality Management* 16, 8 (October/November 2005): 1,023–1,029.

23. Joint Commission Resources. "Using Data Dashboards to Improve Clinical Quality and Safety." *Benchmark* 8 (March/April 2006): 1–11.

24. "Hospital Report Cards." *Consumer Reports. www.consumerreports.org,* retrieved August 11, 2006.

25. "NCQA Health Plan Report Cards." National Committee for Quality Assurance. *http://hprc.ncqa.org/menu.asp,* retrieved August 11, 2006.

26. Chang, Li-Cheng, Stephen W. Lin, and Deryl N. Northcott. "The NHS Performance Assessment Framework: A Balanced Scorecard Approach?" *Journal of Management in Medicine* 16, 5 (2002): 345–358.

27. Department of Health. *NHS Performance Indicators: A Consultation,* 2. London: The Stationary Office, 2001.

28. NHS Executive. *Quality and Performance in the NHS: NHS Performance Indicators*. London: The Stationary Office, 2000.

29. Fottler, Myron D. "Strategic Human Resources Management." In *Human Resources in Healthcare: Managing for Success,* edited by Bruce J. Fried and James A. Johnson, 1–18. Chicago: Health Administration Press, 2002.

30. Fottler, Myron D. "Strategic Human Resources Management," 2.

31. Hernandez, S. Robert, Myron D. Fottler, and Charles L. Joiner. "Integrating Strategic Management and Human Resources." In *Essentials of Human Resources Management in Health Services Organizations,* edited by Myron D. Fottler, S. Robert Hernandez, and Charles L. Joiner, 2. Albany, NY: Delmar Publishers, 1998.

32. Fottler, Myron D., Robert L. Phillips, John D. Blair, and Catherine A. Duran. "Achieving Competitive Advantage Through Strategic Human Resource Management." *Hospital & Health Services Administration* 35 (Fall 1990): 341–363.

33. Discussion adapted from Longest, Beaufort B., Jr. *Managing Health Programs and Projects,* 56–60. San Francisco: Jossey-Bass, 2004.

34. Austin, Charles J., and Stuart B. Boxerman. *Information Systems for Healthcare Management*. Chicago: Health Administration Press, 2003.

35. Carroll, Stephen J., and Dennis J. Gillen. "Are the Classical Management Functions Useful in Describing Managerial Work?" *Academy of Management Review* 12 (January 1987): 38–51.

36. Katz, Robert L. "Skills of an Effective Administrator." *Harvard Business Review* 52 (September/October 1974): 90–102.

37. Mintzberg, Henry. *The Nature of Managerial Work*. New York: Harper & Row, 1973; Mintzberg, Henry. "The Manager's Job: Folklore and Fact." *Harvard Business Review* 53 (July/August 1975): 49–61.

38. Zuckerman, Howard S., and William L. Dowling. "The Managerial Role." In *Essentials of Healthcare Management,* edited by Stephen M. Shortell and Arnold D. Kaluzny, 34–62. Albany, NY: Delmar Publishers, 1994.

39. Swayne, Linda M., W. Jack Duncan, and Peter M. Ginter. *Strategic Management of Healthcare Organizations,* 5th ed., 7. Malden, MA: Blackwell, 2006; Luke, Roice D., Stephen L. Walston, and Patrick Michael Plummer. *Healthcare Strategy: In Pursuit of Competitive Advantage*. Chicago: Health Administration Press, 2004.

40. Vladeck, Bruce C. "Healthcare Leadership in the Public Interest." *Frontiers of Health Services Management* 8 (Spring 1992): 1–26.

41. Asay, Lyal D., and Joseph A. Maciariello. *Executive Leadership in Healthcare*. San Francisco: Jossey-Bass, 1991.

42. Shewchuck, R.M., S.J. O'Connor, and D.J. Fine. "Building an Understanding of the Competencies Needed for Health Administration Practice." *Journal of Healthcare Management* 50, 1 (2005): 32–47, p. 33.

43. Lucia, A.D., and R. Lepsinger. *The Art and Science of Competency Models: Pinpointing Critical Success Factors in Organizations*. San Francisco: Jossey-Bass/Pfeiffer, 1999.

44. National Center for Healthcare Leadership (NCHL). *NCHL Healthcare Leadership Competency Model, version 2.0*. Developed by the National Center for Healthcare Leadership and Hay Group, Inc., © 2004 National Center for Healthcare Leadership. All rights reserved. Chicago: National Center for Healthcare Leadership, 2004.

45. National Center for Healthcare Leadership (NCHL). *NCHL Healthcare Leadership Competency Model, version 2.0,* 5–7. Developed by the National Center for Healthcare Leadership and Hay Group, Inc., © 2004 National Center for Healthcare Leadership. All rights reserved. Chicago: National Center for Healthcare Leadership, 2004.

46. Adapted from Longest, Beaufort B., Jr. "Managerial Competence at Senior Levels of Integrated Delivery Systems." *Journal of Healthcare Management* 43 (March/April 1998): 115–135.

47. Katz, Robert L. "Skills of an Effective Administrator." *Harvard Business Review* 52 (September/October 1974): 90–102.

48. Longest, Beaufort B., Jr. "Managerial Competence at Senior Levels of Integrated Delivery Systems." *Journal of Healthcare Management* 43, 2 (1998): 115–133.

49. Coddington, Dean C., Keith D. Moore, and Elizabeth A. Fischer. "Physician Leaders in Integrated Delivery." *Medical Group Management Journal* 44, 5 (September/October 1997): 90.

50. Hudak, Ronald P., Paul P. Brooke, Jr., Kenn Finstuen, and James Trounson. "Management Competencies for Medical Practice Executives: Skills, Knowledge and Abilities Required for the Future." *Journal of Health Administration Education* 15 (Fall 1997): 219–239.

51. Miles, Raymond E., and Charles C. Snow. "Twenty-First Century Careers." In *The Boundaryless Career: A New Employment Principle for a New Organizational Era*, edited by Michael B. Arthur and Denise M. Rousseau, 261–307. New York: Oxford University Press, 1996.

52. Coddington, Dean C., Keith D. Moore, and Elizabeth A. Fischer. *Making Integrated Healthcare Work*, 119. Englewood, CO: Center for Research in Ambulatory Healthcare Administration, 1996.

53. Schneller, Eugene S. "Accountability for Healthcare." *Healthcare Management Review* 22 (Winter 1997): 45.

54. Longest, Beaufort B., Jr. *Health Policymaking in the United States,* 4th ed. Chicago: Health Administration Press, 2006; Longest, Beaufort B., Jr. *Seeking Strategic Advantage Through Health Policy Analysis.* Chicago: Health Administration Press, 1997.

55. Longest, Beaufort B., Jr. *Health Policymaking in the United States,* 4th ed. Chicago: Health Administration Press, 2006.

56. Kingdon, John W. *Agendas, Alternatives, and Public Policies*, 2nd ed. New York: HarperCollins College Publishers, 1995.

57. Zelman, Walter A. *The Changing Healthcare Marketplace: Private Ventures, Public Interests.* San Francisco: Jossey-Bass, 1996.

58. Mintzberg, Henry. *Power In and Around Organizations.* Englewood Cliffs, NJ: Prentice-Hall, 1983.

59. Orlikoff, James E., and Mark K. Totten. *The Future of Healthcare Governance: Redesigning Boards for a New Era.* Chicago: American Hospital Publishing, 1996.

60. Gamm, Larry D. "Dimensions of Accountability for Not-for-Profit Hospitals and Health Systems." *Healthcare Management Review* 21 (Spring 1996): 74–75.

61. Shortell, Stephen M., and Arnold D. Kaluzny. "Organization Theory and Health Services Management." In *Healthcare Management: Organization Design and Behavior,* 5th ed., edited by Stephen M. Shortell and Arnold D. Kaluzny, 5–41. Clifton Park, NY: Thomson Delmar Learning, 2006.

62. *Raising the Bar: Increased Accountability, Transparency, and Board Performance: 2005 Biennial Survey of Hospitals and Healthcare Systems.* San Diego: The Governance Institute, 2006.

63. Pointer, Dennis D., Jeffrey A. Alexander, and Howard S. Zuckerman. "Loosening the Gordian Knot of Governance in Integrated Healthcare Delivery Systems." *Frontiers of Health Services Management* 11 (Spring 1995): 3–37.

64. Molinari, Carol, Laura L. Morlock, Jeffrey A. Alexander, and Charles A. Lyles. "Hospital Board Effectiveness: Relationships Between Governing Board Composition and Hospital Financial Viability." *Health Services Research* 28, 3 (August 1993): 358–377.

65. Longest, Beaufort B., Jr. *Health Policymaking in the United States,* 4th ed. Chicago: Health Administration Press, 2006; Longest, Beaufort B., Jr. *Seeking Strategic Advantage Through Health Policy Analysis.* Chicago: Health Administration Press, 1997.

66. American Hospital Association. *Ethical Conduct for Healthcare Institutions: Management Advisory,* 1–2. Chicago: American Hospital Association, 1992.

67. National Center for Health Workforce Analysis, Bureau of Health Professions, Health Resources and Services Administration. *What Is Behind HRSA's Projected Supply, Demand, and Shortage of Registered Nurses?* (September 2004). Available at *ftp://ftp.hrsa.gov/bhpr/workforce/behindshortage.pdf.* See also American Hospital Association and Avalere. *Trendwatch Chartbook, 2007.* Chart 5.12. Chicago: American Hospital Association. Reprinted by permission of the American Hospital Association.

6

Managerial Problem Solving and Decision Making

Health services organizations and health systems (HSOs/HSs) are vibrant entities in a fluid environment. The management model in Figure 5.8 reflects this dynamism. HSOs/HSs convert inputs (e.g., human resources, material and supplies, technology, information, and capital) into outputs (individual and organizational work results) to achieve objectives—work results such as delivering health services, educating, and researching. HSO/HS managers produce that conversion when they integrate structure, tasks/technology, and people. In doing so, they are accountable for allocating and using resources and for the outcomes.

Anticipating and preventing problems, or solving them when prevention fails, are traditional and essential management tasks. The new paradigm emphasizes patient safety and relies on permutations of continuous improvement of quality, a proactive approach that assumes that all processes can be improved and that managers must create the environment and give employees the tools to make improvement possible.

Like its title, this chapter distinguishes problem solving from decision making. A problem-solving model is developed, and the factors influencing managerial problem solving and decision making are discussed. The benefits of group problem-solving strategies are identified. A model assists in determining when group, rather than individual, problem solving is more effective.

Problem Analysis and Decision Making

A manager's work revolves around the elements of problem solving—problem analysis and decision making. Problem analysis includes recognizing and defining circumstances that require action (a decision) and implementing and evaluating the alternative that is chosen. Chapter 5 identifies decision making as a managerial function, defined as choosing among alternatives.[1] *Choosing* is key and defines decision making. Simply put, decision making involves two steps: identifying and evaluating alternatives, and choosing an alternative.

Decision making is integral to all management functions, activities, and roles. For example, planning involves making decisions (choosing), whether senior-level managers are formulating strategy or middle-level managers are implementing programs. Decisions about the management function of organizing range from establishing authority–responsibility relationships to designing work systems, procedures, and flows, and from establishing structure–task–people relationships to making job assignments. In the staffing function, managers decide about numbers of staff and their pay, training, and performance appraisal. In leading, motivating, and communicating, managers choose the most effective management style and when, where, and to whom information is imparted.

When managers control, they compare individual and organizational work results with predetermined expectations and standards and decide whether results can be improved or standards can be raised. This means making decisions about what type of information to collect and report and which monitoring systems should be used to measure and compare HSO/HS conversion activities and outputs with expectations and standards. Managers also decide which managerial roles to adopt, choosing among the interpersonal roles of figurehead, liaison, and influencer; the informational roles of monitor, disseminator, and spokesperson; and the decisional roles of entrepreneur, disturbance handler, resource allocator, and negotiator. Figures 5.1 and 5.4 show the interrelationship of decision making with other management functions and with managerial roles, respectively.

TYPES OF DECISIONS

Three types describe most managers' decisions: 1) ends–means, 2) administrative-operational, and 3) nonprogrammable-programmable.

Ends–Means

Ends decisions determine the individual or organizational objectives and results to be achieved. Means decisions choose the strategies or programs and activities to accomplish desired results. For example, a decision to emphasize quality and productivity improvement (means) accomplishes the organizational objectives of enhancing care and service, higher patient or customer satisfaction, and better resource use (ends). Ends are shown as the outputs component of the management model in Figure 5.8. Decisions about ends are inherent in strategic planning, which includes formulating objectives. Health systems may make these decisions at the corporate level. Greater specificity is found in a department's ends–means decision making, which reflects its objectives and the operational programs that contribute to the HSO's/HS's overall mission.

Administrative-Operational

Many administrative decisions that are made by senior executives significantly affect the HSO/HS and have major implications for resource allocation and utilization. *Policy decision* is a synonym for *administrative decision*. Examples include deciding whether to finance facility construction or renovation using debt, recognize a union without demanding a certification election, hire hospital-based physicians, contract for laundry services, reduce the capital equipment budget, or participate in an integrated system of HSOs. In contrast, operational decisions are made about day-to-day activities by middle- and first-level managers. Operational decisions include deciding whether to purchase noncapital equipment, reassign staff, modify work systems, and modify job content.

Nonprogrammable-Programmable

Nonprogrammable decisions are novel, unstructured, and significant.[2] Examples are whether to expand facilities; add, close, or share services; seek Medicare certification of skilled beds; restruc-

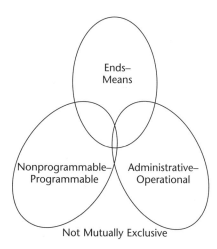

Figure 6.1.   Types of decisions.

ture the organization or align with a network of HSOs; acquire a clinical information system; or add a family practice residency program. Such decisions occur infrequently. Programmable decisions are repetitive and routine; procedures and rules are used to guide them.[3] Patient admitting, scheduling, and billing, and inventory and supply chain procedures are examples.

Overlap of Decision Types

The Venn diagram in Figure 6.1 shows that the three decision types overlap—decisions may include parts of each. For example, merging with another HSO or establishing a satellite urgent care center or primary care preferred provider organization is a means decision because it is a strategy to achieve the organization's objectives. Furthermore, it is an administrative decision because it involves a major commitment of resources, compared with a primarily operational decision about day-to-day activities. Finally, the decision is nonprogrammable because it is unique and occurs infrequently.

Problem Solving

Managers are problem solvers. Problems may be unstructured or structured; complex or simple; major or minor; or urgent or nonurgent; and they may involve varying degrees of cost, risk, and uncertainty. Problem solving involves a series of steps "characterized by intentional reasoning about what the problem is and what the solution should be,"[4] the result of which is to make the current state more closely match the desired state.[5] Using terminology from the management model, problem solving causes change so that actual HSO/HS results or outputs more closely align with those desired. The process by which managers solve problems includes

- Selecting and analyzing a situation that requires a decision
- Developing and evaluating alternative solutions to address the situation
- Choosing an alternative (sometimes called decision analysis)
- Implementing the alternative
- Evaluating the results after implementation

Figure 6.2 shows the relationships among problem solving, problem analysis, and decision making. The terms *problem solving* and *decision making* are often used interchangeably but are not synony-

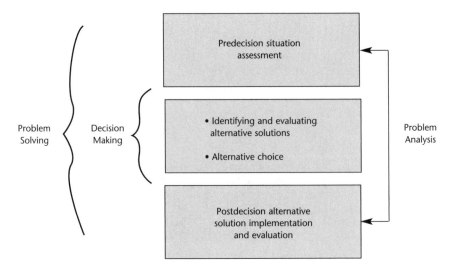

Figure 6.2.   Problem solving and decision making.

mous. All problem solving involves decision making (i.e., choosing among alternatives), but not all decision making involves problem solving.[6] The distinction is that problem solving includes problem analysis—predecision situation assessment and postdecision implementation and evaluation. The discussion here is relevant to both problem solving and decision making, and they are distinguished as necessary.

Managers perform a series of steps when undertaking either problem analysis or decision making. As with all processes, there are variables, conditions, and situations that influence the approach, manner, and style that are used. Problem-solving skills are crucial to managerial success; there are situations in which being an effective problem solver is more important than are communication or interpersonal relationships skills, which is not to diminish their importance, generally. It does mean, however, that problem solving is fundamental to everything that a manager does and to effective managerial performance.

Briefly described, a manager is a problem solver and decision maker. The role of problem solving in managerial effectiveness was demonstrated by a large Canadian study involving 4,000 HSO managers from hospitals, nursing facilities, community health centers, and medical clinics; 2,500 were chief executive officers (CEOs). Almost all of the managers identified problem solving, along with decision making, as among their most important activities.[7] A major finding from research involving 524 U.S. hospital CEOs was the need to improve the process of problem solving. Areas ranked highest in need were external stakeholder (community) relations, business and finance, medical care and medical staff, and staff.[8]

Process and Model

Problem solving is a process by which managers analyze situations and make decisions that cause organizational results to be more like those desired. Prospective problem solving anticipates organizational results that are more or less desirable. Retrospective problem solving identifies and corrects previous causes of deviation from desired results. Concurrent problem solving occurs in HSOs/HSs that are committed to a philosophy of continuously improving quality and performance.

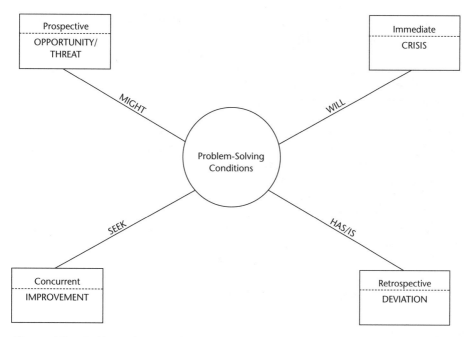

Figure 6.3.   Problem-solving conditions.

CONDITIONS THAT INITIATE PROBLEM SOLVING

Another way to classify problem solving is by conditions that initiate it.[9] Figure 6.3 shows the conditions and corresponding approaches to problem solving. These are

- Opportunity/threat (prospective, might)
- Crisis (immediate, will)
- Deviation (retrospective, has/is)
- Improvement (concurrent, seek)

Opportunity problem solving is prospective and anticipatory. It occurs when a favorable internal or external circumstance enables the HSO/HS to achieve or enhance desired results.[10] For example, technology and consumer expectations permit an acute care hospital to offer obstetrics services at a birth center. Developing the program involves problem analysis, which consists of predecision assessment and postdecision evaluation. The outcome is organizational results (new service) that align more closely with desired results, including improved patient service and satisfaction and increased revenue.

Threat problem solving is also prospective and anticipatory but is the converse of opportunity problem solving. Threats may be internal or external and, if left unaddressed, may cause future results to be less than what is desired. For example, not responding to a competitor's aggressive marketing program may cause loss of market share.

Crisis problem solving is immediate. It responds to a current or predictable threat. Failing to act promptly will cause untoward results, such as a decline in near-term performance. Examples of crisis problem solving are a local natural disaster, a wildcat strike by unionized employees, bypass equipment malfunction during surgery, or a sudden reduction in Medicaid payments. Loss of an essential employee may be a crisis.

Deviation problem solving is retrospective and occurs when actual and desired results differ. Even small deviations may indicate large problems that must be clearly identified and solved.

Improvement problem solving is concurrent and reduces future deviation problem solving or improves performance. The perspective, mind-set, and process of continuous improvement differ from other problem-solving conditions in two important ways. First, continuous improvement is rooted in a philosophy that further improvement is always possible and management's job is to support these efforts. This leads to continuously examining processes and seeking ways to improve them. Second, analysis is concurrent, broad based, and organizationwide and focuses on inputs and the conversion process. The management model in Figure 5.8 shows this relationship. Improvement problem solving involves managers and staff as problem seekers who systematically seek opportunities for improvement.[11]

The condition of deviation is specifically referenced in the problem-solving process model that is depicted in Figure 6.4, but the model is generic and is applicable to all problem solving except that conducted under the condition of improvement, where problem analysis differs. Historically, managers engaged most frequently in problem solving under conditions of deviation[12] and less frequently under conditions of crisis.[13] The contemporary emphasis on quality and performance improvement, which is undertaken without a condition of deviation, is likely to make it the most common type of problem solving. Chapter 7 details improvement problem solving.

PROBLEM-SOLVING ACTIVITIES

Middle- and senior-level managers spend most of their time solving problems. The results of these efforts affect allocation and use of resources as well as work product. The circumstances surrounding problem solving are often complex, unstructured, and nonroutine, thus making the task difficult and time-consuming. Sometimes the situation is beyond the manager's direct control. Except for the condition of improvement, the process is essentially the same regardless of problem type, scope, time involved, intensity of analysis, or the conditions that initiate it. Basic problem solving includes

1. Problem identification—recognizing the presence of a problem (including gathering and evaluating information), and stating the problem
2. Making assumptions
3. Developing tentative alternative solutions and selecting those to be considered in depth
4. Evaluating the selected alternative solutions by applying decision criteria
5. Selecting the alternative that best fits the criteria
6. Implementing the solution
7. Evaluating results

These steps are shown in Figure 6.4, and the numbers in that figure correspond to those noted in the following discussion.

PROBLEM ANALYSIS [1]

Problem analysis is divided into problem recognition and definition, and developing a problem statement. The product of problem analysis is the problem statement. It is the problem statement about which assumptions are made in Step [2].

Problem Recognition and Definition

Problem solving under the condition of deviation begins when actual results are inconsistent with desired results and the manager determines that this constitutes a problem that is in need of a solu-

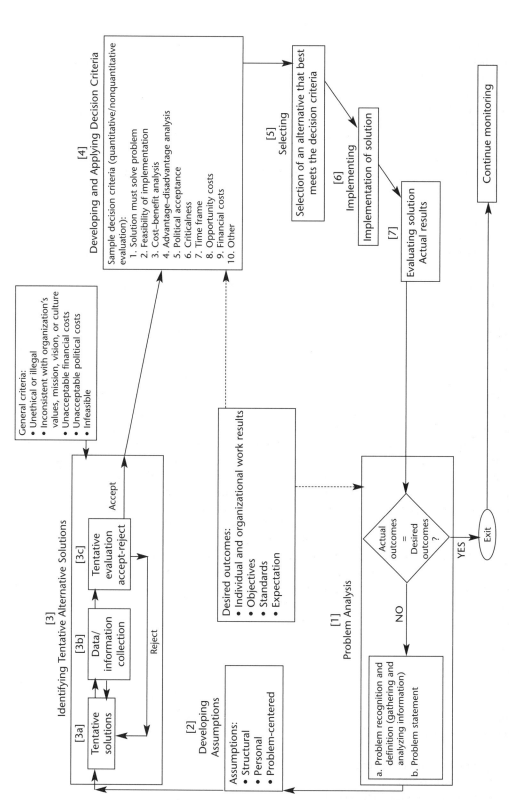

Figure 6.4. Problem-solving process model.

tion. Examples of desired results are 1) organizationwide objectives such as quality of patient care, better client services, and financial solvency; 2) departmental objectives such as increasing customer satisfaction, reducing staff turnover, decreasing surgical infection rates, eliminating mislabeled laboratory specimens and radiograph retakes, and minimizing budget variances; and 3) improving the work of an individual employee. Whether negative deviation indicates the presence of a problem depends on whether it is "common cause" variation or "special cause" variation, a statistical process control concept that is discussed in Chapters 7 and 10. Similarly, positive special cause variation (deviation) should be studied so it can be incorporated into the process.

Applying the theory of problem recognition is not easy. Problem recognition

> Rarely occurs as a completely discrete event. In practice the process occurs through various time intervals (from seconds to years), amidst a variety of ongoing activities and in different ways depending on both situational and individual factors. At times, the process of problem recognition is automatic; at other times, it involves conscious effort. Often, it is a highly objective phenomenon resulting in problem descriptions that most anyone would agree on. At other times it is definitely a subjective process, where the nature of a problem description varies from individual to individual.[14]

Problem recognition occurs in three stages. The first is gestation/latency, in which some cue or triggering event indicates a potential problem. The second is categorization, in which managers become aware that something is wrong but cannot fully and clearly describe it. Third is diagnosis, which involves efforts to obtain the information that will provide greater certainty in problem definition.[15]

Often, symptoms clutter and confuse and make it difficult to recognize a problem and define its parameters. More experienced and expert managers tend to be better problem solvers because they have superior problem recognition and definition skills. Asking the right questions, recognizing limits, and being sensitive to identifying and interpreting cues are skills gained only with experience.

Problem recognition and definition includes gathering, systematically evaluating, and judging the importance of information from sources such as routine reports and data, interviews and observation, information from workgroups, and customer feedback.[16] In this process, it is difficult to overestimate the importance of facts—information derived from consistently applied operational definitions. An essential and difficult job for the problem solver is to distinguish facts from other types of information—a learned and honed ability that permits better problem solving.

In unstructured or complex situations, circumstantial evidence and deductive reasoning are helpful. Exclusionary thinking may be used to "rule out" problems. Once conclusions are reached, the problem is classified by type, nature, and scope. This recognition definition stage is formative because subsequent actions, especially developing alternatives, are derived from it.[17] Ending the problem definition stage too soon may result in a low-quality solution or in solving the wrong problem.[18]

Problem Statement

The problem statement puts what is learned during the definition stage into a brief description of the problem to be solved. Almost always, one sentence is sufficient. Good problem statements have four parts: 1) an invitational stem, 2) an ownership component, 3) an action component, and 4) a goal component.[19] A sample problem statement—In what ways can we improve system response time to reduce how long marketing analysts must wait for an answer to an inquiry?—contains the four parts:

- In what ways can (stem)
- we (ownership)
- improve response time (action)
- to reduce how long marketing analysts must wait for an answer to an inquiry? (goal)[20]

The invitational stem, "In what ways can," encourages a divergent response, unlike the more narrow "How." *Divergent* means thinking in different directions or searching for a variety of answers to a question that may have many right answers.[21]

The problem statement should have other attributes as well. Ideally, the problem definition phase has identified the root cause, which is reflected in the problem statement. If the problem statement reflects only a symptom, then the problem must be "solved" again and again. A clinical simile is the symptomatic relief that aspirin gives flu sufferers; they feel better, but the cause is uncured. Sometimes the root cause of the problem cannot be determined, or even if the root cause is known, resources may be insufficient to solve it. Occasionally, it is politically infeasible to solve the root cause. There may be many reasons why addressing symptoms is the only realistic choice. Doing so, however, must be seen for what it is—a temporary, expedient solution.

The problem statement should be narrow enough so that solving it lies within the problem solver's authority, resource limits, and the like, but not so narrow that only the symptoms are "treated." For example, certain employees seem to be taking too many coffee breaks. A narrow problem statement focuses on the employees. A somewhat broader problem statement addresses coffee breaks or breaks in general. An even broader problem statement, but one that is not too broad, identifies the efficient use of time or the quantity and assignment of work as the focus for action. Focusing on employees addresses only a symptom, not the root cause.

The breadth of the problem statement also determines the clarity of direction that is given the problem solver. A narrow problem statement identifies clearly what problem needs solving but risks addressing only a symptom. Overly broad problem statements may leave the problem solver without clear direction—no understanding of the first step. Sometimes problems are amorphous or lack specificity, especially as to knowing where to start. Organizational malaise or morale problems are amorphous. Here, problem solvers must cast their nets widely and engage in several iterations of problem solving—from the very broad to the more narrow and specific—before the problem is identified. Iterative problem solving is also known as heuristic problem solving.

The psychological stimulus that is provided by an action orientation should not be underestimated. Problem statements include positive goals but may also include limitations. The problem statement regarding coffee breaks described earlier could be: In what ways can I (we) solve the problem of excessive coffee breaks by staff so as to maximize use of staff resources, but without damaging morale? Here, a limitation to be considered in selecting a solution is avoiding damage to morale.

There is more than one correct way to state a problem, but doing it well requires thought and the patience to prepare more than one iteration. The importance of developing a problem statement lies in the discipline of reducing thoughts to writing and the advantages of a written document in communicating to others who are working to solve the problem. As the great American educator John Dewey stated, "A question well put is half answered."[22] The admonition to "Stand there, don't just do something" until a suitable problem statement has been developed has more application than might be generally thought.

FACTS AND REASONING

A fact can be defined as an actuality, certainty, reality, or truth. Facts are highly prized and provide the firmest grounding for problem solving and decision making. Some facts are objectively verifiable. Many "facts" are subject to dispute, however, unless they result from an operational definition. Deming stressed the critical importance of operational definitions.[23] Objectively verifiable facts, or facts that are based on the same operational definition, take precedence over all other types of information.

Once facts have been identified, two other issues arise. One is the weight to be given to them. Obviously, some facts are more important than others, and people who share problem-solving responsibilities must understand how facts are weighted. A second issue is that facts are subject to judgment and interpretation. For example, a tape measure will gauge a room's dimensions. Whether the room is large enough for a certain activity or job is a matter of opinion. The fact that the room has seating does not answer the question of how comfortable the seating is. Decision makers must be able to separate fact from conclusion (judgment), interpretation, and opinion and not allow them to merge.

Rarely are facts sufficient to solve a problem, however. Obtaining facts is necessarily constrained by time and resources. Problem solvers can partly overcome this deficit through inductive and deductive reasoning. Inductive reasoning moves from the single event or fact to a conclusion or generalization based on that event or fact. Inductive reasoning allows one to conclude that the fact of a painted wall means that there was a painter. Deductive reasoning uses the facts of related or similar events to reach a conclusion. Deductive reasoning is employed in a criminal prosecution when circumstantial evidence is used to prove a person's guilt, despite lack of direct evidence such as fingerprints or the testimony of a witness. Circumstantial evidence is based on inferences (deductions) that are drawn from facts. A deduction from finding room after room with half-painted walls is that the work of the painter(s) is undone.

Often, problem solvers and decision makers have the need to consider what weight, if any, to give to information that is hearsay, rumor, or assertion. Hearsay is words attributed to a third party. With a few exceptions, hearsay is inadmissible in court proceedings. Similarly, decision makers should learn to identify hearsay and give it little or no weight. As in all organizations, rumors abound in HSOs; many of them will come to the notice of decision makers. Rumors, too, should be given little weight. Assertions are statements that may be based on fact, hearsay, or rumor. Assertions may also be called judgments or conclusions. Often, assertions are stated forcefully and with a degree of authority that makes them seem credible.

Hearsay and rumor may have an element of truth and, thus, are important to the extent that they suggest potential problems that warrant further investigation. In themselves, hearsay and rumor should never be the basis for action or decision making. Persons who make assertions should be asked to show how they are supported by facts. Absent facts, assertions should be given little or no weight.

DEVELOPING ASSUMPTIONS [2]

The problem statement developed in problem analysis [1] is the focus of the next step, developing assumptions [2]. Assumptions never take the place of facts. When facts are insufficient, however, problem solvers use inductive and deductive reasoning to make assumptions. Only in the most unusual circumstances should problem solvers make assumptions that are unsupported by logic, because doing so means that the assumptions were selected capriciously—certainly not a basis for good management. Assumptions are based on extending what is known. For example, if every time a nurse is disciplined, flyers are distributed that urge nurses to unionize, deductive reasoning tells us that the same thing is likely to happen next time. This, then, is a logically supportable assumption.

Assumptions have a significant effect on the choice and quality of the solution and, as a result, on the quality of problem solving. In general, there are three types of assumptions: structural, personal, and problem centered.[24] Table 6.1 summarizes their attributes.

Structural assumptions relate to the context of the problem—they are boundary assumptions: the problem lies within (or outside) a manager's authority; additional resources are (or are not) available to solve the problem; other departments cause the problem; or the problem is caused by an uncontrollable external factor, such as that high unemployment in the service area means fewer people have employer-based health insurance to pay for elective procedures.

Personal assumptions are conclusions and biases that decision makers bring to the problem. Often, they are based on experience. Managers may have a high or low tolerance for the risk and uncertainty inherent in changes that invariably result from problem solving. A manager's previous experience of being blamed for the problems caused by changes after problem solving may cause an

TABLE 6.1.   ATTRIBUTES OF THE THREE TYPES OF ASSUMPTIONS

Assumptions	Attributes
Structural	Relate to context of problem—boundary assumptions Within (outside) manager's authority Additional resources are (are not) available Other departments cause problem Problem caused by uncontrollable external factor(s)
Personal	Conclusions and biases decision makers bring to problem Risk taker; risk averse Likely reactions of superiors, subordinates, stakeholders Anchoring—adjustments from past starting point Escalating commitment—unwilling to admit past mistakes
Problem Centered	Perceived relative importance of problem Degree of risk from problem How urgently solution is needed Economic cost and benefit Political cost and benefit Degree to which subordinates or superiors will accept solution Likelihood of success if solution implemented

aversion to risk, and this may lead to making assumptions about the problem or alternatives that cause selection of low-risk solutions. Assumptions may be made about the likely reactions of superiors, subordinates, or stakeholders to potential solutions. In addition to risk taking and other types of experiences that cause bias in the decision maker, the personal assumptions referred to as "anchoring" and "escalating commitment" can affect problem solving. Anchoring occurs when the individual "chooses a starting point (an 'anchor'), perhaps from past data, and then adjusts from the anchor based on new information."[25] An inaccurate anchor causes flawed analysis. Despite this, "decision makers display a strong bias toward alternatives that perpetuate the status quo."[26] Escalating commitment occurs when a manager is unwilling to admit earlier mistakes. A manager whose decisions have become a problem will "tend to be locked into a previously chosen course of action."[27] The tendency of decision makers to make decisions in a way that justifies past choices has also been described as the "sunk-cost trap," meaning that old investments of time and resources cannot be recovered, but further commitments are made because it is so difficult for managers to admit past mistakes.[28]

Problem-centered assumptions cover a wide range, including perceived relative importance of the problem, degree of risk posed by the problem, and how urgently a solution is needed. Other problem-centered assumptions include economic and political costs and benefits, the degree to which subordinates or superiors will accept solutions, and the likelihood of success if a solution is implemented.

It is important to emphasize that the three types of assumptions affect the decision maker and the problem-solving process differently. Assumptions differ in at least two ways: qualitatively and in the amount of control that decision makers have over them. For example, a structural assumption that no funds are available to solve a problem will profoundly affect the solutions that can be considered, and there may be little or nothing the decision maker can do to remedy the lack of funds. A personal assumption in which the decision maker recognizes an aversion to risk can be overcome to some extent, even though the decision maker may remain less willing to accept certain solutions or may continue to be reluctant to experience higher levels of discomfort. Problem-centered assumptions are likely to involve more judgment, which is more often based on the decision maker's experience, hunch, or intuition than are structural assumptions.

In summary, making assumptions is necessary to almost all problem solving. Decision makers must use caution in formulating and accepting assumptions, because if assumptions are formulated poorly, they can limit the scope of problem solving or even preclude identifying the best solution.[29]

IDENTIFYING TENTATIVE ALTERNATIVE SOLUTIONS [3]

Once the manager has recognized, defined, and analyzed the problem, established its cause(s) and parameters, prepared a problem statement [1], and made assumptions [2], then tentative alternative solutions are developed [3]. In Figure 6.4, this step includes identifying tentative alternative solutions [3a], collecting data/information if necessary [3b], and evaluating the merits of each tentative alternative [3c] for an initial accept-reject decision. The initial accept-reject decision uses general criteria such as whether the tentative solution is unethical or illegal; is inconsistent with organizational values, mission, vision, and culture; has unacceptable financial or political costs; or is infeasible. If a tentative alternative meets any of these general negative criteria, the step must be repeated. Unique, nontraditional, and creative tentative solutions are identified more readily if structural, personal, and problem-centered assumptions are not overly restrictive.

Identifying tentative solutions is very important because it consumes more resources than any other problem-solving activity and because if creativity is to occur, it must occur here.[30] It is in the tentative alternative loop that creativity is important.[31] Although the terms are often used synonymously, *creativity*—defined as imagination and ingenuity—should be distinguished from the narrower concept of *innovation*—defined as changing or transforming.[32] Figure 6.5 shows this distinction.

Several categories or tactics that can be used to identify ideas for solutions have been described.[33] Regrettably, most do not suggest creativity as a source. "Ready-made" tactics assume that organizations have a store of fully developed solutions—a situation in which solutions wait for problems. "Search" tactics identify solutions from available ideas. Proposals are elicited and compared in order to identify solutions that seem viable. A "design" tactic seeks a custom-made solution—an opportunity for creativity.

Several factors influence the time and resources that are devoted to the tentative alternative solution loop. Most important are the quality and precision of the initial problem definition and the restrictiveness of assumptions. Others include sophistication of the HSO's/HS's information systems, availability of data, and the degree to which the problem is structured. Unstructured problems are more complex, involve many variables, and take longer to solve than problems that are straightforward, relatively obvious, or narrowly defined. Typically, unstructured problems require several iterations of problem solving.

The tentative alternative solution loop has two hazards. Some managers spend excessive time and resources seeking optimal solutions when other solutions are acceptable. In addition, extensive attention to activities in the loop and reiteration may be an excuse for not taking action. "I need more information" may be an excuse to procrastinate and make no decision.[34]

DEVELOPING AND APPLYING DECISION CRITERIA [4]

The alternatives that met the general criteria applied in the tentative alternative solution loop [3] are now ready for formal assessment. To select the best of several alternatives, managers must develop decision criteria that allow alternative solutions to be evaluated and compared [4]. The decision criteria include those in the Desired Outcomes cell in the center of Figure 6.4: individual and organizational work results, objectives, standards, and expectations. At least three other decision criteria are usually applied: effectiveness of the alternative in solving the problem, feasibility of implementation, and acceptability of the alternative based on objective and subjective analyses.[35]

Alternatives that are not effective in solving the problem should be rejected. Examples are alternatives that solve only part of a problem, address only symptoms, or are not permanent. Exceptions may be necessary, however. For example, if the need for action is critical, then it may be appropriate to select and implement a less-than-optimal solution because the consequences of doing nothing or waiting for a better solution are worse.

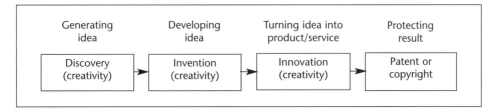

Figure 6.5. Differentiation of discovery/invention/innovation. (Adapted from Cougar, Daniel J. *Creative Problem Solving and Opportunity Finding,* 18. Danvers, MA: Boyd & Fraser, 1995; reprinted by permission.)

The feasibility of implementing an alternative is the second common decision criterion. Alternatives that are infeasible will be rejected in the tentative alternative solution loop. Those that survive may be implemented to varying degrees in terms of effort; structural boundaries and constraints; dependence on other people, departments, or both; and costs. Managers are less likely to select an alternative that depends on people and departments beyond their control. This is especially true if high political costs are associated with forcing implementation.

The third common criterion judges the effective use of resources through quantitative (objective) cost–benefit analysis and assessment of nonquantitative (subjective) advantages and disadvantages. Lowest cost should not be a sole criterion—costs and benefits of alternatives must be considered, as should the opportunity costs of doing nothing. *Objective evaluation* means quantifying costs and benefits and should be attempted, despite the difficulty of estimating some data. *Subjective evaluation* means understanding advantages and disadvantages that may be impossible to quantify but cannot be ignored. Both types of assessment should be considered when evaluating and comparing alternatives. If an alternative is costly but the problem solver concludes that subjective considerations are more important, then a rational decision has been made. Here, it might be useful to list nonquantitative advantages and disadvantages, which will add the useful dimension of subjective judgment to the decision-making process.

Some decision criteria are likely to be more important than others in a given situation; several methods may be used to differentiate them. One method ranks decision criteria using decision-maker judgments. Another method divides criteria into "mandatory" (must be met) and "wanted." A solution that does not meet a mandatory criterion is discarded. Wanted criteria are weighted by degree of desirability. The resulting weighted scores determine which solution is selected.[36] A third method assumes that all decision criteria are equally important (which is unlikely) and judges how closely or well each alternative meets them and assigns a numerical value. The highest total determines which alternative is chosen. A decision matrix is an excellent tool for arraying and comparing decision criteria and solutions. Table 6.2 presents a sample decision matrix.

The virtues of numerically weighting decision criteria include forcing decision makers to compare and evaluate the criteria and providing a basis for discussion in group decision making. It is important that the numbers are understood to be the results of judgments by decision makers, judgments that could be challenged by reasonable people. This basis in subjectivity means that the numbers are, at best, approximations. This must be borne in mind during analysis.

As noted earlier, this step is sometimes called decision analysis. Most often, decision makers have several alternative solutions that can be used; it is a matter of determining which one best (fully or partially) meets the decision criteria. There are, however, other variations of decision analysis. Sometimes, there is only one solution and a yes-no, accept-reject decision must be made. Here, the analysis compares the proposed solution to a reasonable (perhaps idealized) model of what could or should be done, to determine whether the solution is acceptable. At other times, there are no alternatives and the decision maker must decide how to accomplish a desired result. Here, the first step

TABLE 6.2. DECISION MATRIX FOR EVALUATING ALTERNATIVE SOLUTIONS[a]

Decision criteria	Alternative solution 1	Alternative solution 2	Alternative solution 3
Must meet these requirements			
1. Solution effectively solves the problem	3	5	5
2. Feasibility of implementation	5	3	5
3. Cost–benefit analysis	5	5	3
4. Advantage–disadvantage analysis	3	3	5
Want to meet these requirements			
5. Political acceptability	1	3	3
6. Criticalness	1	3	5
7. Time frame	1	3	5
8. Opportunity costs	5	1	3
9. Monetary costs	3	5	5
Total score	27	31	39

Conclusion: Alternative solution 3 accepted.
Adapted from Arnold, John D. *The Complete Problem Solver: A Total System for Competitive Decision Making,*
62. New York: John Wiley & Sons, 1992.
    [a]Key:
    5 = Solution *fully* meets decision criterion.
    3 = Solution *partially* meets decision criterion.
    1 = Solution *fails* to meet decision criterion.

is to clearly define the objectives. Then, a set of components that will most feasibly and effectively meet those objectives is selected from all of the available components.[37]

SELECTING, IMPLEMENTING, AND EVALUATING THE ALTERNATIVE SOLUTION [5, 6, AND 7]

Almost always, a manager selects an alternative (makes a decision) [5]. This does not end the problem-solving process, however. Implementation [6] and evaluation [7] must be planned. Implementation [6] usually requires that resources are made available. The effects of intervention (change) that has been implemented must be evaluated (monitored) [7] to determine that they are consistent with desired results [1]—the problem has been solved. Effective implementation and evaluation require that who will do what, how, and in what time frame are determined prospectively. It is desirable for evaluation to be integral to (built into) implementation. Data collection must be specific, especially as to where in the organization intervention will be done and with whom responsibility lies.

Evaluation is the most often neglected part of problem solving—busy managers assume that the solution selected and implemented will be effective, and they turn to solving other problems. The solution, however, may solve the problem completely, partially, or not at all. Effectiveness of the solution can only be known if data are collected.

If the problem is not solved, the problem-solving process begins again, perhaps with fine-tuning of the alternative implemented, reconsidering alternatives previously rejected, or developing new alternatives. Furthermore, solving one problem often causes others. For example, decreasing the average length of a hospital stay may reduce revenue, necessitate higher staffing ratios using more skilled providers, and put higher demands on postacute care services, such as home health. This ripple effect necessarily leads to new rounds of problem solving.

IMPLICATIONS FOR THE HEALTH SERVICES MANAGER

Problem solving is a major responsibility of health services managers. When problem solving is done effectively, resource allocation and consumption are superior, and results are more consistent with those desired. Managers' skills in problem solving, including decision making, are directly reflected in the quality of solutions and interventions.

Influencing Problem Solving and Decision Making

Problem solving and decision making do not occur in a vacuum; many factors shape how they are performed, the style that is used, and the outcome. Figure 6.6 shows three groups of factors: 1) attributes of the problem solver, 2) nature of the situation, and 3) characteristics of the environment.[38] These affect all steps of problem solving and decision making.

PROBLEM-SOLVER ATTRIBUTES

Knowledge, Experience, and Judgment

Among the most important attributes affecting problem solving are the decision maker's knowledge, experience, and judgment. Trained and experienced clinical staff such as physicians, nurses, and pharmacists are essential to high-quality patient care, and these attributes are recognized by licensing and certification. Health services managers are formally educated in graduate programs and informally educated through continuing education and in-service training. Their education is tempered and tested in administrative residencies and by the experience gained in the first several years of work. Knowledge and experience are not sufficient, however. Sound judgment must be added to the mix to achieve effective problem solving. Sometimes, intuition and hunch are important.[39]

Perspective, Personality, and Biases

The problem solver's perspective and personality influence problem solving and decision making. Decision-maker biases were discussed in the previous section on assumptions, but they warrant further attention here.

Perspective determines how the problem solver views a problem or situation. Problem solvers with narrow perspectives (tunnel vision) and those who think vertically rather than horizontally approach problems differently and are likely to make lower quality decisions.[40] The conclusions and biases that were discussed in the section on personal assumptions are extensions of perspective. Perspective is managers' general outlook—their Weltanschauung. Similarly, biases affect problem solving, and making assumptions allows decision makers to understand their effects on specific situations.

Personality traits such as temperament, aggressiveness, self-centeredness, self-assurance, and self-confidence, as well as demeanor (introvert or extrovert) and tolerance for risk, change, uncertainty, or instability, influence how managers solve problems and the quality of their decisions. Nonassertive, introverted, procrastinating people who are averse to risk and fearful of change are likely to make assumptions or select solutions that limit the range of problem solving. Such managers are less creative in the tentative alternative solution loop, stay in it longer as they search for the best solution (or implicitly hope the problem will dissipate), and make compromises or less bold decisions. Often, such people are reactive and must be forced to act. Conversely, proactive people take the initiative, anticipate problems, manage events rather than being managed by them, and get the job done. This type of manager is more inclined to make difficult, bold, progressive, or nontraditional decisions that include higher levels of risk.

Values and Philosophy

One's value system and personal ethic influence problem solving by affecting problem definition, formulation of assumptions, and selection of acceptable alternatives. For example, solutions inconsistent with the problem solver's value system are likely to be excluded. Managers whose value system is ego-centered are likely to select solutions that are short-term and self-serving but that may be inconsistent with, or even detrimental to, the long-term good of the HSO/HS. A manager's value system includes views on politics and policy issues, as well as on leadership and motivation. Effective problem solvers have a clear understanding of their personal ethic and the values from which that ethic is derived.

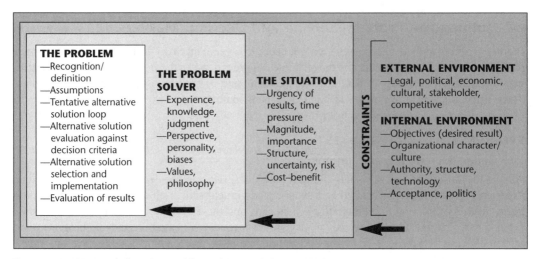

Figure 6.6.   Factors influencing problem solving and decision making.

THE SITUATION

The circumstances and facts of a problem influence the problem-solving process and outcome. Those identified in Figure 6.6 are the urgency of results and time pressure; magnitude and importance of the problem; degree of structure, uncertainty, and risk; and costs versus benefits.

Urgency of Results and Time Pressure

Sometimes immediate decisions are required because delay is costly. Trauma or medical crises are examples. An impending work stoppage, a major initiative by a competitor, or inadequate cash flow to meet payroll require action quickly because such problems have significant consequences. They necessitate rapid use of the tentative alternative solution loop and an evaluation process that is likely to be less thorough. In situations with little time pressure such as problem solving under conditions of opportunity, noncrisis deviation, or improvement, problem solvers use a decision style that involves consultation, collecting more information, and thoroughly evaluating alternatives.

Magnitude and Importance

The problem's magnitude and importance directly affect the time, energy, and resources spent in assessing it and making a decision. For example, administrative decisions warrant greater attention and more intense evaluation than do operational decisions. The cost implications of resource commitment and opportunity costs of delay are other measures of importance.

Problems with high cost or resource commitment (e.g., those being addressed under conditions of opportunity or improvement) justify spending more time and collecting more information in the tentative alternative solution loop than do low-cost problems. The same is true for unstructured problems. A potential hazard for managers is that resources such as time consumed to find the best solution may approach or exceed the cost consequences of the problem. It is senseless to spend $15,000 on staff time for feasibility studies and collection of nonroutine data to solve a medical records storage problem when old records can be stored off-site. Obviously, the cost of developing alternatives must not exceed the benefits of the one that is selected. Conversely, a freestanding HSO in financial distress would appropriately spend more time and resources evaluating an acquisition offer by an HS.

Structure, Uncertainty, and Risk

From a problem-solving perspective, structure is the clarity of the situation—the degree to which the scope and nature of problem and alternatives are precise.[41] Ends–means, administrative, and non-programmable decision situations are less structured than are operational or programmable situations. Problems regarding equipment and supplies, job design, and process flow are more structured than are those with behavioral dynamics or with external stakeholders and competitors. Risk is a function of certainty. A problem that is certain is one for which the manager has complete information and can predict the outcomes of alternative solutions. Less information means greater risk because even carefully derived estimates have a degree of uncertainty. For example, certainty of negative results approaches 100% if mismatched blood is transfused. Certainty is much less than 100% if the problem-solving process determines that establishing a freestanding family practice center will provide inpatient referrals to a hospital. The more unstructured and uncertain the situation, the greater the time spent and resources allocated and the more participative the problem-solving and decision-making processes are likely to be.

Cost–Benefit

Ultimately, problem solving means selecting an alternative, which will be based partly on quantitative cost–benefit or nonquantitative advantage-disadvantage criteria, or both. Many problems are suited to cost–benefit analysis: What equipment most improves productivity and decreases patient waiting time? Which new service will increase revenues most? Will more nursing staff (cost) decrease length of stay (benefit)? Sometimes costs and benefits cannot be measured, or nonquantitative criteria may be more important. In fact, an alternative should be chosen only when both quantitative and nonquantitative decision criteria are used. Excluding either diminishes the quality of the decision.

THE ENVIRONMENT

The HSO's/HS's environments influence managerial problem solving by imposing variables that management may be unable to control, affecting the feasibility of alternatives and constraining implementation of the solution selected.

External

Policy, political, economic, cultural, stakeholder, competitive, and similar external forces are always present. A requirement to obtain a certificate of need for facility expansion or a new service constrains alternatives. High local unemployment with loss of employer-paid health insurance adversely affects revenues and increases bad debt. Unfunded federal mandates and regulations constrain health systems with a managed care component or a hospital with an emergency department. Changes in Medicare and Medicaid payments may limit the organization's ability to add technology and equipment.

Internal

Environmental factors within the HSO/HS affect problem solving more directly. Organizational objectives restrict which alternatives can be considered. Influential but less precise is organizational character/culture—the embedded and permeating values and beliefs. Each organization's culture is unique. It may be creative or traditional, assertive or restrained, proactive or reactive, friendly or distant. Such characteristics influence problem solving. Managers in a reactive, tradition-bound culture are unlikely to select bold solutions. Similarly, managers in an action-oriented culture tend to act quickly, with less preparation. Finally, any alternative that is considered must be consistent with the organization's character/culture.

As managers apply decision criteria to the alternatives, they must consider implementation, which is affected by an array of factors ranging from resource availability to organizational commitment. Noteworthy factors are authority, structure, and technology. An alternative whose implementation is beyond the scope of the manager's authority may not be feasible. The president of the professional staff organization has no authority to change the HSO/HS information system; the CEO has no authority to discharge a patient.

Organizational configuration (structure) may make implementing one alternative infeasible; absence of a technology may eliminate another. For example, physical plant layout may preclude changing patient flow and the logistics of managing the supply chain, union contracts may constrain job definition and design, or the computer system may not allow online connection to nursing units.

Another influence essential to successfully implementing an alternative is acceptance by superiors, peers, and subordinates. A decision to decrease inpatient length of stay by reducing turnaround time for diagnostic testing will be difficult to implement if those who read and interpret tests are resistant. Involving others in problem solving is influenced by how important their acceptance is to implementation. Moreover, organizational politics influence problem solving and its results. The degree of informal influence, conflict, and competition among factions may cause a manager to negotiate, collaborate, compromise, or "satisfice" (find a workable, if imperfect, solution) when solving problems.

IMPLICATIONS FOR THE HEALTH SERVICES MANAGER

Problem-solver attributes, the nature of the situation, and the environment influence problem solving—how it is done, the time and resources consumed, and quality of the decision. These influences are not mutually exclusive; one may supersede or preempt others. An urgent situation can force the manager who usually seeks input, develops a range of alternatives, and does extensive evaluation to act quickly and unilaterally.

Health services managers should recognize and be sensitive to the factors that affect problem solving, change their methods as appropriate, modify and mitigate detrimental influences when possible, and learn to cope with those factors that cannot be changed. Doing so will improve the quality of problem solving.

Unilateral and Group Problem Solving

In meeting their accountability for resource allocation and utilization, managers may solve problems and make decisions unilaterally, or they may involve superiors, peers, or subordinates on a continuum from minimal or consultative to group participation. Both methods have advantages and disadvantages. Consultative problem solving is intraorganizational in a freestanding HSO and interorganizational in an HS. Chapter 4 discusses the ethical aspects of problem solving and decision making.

Unilateral problem solving is efficient, whereas group problem solving raises overhead costs considerably.[42] Unilateral action avoids "groupthink" (extreme group conformity) and "risky shift," which are negative aspects of group problem solving. Anchoring and escalating commitment are more likely in unilateral than group decision making.

Groups exert social pressure to conform and concur with decisions. Groupthink occurs when team members discount warnings about what others (competitors) may do, fail to examine critical and underlying assumptions, stereotype others, put heavy pressure on dissenters, self-censor, share an illusion of unanimity, and stop the flow of information contrary to the group's position through self-appointed "mindguards."[43]

Others have observed that "groupthink has been a primary cause of major corporate- and public-policy debacles. And although it may seem counterintuitive, . . . the teams that engaged in healthy conflict over issues not only made better decisions but moved more quickly as well."[44] The Watergate political scandal of the 1970s is the classical example of political groupthink.[45] The phenomenon of risky shift is a hazard of group problem solving. It occurs because the diffused responsibility of a group encourages acceptance of riskier decisions than would be acceptable to one person who is responsible for a decision.[46]

As a general rule, group problem solving produces better-quality solutions. The reasons are numerous. Multiple perspectives and more information and experience are brought to bear. Knowledgeable staff, especially subordinates, can help define a problem and identify tentative alternative solutions. Involving staff with process knowledge is essential to successful quality improvement. Group problem solving results in consideration of more alternatives because overly restrictive assumptions are likely to be challenged. Furthermore, involving others enhances acceptance and facilitates implementation because those involved take ownership and usually are more committed to implementation. Finally, group problem solving heightens communication and coordination because those involved in implementation have greater knowledge about the solution and the process that produced it.

The benefits of employee participation in problem solving and decision making are well documented in behavioral science literature. Involved employees identify with the HSO/HS and its actions. Kaluzny's model of involvement and commitment has two foci that are especially useful in quality improvement.[47] First, senior-level managers must rethink problem-solving activities to increase the roles, responsibilities, and authority of middle-level managers. Second, middle-level managers must rethink superior–subordinate relationships so that greater involvement of subordinates in problem solving will increase their commitment to HSO/HS objectives. Staff participation in complex decisions adds expertise, which facilitates work unit performance and enhances commitment to the organization.[48]

GROUP PROBLEM-SOLVING AND QUALITY IMPROVEMENT TECHNIQUES

Certain conditions must exist for group problem solving to be effective. First, a climate of openness must permit the free expression of ideas; the focus must be on reaching solutions rather than finding fault.[49] Second, participation must be legitimate—subordinates involved in problem solving must believe that managers are truly interested in the group's reasonable recommendations. This is called "empowering" because subordinates actually influence decisions.[50] Problem solving based on staff expertise about their work will result in better solutions; greater employee involvement and commitment to the HSO/HS will lead to higher motivation, morale, and job satisfaction.[51] Given the opportunity, employees can and do contribute significantly to solving problems.

Quality Circles

A failed group problem-solving method that held significant promise for improving productivity and quality in health services delivery was quality circles, which were especially common in nursing.

The quality circle is a parallel-structure approach to involving employees in problem solving. A parallel structure is one that is separate and distinct from the regular, ongoing activities of an organization and, as such, operates in a special way. In quality circle programs, groups are composed of volunteers from a work area who meet with a special type of leader and/or facilitator for the purpose of examining productivity and quality problems.[52]

Effective quality circles required senior-level management to be committed to both the process and its outcomes. Staff time and employee training in problem solving were some of the substantial resources required. Management had to be willing to act on appropriate recommendations. It is generally understood that quality circles failed because management made no commitment to them and that this suggested staff's efforts were unimportant and a waste of time.

Other Group Formats

Quality circles were one type of group problem solving. Ad hoc task forces may be formed to solve significant organizationwide problems or to address unstructured, major problems under conditions of opportunity or threat. Focus group teams[53] or quality improvement teams can be used. These teams may be departmental or cross-functional. As their name suggests, departmental teams are active in processes exclusive to a department, much as were quality circles. Cross-functional teams improve processes or undertake other quality improvement initiatives that may span the organization and hierarchical levels. Chapter 7 provides detail on quality improvement teams. Finally, managers should encourage ad hoc problem solving by subordinates and assist them, as necessary. This may involve one or several subordinates in a group; it need not be formalized or institutionalized, as are quality circles and quality improvement teams.

Problem-Solving and Decision-Making Styles

The manager's problem-solving and decision-making styles may involve individuals or groups. Style is influenced by the problem's nature and importance, how clearly it can be defined, and whether acceptance by organization members is key to implementation.

INVOLVING OTHERS—A CONCEPTUAL MODEL

A conceptual model of problem-solving/decision-making styles developed by Vroom is useful in determining the degree and conditions of involvement by others.[54] The five problem-solving and decision-making styles shown in Table 6.3 specify subordinate involvement, but they have application to peers and superiors, as well. Each style describes a different degree of subordinate involvement.[55] Style AI is unilateral (autocratic)—subordinates are not involved in predecision assessment or choosing the solution. AII is a variant of AI—subordinates only provide information. Managers using consultative styles CI or CII elicit and consider subordinates' opinions. GII is a group style that involves subordinates fully, and the manager accepts the group's decision. There are situations in which the quality of a decision and its acceptance by subordinates are enhanced with group problem solving.

SITUATIONAL VARIABLES (PROBLEM ATTRIBUTES)

The situational variables influencing style are characterized by the seven different problem attributes (a–g) at the top of Figure 6.7. The problem-solving style outcomes in Figure 6.7 have capital letter notations AI, AII, CI, CII, and GII. The first four problem attributes, a–d, denote the importance of decision quality and acceptance by others. The last three problem attributes, e–g, moderate the effects of subordinate participation on quality and acceptance (a–d). The seven problem attributes in Figure 6.7 are repeated in Table 6.4, along with diagnostic questions requiring yes-or-no answers.

SITUATIONS AND STYLES

Answers to the diagnostic questions for the seven problem attributes in Table 6.4 produce 14 possible situations, which are identified as 1–14 in Figure 6.7. Each is linked with the appropriate

TABLE 6.3. MANAGEMENT PROBLEM-SOLVING AND DECISION-MAKING STYLES

AI	The manager solves the problem or makes the decision unilaterally, using information available at that time.
AII	The manager obtains necessary information from subordinate(s), then develops and selects the solution unilaterally. Subordinates may or may not be told what the problem is when the manager gets information from them. Subordinates provide necessary information rather than generating or evaluating alternative solutions.
CI	The manager shares the problem with relevant subordinates individually, getting their ideas and suggestions without bringing them together. The manager's decision may or may not reflect the subordinates' contribution.
CII	The manager shares the problem with subordinates as a group, obtains their ideas and suggestions, and then makes the decision that may or may not reflect the subordinates' contribution.
GII	The manager shares the problem with subordinates as a group. Together they generate and evaluate alternatives and attempt to reach agreement (consensus) on a solution. The manager's role is much like that of chairperson—not trying to influence the group to adopt a particular solution. The manager is willing to accept and implement any solution supported by the group.

Adapted from Vroom, Victor H. "A New Look at Managerial Decision Making." *Organizational Dynamics* 1 (Spring 1973): 66–80; reprinted by permission from Elsevier. © 1973. American Management Association, New York. All rights reserved.

problem-solving/decision-making style AI–GII. Vroom assumes that managers wish to minimize the time that is required to solve a problem; thus each style is the most restrictive for that set of problem attributes. For example, a manager with Situation 1 could use Styles AII, CI, CII, or GII, but they require more time. Therefore, the problem attributes suggest that AI is appropriate and saves time compared with less restrictive styles.

USING THE MODEL

The manager assesses the situation by examining problem attributes a–g and answering yes or no to the questions. The model indicates which decision style (AI–GII) is most appropriate. The following discussion analyzes the branching for Situations 1, 2, 3, 11, 12, 13, and 14 to show how managers could use the model.

Situations 1, 2, and 3

Situations 1, 2, and 3 assume that there is no decision quality requirement [a]. The presence of several obvious, relatively meritorious alternatives implies that the decision maker has sufficient information [b] to solve the problem unilaterally. Thus, the problem must be relatively structured [c]. If subordinate acceptance of the decision is not critical to implementation [d], the manager is correct in using unilateral Style AI for Situation 1 (1-AI in Figure 6.7). If subordinate acceptance is critical to implementation, Attribute e is evaluated. If subordinates are likely to accept the unilateral decision, the manager can use Style AI for Situation 2 (2-AI in Figure 6.7).

If subordinates are unlikely to accept the manager's decision, as in Situation 3, the Style GII is appropriate (3-GII in Figure 6.7) because participation increases acceptance. Also, the manager is indifferent as to which alternative solution is chosen, because there is no quality requirement and all are relatively meritorious [a].

Situations 11, 12, 13, and 14

Situations 11, 12, 13, and 14 assume that there is a quality requirement [a], meaning that alternatives are not equally acceptable because one is more rational. Situations 11, 12, 13, and 14 also assume that the manager has insufficient information to make high-quality decisions [b] and that the problem is not structured [c].

If the attribute of subordinate acceptance [d] is critical to implementation, then the manager

TABLE 6.4.   PROBLEM ATTRIBUTES USED IN THE PROBLEM-SOLVING AND DECISION-MAKING STYLE MODEL (FIGURE 6.7)

Problem attributes	Diagnostic questions
a. Importance of the quality of the decision	Is quality requirement such that one solution is likely to be more rational (better) than another? (Another way of discerning the quality is: If the alternatives are *not* equally meritorious—some are or can be much better than others—there is a quality requirement.)
b. Extent to which the decision maker possesses sufficient information/expertise to make a high-quality decision unilaterally	Do I have sufficient information to make a high-quality decision?
c. Extent to which problem is structured	Is problem structured? (Does decision maker know what information is needed and where to find it?)
d. Extent to which acceptance or commitment of subordinates is critical to effective implementation	Is acceptance of decision by subordinates critical to effective implementation?
e. Prior probability that a unilateral decision will receive acceptance by subordinates	If decision is made unilaterally, will it probably be accepted by subordinates?
f. Extent to which subordinates are motivated to attain organizational goals as represented in objectives explicit in statement of problem	Do subordinates share organizational goals to be obtained in solving problems?
g. Extent to which subordinates are likely to be in conflict over preferred solutions	Is conflict among subordinates likely to occur in preferred solutions?

Adapted from Vroom, Victor H. "A New Look at Managerial Decision Making." *Organizational Dynamics* 1 (Spring 1973): 66–80; reprinted by permission from Elsevier. © 1973. American Management Association, New York. All rights reserved.

determines whether subordinates would be likely to accept a unilateral decision [e]. If subordinates would accept a unilateral decision, then Style CII is appropriate for Situation 11 (11-CII in Figure 6.7). If subordinates are unlikely to accept a unilateral decision (i.e., the answer to Attribute e is no), then the manager assesses whether subordinates share the organizational goals met by solving the problem—Attribute f. If the answer is yes, Style GII is appropriate (12-GII in Figure 6.7). Group involvement is appropriate because the acceptance that is critical to implementing the alternative is enhanced. Because all participants have the same goals, the group cannot make a decision that is different from the decision the manager would have made. However, if the answer to Attribute f is no (i.e., subordinates do not share the organizational goals met by solving the problem), then Style CII is appropriate for Situation 13 (13-CII in Figure 6.7).

If the attribute of subordinate acceptance [d] is not critical to implementation, then the consultative Style CII is appropriate for Situation 14 (14-CII in Figure 6.7). Here, sharing the problem with subordinates and obtaining their ideas and suggestions provide information that the manager needs, yet the decision that is made need not reflect subordinates' influence.

IMPLICATIONS FOR THE HEALTH SERVICES MANAGER

The problem-solving and decision-making style model in Figure 6.7 is an algorithm to assist in selecting the decision style that is appropriate for different conditions. Although linked here to the degree of subordinate involvement in problem solving, the same model could be used in analyses of peer or superior involvement. In addition, it is important to remember that individual, situational, and environmental variables influence decision style. Vroom's model provides a systematic way to determine the involvement of others in decision making and how that involvement affects the quality of the solution and the success of implementation.

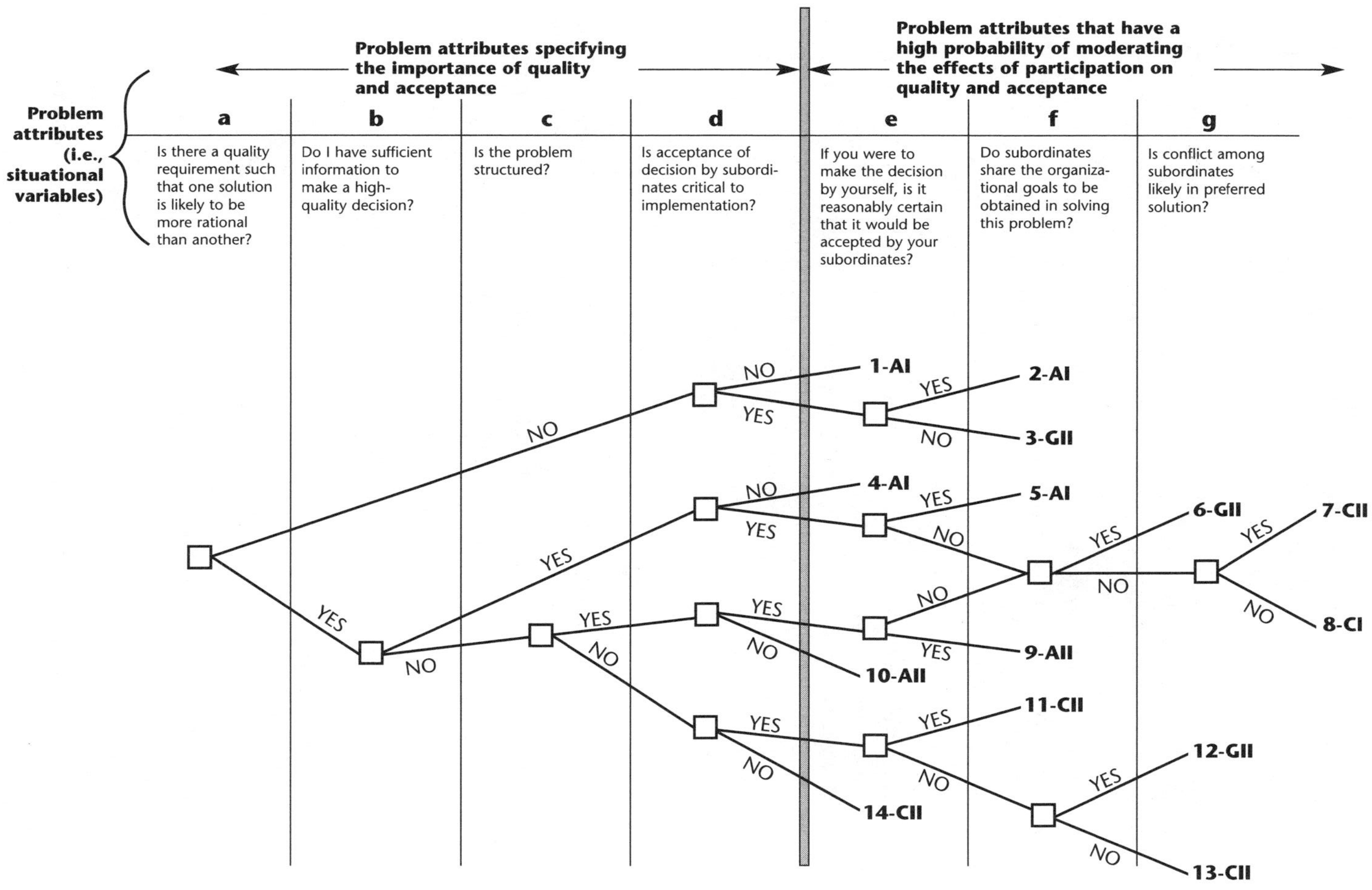
Problem attributes (i.e., situational variables)
Problem attributes specifying the importance of quality and acceptance
Problem attributes that have a high probability of moderating the effects of participation on quality and acceptance
a
Is there a quality requirement such that one solution is likely to be more rational than another?
b
Do I have sufficient information to make a high-quality decision?
c
Is the problem structured?
d
Is acceptance of decision by subordinates critical to implementation?
e
If you were to make the decision by yourself, is it reasonably certain that it would be accepted by your subordinates?
f
Do subordinates share the organizational goals to be obtained in solving this problem?
g
Is conflict among subordinates likely in preferred solution?
YES
NO
1-AI
2-AI
3-GII
4-AI
5-AI
6-GII
7-CII
8-CI
9-AII
10-AII
11-CII
12-GII
13-CII
14-CII

Figure 6.7. Problem-solving and decision-making style model. (Adapted from Vroom, Victor H. "A New Look at Managerial Decision Making." *Organizational Dynamics* 1 [Spring 1973]: 66–80; reprinted by permission from Elsevier. © 1973. American Management Association, New York. All rights reserved.)

DISCUSSION QUESTIONS

1. Explain why decision making is a distinct management function and why it is linked to all other management functions. Identify the three managerial decision classifications, and give examples of each.
2. What conditions initiate problem solving? Discuss how problem solving under the condition of improvement is related to problem solving under the condition of opportunity.
3. How are problem solving and decision making related? What predecision and postdecision activities are inherent in problem solving? What are the steps of problem solving?
4. Using the problem-solving process model in Figure 6.4, discuss and give examples of the following: How do assumptions affect problem solving? What are some positive and negative results that can occur in the tentative alternative solution loop? Why are both quantitative and nonquantitative criteria important when evaluating and choosing an alternative?
5. Distinguish facts and assumptions. Give examples of the role of inductive and deductive reasoning in making assumptions.
6. Identify the factors that influence problem solving. Describe three situations, and indicate which factors were influential in shaping the outcomes.
7. What are the advantages of group problem solving? List reasons why it is critical to the success of organizationwide quality improvement. Describe a situation from your experience in which the phenomenon of groupthink occurred.
8. Identify the types of problem-solving and decision-making styles. Use Figure 6.7 and Table 6.4 to describe situations that show the following styles: AI, CI, and GII.

Case Study 1: The Nursing Assistant

You are the supervisor on the day shift at a 100-bed nursing facility. In one 20-bed unit, the workload relative to other units has been very heavy for the past month. In that unit, you observed family members of a bed-bound resident turning the resident. When you asked why they were doing that, one of the family members said, "Nursing assistant Johnson told us that the staff is too busy. If we want our father turned, we have to do it ourselves or wait 3 or 4 hours before the staff can help." On several occasions in the past week, you saw nursing assistant Johnson sitting in the utility room for what seemed to be long periods of time.

QUESTIONS

1. Identify the facts present in this case.
2. State the problem.
3. Make assumptions of the three types described in the chapter. List them in order of declining certainty.
4. Develop five solutions that should be considered. Which one should be chosen? Why?

Case Study 2: The New Charge Nurse

You are a third-shift (11:00 p.m. to 7:00 a.m.) nurse supervisor to whom several charge nurses report. Each charge nurse is responsible for a nursing unit. Six months ago, you promoted Sally Besnick to be one of the charge nurses. Six months before she was promoted, Besnick had earned a bachelor of science in nursing (B.S.N.) from an out-of-state university. She is the same age as the five registered nurses (RNs) she supervises, all of whom graduated from a two-year associate of arts (A.A.) nursing degree program at a local technical college. B.S.N. programs are generally considered the "gold standard" of nursing preparation. Sally is the only charge nurse with a B.S.N. who reports to you.

Besnick received the same in-service training in supervision as the other charge nurses, but there are major problems on her unit. Morale among her nursing staff is low, absenteeism is high, and not all of the administrative work on her unit is getting done. There are no indications that the quality of care on her unit is below acceptable levels, however. You think Besnick's main difficulty is that she cannot control, lead, discipline, or correct her subordinates. She seems easygoing; her subordinates call her Soft Sally behind her back. Given their hands-on training and greater experience, they feel that they can deliver technically better patient care than she can.

Besnick is personable and well liked by you and by the other charge nurses. She socializes with them after hours and, like them, Besnick participates in American Nurses Association professional activities. Besnick and her husband recently bought a new house in town after renting for the year that she has worked at the hospital. They adopted a baby 2 months ago.

You are concerned that if you demote Besnick, her pride will be hurt and she will quit. You do not want to lose a good RN, especially one with a bachelor's degree.

QUESTIONS

1. Describe the education and training received by nursing assistants, licensed practical (licensed vocational) nurses, and the RNs of the various types. Referring to the discussion of nursing in Chapter 1 may be helpful.
2. Develop a problem statement. Identify several tentative alternative solutions.
3. Which solution is best? Why?
4. Describe how you would implement the solution chosen. How would you evaluate the results?

▨ Case Study 3: Listening

Billy and Bobbie are retired, and they regularly go to the nearby hospital cafeteria for their noon meal. The cafeteria is open to the public, has a variety of healthy food choices, and is reasonably priced. At the end of the cafeteria line is a table that has condiments, paper napkins, and plastic silverware for carryout. In addition, there is a toaster on the table. Bobbie likes her bread toasted and expressed dissatisfaction with the toaster for several months. The toaster heated the bread, but it wasn't hot enough, so the bread dried out instead of being toasted. Billy mentioned the toaster problem to the cafeteria cashier and other cafeteria staff on several occasions. The staff was always polite and promised to tell management about the toaster. Nothing changed, however. Finally, Billy's patience reached its limit, and he asked to see the cafeteria manager. The manager met Billy and Bobbie in the cafeteria. She seemed surprised to learn about the toaster problem but thanked Billy and promised action. In less than a week, a new commercial-grade toaster appeared on the condiment table. The next time Billy and Bobbie came to the cafeteria, several of the staff came to their table and told them how pleased they were that management had replaced the old toaster. They said that other patrons had complained about the toaster, too. The staff members said that despite their telling the manager about the problem numerous times, no action had been taken. They were frustrated that it had taken so long to correct the problem with the toaster.

QUESTIONS

1. Develop a problem statement.
2. Characterize the manager's management style and the cafeteria staff's view of their role in serving the cafeteria's patrons.

3. How is customer satisfaction factored into efforts to improve performance?
4. Develop three solutions to solve the kind of problem that Billy and Bobbie had.

■ Case Study 4: Ping-Ponging

You are the CEO of a hospital. The vice president for medical affairs (VPMA) has just left your office. In broad detail, she described some referral patterns that she characterized as very unusual, even strange. Several "cliques" of physicians appear to have developed a system of referring to one another in ways that result in overtesting and excessive consultations, to the point that their patients, most of whom are older, have longer lengths of stay. The hospital has experienced above-average denials for Medicare reimbursement for the care of these types of patients. The various cliques of physicians seem to be connected by culture, ethnicity, and social relationships. The VPMA called the referrals among those in the cliques "ping-ponging" and said that she would collect some more data.

QUESTIONS

1. What are the clinical implications of patients receiving unneeded tests and having overlong lengths of stay?
2. Develop a statement of the problem from the perspective of the VPMA.
3. What weight should be given to the ethical and legal implications, compared with the economic implications?
4. What, if anything, should you as CEO do about the problem described by the VPMA, as stated in the answer to Question 2 above?

Notes

1. Drucker, Peter F. *An Introductory View of Management,* 396. New York: Harper's College Press, 1977; Pearce, John A., III, and Richard B. Robinson, Jr. *Management,* 62. New York: Random House, 1989.
2. Simon, Herbert A. *The New Science of Management Decision,* rev. ed., 46. Englewood Cliffs, NJ: Prentice-Hall, 1977.
3. Pearce, John A., III, and Richard B. Robinson, Jr. *Management,* 63–64. New York: Random House, 1989.
4. Gallagher, Thomas J. *Problem Solving with People: The Cycle Process,* 9. New York: University of America Press, 1987.
5. Vroom, Victor H., and Arthur G. Jago. *The New Leadership: Managing Participation in Organizations,* 56. Englewood Cliffs, NJ: Prentice-Hall, 1988.
6. Higgins, James M. *The Management Challenge: An Introduction to Management,* 70–71. New York: Macmillan, 1991.
7. Hastings, John E.F., William R. Mindell, John W. Browne, and Janet M. Barnsley. "Canadian Health Administrator Study." *Canadian Journal of Public Health,* 72 (March/April 1981, suppl. 1): 46–47.
8. American College of Hospital Administrators. *The Evolving Role of the Hospital Chief Executive Officer.* Chicago: The Foundation of the American College of Hospital Administrators, 1984.
9. Cowan, David A. "Developing a Process Model of Problem Recognition." *Academy of Management Review* 11 (Spring 1986): 763–764.
10. Gallagher, *Problem Solving,* 77; Pearce and Robinson, *Management,* 65.
11. Postal, Susan Nelson. "Using the Deming Quality Improvement Method to Manage Medical Record Department Product Lines." *Topics in Health Record Management* 10 (June 1990): 36.
12. Cowan, "Developing a Process," 764.

13. Nutt, Paul C. "How Top Managers in Health Organizations Set Directions that Guide Decision Making." *Hospital & Health Services Administration* 36 (Spring 1991): 67.

14. Cowan, "Developing a Process," 764.

15. Cowan, "Developing a Process," 766.

16. Andriole, Stephen J. *Handbook of Problem Solving: An Analytical Methodology,* 25. New York: Petrocelli Books, 1983.

17. Nutt, "How Top Managers," 59.

18. For a discussion on problem definition, see Chow, Chee W., Kamal M. Haddad, and Adrian Wong-Boren. "Improving Subjective Decision Making in Health Care Administration." *Hospital & Health Services Administration* 36 (Summer 1991): 192–193.

19. Evans, James R. *Creative Thinking in the Decision and Management Sciences,* 104. Cincinnati: South-Western, 1991.

20. Couger, Daniel J. *Creative Problem Solving and Opportunity Finding,* 184. Danvers, MA: Boyd & Fraser, 1995.

21. Couger, *Creative Problem Solving,* 113.

22. Dewey, John. *How We Think: A Restatement of the Relation of Reflective Thinking to the Educative Process,* 108. Boston: D.C. Heath, 1933.

23. "There is no true value of any characteristic, state, or condition that is defined in terms of measurement or observation. Change of procedure for measurement (change in operational definition) or observation produces a new number. . . . There is no true value for the number of people in a room. Whom do you count? Do we count someone that was here in this room, but is now outside on the telephone or drinking coffee? Do we count the people that work for the hotel? Do we count the people on the stage? The people managing the audio-visual equipment? If you change the rule for counting people, you come up with a new number. . . . There is no such thing as a fact concerning an empirical observation. Any two people may have different ideas about what is important to know about any event. Get the facts! Is there any meaning to this exhortation?" (Deming, W. Edwards. *The New Economics for Industry, Government, Education,* 2nd ed., 104–105. Cambridge, MA: MIT-CAES, 2000.)

24. A useful discussion of problem-solving constraints, including assumptions, is found in Chapter 3 of Brightman, Harvey J. *Problem Solving: A Logical and Creative Approach.* Atlanta, GA: Business Publication Division, College of Business Administration, Georgia State University, 1980.

25. Chow, Haddad, and Wong-Boren, "Improving Subjective Decision Making," 194.

26. Hammond, John S., Ralph L. Keeney, and Howard Raiffa. "The Hidden Traps in Decision Making." *Harvard Business Review* 84, 1 (January 2006): 120.

27. Chow, Haddad, and Wong-Boren, "Improving Subjective Decision Making," 202.

28. Hammond, Keeney, and Raiffa. "The Hidden Traps in Decision Making," 122.

29. Chow, Haddad, and Wong-Boren, "Improving Subjective Decision Making," 192.

30. Nutt, Paul C. "The Identification of Solution Ideas During Organizational Decision Making." *Management Science* 39 (September 1993): 1,071.

31. An excellent discussion of techniques for generating solutions is found in Chapter 8 of Couger, *Creative Problem Solving.*

32. Couger, *Creative Problem Solving,* 18.

33. Nutt, "The Identification of Solution Ideas," 1,072.

34. Etzioni, Amitai. "Humble Decision Making." *Harvard Business Review* 67 (July/August 1989): 125.

35. Pearce and Robinson (*Management,* 75) describe these criteria as Will the alternative be effective?, Can the alternative be implemented?, and What are the organization consequences?, respectively.

36. Kepner, Charles H., and Benjamin B. Tregoe. *The New Rational Manager,* 94–99. Princeton, NJ: Kepner-Tregoe, 1981.

37. Kepner and Tregoe, *The New Rational Manager,* 103–137.

38. Good discussions of problem solving and factors influencing problem solving are found in Ackoff, Russell L. *The Art of Problem Solving.* New York: John Wiley & Sons, 1978; Ivancevich, John M., James H. Donnelly, Jr., and James L. Gibson. *Management Principles and Functions,* 4th ed. Homewood, IL: Irwin, 1989; Kepner and Tregoe, *The New Rational Manager;* and Nutt, "How Top Managers."

39. "Decision Making: Better; Faster; Smarter." *Harvard Business Review* 84, 1 (January 2006, Special Issue).

40. Brightman, *Problem Solving*, 83–84.

41. Vroom and Jago, *The New Leadership,* 56.

42. Vroom and Jago, *The New Leadership,* 28.

43. Brightman, Harvey J. *Group Problem Solving: An Improved Managerial Approach,* 51. Atlanta, GA: Business Publishing Division, College of Business Administration, Georgia State University, 1988. Pages 63–69 discuss techniques for overcoming groupthink.

44. Eisenhardt, Kathleen M., Jean L. Kahwajy, and L.J. Bourgeois, III. "How Management Teams Can Have a Good Fight." *Harvard Business Review* 75, 4 (July/August 1997): 85.

45. Ways, Max. "Watergate as a Case Study in Management." *Fortune* 88 (November 1973): 196–201. Watergate is the residential and commercial complex in Washington, D.C., that housed the Democratic National Committee during the 1972 presidential election campaign. Operatives of the (Republican) Committee to Re-elect the President (Richard M. Nixon) were arrested there during a failed burglary. The political stonewalling, resulting scandal, and Nixon's resignation are collectively called Watergate. The problem-solving process and mind-set of the people who were involved exemplify groupthink.

46. Higgins, *The Management Challenge*, 87.

47. Kaluzny, Arnold D. "Revitalizing Decision Making at the Middle Management Level." *Hospital & Health Services Administration* 34 (Spring 1989): 42.

48. Kaluzny, "Revitalizing Decision Making," 45.

49. Crosby, Bob. "Why Employee Involvement Often Fails and What It Takes to Succeed." In *The 1987 Annual: Developing Human Resources,* edited by J. William Pfeiffer, 179. San Diego: University Associates, 1987.

50. Crosby, "Why Employee Involvement," 181.

51. Kahn, Susan. "Creating Opportunities for Employee Participation in Problem Solving." *Health Care Supervisor* 7 (October 1988): 39.

52. Lawler, Edward E., III, and Susan A. Mohrman. "Quality Circles: After the Honeymoon." In *The 1988 Annual: Developing Human Resources,* edited by J. William Pfeiffer, 201. San Diego: University Associates, 1988.

53. Dailey, Robert, Frederick Young, and Cameron Barr. "Empowering Middle Managers in Hospitals with Team-Based Problem Solving." *Health Care Management Review* 16 (Spring 1991): 55.

54. Vroom, Victor H. "A New Look at Managerial Decision-Making." *Organizational Dynamics* 1 (Spring 1973): 66–80.

55. See also Vroom, Victor H., and Philip W. Yetton. *Leadership and Decision-Making*. Pittsburgh: University of Pittsburgh Press, 1973; Vroom and Jago, *The New Leadership*.

7

The Quality Imperative

The management model in Figure 5.8 shows how health services organizations (HSOs) and health systems (HSs) convert inputs into outputs. The inputs of structure, tasks and technology, and people are integrated to achieve individual and organizational outputs (productivity). The types and nature of inputs and the conversion process determine the quality of output.

This chapter discusses the two dimensions of quality. The first is the theory of continuous quality improvement (CQI), which is drawn primarily from the work of W. Edwards Deming and his mentor Walter A. Shewhart. Dr. Deming's contributions to quality and performance improvement, especially his 14 points for quality, receive special attention. The contributions of Joseph M. Juran and Philip B. Crosby are outlined. The second dimension of quality is process improvement. Improved quality enables HSOs to become more productive and cost-effective, which gives them a competitive advantage.

Quality improvement (QI) focuses on doing the right things and doing the right things right. The chapter introduces a CQI process improvement model and the relationship between problem solving and the use of teams in process improvement. The contributions of benchmarking, six sigma, lean manufacturing, and reengineering are discussed. Accreditation and registration, through organizations such as The Joint Commission on Accreditation of Healthcare Organizations (The Joint Commission) and the International Organization for Standardization (ISO), respectively, are addressed. Productivity improvement* (PI) methods to improve work systems and job design; capacity and facilities layout; and production control, scheduling, and materials handling are described.

Strategic quality planning links QI to the strategic plans of the HSO/HS. Steps include choosing the organization's strategic direction and prioritizing the key processes needed to attain and maintain a competitive position. Organizational alignment and implementation are discussed. The chapter con-

---

*Productivity improvement and performance improvement are similar concepts, although not synonymous. The quality improvement literature uses the former, The Joint Commission the latter.

cludes by considering the necessity of, and means by which to achieve, physician involvement in CQI and the next iteration of the quality movement—interorganizational and communitywide initiatives.

Background

There has been a shift in the health services paradigm with respect to quality:[1] "It represents a 'new order of things' in the provision of healthcare."[2] This shift has occurred at two levels: the definition of quality output and the means of achieving it. First, the traditional definition of quality of care and service—its output—has expanded beyond meeting specifications or standards to incorporate conformance to requirements and fitness for use, both of which include meeting or exceeding patient (customer) expectations. Second, there is recognition of a need to focus on improving the inputs and processes that generate the outputs of product and service.[3] This expanded definition of quality output and the focus on improving inputs and processes are the twin pillars of CQI. Adopting the philosophy and methods of CQI will positively affect HSO/HS management and organizational arrangements; resource allocation, utilization, cost-effectiveness, and PI; the quality of services provided (i.e., conformance to requirements and customer satisfaction); and the HSO's/HS's competitive position.

International competition and increased consumer demands and expectations for quality products and services profoundly affected American industry in the last decades of the 20th century. Industry was found wanting. The quality awakening in the 1980s and 1990s increased awareness of the importance of quality and the need to satisfy customers; initiatives to improve the quality of outputs to be globally competitive; and, as described by Deming, the beginning of the transformation of American business[4] that is ongoing.

Like industry, the health services system continues to undergo profound change. The last two decades of the 20th century were tumultuous for HSOs/HSs. The effects of environmental forces and the changes that occurred then have continued into the 21st century. Changes include revenue and cost pressures; competition from alternate forms of delivery, such as managed care; and restructuring because of closures, mergers, consolidations, and other actions of HSs.[5] The turbulent health services environment and increasing demands from, and accountability to, customers for lower cost care with improved quality put HSOs/HSs at risk. The concept of customers has expanded beyond patients to include third-party payers of all types.[6] To survive and thrive, HSOs/HSs must respond effectively to these customers' and stakeholders' expectations.

Quality—Two Dimensions

Traditionally, quality in HSOs/HSs focused on the product or service content[7] and meeting specifications or standards. Quality was evaluated retrospectively; the product or service was assessed using predetermined criteria. Examples are accuracy of diagnosis, physiological change and improvement in patients at discharge, mortality and morbidity rates, and the efficacy of medical procedures and drugs. Methods of quality evaluation include inspection, peer review, and quality assurance, as well as tracking indicators such as infection rates, unanticipated readmissions after discharge, and accuracy and timeliness of diagnostic tests.

The contemporary view of health services quality includes conformance to requirements and fitness for use—both of which incorporate satisfying customer needs and meeting or exceeding expectations. The American Society for Quality defines quality as "1. The characteristics of a product or service that bear on its ability to satisfy stated or implied needs; 2. A product or service free of deficiencies."[8]

Quality judgments occur when the HSO or individuals within it generate outputs.[9] Judging quality includes asking questions such as Are there defects? Does the product work? Was the service appropriate? Is treatment reliable? Was the service on time? Was it delivered in a friendly manner? Was it the right service? Did it meet the customer's needs? Was the customer delighted? Did product or service attributes exceed the customer's expectations?[10] The answers to such questions about expectations by customers are influenced by their experiences, perceptions, and values.

The American Hospital Association's Hospital Research and Educational Trust (HRET) Quality Management for Health Care Delivery (QMHCD) report termed this *delivery quality*. Delivery quality covers all aspects of the customer's satisfaction with the HSO.[11] Conformance and expectation quality monitoring and improvement must be directed at every level and at every process.[12] Customers are not only patients; others include physicians and other internal customers (downstream users of a unit's output) and external customers such as payers and the community. For example, nursing is a customer of pharmacy in terms of medications and a customer of dietary services in terms of patients' dietary needs; physicians are customers of diagnostic testing; the intensive care unit is a customer of the emergency department (ED) when trauma patients are admitted; third-party payers are customers of patient billing; and, to some degree, all HSO departments and units are customers of administration. Depending on the transaction, the process, department, unit, or staff member commonly changes from customer to processor to supplier.[13] It is essential that all persons in a process understand their roles as customer, processor (person who adds value), and supplier. They must know how what they do contributes to the aim of the organization. Figure 7.1 is a simplified representation of a customer–processor–supplier relationship. In vertically integrated HSs, the skilled nursing facility is the customer of the acute care hospital. Figure 7.2 shows the internal and external customers of a hospital's functional departments.

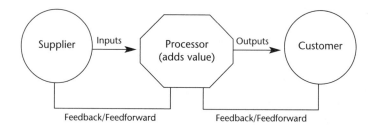

Figure 7.1.   The customer–supplier relationship.

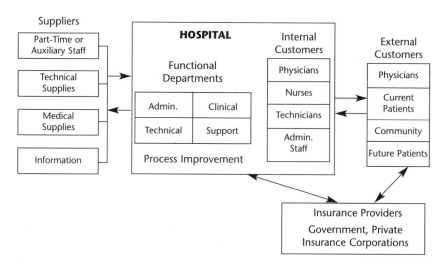

Figure 7.2.   Internal and external customers of hospital functional departments. (From Carol Greebler, TQM Plus, San Diego, CA, 1989; reprinted by permission.)

▄ Taking A CQI Approach

BACKGROUND

The now pervasive philosophy about quality in healthcare that gained wide acceptance from the late 1980s draws on the work of industrial quality experts W. Edwards Deming,[14] Joseph M. Juran,[15] and Philip B. Crosby.[16] The CQI philosophy has four attributes. First, output quality includes meeting or exceeding customer needs and expectations. Second, monitoring and evaluating quality is retrospective; it is prospective in that poor quality can be prevented. Third, "quality is not the responsibility of just one department or individual";[17] it is organizationwide and involves everyone. Fourth, quality and CQI focus on both process (and inputs) and outcomes, not just outcomes.[18] The Joint Commission's *Specifications Manual for National Hospital Quality Measures, version 2.2,* recognizes the need for outcome and process quality.[19] The philosophical context of The Joint Commission's manual is CQI:

- *Quality as a central priority:* organizationwide devotion to quality, leadership involvement in promoting and improving quality
- *Customers:* attention to customer needs, feedback from internal and external customers, customer–supplier dialogue
- *Work processes:* describing key clinical and managerial processes, systems approach, and cross-disciplinary teams
- *Measurement:* use of data, understanding of variation, search for underlying causes
- *Improvement:* never-ending commitment to improving performance[20]

Improving quality may use several names: *quality management,*[21] *total quality management (TQM),*[22] *total quality care,*[23] or *QI.*[24] CQI is preferred because it reflects the major break from previous efforts to achieve quality, is the most positive way to state the concept, and minimizes any suggestion that quality is the job only of one group in an organization.

CQI is defined as an ongoing, organizationwide framework in which HSOs and their employees and clinical staff are committed to, and involved in, monitoring and evaluating all aspects of the organization's activities (inputs and processes) and outputs for the purpose of continuously improving them.[25] The essential elements of this definition are

- *CQI is organizationwide.* CQI can be successful only if the organization is transformed to seek quality in all that it does. It requires a total commitment to quality—a philosophical transformation—by the governing body and senior-level management; it involves all HSO/HS employees, including clinical staff;[26] and it is rooted in a cultural setting that supports quality initiatives, teamwork, adaptability, and flexibility.[27]
- *CQI is process focused.* CQI seeks to understand processes, identify process characteristics that should be measured, and monitor processes as changes are made to determine the effects of those changes. The result is improved processes that enhance productivity through more efficient and effective use of resources. In sum, CQI improves conversion processes, thus generating higher quality products and service (outputs).
- *CQI is staff focused.* Process understanding and improvement require a team-based approach that involves and empowers employees to effect change.
- *CQI uses output measures.* Outcomes of care (indicators) provide macro-level data to determine how well groups of processes and the organization as a whole are per-

forming. Indicators allow time-series as well as inter-HSO/HS comparisons. These crude arrows may point to a need for specific foci for process improvement.

- *CQI is customer driven.* The goal is to meet or exceed the expectations of customers, who are defined broadly and include internal and external customers.

The literature is replete with CQI applications in HSOs.[28] Examples include hospitals[29] and integrated health systems.[30] There are success stories in disparate areas: clinical medicine,[31] laboratory,[32] radiology,[33] medical records,[34] ED,[35] pharmacy,[36] and adverse drug events.[37] The examples extend internationally to applying CQI in small general medical practices (Netherlands)[38] and a multisite teaching hospital (Canada).[39] A survey of U.S. and Canadian hospitals found that approximately 90% of those responding had implemented CQI and 65% had undertaken six or more CQI projects. The study found that larger teaching hospitals were more likely to be involved in CQI than smaller nonteaching hospitals.[40]

CQI MODEL

CQI fundamentally shifts organizational thinking because it is customer driven and focuses on internal and external customers. CQI is systematic and organizationwide, with top management commitment to improving processes (and inputs) through employee empowerment. The result is improved quality and customer satisfaction, PI, and enhanced competitive position.

The HRET QMHCD described the CQI challenge: "Continuous Quality Improvement demands that healthcare providers answer three questions. Are we doing the right things? Are we doing things right? How can we be certain that we do things right the first time, every time?"[41] Figure 7.3 answers these questions in the context of a CQI model. The following discussion references the numbers in that model.

Are We Doing the Right Things?

The first pillar of CQI, output quality [3], determines whether the HSO is doing the right things. Products and services that are in conformance and that meet or exceed customer expectations mean the organization is doing the right things. From the CQI perspective, customers are not only patients and external stakeholders but also internal users of a department, a unit, or an individual's outputs. The customer is the next person or process that relies on another person or process for inputs. Output that is in conformance and meets customers' needs and expectations is a quality product or service and means that the HSO is doing the right things.

Are We Doing Things Right?

Process improvement [2] is the second pillar of CQI. Output quality can be improved only by improving the processes that produce it. All processes can be improved. Because of their high degree of human dependency, patient care systems can always be improved.[42] CQI means that even a process that functions well can be improved.[43] "If it isn't perfect, make it better."[44]

The final element of "doing things right" is that monitoring, evaluating, and intervening to improve processes are continuous. Requisite to continuous improvement is developing a systematic understanding and documentation of processes. All staff must be trained in process improvement and encouraged to seek opportunities to improve work results by improving the way they are produced. The outcome is not only improved output quality [3] but also improved productivity [4], in which there is more effective resource use, and enhanced competitive position [5]. Crosby urged organizations to establish a goal of "do it right the first time."[45] This goal may be unattainable, but HSOs that continuously improve processes are moving in the "right" direction.

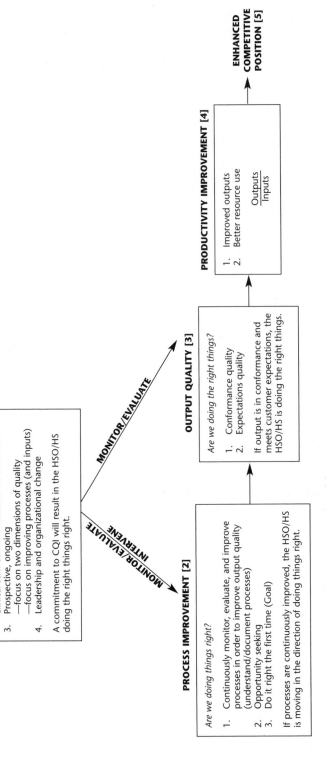

CONTINUOUS QUALITY IMPROVEMENT [1]

GOAL: How can we be certain we do things right the first time, every time?

1. Organizational philosophy
   (organizationwide, all levels)
2. Governing body, management, staff, and
   clinical staff commitment and involvement
3. Prospective, ongoing
   —focus on two dimensions of quality
   —focus on improving processes (and inputs)
4. Leadership and organizational change

A commitment to CQI will result in the HSO/HS
doing the right things right.

MONITOR/EVALUATE

MONITOR/EVALUATE/INTERVENE

PROCESS IMPROVEMENT [2]

Are we doing things right?

1. Continuously monitor, evaluate, and improve
   processes in order to improve output quality
   (understand/document processes)
2. Opportunity seeking
3. Do it right the first time (Goal)

If processes are continuously improved, the HSO/HS
is moving in the direction of doing things right.

OUTPUT QUALITY [3]

Are we doing the right things?

1. Conformance quality
2. Expectations quality

If output is in conformance and
meets customer expectations, the
HSO/HS is doing the right things.

PRODUCTIVITY IMPROVEMENT [4]

1. Improved outputs
2. Better resource use

$$\frac{Outputs}{Inputs}$$

**ENHANCED
COMPETITIVE
POSITION [5]**

Figure 7.3. Continuous quality improvement model.

How Can We Be Certain that We Do Things Right the First Time, Every Time?

CQI has the goal of doing things right the first time, every time. If there is quality output (the right things) and process improvement (doing things right) with CQI, the HSO/HS will move in the direction of doing things right the first time, every time (goal).[46] The essential attributes of CQI [1] are as follows (see Figure 7.3):

- CQI is an organizational philosophy that becomes pervasive in the culture—the ingrained beliefs and values of the HSO/HS. It is customer driven and requires the transformation of the existing beliefs and values regarding quality.
- CQI requires the total commitment and involvement of everyone in the HSO/HS. Management must nurture the value system and commit the resources that support continuous improvement as integral to the work of everyone in the organization.[47] Staff must participate in, and be committed to, continuously improving their work results and the way those results are achieved. This requires collaboration and cross-functional coordination among work units and departments.[48] All staff must be involved in problem solving, especially to seek and identify opportunities for improvement.
- CQI is prospective and ongoing. The focus on output quality must be prospective, not just retrospective; it must be continuous, not intermittent.[49] The aim is to prevent poor quality before it happens and to seek opportunities to improve processes in an organized fashion.
- CQI requires management to meet its leadership responsibility to train employees; encourage innovation, worker participation, and empowerment and build teams so that employees can contribute to process improvement problem solving; and facilitate organizational change that leads to improvement.

CQI, Productivity Improvement, and Competitive Position

The CQI paradigm is the reciprocal of the conventional cost-containment initiatives prevalent during the 1970s and into the 1980s. In the context of the management model in Figure 5.8, the emphasis then was to increase the ratios of outputs to inputs. The resulting initiatives were narrowly applied, episodic, and short-term. Typically, these initiatives had little worker involvement and commitment and focused on reducing input costs rather than enhancing output quality. By contrast, rather than simply reducing costs, CQI improvement initiatives are broad-based, long-term, and ongoing; have extensive management and employee involvement and commitment; are customer driven; and focus on improving both process and output quality.

Figure 7.3 depicts the ways CQI improves quality and productivity improvement [4], leading to enhanced competitive position [5]. Deming asserted that productivity improvement does not improve output quality. Rather, improved quality results in productivity improvement. The Deming Chain Reaction shown in Figure 7.4 suggests this relationship: Better quality decreases costs, which improves productivity. In turn, this leads to decreased prices and increased market share; thus the organization stays in business, provides jobs, and yields greater returns. Consequently, competitive position is enhanced. Deming argued that improved quality results in better resource use (lower costs) because improved processes mean less rework (readmissions), fewer mistakes (repeats of tests), and fewer delays (waiting for service). These results occur because the prospective and continuous assessment of, and changes made to, work processes and inputs yield both improved quality and improved productivity.[50]

The Malcolm Baldrige National Quality Award (MBNQA), named for a U.S. secretary of commerce who died while in office, was created in 1987 and has been awarded since 1988. The appli-

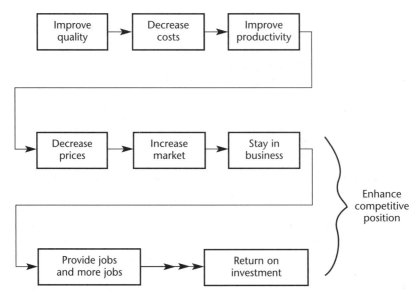

Figure 7.4.   Deming chain reaction. (Adapted from Joiner, Brian L. *Fourth Generation Management: The New Business Consciousness,* 23. New York: McGraw-Hill, 1994; reprinted by permission of the McGraw-Hill Companies, Inc.)

cation process is rigorous, the award prestigious. Its purpose is to promote quality excellence; recognize organizations that have made significant improvements in product, service, and competitive position; and foster information sharing among organizations. Criteria for the Baldrige award in healthcare are leadership; strategic planning; focus on patients, other customers, and markets; measurement, analysis, and knowledge management; workforce focus; process management; and results.[51]

Theory of CQI

THE PIONEERS

Modern history is replete with those who have striven to improve the quality of care. The eminent English physician Thomas Percival (1740–1804) lived and worked in Manchester, where he was active in improving clinical practice and public health. Percival's experiences caused him to write two pamphlets—"Internal Regulation of Hospitals 1771" and "A Scheme of Professional Conduct Relative to Hospitals and Other Medical Charities 1772"—that sought to stimulate reform.[52] In 1803, Percival presented the idea of a hospital register to help physicians improve the quality of their care.[53] The concept must have been startling to his medical colleagues, and little apparent interest resulted. Chapter 4 notes that the AMA's "Principles of Medical Ethics" reflects Percival's influence.

In 1847, the Austro-Hungarian physician Ignaz Semmelweis (1818–1865) sought to reduce the incidence of puerperal (childbed) fever, an often fatal bacterial infection rampant among newly delivered women at the Vienna General Hospital. Semmelweis used mortality statistics to show that washing hands and instruments in carbolic acid (a solution of chlorinated lime) stopped the causative bacterium from spreading and virtually eliminated puerperal fever from his ward. Medical colleagues rejected his findings and so ridiculed him that he left Vienna.[54] Only when the French bacteriologist Louis Pasteur (1822–1895) demonstrated the germ theory of disease causation in 1862 was Semmelweis vindicated.

Florence Nightingale (1820–1910) demonstrated the value of good organization, cleanliness, and properly trained nurses in treating British soldiers during the Crimean War in 1854–1856. She used data to significantly improve clinical outcomes, including development of a "model hospital statistical form" to collect and generate consistent data and statistics.[55] Nightingale applied epidemiological principles, including the polar-area diagram, which she invented, to understand the morbidity and mortality of soldiers who had been wounded or were ill from disease.[56] Later, she led in establishing nursing as a profession in England. Nightingale's work to organize hospital-based care qualifies her as the first hospital administrator.[57]

In 1877, the English surgeon Joseph Lister visited New York City and reported on the benefits of antisepsis in preventing the spread of microorganisms by disinfecting surgical instruments, gowns, and drapes with carbolic acid, as well as using it copiously throughout the operating theater. William S. Halsted, who later became an eminent surgeon at The Johns Hopkins Hospital, was beginning his career and sought to introduce antisepsis at Bellevue Hospital in New York. Most surgeons opposed the concept, and there was such resistance to his use of antisepsis that he was forced to perform surgery in a tent outside the main hospital building. Halsted's results were so startling, however, that surgeons throughout New York soon followed suit.[58]

Reformers such as these were vindicated—some sooner, some later. Their struggles against medical orthodoxy, however, reflect the difficulties of changing a profession's trajectory, even when the evidence clearly supports a need for change. Their like-minded successors fared somewhat better.

Ernest A. Codman (1869–1940)

Dr. Ernest Codman, a surgeon, was an advocate of hospital reform and is the acknowledged founder of what is known today as outcomes management in patient care. It was his lifelong pursuit to establish an "end results system" that tracked the outcomes of patient treatment to identify clinical misadventures that could provide a foundation to improve care for future patients.[59] Codman is credited with a number of firsts in medical care. As a prominent surgeon on staff at Massachusetts General Hospital in the early 1900s, he organized morbidity and mortality (M&M) conferences at which physicians discussed cases openly for the purpose of learning about the care received by patients and whether it contributed to good results. M&M conferences became ubiquitous in hospitals and are required in hospitals that have an accredited graduate medical education program. Codman was one of several leading American surgeons who organized the American College of Surgeons (ACS) in 1913.[60] The "end result system of hospital standardization" became the stated objective of the ACS, whose Hospital Standardization Program became the Joint Commission on Accreditation of Hospitals, now known as The Joint Commission on Accreditation of Healthcare Organizations, or The Joint Commission. In 1920, Codman established the first bone tumor registry in the United States, which was the precedent for a national exchange of information on bone tumor cases.[61]

The failure of Massachusetts General Hospital to adopt outcomes evaluation, or end results, led to Codman's resignation. In 1911, he established his own private hospital, the Codman Hospital, at which he instituted a program of monitoring surgical performance. He tracked patients after hospital treatment, to understand their long-term benefits and to learn how care could be improved—the "end results" of care. The data, both negative and positive, were made public, and Codman challenged hospitals everywhere to do the same. Codman's review of his own clinical outcomes found that one error occurred for every three patients treated.[62]

It is useful to recall that in the late 19th century, the modern hospital was just emerging from the darkness of scientific ignorance. Supported by technologies such as asepsis, laboratory and x-ray services, and inhalation anesthesia, hospitals became a temple of healing that was largely based on efficacious surgery. Codman's proposal must have been startling and intimidating to clinicians and administrators alike. Making outcomes evaluations public could be embarrassing and even politically and economically dangerous for hospitals and their physicians; it is easy to understand the reluctance to publicize the "end result." Codman's reforming efforts brought him mostly ridicule, poverty, and censure, but he never stopped his efforts to link care, errors, and end results and to measure, report, and improve.[63] Except for the work of the ACS in its Hospital Standardization Program, Codman's "end results system" died with him.

Notably, public reporting of hospital outcome data is only now becoming commonplace and is the result of intense pressure from public interest groups, third-party payers, and government. Although Percival's idea to establish a hospital register of "end results" predated Codman's work by almost a century, Codman must be credited with beginning the long, often interrupted 100-year journey to the current emphasis on quality and performance improvement in health services delivery. Codman's application of elements of classic CQI methodology occurred well before the work of Walter A. Shewhart and his successors.

Walter A. Shewhart (1891–1967)

Walter A. Shewhart and Ernest A. Codman were contemporaries, although there is no evidence that they ever met—regrettably. Dr. Shewhart was the trail-blazing American statistician who developed the basic theory and application of statistical process control (SPC) and the precursor to the Plan, Do, Study, Act (PDSA) cycles that provide the methodological underpinnings for CQI. Shewhart's theories of SPC were applied in the 1920s at the Hawthorne Works of Western Electric, a facility near Chicago that manufactured telephones. W. Edwards Deming was one of Shewhart's students and colleagues during the 1920s and 1930s. Shewhart's book *Statistical Method from the Viewpoint of Quality Control,* published in 1939, was edited by Deming and contained the first version of the "Shewhart cycle." The Shewhart cycle evolved during the next four decades and is known as the PDSA cycle (as Shewhart and Deming developed it) and the Plan, Do, Check, Act (PDCA) cycle in Japan, primarily because of a misunderstanding in translation.[64]

The success of Shewhart's efforts is reflected in the slogan "alike as two telephones," which suggests that quality can be improved by reducing variation. Shewhart's SPC and PDSA were applied extensively and very successfully to military production during World War II. The PDSA

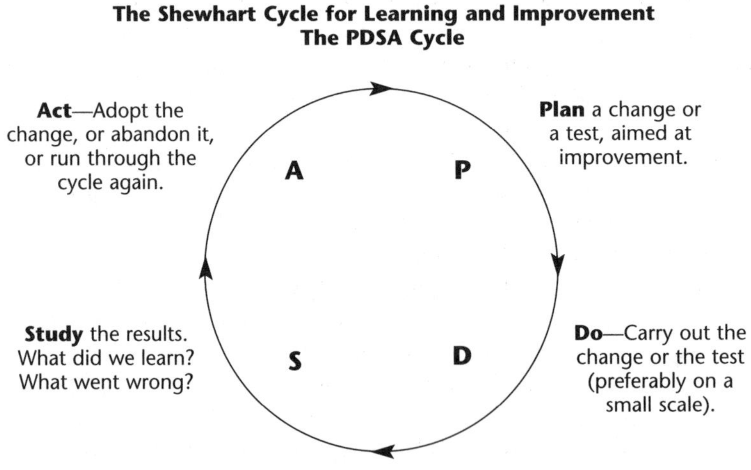

The Shewhart Cycle for Learning and Improvement
The PDSA Cycle

Act—Adopt the change, or abandon it, or run through the cycle again.

Plan a change or a test, aimed at improvement.

Study the results. What did we learn? What went wrong?

Do—Carry out the change or the test (preferably on a small scale).

A   P
S   D

Figure 7.5. The Shewhart Cycle for Learning and Improvement. The PDSA Cycle. (From Deming, W. Edwards. *The New Economics for Industry, Government, Education,* 2nd ed., p. 132. Shewhart Cycle © 2000 W. Edwards Deming Institute, by permission of MIT Press.)

cycle is also known as the Shewhart cycle.[65] Figure 7.5 shows the PDSA cycle, with a description for each step. When World War II ended in 1945, the American industrial base was undamaged; Germany's and Japan's lay in ruins. This fact, plus the pent-up demand for consumer goods after almost 4 years of total focus on war production, allowed American manufacturers to be less concerned about quality—there were buyers for everything they could produce, regardless of how well it was made. Thus, quantity gained the ascendancy over quality. It was not until the 1980s that the focus returned to quality, prompted by declining markets for American products. Attention to service quality soon followed.

THE BUILDERS

Deming, Juran, and Crosby

Three contemporary theorists, educators, and practitioners of quality—W. Edwards Deming, Joseph M. Juran, and Philip B. Crosby—advocated CQI and greatly influenced its philosophy and practice. Their work provides philosophies and methodologies to establish a quality culture. In varying degrees and a variety of forms, their principles have been adopted by HSOs/HSs.[66] The three were not of like mind on some of the specifics of how to achieve quality, however.

The emphasis here is on Deming, who developed a philosophy applicable to life and to management, much of which applies to improving quality in product and service. His theory of "profound knowledge" is a conceptualization of what is necessary for quality to be improved. Juran developed numerous models and statistical methods that support the managerial and applications perspectives. Crosby was more the organizational behaviorist and motivator and less the philosopher or technician. Their routes differ, but they have the same destination of improved quality.[67]

W. Edwards Deming (1900–1993)

W. Edwards Deming earned his doctorate in mathematical physics and was Shewhart's protégé at the Hawthorne Works. Deming made extensive use of Shewhart's theories of SPC and PDSA in his own approach to improving quality.[68] Deming went to Japan in 1947 to assist in a census. Because of his work in quality improvement, he was again invited to Japan in 1950 to lecture to Japanese manufacturers about how to improve their consumer products, which had inferior quality and were poorly regarded before and after World War II. Deming's lectures were widely attended and highly influential as Japan rebuilt its industrial base that transformed it into the major economic power that it became. Dr. Deming's work is considered so important that Japan's highest award for quality is the Deming Prize. Because Deming introduced Shewhart's PDSA cycle to Japan, it is known as the Deming cycle there. It was only in the 1980s that Deming's work began to be appreciated in the United States.[69] Deming's most significant book, *Out of the Crisis,* was published in 1986, when he was 86 years of age.

Deming defined quality broadly: "A product or service possesses quality if it helps somebody and enjoys a good and sustainable market."[70] Key to understanding how to improve quality is his view that poor quality results from badly designed or malfunctioning processes—not worker actions. Workers work in processes over which they have little or no control and are, therefore, able to do only what the process allows them to do. The process, not the worker, produces good or poor quality. Thus, better quality can be reached only by improving the process. Management controls processes; thus, it must lead in quality improvement. This view is reflected in Deming's emphasis on monitoring and evaluating processes through SPC and searching for ways to improve them. The Deming Chain Reaction in Figure 7.4 shows how improving quality will decrease costs, increase productivity, and enhance competitive position. This sequence is incorporated in the CQI model in Figure 7.3.

The Deming method has two distinct components. The first is critical: Managers must establish and maintain an environment in which quality is integral to all work. This means a transformation—a major philosophical shift and commitment that HSOs/HSs will improve quality. This philosophy is reflected in Deming's 14 points (see below). The second, concurrent component is that efforts to improve quality must be supported by SPC—management must have data that show what processes are doing and how well they are doing it. Analysis of these data allows managers to identify and correct problems. More importantly, the data support improvement of processes.

Deming's theory of profound knowledge includes four elements: knowledge of a system, knowledge of variation, theory of knowledge, and psychology.[71] *Appreciation for a system* means that management must understand the need for interdependent components to work together to try to accomplish the aim of a system. The greater the interdependence among components, the greater is the need for cooperation and communication. Some components of the system may have to suboptimize if doing so allows optimization of the whole system. *Knowledge about variation* means that management must understand that there is variation in every activity and in every process. Management must collect data to know if a process is in statistical control; a process "in control" has a definable capability and can be improved. Deming's *theory of knowledge* teaches us that a statement, if it contains knowledge, predicts future outcome. Rational prediction requires theory and builds knowledge through systematic revision and extension of theory based on comparison of prediction with observation. In this regard, management is prediction. The fourth element, *psychology*, helps us to understand people, interactions of people and circumstances, and those between a manager and staff in any system of management. Managers must be aware that people are different and learn differently and that there are intrinsic and extrinsic sources of motivation. In total, Deming's system of profound knowledge challenges managers to understand themselves and their jobs and staffs in ways that will enhance their effectiveness.

Deming's 14 points for improvement of management are complementary to CQI and its application, but they are essential to creating an environment in which quality can be achieved. The 14 points for quality[72] have been discussed extensively[73] and have been applied to HSOs by Batalden and Vorlicky, as cited in Deming[74] and Darr.[75]

1. *Create constancy of purpose toward improvement of product and service with the aim to become competitive, to stay in business, and to provide jobs.*[76] This means identifying customers, giving good-quality service to them, and ensuring organization survival through innovation and constant improvement.

2. *Adopt the new philosophy.* Commonly accepted levels of nonquality are unacceptable.

3. *Cease dependence on inspection to achieve quality.* Health services should

   require statistical evidence of quality of incoming materials, such as pharmaceuticals, serums, and equipment. Inspection is not the answer. Inspection is too late and is unreliable. Inspection does not produce quality. . . . Require corrective action, where needed, for all tasks that are performed in the hospital or other facility, ranging all the way from bills that are produced to processes of registration. Institute a rigid program of feedback from patients in regard to their satisfaction with services.[77]

4. *End the practice of awarding business on the basis of price tag.* The intent is to develop long-term relations with suppliers so that they can improve the quality of the products (and services) they provide as an input to the HSO/HS.

5. *Improve constantly and forever the system of production and service, to improve quality and productivity, and thus constantly decrease costs.* Improvement is not a one-time effort. Management is obligated to continually look for ways to reduce waste and improve quality.

6. *Institute training on the job.* Too often, workers learn their jobs from other workers who were never trained properly. They cannot do their jobs well because no one tells them how.

7. *Institute leadership.* A supervisor's job is not to tell people what to do or to punish them, but to lead.

   Supervisors need time to help people on the job. Supervisors need to find ways to translate the constancy of purpose to the individual employee. Supervisors must be trained in simple statistical methods for aid to employees, with the aim to detect and eliminate special causes of mistakes and rework.[78]

8. *Drive out fear so that everyone may work effectively for the company.* Many workers are afraid to take a position or ask questions, even when they do not understand the job or what is right or wrong.

   We must break down the class distinctions between types of workers within the organization— physicians, nonphysicians, clinical providers versus nonclinical providers, physician to physician. . . . Cease to blame employees for problems of the system. Management should be held responsible for faults of the system. People need to feel secure to make suggestions.[79]

9. *Break down barriers between departments.* Often, areas compete with one another or have conflicting goals. They do not work as a team to solve or foresee problems. Worse, one department's goals may cause trouble for another department.

10. *Eliminate slogans, exhortations, and targets for the workforce asking for zero defects and new levels of productivity.* "Instead, display accomplishments of the management in respect to assistance to employees to improve their performance."[80]

11. *Eliminate work standards (quotas) on the factory floor.* Quotas that represent measured day work or output alone without regard to quality should be eliminated. "It is better to take aim at rework, error, and defects [all measures of quality], and to focus on [helping] people to do a better job."[81]

12. *Remove barriers that rob the hourly worker of the right to pride of workmanship.* People are eager to do a good job and distressed when they cannot. Too often, misguided supervisors, faulty equipment, and defective materials stand in the way. These barriers must be removed.

13. *Institute a vigorous program of education and self-improvement.* "Institute a massive training program in statistical techniques. Bring statistical techniques down to the level of the individual employee's job, and help him to gather information in a systematic way about the nature of his job."[82] Also, the training "program should keep up with changes in model, style, materials, methods, and if advantageous, new machinery."[83]

14. *Put everyone in the company to work to accomplish the transformation.* As observed by Darr, "taking action to accomplish the transformation . . . will take a special top management team with a plan of action to carry out the quality mission. Workers can't do it on their own, nor can managers."[84]

An interpretation of Deming is useful:

   Quality must become a central focus of the corporation. The emphasis must shift from inspection to prevention. Preventing defects before they occur and improving the process so that defects do not occur are goals for which a company should strive.

   Training and retraining of employees [are] critical to the success of the organization. Deming believes that it is management's job to coach employees. Education and training are investments in people. They help to avoid employee burnout, [reenergize] employees, and give a clear message to employees that management considers employees to be a valuable resource. Finally, Deming also believes that management must pay attention to variability within processes. He advocates systematic understanding of variation and reduction of variation as a strategy to improve processes.

Deming believes that the road to enhanced productivity is through continuous quality improvement called the Deming Chain Reaction. Improving quality through improving processes leads to a reduction of waste, rework, delays, and scrap. This reduction causes productivity as well as quality to improve.[85]

Even in the last years of his life, Deming worked with an intensity improbable for a man his age. He continued his worldwide consulting practice and writing until his death at age 93. At his death, he was working on his last book, *The New Economics,* which was published posthumously. Deming was impatient to see his philosophy and methods implemented in his homeland, where until very late in life, he was, as the aphorism states, "a prophet without honor."

Joseph M. Juran (1905–2008)

Joseph M. Juran, consultant and founder and chairman emeritus of the Juran Institute, is an advocate of total quality management (TQM). In his career, he was an engineer, industrial executive, government administrator, university professor, corporate director, and management consultant.[86] Juran worked at the Hawthorne Works in the mid 1920s,[87] making him a contemporary of Deming's. Juran, too, worked with the Japanese after the war but did so several years later and did not achieve the prominence of Deming.

Juran defined quality as fitness for use, which includes being free from deficiencies and meeting customer needs.[88] Juran's Quality Trilogy is a generic way to think about quality. It is applicable to all functions, levels, and product lines.[89] The quality trilogy's parts are quality planning, quality control, and quality improvement.

> *Quality Planning.* At the initial stage, products and services that will meet customers' needs are developed. Its steps are as follows:
> 1. Determine who the customers are.
> 2. Determine the needs of customers.
> 3. Develop product features that respond to customers' needs.
> 4. Develop the processes that are able to produce those product features.
> 5. Transfer the resulting plans to the operating forces.
>
> *Quality Control.* This activity has three steps:
> 1. Evaluate actual quality performance.
> 2. Compare actual performance to quality goals.
> 3. Act on the differences.
>
> *Quality Improvement.* This is a means of raising quality performance to unprecedented levels ("breakthrough"). The methodology has several steps:
> 1. Establish the infrastructure that is needed to secure annual quality improvement.
> 2. Identify the specific needs for improvement—the improvement projects.
> 3. For each project, establish a project team with clear responsibility for bringing the project to a successful conclusion.
> 4. Provide the resources, motivation, and training that are needed by teams to diagnose the causes, stimulate the establishment of a remedy, and establish controls to hold the gains.[90]

Juran asserted that there is a cost to nonquality, including reworking defective products, scrap, liability from lawsuits, and lost sales from dissatisfied previous customers or customers who purchase competitors' products or services because their quality is better.[91] Figure 7.6 depicts the trilogy, which Juran described as follows:

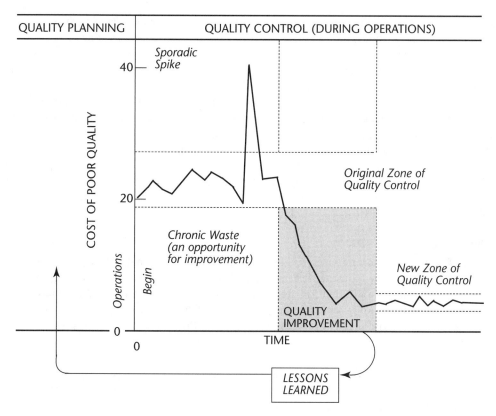

Figure 7.6. Juran quality trilogy. (From Juran, Joseph M. "The Quality Trilogy." *Quality Progress* 19 [August 1986]: 20; reprinted by permission.)

The Juran Trilogy diagram is a graph with time on the horizontal axis and cost of poor quality (quality deficiencies) on the vertical axis. The initial activity is quality planning. The planners determine who are the customers and what are their needs. The planners then develop product and process designs that are able to respond to those needs. Finally, the planners turn the plans over to the operating forces.

The job of the operating forces is to run the processes and produce the products. As operations proceed it soon emerges that the process is unable to produce 100 percent good work. [Figure 7.6] shows that 20 percent of the work must be redone as a result of quality deficiencies. This waste then becomes chronic because the operating process was designed that way.

Under conventional responsibility patterns, operating forces are unable to get rid of that planned chronic waste. What they do instead is carry out quality control—to prevent things from getting worse. Control includes putting out the fires, such as that sporadic spike.

The chart also shows that in due course the chronic waste is driven down to a level far below the level that was planned originally. That gain is achieved by the third process of the trilogy: quality improvement. In effect, it is realized that chronic waste is also an opportunity for improvement, and steps are taken to seize that opportunity.[92]

The third part of the Juran Trilogy uses CQI to improve an existing process (redesigned, if necessary) so that the chronic waste associated with the "original zone of quality control" can be reduced and quality increased. The result is the "new zone of quality control" shown in Figure 7.6.

Juran viewed CQI as seeking and finding opportunities for improvement that result in achieving the new zone. In earlier writings, Juran called this the "breakthrough" zone, consisting of a new and better level of performance and quality. A breakthrough necessitates accepting the premise that current performance is not good enough and can be improved, as well as making an attitudinal change about quality that becomes part of the organization's culture.[93]

Juran described the triple role of the worker shown in Figure 7.1. Workers in a process have three basic functions: being customers by receiving work products that come to them, being processors who add value to the input supplied, and in turn, being suppliers to the customers in the next step in the process. Juran also formulated the criteria that must be present for workers to be in a state of self-control, which allows management to hold the worker, rather than the process, responsible for quality: Workers must have 1) knowledge of what they are supposed to do, 2) knowledge of what they are doing, and 3) the means to regulate what they are doing if they fail to meet goals.[94] Juran guided managers to apply quality control principles in the workplace.

Philip B. Crosby (1926–2001)

Philip B. Crosby was a former vice president of quality at International Telephone and Telegraph and a consultant to many industrial organizations. Crosby emphasized understanding nonquality: "Quality is free. It's not a gift, but it is free. What costs money are the nonquality things—all the actions that involve not doing jobs right the first time."[95] Crosby defined quality as "conformance to requirements" and said that an organization's goal should be to "satisfy the customer first, last, and always."[96]

> Crosby strongly advocates a system of quality improvement that focuses on prevention rather than appraisal. Prevention involves careful understanding of the process and identification of problem areas, followed by improvement of the process.
>
> Crosby strongly advocates the ultimate goal of quality as "Zero Defects" and that a company should constantly strive to achieve this goal. He believes that the best measure of quality is "cost of quality" and that this cost can be divided into two components: the price of nonconformance, and the price of conformance. The price of nonconformance includes the cost of internal failures (i.e., the cost of reinspection, retesting, scrap, rework, repairs, and lost production) and external failures (i.e., legal services, liability, damage claims, replacement, and lost customers). Crosby estimates that an organization's *cost of nonconformance can be as high as 25 to 30 percent of operating costs* [emphasis added]. The price of conformance, on the other hand, includes the cost of education, training, and prevention as well as costs of inspection and testing. An organization must minimize the sum of both costs. The focus on process improvement, error-cause removal, employee training, management leadership, and worker awareness of quality problems are all important tenets.[97]

Crosby emphasized that organizations must identify the hidden costs of poor quality. In health services, malpractice is one such cost. Seven eighths of an iceberg is below the waterline, and Figure 7.7 uses this simile to suggest the visible and hidden costs of poor quality for an HSO/HS. Crosby's goals were "do it right the first time" and the derivative concept of "zero defects."[98] These ultimate quality goals may be unattainable but give important direction to the organization, nevertheless.[99] To move toward improved quality, the HSO/HS must go through a maturation process with respect to a philosophy about quality and then use Crosby's 14 steps of CQI (see below).

Crosby's organizational maturity model includes the stages of uncertainty, awakening, enlightenment, wisdom, and certainty.[100] Enlightenment occurs when management's understanding and attitude about CQI are heightened and it is supportive of and accepts CQI; problems are faced openly

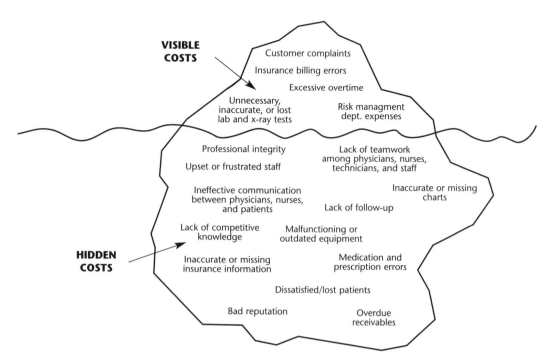

VISIBLE COSTS

Customer complaints

Insurance billing errors

Excessive overtime

Unnecessary, inaccurate, or lost lab and x-ray tests

Risk managment dept. expenses

Professional integrity

Upset or frustrated staff

Lack of teamwork among physicians, nurses, technicians, and staff

Ineffective communication between physicians, nurses, and patients

Inaccurate or missing charts

Lack of follow-up

Lack of competitive knowledge

Malfunctioning or outdated equipment

HIDDEN COSTS

Inaccurate or missing insurance information

Medication and prescription errors

Dissatisfied/lost patients

Bad reputation

Overdue receivables

Figure 7.7. The iceberg of visible and hidden costs of poor quality. (From Carol Greebler, TQM Plus, San Diego, CA, 1989; reprinted by permission.)

and resolved in an orderly manner; and there is implementation of Crosby's 14 steps to quality. Crosby states that in the last stage, certainty, CQI is ingrained in the organization's culture.

Crosby's 14 steps of CQI are not necessarily sequential; many are parallel:

1. Management commitment to and involvement in quality
2. Use of QI teams composed of people with process knowledge and a commitment to action
3. Quality measurement so that areas for improvement can be identified and action can be taken
4. Measuring the cost of quality, meaning the cost of nonquality
5. Quality awareness by all organization members
6. Corrective actions—seek opportunities for improvement
7. Zero defects planning—striving to "do it right the first time"
8. Employee education, with formal orientation at all levels of management (and employees), about the 14 steps
9. Zero Defect Day, which is management's demonstration of its commitment to quality
10. Goal setting—the ultimate is zero defects, but "intermediate goals move in that direction"
11. Error-causal removal, in which people describe problems that prevent error-free work
12. Recognition of those who meet their goals
13. Quality councils composed of quality professionals assisting others in QI
14. Doing it all (Steps 1–13) over again[101]

Crosby stated that his 14-step program is "a systematic way of guaranteeing that organized activities happen the way they are planned."[102] It results in doing the right things the right way and doing them right the first time.

TABLE 7.1. DIFFERENCES AND SIMILARITIES IN THE APPROACHES TO QUALITY OF DEMING, JURAN, AND CROSBY

Dimension	Deming	Juran	Crosby
Definition of quality	A product or service that helps someone and has a good, sustainable market	Fitness for use—free of deficiencies and meeting customer needs	Conformance to requirements, including "satisfy the customer"
Poor quality	Overwhelmingly caused by process, not workers; common cause variation	Caused by poor planning/design (chronic) and sporadic spike (see Figure 7.6, p. 315)	Nonconformance; there are (hidden) costs of nonquality (see Figure 7.7)—quality is free
Quality objective	Error-free (reduce common cause variation); hit target every time	Reduce chronic poor quality and sporadic spike; move to "new zone" of quality control	Zero defects (objective); "do it right the first time"
Customer orientation	Yes, transformation—improve quality (so customers buy products) to improve competitive position (see Figure 7.4, p. 308)	Yes, meet customer needs	Yes, satisfy the customer
General approach to quality	Prospective prevention in all processes, not retrospective inspection; understand and reduce variation through statistical process control; transform organization (change culture)	General management approach; find opportunities for improvement; "breakthrough"; change culture regarding quality	Managerial approach: QI teams, project basis for improvements, move to "certainty" stage, prevention and error-cause removal
Method for quality improvement	14 points for QI	Trilogy (quality planning, quality control, QI)	14 steps to QI
Management responsibility	Commitment to quality control (central focus); cause transformation; establish and perpetuate environment in which quality is integral to work of all employees; don't blame employees; drive out fear; break down barriers; and train, coach, and teach statistical methods to employees	Commitment to quality, especially design; instill quality culture; support operating forces and QI project teams	Commitment, leadership, and involvement in QI; worker training; promote quality awareness by all employees and management

Table 7.1 shows the differences and similarities among Deming, Juran, and Crosby, including their definitions of quality, objectives for CQI, general approaches to quality, methods for CQI, and views of management responsibilities. For Crosby, the journey toward zero defects is attaining and surpassing the enlightenment stages of his organizational maturity model and moving to the certainty stage.

Statistical Process Control

Deming and Juran asserted that poor quality is almost always caused by processes, not by workers. They emphasized use of statistical methods for quality control and to identify process variation.[103] Deming was adamant that variation in processes causes poor quality. There is ample empirical evidence that he was correct. Many consider the world's finest violins to be those crafted by Antonio Stradivari in the 17th and 18th centuries. These instruments were made to a perfect thickness at all parts; the result was an incomparable quality of sound. The seven-time world champion Formula One driver, Michael Schumacher, best known as a driver for Ferrari, determined the fastest line around a race track at practice. During the race, he deviated from that line as little as possible, thus earning him the best time and 91 victories.

For the purposes of SPC, Deming defined variation as "performance within three standard deviations of the mean—a generous amount of variation, although management can set more stringent limits."[104] Depending on the process and the amount of variation in it, HSOs/HSs may set control limits at two standard deviations. However, narrowing control limits risks increasing the number of false positives—common cause variation (caused by unknown factors) that appear to be special cause variation (caused by known factors) but are not. Thus, management may undertake to find the source of the "special cause" variation, which will be impossible because the false positive is actually common cause variation that is, by definition, nonassignable to any source.

Variation within control limits is common cause variation and produced by the process itself. Variation beyond the control limits is special cause variation. Shewhart called this variation "assignable" because it could usually be attributed to a cause from outside the process. Special cause variation can be negative or positive. Reasons for negative special cause variation must be identified and prevented, if possible.[105] Examples are an act of nature, such as a hurricane, or delays in service because of an unanticipated surge in arrivals in the ED. Special cause variation for Juran is the "sporadic spike," which causes the process to not be "in control." Deming and Juran asserted that only processes "in control," meaning those affected by only common cause variation, can be improved. Juran refers to this process improvement as moving to the "new zone of quality control." Deming terms this improving the process by decreasing common cause variation around the mean. For Crosby, it is moving through the organizational maturity stages toward certainty and striving for the goal of "do it right the first time." Deming used control charts to determine whether a process was stable and, therefore, its performance was predictable and process improvement could be undertaken.

The most important reason for process improvement is to reduce common cause variation around the mean in a process that is in statistical control. To be in statistical control means that, in a control chart with control limits of $+/-$ 3 standard deviations, there is a 99.74% probability that the next data point (process output being measured) will fall within the control limits, even though it is impossible to know exactly where within the control limits the data point will fall.

Deming asserted that all processes in control can be improved and that initiatives to reduce variation will result in higher quality, which in turn means improved productivity. Juran called this moving to the new zone of quality control. For Crosby, this is moving toward the goal of zero defects.

▬ Process Improvement Models ▬

CQI uses data to understand the performance of processes. Monitoring data allows managers to identify the parts of a process that will benefit most from improvement efforts. There are many variations on Shewhart's PDSA cycle, but it remains the methodologic core of quality/productivity improvement (Q/PI). One widely used variation has been FOCUS-PDCA, which was developed in the 1980s by for-profit Columbia/HCA (formerly the Hospital Corporation of America).

> (F)ind a process to improve.
>
> (O)rganize a team that knows the process.
>
> (C)larify current knowledge of the process.
>
> (U)nderstand sources of process variation.
>
> (S)elect the process improvement.
>
> (P)lan the improvement.
>
> (D)o the improvement.
>
> (C)heck the effect of the change.
>
> (A)ct to hold the gain.

Data collection is essential to allow managers to monitor and evaluate, to determine if an opportunity for improvement is present, to clarify current knowledge about a process to be improved, to uncover causes of variation, to determine effects of improvement, and to continue monitoring.

In 2005, HRET published *Quality Management for Health Care Delivery* (QMHCD), an evolution of the 1989 Quality Measurement and Management Project research initiative that directly linked CQI to HSOs. QMHCD is a CQI model similar to the FOCUS-PDCA model.[106] The QMHCD emphasizes the need for high quality through a structured approach ultimately affecting competition, quality, and cost and system synergy.[107]

HRET's QMHCD model includes the following:[108]

1. *Find a process that needs improvement.*
2. *Assemble a team that knows the process.* In general, those who understand it best are the employees involved in it. "Through its members, the team must also have an understanding of continuous quality improvement principles, statistical quality control, the use of data management systems, and access to management so that organizational roadblocks to improvement can be overcome."
3. *Identify customers and process outputs, and measure customer expectations* regarding outputs. Different processes have different outputs, and "the team's first task is therefore to list the outputs of the process, identify its customers, and measure expectations of outputs." Customers may be patients, external stakeholders, or an internal downstream process.
4. *Document the process.* A process consists of a series of steps that convert inputs into outputs. They are usually hierarchical; that is, the main process may be broken down into subprocesses, each with subinputs and suboutputs. The hierarchical chain may be followed to that level of detail necessary to understand the process.
5. *Generate output and process specifications.* "A specification is an explicit, measurable statement regarding an important attribute of an output (a customer expectation) or the (sub)process that produces it."
6. *Eliminate inappropriate variation (implement).*

7. *Document continuous improvement (innovate).* The team can select those ideas that seem most promising and then apply them on a test basis within their process. . . . The proposed change can then be discarded, implemented, or modified and tried again, based on the results of the test.

As noted earlier, the QMHCD report credits Deming with providing the framework and inspiration for improvement of quality in health services.[109]

Organizing for Improvement

ROLE OF GOVERNANCE AND SENIOR MANAGERS

The governing body (GB) sets the overall direction of the HSO/HS. In this leadership position, the GB, through senior management, determines the level of commitment to quality and quality improvement. The GB's decisions regarding strategic direction, selection of the chief executive officer (CEO) and approval of other senior leadership, and expectations regarding quality improvement are key. The GB must support its commitment to quality with resources sufficient to ensure success. In addition, the GB sets a moral tone that ultimately affects the organization's culture and its focus on quality. Thus, in Dr. Deming's words, the transformation of the HSO/HS begins at the top. It is there that constancy of purpose and adoption of the new philosophy toward improvement of product and service that are hallmarks of CQI must be found.

Typically, GB members are unlikely to be conversant with quality and performance improvement theory and applications in health services. It rests with the CEO and other senior leadership to educate GB members and instill the commitment to CQI. Failure to educate them as to the long-term commitment needed to transform the organization will cause quality efforts to falter long before they are integral to the organization's culture and are the focus of all that is done. The need to reinforce the GB's commitment cannot be overstated. Special attention should be directed to educating and involving members of the GB's quality committee because it will be most closely linked to operationalizing CQI.

QUALITY IMPROVEMENT COUNCIL

Reporting to the GB's quality committee is the quality improvement council (QIC). The QIC is the implementation arm of Q/PI. The QIC's core membership is typically 12 to 15 and includes senior managers (including medical staff leadership), assorted middle managers, and specialists and consultants in QI. Ad hoc participants are those reporting on QI activities, including service line managers, "owners" of cross-functional processes, department heads, and staff such as those monitoring infectious disease, those doing utilization review, and patient educators.

The QIC's important roles include using customer satisfaction, quality, and performance data to set priorities for improvement efforts; sanctioning and monitoring cross-functional quality improvement teams (QITs); reviewing performance and patient satisfaction data; and setting education and staff involvement goals.

QUALITY IMPROVEMENT TEAMS

There are several types of QITs. The most common and simple are those in functional areas or departments, each of which should have several QITs undertaking internal improvement efforts at any one time. The processes being improved are those almost entirely internal to the functional area and over which the functional area manager has authority. Typically, the process improvements these teams recommend can be approved and implemented by the department head or functional area manager without review by more senior management. Only when other areas are affected or additional resources are required must higher authority be involved. Such efforts are the grassroots of Q/PI.

QITs for processes that cross functional area lines or are interdepartmental must be sanctioned by the QIC. Complex HSOs such as hospitals have scores of cross-functional processes; improving them will provide the greatest return of improved quality and reduced costs. The QIC sanctioning process must identify a process owner, who is usually the manager whose work most depends on the process's performance. Although the process owner will lead the team in its quest for quality improvement, the QIC must be sure that team members are adequately educated to effectively participate. Often, QITs include a facilitator who is part of the HSO's quality resources department. Facilitators meet with the team but are not team members. They assist with group process, application of QI tools, and efficient use of meeting time.

▬ Undertaking Process Improvement ▬▬▬▬▬▬▬▬▬▬▬▬▬

Quality improvement begins by selecting a process to improve and choosing the members of the QIT. Improving quality consumes significant staff time, for both team members and those who provide support. This means that the HSO is best served if high-value processes are improved first. Success in improving simple but important processes—picking the low-hanging fruit—will produce results quickly, demonstrate the value of CQI, and help convince skeptical staff of CQI's usefulness.

Figure 7.8 shows the flow of QI activities. Data sources (many of them outcome indicators) focus the attention of the coordinating body—the QIC, or quality improvement council. The QIC approves formation of cross-functional QITs, or quality improvement teams, to analyze processes and recommend changes to improve them. Intradepartmental QITs are established by departments and monitored by them and by the QIC. In addition, departments may assign individual workers who are process owners to monitor and improve processes. The QIC may have authority to approve major changes and expenditures resulting from QIT recommendations, or CEO and/or GB approval may be required.

QITs

The basic component for undertaking quality improvement is the QIT, sometimes known as a process improvement team (PIT), despite the latter's less than desirable acronym. As noted, QITs may be internal to a function or department or may be cross-functional. The PDSA cycle is the basic methodology applied by the QIT.

QITs are composed of persons who have process knowledge and who can document the process as it functions *currently*. The QIT identifies the key quality characteristic (KQC) of the process—an outcome that can be used to measure quality, such as patient satisfaction, waiting time, or accuracy of medication. Sometimes, there is more than one KQC. Next, the QIT develops an understanding of the process. Flowcharts, also known as flow diagrams or process maps, are used to visualize and understand the process. This visualization must show the process in all its complexity if it is to be useful. Process complexity and the handoffs from one step to the next are common sources of delay, error, and rework. Only by understanding process complexity can one effect improvement.

After the process in all its complexity is understood, data can be collected to determine whether the process is in control, i.e., whether only common cause variation (within 3 standard deviations [*SD*]) is present. A process that is not in control must be brought into control. This means eliminating special cause variation, defined as beyond 3 *SD*, or what Shewhart called assignable variation. Once a process is in control, key process variables (KPVs) can be identified and measured, and the data can be used to determine where to make changes that will help the process meet the KQC(s). The process should be changed in only one way at a time so that the effects of a change can be mea-

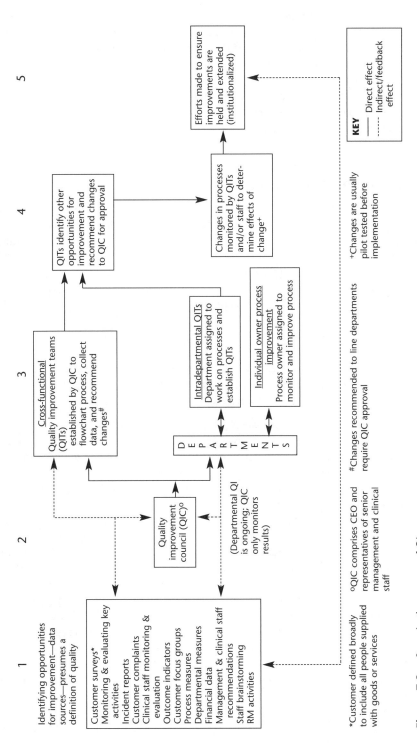

Figure 7.8. Steps in the process of QI.

1

Identifying opportunities for improvement—data sources—presumes a definition of quality

Customer surveys*
Monitoring & evaluating key activities
Incident reports
Customer complaints
Clinical staff monitoring & evaluation
Outcome indicators
Customer focus groups
Process measures
Departmental measures
Financial data
Management & clinical staff recommendations
Staff brainstorming
RM activities

2

Quality improvement council (QIC)°

(Departmental QI is ongoing; QIC only monitors results)

3

Cross-functional
Quality improvement teams (QITs)
established by QIC to flowchart process, collect data, and recommend changes#

D
E
P
A
R
T
M
E
N
T
S

Intradepartmental QITs
Department assigned to work on processes and establish QITs

Individual owner process improvement
Process owner assigned to monitor and improve process

4

QITs identify other opportunities for improvement and recommend changes to QIC for approval

Changes in processes monitored by QITs and/or staff to determine effects of change+

5

Efforts made to ensure improvements are held and extended (institutionalized)

KEY
——— Direct effect
------- Indirect/feedback effect

*Customer defined broadly to include all people supplied with goods or services

°QIC comprises CEO and representatives of senior management and clinical staff

#Changes recommended to line departments require QIC approval

+Changes are usually pilot tested before implementation

sured. Data collected after the change measure the effects of the change. Understanding cause and effect is key to further improvement. A pilot project or experimental design should be utilized so that change(s) in processes used elsewhere in the HSO can be understood before they are implemented generally. For example, changes in a nursing care process should be piloted (tested) in one unit before wider implementation.

Figure 7.3 shows that monitoring and evaluating are key to successful process improvement. Formal sources of data include routine reports, run and control charts, and customer and staff surveys. Informal sources include customer complaints and suggestions solicited from staff. These data must be organized to become information usable for decision making.

▬ Other Improvement Methodologies ▬▬▬▬▬▬▬▬▬

Since the concepts of CQI, including PDSA, were first applied to health services in the 1980s, there have been numerous permutations of its basic content. Some, such as the ISO standards, predate the health services applications but not the basic concepts, such as SPC developed in the 1920s. Others are "old wine in new bottles," meaning that they are posited as more useful or effective than CQI but are primarily repackaged variations on the same theme. This is not to denigrate their usefulness but is only to suggest that basic CQI and its corollaries are intrinsic to them. Someone well versed in the fundamentals of CQI will find a familiar landscape.

LEAN AND SIX SIGMA

The lean concept focuses on reducing waste and eliminating unnecessary steps to increase speed and productivity. The six sigma methodology focuses on reducing variation to improve quality.[110] Typically, lean and six sigma are used as complements.

Lean. The concept of lean is derived from the Toyota production system, or just-in-time production. Lean's antecedents can be traced to Eli Whitney's development of interchangeable parts for musket manufacturing in 1799 and Henry Ford's development of the assembly line for manufacturing the Model T in 1910. Ford may be considered the first practitioner of just-in-time and lean manufacturing. After World War II, Taichi Ohno and Shigeo Shingo began to apply Ford production, SPC, and techniques such as quality circles at Toyota.[111]

The true benefits of lean can only come from strategic planning. A lack of governing body and senior management commitment and knowledge is often to blame for failure of the transformation to lean. Short-term solutions are not the answer,[112] a theme repeatedly sounded by Deming. In health services, the theories of lean can be applied effectively as the concept of lean processes.[113]

Lean's goal is to eliminate activities that do not add value, defined as something for which customers are willing to pay. Lean relies on various methods and tools, including problem-solving diagrams and statistical techniques, to find waste.[114] Typically, waste results from processing, correction, overproduction, motion, material movement, waiting, and inventory. Preventive error proofing is needed because lean implementation frequently results in *reduction* of automation and an increase in manual labor, because for some processes automation is less flexible than an operator performing a variety of tasks. When automation is reduced, the opportunity for error increases even when the work is standardized.[115]

Staff empowerment is integral to lean because as staff decreases, those remaining are challenged to find ways to overcome the deficiency. This approach allows the intellect of staff to be applied in problem solving, encourages buy-in, and allows self-actualization.

Six Sigma. Lean is often a precursor to application of six sigma, which is a statistical description of performance. Some literature combines the two as "lean six sigma." Six sigma originated with the work of mathematician Carl Frederick Gauss (1777–1855), who introduced the concept of the "normal curve." Shewhart (and Deming) used three sigma to distinguish nonassignable from assignable variation and to guide decision making about actions to be taken. The term *six sigma* originated with Motorola engineer Bill Smith (1929–1993) and has been refined since the 1970s into a change-management and data-driven methodology focusing on business excellence.[116] The objective of six sigma is to reduce process output variation so that over the long term, there are no more than 3.4 defects per million opportunities (for defects). As the process sigma value increases from zero to six, the variation of the process around the mean value decreases. With a high enough value of process sigma, the process approaches zero variation and is known as "zero defects." Decreasing process variation will increase the sigma of the process, resulting in higher customer satisfaction and lower costs.[117] A framework to apply six sigma to reduce variation has the acronym DMAIC—for define, measure, analyze, improve, control—a method that is being used in health services.[118]

ISO 9000 AND ISO 14000

The International Organization for Standardization, headquartered in Geneva, Switzerland, began developing voluntary technical standards for almost all sectors of business, industry, and technology in 1947. ISO 9000 and ISO 14000 are two families of generic management systems standards that can be applied in the health services field. *Generic* means that the standards can be applied to any sector of activity, whether product or service based; *management system* means what the organization does to manage its processes or activities. ISO 9000 is concerned with *quality management,* which means what the organization does to enhance customer satisfaction by meeting customer and applicable regulatory requirements and to continually improve its performance. ISO 14000 is primarily concerned with environmental management and what the organization does to minimize harmful effects on the environment caused by its activities and to continually improve its environmental performance.[119] Thus, ISO 9000 and ISO 14000 standards are suitable for HSOs.

Once the standards are implemented, the organization seeks certification and is audited by an independent auditor, who determines whether the management system conforms to the requirements specified in the standard. If the management system conforms, the certification is recorded by the auditing body, which constitutes registration of the management system.[120] Like The Joint Commission accreditation, the ISO 9000–compliant organization has met minimum standards with regard to a quality system. ISO neither carries out certification to its standards nor controls the certification business sector.[121]

ISO 9000 standards do not define quality—the organization does that. However, the 150 guidelines in the standards provide the structure for developing and maintaining a quality system. Organizations that become registered must follow procedures in more than 20 areas, some of which are management responsibility, quality system, process control, inspection and testing, corrective and preventive action, control of quality records, training, and statistical techniques.[122] Customers are aware that the organization is structured to produce consistent results. The organization may extend the quality system requirements backward and require ISO registration of its suppliers to ensure their conformance to requirements.

The eight quality management principles of ISO 9000 in its year 2000 standards are as follows:

1. *Customer focus*. Organizations depend on their customers and therefore should understand current and future customer needs, meet customer requirements, and strive to exceed customer expectations.
2. *Leadership*. Leaders establish unity of purpose and direction of the organization. They should create and maintain the internal environment in which people can become fully involved in achieving the organization's objectives.

3. *Involvement of people.* People at all levels are the essence of an organization, and their full involvement enables their abilities to be used for the organization's benefit.

4. *Process approach.* A desired result is achieved more efficiently when activities and related resources are managed as a process.

5. *System approach to management.* Identifying, understanding, and managing interrelated processes as a system contribute to the organization's effectiveness and efficiency in achieving its objectives.

6. *Continual improvement.* Continual improvement of the organization's overall performance should be a permanent objective of the organization.

7. *Factual approach to decision making.* Effective decisions are based on the analysis of data and information.

8. *Mutually beneficial supplier relationships.* An organization and its suppliers are interdependent, and a mutually beneficial relationship enhances the ability of both to create value.[123]

By the late 1990s, registration to ISO 9000 standards had made few inroads into the predominant position in health services accreditation enjoyed by The Joint Commission. In 2005, it was estimated that only 150 U.S. hospitals were ISO certified.[124] This is likely to change with increased recognition of ISO standards in the health services field. The consulting firm TUV Healthcare Specialists has applied for deeming status from the Centers for Medicare and Medicaid Services, using ISO standards. If TUV obtains deeming status, being registered to ISO standards through TUV will make HSOs eligible to receive Medicare reimbursement.[125] This alternative will challenge The Joint Commission as the preeminent voluntary accrediting body for HSOs and have far-reaching implications for the health services field.

REENGINEERING

Reengineering is more technique, less philosophy, and can complement CQI. It is "plan" in the PDSA cycle, and quality planning in the Juran Trilogy. CQI and reengineering share an orientation toward process, a dedication to improvement, and the dogma that one begins with the customer.[126] Reengineering is another approach in the continuum of improvement that builds on the principles and tools of CQI.[127] It includes additional features—radical change and process redesign.

Hammer and Champy defined reengineering as "the fundamental rethinking and radical redesign of business processes to achieve dramatic improvements in critical, contemporary measures of performance such as costs, quality, service, and speed."[128] Sometimes termed "process innovation" or "core process redesign,"[129] reengineering as applied to health services seeks fundamental and radical change in processes and in how healthcare is arranged and delivered, including time and place.[130]

Outward-In, Right to Left. Creating quality and enhancing competitive position require an outward-in orientation. To obtain the high-quality service that enhances competitive position, HSOs/HSs must work backward, thinking right to left, to improve processes. The CQI model in Figure 7.3 focuses on market changes and customer needs that result in an enhanced competitive position [5]. This is done through quality outcomes that conform to requirements and meet or exceed customer expectations [4]. CQI changes existing processes incrementally to improve quality.[131] Sometimes, a change in customers' needs or in competition causes a performance gap.

> If the world has changed dramatically since the process was (or most recently [was]) redesigned, the current design may be fundamentally flawed and incapable of delivering the required performance. Reengineering is then called for. Reengineering does not merely enhance the individual steps of the process but entirely reconsiders how they are put together.[132]

The transition from inpatient to outpatient care in HSOs,[133] including support mechanisms, apparatus, facilities, and staffing, is an example of a radical change in the process of patient care delivery. Formation of HSs is an example of redesigning integration and delivery of care among entities. Prospective pricing and managed care required rethinking how HSOs/HSs do business, because of a fundamental shift that increased the bargaining power of the payer.

Elements. The critical elements of reengineering are

1. Outside-in, customer focus, putting the organization in the shoes of the customers to understand and meet their needs
2. Focus on cross-functional end-to-end processes, versus intradepartmental processes
3. Understanding of processes and customer requirements, leading to recognition of the weaknesses of the existing process and the performance requirements of the new one[134]
4. Articulated vision of where the HSO/HS wants to be in the future, with that vision communicated and understood by all organization members
5. Top-down rather than bottom-up leadership initiated with committed senior-level management who elicit and obtain acceptance by process owners
6. Identification and questioning of underlying assumptions about processes
7. Design of new processes, including piloting (small-scale use) to see if they work, and redesigning and rolling out the new processes in rapid fashion
8. An organizational environment that supports reengineering, including communication throughout the organization, supportive leader personal behavior, measurements, rewards, and "selling the new way of working and living to the organization as a whole"[135]

Additional elements to be implemented are senior management's commitment to and championing of the reengineering effort; identification of process owners—those with direct interest in and responsibility for processes—and empowering them to initiate change; formation of reengineering teams—groups that diagnose existing processes, oversee their redesign, and implement new processes; and use of a steering committee—"a policy-making body of senior managers who develop the organization's overall reengineering strategy and monitor its progress."[136]

What Reengineering Is Not (Reengineering and CQI). A major criticism of reengineering is that it is downsizing, a term that encompasses cost reduction strategies of reducing labor costs, outsourcing work previously done in-house, replacing permanent employees with temporary employees,[137] or discontinuing programs or services. Reengineering can be differentiated by what it is not. It is not automating, restructuring or downsizing, or reorganizing, de-layering, or flattening the organization. However, these results often occur with use of the "clean sheet of paper" radical, cross-functional redesign with a customer focus. Further, reengineering is not the same as CQI. "Quality improvement seeks steady incremental improvement to process performance. Reengineering . . . seeks breakthroughs, not by enhancing existing processes, but by discarding and replacing them with entirely new ones."[138]

CQI improves processes and performance on a consistent upward slope. At some point, however, performance gaps, such as diminished or weakened competitive position and changed customer needs and demands, necessitate replacement of some processes through reengineering, which may be conceptualized as a step increase, rather than a slope. Once reengineering occurs, CQI—improvement of the new, redesigned process—continues until external forces require another breakthrough change. This relationship is similar to the Juran Quality Trilogy of quality planning (reengineering), quality control (preparatory to CQI), and quality improvement (CQI).

The triggers or drivers of reengineering efforts may include a strategy of retrenchment because the HSO/HS no longer has a competitive advantage or market strength for a program or service (see

Chapter 8); because of limited resources that can be more effectively allocated to other existing or new services; or because of changing needs of patients/customers, including shifts in market demand or composition. Examples include a decision to exit a product or service line, based on assessment of external threats and opportunities and internal strengths and weaknesses, or a situation in which the HSO/HS cannot maintain or cannot attain a comparative advantage. Reengineering as the organization's response to a changing marketplace can be viewed as strategic in nature, whereas CQI is tactical.[139]

Applications. Various reengineering applications in HSOs/HSs are described in the literature. Among them are service decentralization, clinical resource management, patient aggregation, skill-mix changes, and alterations to noncore processes. In their research based on interviews with 255 senior managers, physicians, and staff at 14 hospitals, Walston and Kimberly found that service decentralization occurred in 13 of the HSOs examined. They reported that ancillary services such as respiratory therapy, physical therapy, and dietary, laboratory, and radiology services were segmented departments in hospitals. To decrease multiple patient handoffs and "throwing services over the wall" to other departments, which resulted in scheduling complications and increased waiting time, a redesign was undertaken that resulted in initiating responsibility for some support services, such as phlebotomy and respiratory services, on the nursing unit. "Housekeeping, dietary, and EKGs were often combined into new patient services positions titled patient care associates, patient care partners, or support partners."[140] Clinical resource management initiatives involved the creation of clinical protocols to lessen treatment variation and to provide a day-to-day schedule for each different type of patient by diagnosis using physician "best practices." Only modest success was reported, however.[141]

Patient aggregation and redesign involves combining patients who require similar skills and resources. After examination of historical admitting locations of patients, the reallocation of beds by specialty and aggregation of patients with common resource needs will result in better care. Homogeneous patient populations requiring similar clinical resources enable dedicated delivery teams to enhance their skills, provide for coordination and continuity of care, decrease unnecessary clinical variation, and enhance outcomes of quality and customer satisfaction.[142] Skill-mix changes reported included using nursing assistants rather than licensed practical nurses and also abandoning primary care nursing. Nonpatient care reengineering examples were increasing charge capturing, improving materials contracts, and modifying employee benefits.[143]

Finally, although advocates of reengineering indicate that downsizing and de-layering are not its focus, Walston and Kimberly report "it was our experience that downsizing through layoffs was specifically a focus of many executives,"[144] in part because of situations of decreased inpatient census and diminished competitive position. Others are critical of reengineering, citing its use to absolve HSOs from blame if layoffs are perceived negatively.[145]

Facilitators and Barriers to Improvement

Change is threatening. CQI and PI require change, and managers must recognize the necessity of change if improvement is to occur. Resistance to change may be political in nature, or it may come from those who will be adversely affected, have low tolerance for change and prefer the status quo, or are unconvinced that change is needed. Resistance may be overt and explicit or covert and indirect. Managers should uncover resistance to change, understand the motivation, provide incentives for accepting and disincentives for not accepting change, and deal with people's concerns.[146]

Vision, organizational philosophy, senior-level management commitment, physician participation, process design and implementation, and performance measures will help ensure success. Complete and open communication lessens fear and dispels uncertainty; employee involvement can lead to co-optation and accepting ownership. Chapter 8 discusses resistance as a natural reaction to

TABLE 7.2.   REENGINEERING FACILITATORS AND BARRIERS

Facilitators	Barriers
Establish and maintain a constant, consistent vision	Lack of continuity of vision/purpose Disconnection of vision with environment
Prepare smooth transitions for the reengineering effort	Poor transition between project phases Planning to implementation Implementation to a continued process
Prepare and train for reengineering changes	Inadequate administrative skills Inadequate clinical/technical skills
Establish continual, multiple communication methods	Historical practices Lack of continuity of communication Little or inadequate feedback Perceived dishonest communication
Establish strong support and involvement	Inconsistent support and involvement Lack of consistent and even administrative support Lack of equitable departmental participation
Establish mechanisms to measure reengineering's progress and outcomes	Inability to measure progress Complexity of changes without understanding causal mechanisms
Effectively establish both new authority and responsibility relationships	Inadequate authority/responsibilities assigned
Find methods to involve physicians	Lack of time and interest

From Walston, Stephen L., and John R. Kimberly. "Reengineering Hospitals: Evidence from the Field." *Hospital & Health Services Administration* 42 (Summer 1997): 153; reprinted by permission from Health Administration Press.

change. Table 7.2 shows facilitators and barriers to reengineering. This depiction mirrors facilitators and barriers to CQI initiatives.

Improvement and Problem Solving

Process improvement problem solving uses the problem-solving model in Figure 6.4. Conditions that initiate problem solving are deviation (actual results inconsistent with desired results), crisis, opportunity or threat, and improvement (see Figure 6.3). As with the other categories, problem solving under the condition of improvement involves 1) problem analysis, including stating the problem, 2) developing assumptions, 3) identifying tentative alternative solutions, 4) developing and applying decision criteria, 5) selecting the alternative that best fits the criteria, 6) implementing the solution chosen, and 7) evaluating the solution. Postchange performance is compared with the results desired.

The PDSA cycle is conceptually similar to the steps of problem solving. CQI can also involve problem solving under the condition of deviation, as when special cause variation is investigated. However, CQI enhances performance primarily by improving processes. The situation analysis step is different when the problem-solving model is applied to opportunities for improvement. It involves collecting and evaluating data about a process that is "in control" so that improvement opportunities can be identified. The purpose is to make the acceptable better. Improvement problem solving for Deming is reducing common cause variation; for Juran, moving a process to the new zone of quality control; and for Crosby, moving toward the goal of doing it right the first time.

The discussion in Chapter 6 of making assumptions states that narrow, overly restrictive structural, personal, and problem-centered assumptions result in lower-quality solutions. Less adequate solutions result because restrictive assumptions limit the range of alternatives that can be considered. The same concern arises in process improvement.

The advantages of group problem solving discussed in Chapter 6 are even more applicable to process improvement. The participation of persons with process knowledge is essential for a QIT to be effective.[147] In addition, QIT members learn new tasks and become aware of others' problems and more attuned to the triple role of customer, processor, and supplier. Team members are likely to be more eager to assist each other in solving problems, team spirit will develop, and motivation and a sense of worth will be enhanced.[148] An important benefit, especially for cross-functional QITs, is that staff will more clearly see how their work fits into the whole system of delivering services and how what they do can optimize the system.

Management must show its commitment to CQI by allocating resources for education, staff, and software, implementing a participative philosophy, and encouraging employee team building. Deming, Juran, and Crosby advocated giving employees the authority to act. Others call it empowerment.[149] The knowledge of QIT team members allows systematic dissection of a process so it can be fully understood, as requisite to improvement.

▬ Tools for Improvement ▬▬▬▬▬▬▬▬▬▬▬▬▬▬▬▬▬▬▬▬▬

CONTROL CHARTS

Control charts are essential to SPC and successful Q/PI. The theoretical basis supporting the importance of control charts was presented above in the discussion of SPC. Control charts are essential to being able to distinguish common cause variation from special cause variation, an ability indispensable to effectively managing. Special cause variation *cannot be identified* only by looking at a set of numbers, even if arrayed on a run chart. Control limits must be calculated.

Run charts are a simple data collection tool. Figure 7.9 is a run chart of data reflecting performance on one aspect of inpatient food service on a nursing unit. Run chart data are used to calculate the standard deviation. As noted above, 3 *SD* are commonly used in SPC. Drawn on the run chart, the upper and lower control limits of 3 *SD* transform it into a control chart such as Figure 7.10. Thus, the process itself establishes the limits that distinguish common cause from special cause variation. As a corollary, it is wrong to set an arbitrary number that the process (and its workers) is expected to produce. Process capability—the capacity of the process—is inherent in it and necessarily limits performance of the process.

Both run charts and control charts array data on two axes: The vertical axis is the performance being measured; the horizontal axis shows time. Control charts can be used to monitor any process, such as customer waiting time in patient admitting, units of laboratory output, or utilization of diagnostic equipment.

The control chart in Figure 7.10 shows that the average time between when noon meal food trays leave the kitchen and receipt of a tray by the first patient on unit 2W is 28 minutes. There is wide common cause variation around the mean, however, with a range of 23 to 35 minutes. This process is not "in control," because there are four special cause variation data points—two well below the lower control limit (LCL) and two well above the upper control limit (UCL). As a first step, SPC requires that the process be brought "in control" by investigating special causes of variation to determine their sources. Delivery times of 40 minutes will almost certainly diminish customer satisfaction. Negative special causes should be identified and eliminated, if possible, or if not, their effects on the process must be minimized. Positive special cause variation is present in delivery times that were much shorter than the mean of 28 minutes. Early delivery times are not necessarily better, because nurses and patients might not be ready. They do, however, show that faster delivery is possible. Reasons for the positive special cause variation should be identified and, if possible, should be incorporated into the process because it is almost certain that food delivered sooner will be more palatable and, therefore, of higher quality. Once the process is "in control," process improvement can be undertaken to reduce variation around the mean and, if desirable, move the mean toward a shorter delivery time.

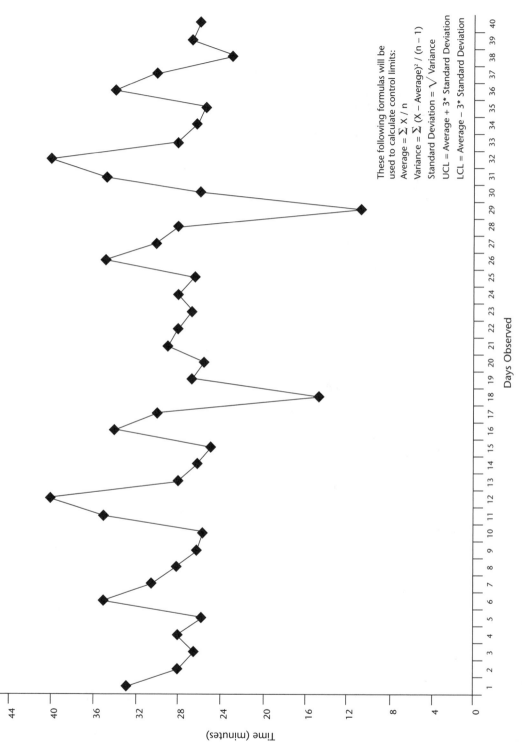

Figure 7.9. Run Chart: Time elapsed between noon meal food trays leaving kitchen and first patient receiving tray on unit 2W, by day, in minutes. Source for formulas: Dunn, Oliver Jean. *Basic Statistics: A Primer for the Biomedical Sciences.* New York City: John Wiley & Sons, Inc., 1964, 38.

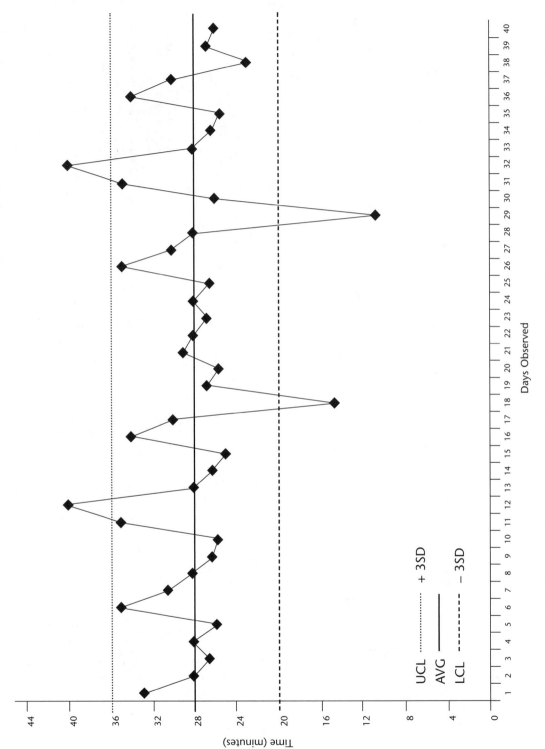

Figure 7.10. Control Chart: Time elapsed between noon meal food trays leaving kitchen and first patient receiving tray on unit 2W, by day, in minutes.

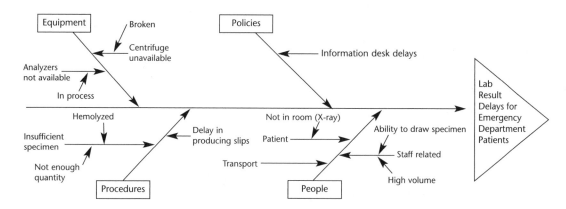

Figure 7.11. A fishbone, or cause-and-effect, diagram examining reasons for delays in laboratory test results for emergency department patients. The fishbone diagram is drawn after a brainstorming session. The central problem is visualized as the head of the fish, with the skeleton divided into branches showing contributing causes of different parts of the problem. (From Merry, Martin D. "Total Quality Management for Physicians: Translating the New Paradigm." *Quality Review Bulletin* 16 [March 1990]: 102; reprinted by permission. Copyright 1990 by Joint Commission Resources.)

Because nursing is involved in delivering trays to patients, one KPV will be predictability. If nurses know that trays will arrive within a narrow range of variation, they can be ready to serve them to patients. This will invariably lead to greater customer satisfaction. In this process, both nurses and patients are customers.

FISHBONE, OR ISHIKAWA, DIAGRAM

Often, a QIT's first step is to brainstorm perceived causes of problems in a process and develop a cause-and-effect diagram like that shown in Figure 7.11. The cause-and-effect diagram is also known as the fishbone diagram, because of its shape, or the Ishikawa diagram, after its originator Kaoru Ishikawa. An effect is a desirable or undesirable situation, condition, or event produced by a system of causes. Figure 7.11 shows reasons for laboratory test delays for patients in an ED. Primary process variables (components) are shown by the long arrows; minor process variables are shown by the short arrows and are elements of the primary variables. Brainstorming to identify the problems in a process suggests the directions for collecting confirmatory data, which, in turn, will suggest the solutions to the problem(s).

PARETO ANALYSIS

Another contribution of Juran was discovering the work of an Italian economist, Vilfredo Pareto. Often cited as separating the "vital few" from the "trivial many," Juran came to realize that the many are still useful and cannot be ignored.[150] Also known as the 80/20 rule, the Pareto principle is commonly applied in marketing where, for example, 80% of sales are derived from 20% of products or services. In QI, it means that 80% of defects—errors, delays, rework, and the like—are typically caused by 20% of the variables in a process. Applied to a hospital operating rooms (OR) schedule, Pareto analysis might find that 80% of delays are caused by 20% of surgeons. The 80/20 ratio is neither fixed nor magical; rather, it helps decision makers understand relationships. Pareto analysis can show the relative importance of variables in a process and their contributions to a result, thus assisting to develop priorities in CQI. The Pareto diagram in Figure 7.12 shows that physicians' untimed

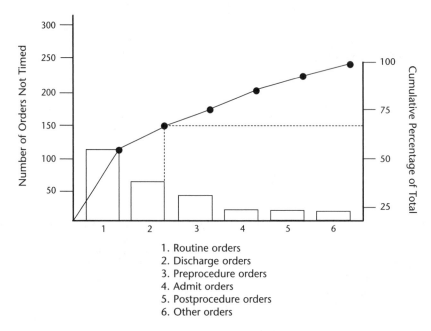

1. Routine orders
2. Discharge orders
3. Preprocedure orders
4. Admit orders
5. Postprocedure orders
6. Other orders

Figure 7.12.   Pareto diagram showing the rank order of untimed physicians' orders in a major hospital. This diagram ranks classes of orders that failed to be timed with a plot line showing that the correction of the first two classes of orders would lead to a greater than 50% improvement in all untimed orders. (From Re, Richard N., and Marie A. Krousel-Wood. "How to Use Continuous Quality Improvement Theory and Statistical Quality Control Tools in a Multispecialty Clinic." *Quality Review Bulletin* 16 [November 1990]: 394; reprinted by permission. Copyright 1990 by Joint Commission Resources.)

routine and discharge orders are the two areas in which most improvement can occur. QITs should focus there.

SCATTER DIAGRAMS

Scatter diagrams, also known as scatter plots, show the relationship between two variables. Figure 7.13 depicts the relationship between the number of coronary artery bypass grafting (CABG) surgeries per year on the horizontal axis and the percent of operated patients who died (mortality)—a strong indication of quality—on the vertical axis. The data show an inverse relationship between mortality and the number of CABG procedures. The learning, or experience, curve for surgeons and staff is often cited as the reason for this relationship.

The statistical technique of least squares linear regression can be applied to scatter diagrams to show a "best fit line." UCLs and LCLs are calculated using the variation of data points from the best fit line. Control limits of 3 *SD* mean that there is a 99.74% confidence level that a data point beyond the UCL or LCL is not due to chance alone. Figure 7.13 shows one data point above the UCL and two below the LCL. These points comprise Deming's special cause variation, Juran's sporadic spike, and Shewhart's assignable cause. All three data points showing special cause variation are of interest. The cause of the data point above the UCL should be determined so that recurrence of this undesirable result can be prevented. Data points below the LCL should be investigated to understand why these positive results occurred so they can be studied and replicated to the extent possible. For example, a surgical team with superior results (positive special cause variation) should be studied and the lessons applied to other surgical teams. Positive special cause variation may result from input dif-

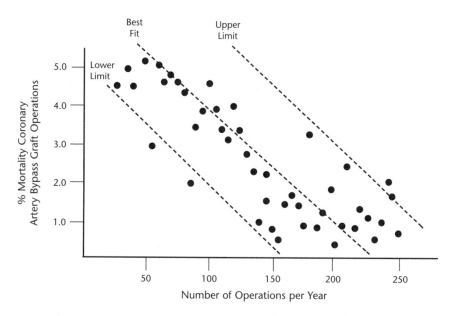

Figure 7.13. Scatter diagram used to determine a possible relationship between two variables: the mortality rate for a surgical procedure and the number of times the procedure is performed during a 12-month period. Each dot represents one surgical team. (From Merry, Martin D. "Total Quality Management for Physicians: Translating the New Paradigm." *Quality Review Bulletin* 16 [March 1990]: 103; reprinted by permission. Copyright 1990 by Joint Commission Resources.)

ferences such as surgeons' skills and training or the acuity levels of patients operated. Or, the process of performing the surgery may be the cause of positive special cause variation.

FAILURE MODE EFFECTS ANALYSIS

Failure mode effects analysis (FMEA) was developed by the National Aeronautics and Space Administration (NASA), the civilian agency of federal government responsible for space travel. The complexities of NASA's systems required a technique to identify the root causes of potential problems so that those causes could be designed out of processes or processes could be modified to prevent them from occurring. FMEA is proactive because it prevents problems—the failure mode—from occurring when the process becomes operational. This makes FMEA part of Juran's quality planning. FMEA is commonly applied after problems have arisen, too.

FMEA is generally applicable to HSOs. It uses a template that enables team members to work through the failure mode and its effects. After identifying a service feature or a process, the team brainstorms to identify potential failure modes, potential effects of each failure, the severity rating for each failure, potential causes of failure, likelihood of the failure occurring, and likelihood of detection by current process controls; finally, the team assigns priority numbers to identify the issues that should receive most attention. The second half of the template addresses how the potential problems will be prevented.[151] Applications of FMEA in health services have included the blood product transfusion process.

CREW RESOURCE MANAGEMENT

Crew resource management (CRM) is a generalized application of cockpit resource management, a concept developed jointly by the Federal Aeronautics Administration and the airline industry in the

1980s to enhance the quality of responses to emergencies involving the crews of commercial aircraft. The study of human factors in aviation emphasizes the role of human beings in high-stress, high-risk environments. An estimated 80% of airplane accidents are caused by human factors. The purpose of CRM is to develop techniques and procedures to catch mistakes before they cause problems.[152] The similarities between the cockpit of a commercial aircraft and a hospital's OR or ED are striking. CRM can be applied to any area in which a team provides care.[153] Since the late 1990s, CRM has been applied in hospital EDs, ORs, and intensive care units. Unlike CQI, CRM is not data driven.

CRM seeks to enhance patient safety and quality of care by improving teamwork through better cooperation, coordination, and communication. Techniques include presurgical briefings, preoperative assessments, and methods to ensure that handoffs from one part of the process or staff member to another are effective. These safety measures (tools) ensure the staff's daily use of the teamwork and communication skills learned in the training classes. The purpose is to achieve a permanent change in behavior.[154] Specific examples of applying safety tools in the OR include the OR time out, which requires confirming vital information about a patient, and surgical site verification, which confirms the surgical site before surgery begins and may include asking a patient to state what is to be done.

Hospitals that have applied CRM report significant positive results, including lower costs of malpractice, higher staff satisfaction levels and less turnover, and far fewer "wrong" surgeries— wrong patient, wrong site, wrong device.[155] The evidence of CRM's value remains anecdotal, however, and it has been argued that while CRM is worth further investigation in healthcare, it is too soon to conclude that it can reduce medical errors.[156] Others have raised questions about the extent of behavior change[157] and the link between attitudes about teamwork and patient outcomes.[158]

BENCHMARKING

Organizationwide or macro-level data collection permits management to prioritize the order in which processes will be improved. Micro- or process improvement–level data collection enables QITs to measure process variables, which is requisite to improvement. Benchmarking allows comparisons by providing norms, standards, and measures for various processes and outcomes such as patient admitting, customer satisfaction, quality of care, and financial performance.

There are several types of benchmarking. Internal benchmarking compares similar activities or processes within the HSO. External benchmarking compares the HSO's performance with similar activities and processes in comparable organizations both in and outside health services. Competitive benchmarking involves comparisons with competitors who provide the same service in similar markets. Its most aggressive application identifies the "best patient outcomes for each service measured by such factors as mortality rates, nosocomial (HSO-acquired) infections, [and] patient mobility" as well as the practice patterns and resource consumption profiles of competitors.[159] World-class benchmarking compares the HSO/HS to organizations in or outside the health services industry that excel in similar processes. Examples common to a wide variety of organizations are order fulfillment, supplier relations, and billing and collection processes.[160]

It must be understood that benchmarks are only guidelines. Achieving the same results as a world-class performance benchmark, for example, requires that the HSO have an exact replica of everything that is present in the benchmark organization, including its culture. Regardless, knowing what can be accomplished might stimulate the HSO to achieve higher quality or even to achieve at a level higher than the benchmark.

Benchmarking includes determining what to benchmark, collecting internal and external data, and applying the conclusions reached to improve existing processes. Examples of processes that HSOs benchmark are admitting, billing, patient transport, and surgical scheduling and OR use. Control is another application of data obtained about other HSOs/HSs. Chapter 10 identifies databases that contain peer organization performance and financial outcomes and resource consumption data.

The data provide comparative benchmarks for "best in class" performance and allow HSOs/HSs to understand the extent to which improvement in competitive position is possible, if resources are adequate. Chapter 8 considers external environmental analysis that enables the HSO to attain and sustain competitive position by knowing its competitors' performance levels.

Productivity and Productivity Improvement

Cost-efficiency and PI result from CQI. Figure 7.3 suggests that process improvement [2] leads to higher quality outputs [3], which lead to PI and better resource use [4] and, thus, enhanced competitive position [5]. The Deming Chain Reaction shown in Figure 7.4 connects improved quality, decreased costs, improved productivity, and the organization's ability to decrease prices, increase market share, and stay in business. CQI and PI are integral and inseparable. Similarly, input resource costs and quality are conjoined with output quality; neither can be considered in isolation from the other.

Productivity is the index of outputs relative to inputs.[161] Alternatively, productivity is the results achieved relative to resources consumed:[162]

$$\text{Productivity} \quad = \quad \frac{\text{Outputs}}{\text{Inputs}} \quad = \quad \frac{\text{Results achieved}}{\text{Resources consumed}}$$

Productivity is increased by any change that increases the ratio of outputs to inputs, which is achieved by altering either the conversion process (structure, tasks/technology, people; see Figure 5.8) or the inputs. For example, fewer nurses caring for the same number of patients increases productivity: fewer inputs, same output. More radiographic procedures per day with the same staff and equipment has the same result. However, while increasing productivity (output) without maintaining or enhancing the level of quality (defined as conformance to requirements and patient satisfaction) may lead to higher output, the lower quality of this higher output actually causes a diminution in productivity because it results in errors, rework, and dissatisfaction of customers and staff. Producing poor quality radiographs or performing unnecessary radiographic procedures (nonconformance output) is not productivity improvement. Neither is decreasing the number of surgical assistants and increasing patient and physician wait times, because they lessen customer satisfaction. productivity improvement occurs only when the index ratio of outputs to inputs increases and conformance and expectation quality is maintained or enhanced. This is denoted in the following formula:[163]

$$\text{Productivity improvement} \quad = \quad \frac{\text{Outputs}}{\text{Inputs}} \quad = \quad \frac{\text{Quantity}}{\text{Inputs}} + \text{Quality} \quad = \quad \frac{\text{Results achieved}}{\text{Resources consumed}}$$

CQI AND PI

Figure 7.14 shows the relationship of the PI triangle to CQI. PI occurs only when lowest costs (inputs) are consistent with appropriate quality (outputs). The original *Quality Measurement and Management Project* report called this the "value of healthcare."[164] Because PI focuses on the relationship of inputs and costs to outputs and quality, both inputs and processes are investigated in PI, as they are in CQI.

HSOs are service organizations that have high levels of customer interaction. Some, such as acute care hospitals, must have flexible capacity to meet surges in demand. At the other end of the spectrum, HSOs such as nursing facilities have little need for flexible capacity because their customers are usually long-term residents and occupancy is commonly near 100%.

CQI focuses on improving processes (see Figure 7.8), which necessitates evaluating inputs. For example, the QIT may determine that higher quality will result from a process if better-skilled employees are recruited or if employees are cross-trained so work assignments can be more flexible

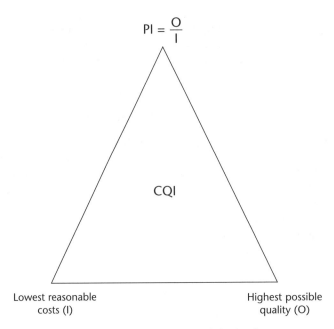

Figure 7.14.   Productivity improvement (PI) triangle.

as workloads change. Enhancing technology inputs can improve work systems and substitute equipment for people. Magnetic resonance imaging improves clinical diagnosis, and personal computers enhance accuracy and productivity in billing and admitting. Other techniques may be used to add efficiency to inputs: increasing the quality of materials and supplies by working closely with suppliers (Deming advocates developing long-term relationships with suppliers and even suggests that sole-source suppliers will improve quality); using a just-in-time inventory system to eliminate inventory other than that needed for safety stock; and using ABC inventory analysis,[165] which is similar to Pareto analysis, to identify the supplies that are most expensive or critical and that require special attention. Management information systems provide data for control and utilization evaluation; successful forecasting enables managers to anticipate demand and alter capacity. Use of work measurement to monitor employee utilization and workloads and information from a patient acuity classification system permits efficient nurse staffing patterns.

Productivity may be improved in numerous ways other than by analyzing inputs. Examination of a process or work system in a CQI framework should ask questions such as Is what we do really necessary? Are we doing the right things? Can the work be done in another way with the same or better quality? How are the work results of one job interdependent with other jobs, materials, or processes? Can we improve the process with a different mix of resources that will improve quality, decrease costs, or both? These questions can be answered by the following methods: 1) analysis and improvement of work systems and job design; 2) capacity planning and facilities layout; and 3) production control, scheduling, and supply chain. Inputs are integral to each. These methods are described in the following sections.

WORK SYSTEMS AND JOB DESIGN

Analysis and improvement of work systems and job design are integral to CQI process improvement and will lead to PI. The basic objectives are to find better ways to work in general, improve specific jobs in particular, and increase the ratio of quality relative to costs—with the same, fewer, or a less costly mix of inputs.

Work systems (processes) are interrelated jobs that form an integrated whole. Hospitals, for example, have hundreds of systems and subsystems: nonpatient care systems include admitting, discharge, accounts receivable and accounts payable, transportation, inventorying and distributing material, patient food delivery, and medication order fulfillment; direct patient care systems include nursing service, clinical support services (e.g., laboratory, radiology, and respiratory therapy), and therapeutic activities such as perioperative services. Analysis of a system can be exclusive (how it functions) or inclusive (how it interrelates with other systems). The purpose is to improve systems to enhance output quality and productivity. Process and methods analyses are techniques used to evaluate systems.[166] In health services, processes are the series of operations, steps, or activities through which patients, material, or information flow. Documenting this flow permits evaluation of each activity in the sequence,[167] which allows deciding whether altering the flow, combining or eliminating operations, or methods redesign will result in higher quality outputs and PI.[168] As noted, one of the first activities of a QIT is to prepare a flow diagram (process map) of the process.

Figure 7.15 is a flowchart (flow diagram) that outlines the process used to implement physicians' orders. Understanding the steps in a process will show that improvements may be made by

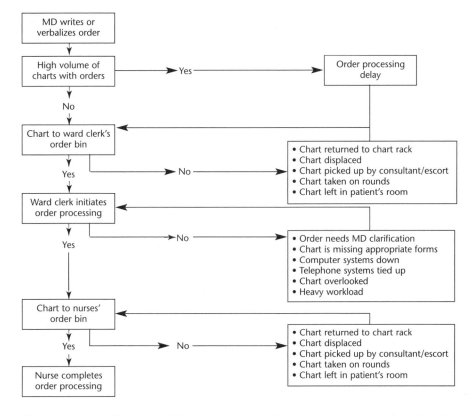

Figure 7.15. Flowchart outlining the initial steps in implementing physicians' orders, clearly identifying points of consumer–producer interchange (e.g., the interaction of physician and ward clerk) and sites of possible system failure or delay. (From Re, Richard N., and Marie A. Krousel-Wood. "How to Use Continuous Quality Improvement Theory and Statistical Quality Control Tools in a Multispecialty Clinic." *Quality Review Bulletin* 16 [November 1990]: 393; reprinted by permission. Copyright 1990 by Joint Commission Resources.)

eliminating bottlenecks, delays, or even steps. Flow analysis is used for processes with high customer interaction, to indicate where and how interactions may be enhanced or lessened, whichever is likely to result in higher patient satisfaction.

HSO work systems are interdependent, and multisystem process flow analysis is necessary to identify areas for improvement. For example, timely reading and reporting of test (radiology, electrocardiography, electroencephalography, and laboratory) results positively affect patient care and shorten lengths of stay; delayed reading or reporting negatively affects patient care and increases lengths of stay. Knowledge about and improvement of system or process outputs that become inputs elsewhere in the HSO positively affect productivity.

Methods analysis involves evaluating how work is done—the specific operations, steps, or activities performed. Such analyses include evaluating appropriateness of the operations, steps, or activities; considering alternative inputs, such as personnel and equipment substitution or redesigning jobs; or evaluating information flow and the media used.

At a micro level, job design improvement evaluates the tasks in a job or a cluster of jobs that constitute an operation or activity in a process. Included are the sequence of job tasks, design of physical layout, and employee–machine relationships, including with equipment, material, and supplies used. Job design improvement or a variant—work simplification—is used to eliminate unnecessary tasks, reduce time between tasks, reallocate tasks among different jobs, combine jobs, or centralize common tasks in one job, that is, use specialization.

Finally, work simplification, which involves dividing work into specific tasks and making it easier, is a way to evaluate and improve jobs and enhance work results. User friendly, menu-driven computers in the admissions department enable employees to admit patients faster and with greater accuracy; both improvements increase quality as well as productivity.

CAPACITY PLANNING AND FACILITIES LAYOUT

Facilities analysis is an important dimension of process improvement. It focuses on the physical aspects of a process, the need for flexibility in meeting variable demand, and balancing timeliness of service and idle resources. Facility layout is the arrangement of equipment and work areas. Facilities, process flow, equipment, and workstations may be rearranged to improve sequence and flow, decrease unnecessary worker movement and material transportation, eliminate bottlenecks and congestion, and yield faster patient throughput. Layout analysis can be accomplished by using drawings, proximity charts, templates, or three-dimensional models. Computer simulation can be used to design the physical layout of a facility within predetermined constraints and assumptions.

The analysis of traffic patterns and material flows consists of observing and recording movement to decrease travel, eliminate or reduce delays, or substitute alternate material handling or delivery methods. For example, the analysis of traffic patterns may reveal that restricting the use of certain elevators to patients, staff, and movement of equipment reduces delays in clinical activities. Similarly, a materials and supplies flow analysis may justify an exchange cart system to improve logistics, decrease inventory and staffing, and ensure that patient care supplies and medications are on units when needed.

PRODUCTION CONTROL, SCHEDULING, AND SUPPLY CHAIN

Production control in HSOs involves matching workload with capacity through work scheduling and is applicable to areas such as admitting, ORs, diagnostic testing, clinics, physician offices, and outpatient services. Production-smoothing techniques are used to spread the workload throughout a shift. For example, if all patients were brought to radiology or all outpatients arrived at 9:00 a.m., waiting lines would build, staff would be overworked, and quality such as patient satisfaction would be reduced because of increased waiting time. In the afternoon, staff would be underutilized. Workload spread throughout the day minimizes patient waiting time, and staff is productive during the entire shift. If demand cannot be controlled through scheduling, part-time staff may be used or other adjustments made to meet peak load demands.

Workload balancing through scheduling of demand or capacity ensures that staff, equipment, and facilities are used efficiently and customer waiting time is lessened. Manual and computerized scheduling techniques are available, including short-interval scheduling, multiple-activity charts, and work distribution analysis. Another technique, simulation, is discussed in Chapter 10.

Effective supply chain management and timely distribution of materials and supplies are important to downstream processes. Improvement techniques are as simple as using exchange carts to deliver supplies to nursing units. On alternate days, one cart is filled and the other is used. Once a day, carts are exchanged. A case cart system may be used in the OR. Each surgeon has a list of instruments, devices, and supplies needed by type of procedure. Before surgery, the case cart for that procedure is packed and delivered to the OR. The unit dose system is used to distribute drugs. Medications are purchased individually prepackaged or are packaged in the pharmacy and distributed to nursing units. Costs are higher, but the risk of medication errors is reduced because each dose is available as needed by the patient.

Strategic Quality Planning: Hoshin Planning[169]

The Japanese word *hoshin* means "shining metal compass" or "pointing direction." Used in planning, hoshin is a strategic approach to quality that is also known as focused planning, policy deployment, or strategic quality planning. Hoshin planning is customer oriented, is externally focused, and seeks to achieve breakthroughs in performance, quality, and competitive position. It is a way of linking quality planning, such as that in CQI and reengineering, to the overall strategic planning process discussed in Chapter 8. Hoshin planning identifies and focuses improvement activities on a few key areas that are strategic priorities to meet customer needs and enhance competitive position.[170]

Hoshin planning has six attributes:

1. *A focus for the organization* in the form of a few breakthrough goals that are vital to the organization's success
2. *A commitment to customers,* including targets and means at every level of the organization that are based on meeting the needs and expectations that customers rank as most important
3. *Deployment of the organization's focus* so that employees understand their specific contributions to it (referred to as the "golden thread" that links employees to what is important to customers and to one another)
4. *Collective wisdom to develop the plan* through a top-down, bottom-up communication process called catchball
5. *Tools and techniques* that make the hoshin planning process and the plan helpful, clear, and easy to use
6. *Ongoing evaluation of progress* to facilitate learning and continuous improvement, that emphasizes both results and the processes that are used to achieve results[171]

Hoshin planning is vertical, as opposed to the horizontal planning of CQI, is based on the strategic vision of the organization in conjunction with its values and mission, and is a systematic way of prioritizing and integrating key success factor process improvement initiatives.[172] It allocates resources and aligns or restructures the organization so that "all units attempt to achieve or contribute to the same few key organizational goals or objectives."[173]

As delivery of health services evolves from focusing on illness to supporting wellness and

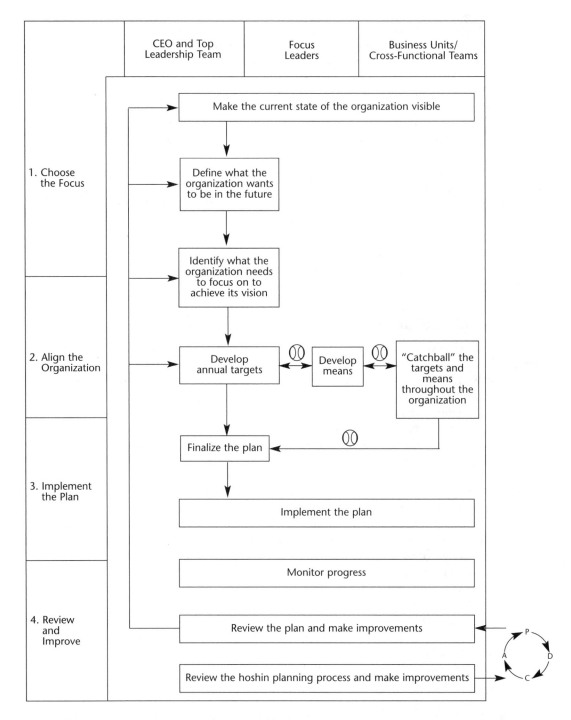

Figure 7.16. Hoshin planning system overview. (From Melum, Mara Minerva, and Casey Collett. *Breakthrough Leadership: Achieving Organizational Alignment Through Hoshin Planning,* 127. Chicago: American Hospital Publishing, 1995; reprinted by permission.)

from independent organizations to aggregations of HSOs in systems, managers must address critical questions:

- How do we plan a successful integrated system?
- What are the right things for people to focus on to ensure long-term success of the system?
- How do we align many different people, departments, and organizations to work together toward the success of the whole system?
- How can we increase employee understanding of the system's priorities and plans?
- How can we balance the need for organizational direction with opportunities for employee initiative and creativity?
- How can we promote breakthrough thinking and results?[174]

Strategic quality planning, or hoshin planning, answers these questions.

Hoshin planning is summarized in Figure 7.16. Components include 1) choosing the focus (defining the future organization), 2) aligning the organization to review and improve performance, 3) finalizing and implementing the plan and monitoring performance against it, and 4) reviewing the plan and making improvements in it to enhance competitive position.

CUSTOMERS AND FOCUS

Choosing the focus includes the tasks inherent in strategic planning discussed in Chapter 8: integrating values, mission, and strategic vision into the plan; analyzing external environment opportunities and threats, including customers, markets, and competitive position; and assessing the HSO's/ HS's internal environment to identify strengths and weaknesses. Hoshin planning focuses on strategic vision—identifying and articulating what the HSO/HS seeks to do: become the highest value provider in the service area; integrate delivery to enhance community health; expand delivery capacity and capability; and provide information on demand for customers.[175]

ALIGN THE ORGANIZATION

The alignment component of Figure 7.16 identifies the performance targets for key success factors that meet customers' needs. Gap analysis using survey data from customers and management will reveal discrepancies between expectations and actual performance in service delivery.[176] An organizationwide iterative process known as catchball develops, negotiates, and communicates targets for key process performance.[177]

> In the catchball process, one level of management throws the ball—the tasks to be accomplished— to the next level of management or another planning team. [There is] input to the development of means to achieve the targets. Dialogue about targets and means proceeds within and across departments, down to the next level of the people closest to the relevant customers and work processes, until the plan is developed in sufficient detail. Then, the process reverses itself. As the plan is finalized, it is rolled back up the organization and checked for gaps, overlaps, and feasibility.[178]

The staff's collective wisdom is applied as the iterative process develops specific targets at all organizational levels and the plans to achieve them. The process includes top-down, horizontal, and bottom-up cascades throughout the HSO/HS. Important outcomes are an understanding of how targets and plans relate to other organizational processes and how they are interconnected. Including employees in planning and implementation enhances acceptance of the strategic plan, and their commitment and motivation to succeed. Furthermore, "catchball" and the resulting understanding of interrelationships facilitate teamwork. The "golden thread" is the concept that interconnected performance targets from all levels tie the organization together.

IMPLEMENT THE PLAN AND REVIEW AND IMPROVE.

Steps 3 and 4 in Figure 7.16 show that implementation of the plan, reviewing, and improving involve the same steps as those in the PDSA cycle. Implementation is based on targets for the processes critical to success and the resulting plan(s). Data track performance for each target. Reviewing and improving the plan are concurrent and interactive with implementation. It is essentially a problem-solving and control activity. If desired results are not attained in key processes, assessment will determine how deviations can be corrected. Assessment may also indicate no deviation but that further improvement is possible. As in the PDSA cycle, lessons learned can be communicated. This can be done with reviews by QITs, the next level of management, and senior management. These activities will facilitate achieving the vision developed in the focus stage.

Physicians and CQI

HSOs/HSs are unique because they are structural blends of administrative and patient care activities in which clinicians are accorded significant autonomy. Historically, the blended structure created conflict between the two. The quality philosophy is changing this relationship, however, by demanding greater collective managerial and clinical accountability for quality, more collaborative participation in quality initiatives, and a mutual interest in both retrospective and concurrent process performance.[179] Both HSO/HS managers and physicians realize they must respect each other's competencies and collaborate to succeed in providing quality services and introducing organizational change, such as improved processes, reengineering, or strategic quality planning. One such change has been the greater use of practice guidelines.

PRACTICE GUIDELINES

Practice guidelines have been developed by various public and private organizations. "Practice parameters (guidelines) is a generic term for acceptable approaches to the prevention, diagnosis, treatment, or management of a disease or condition, as determined by the medical profession based on the best medical evidence currently available."[180] This means practice guidelines stem from evidence-based medicine. Various names are used to express the concept of practice guidelines: critical paths, practice parameters, clinical guidelines, clinical protocols or algorithms, care or target tracks, case management, and clinical pathways. The names differ, but all are meant to assist physicians and other licensed independent practitioners (LIPs) in clinical decision making. HSOs/HSs may define practice guidelines differently and with various degrees of precision. Implementing them is stimulated by a commitment to improve quality and lessen costs by reducing *unnecessary* variation in clinical decision making. This is not "cookbook medicine," as opponents of practice guidelines allege, because deviations can and must be made *if* they are clinically justifiable.

Practice guidelines are not the same as clinical indicators, but they lead to measurable indicators. Practice guidelines describe what should be done; indicators measure what was done.

The American Academy of Pediatrics was the first organization to develop practice guidelines, in 1938. It was not until the late 1970s that such efforts gained momentum, however. By 1990, there were 26 physician organizations that had developed practice guidelines for their specialties;[181] by 1995, approximately 1,800 medical practice guidelines had been cataloged.[182] In 2007, the National Guideline Clearinghouse had over 2,000 practice guidelines. In the late 1990s, 81% of hospitals were using practice guidelines; many others were planning to use them.[183] There is significant evidence, however, of poor adherence to clinical established guidelines.[184]

Clinical CQI initiatives such as practice guidelines can reduce costs while improving quality. Both dimensions are especially important in a provider-at-risk environment that includes capitated and per case revenues, as well as managed care cost limits. Practice guidelines are also an analytical tool to identify optimal timing for clinical interventions by diagnosis and to obtain more effective resource use and better outcomes.[185] Another use of practice guidelines is to promote more consistent clinical decision making—reducing variation around the mean. Better physician decisions and less unnecessary variability in diagnosis and treatment from physicians' and other LIPs' "best practices" will enhance quality initiatives regarding inputs consumed and outcomes attained.

The clinical practice guideline in Figure 7.17 suggests hospital-based ED treatment responses for mild exacerbation of asthma in patients older than 2 years of age. This guideline can assist physician decision making at initial assessment and treatment and in continued assessment and treatment, as well as suggest alternatives ranging from discharge to treatment with a guideline for asthma of greater acuity. HSs that have multiple units providing services on the same continuum of care should monitor practice guidelines for "best practices" consistency.[186] Proof of the value of using practice guidelines is readily available. For example, practice guidelines for congestive heart failure developed by the U.S. Agency for Health Care Policy and Research resulted in fewer readmissions and decreased costs and lengths of stay by boosting the use of recommended posthospital medications.[187] Practice guidelines for intraoperative monitoring (monitoring during surgery) developed by the American Society of Anesthesiologists have been credited with virtually eliminating hypoxic (insufficient oxygen) injury lawsuits and causing a significant reduction in medical malpractice insurance premiums.[188] Another important potential benefit of practice guidelines is major reductions in losses per malpractice claim in high-risk areas such as the EDs, obstetrics, and ORs, with one study reporting a 96% reduction when practice guidelines were used in all three areas.[189]

Beyond offering guidance to physicians and other LIPs, practice guidelines will help establish the legal standard of care. During litigation, physicians will be able to explain deviations from practice guidelines. Deviations are likely because practice guidelines are meant to assist providers, not replace individualized patient treatment plans.[190] It is possible, however, that practice guidelines will become the presumed standard of care and that this will shift the burden to the LIP to prove deviations were justified.

INVOLVING PHYSICIANS

To gain physician support in clinical CQI, there must be physician involvement and ownership.[191] There must be physician champions, and physicians must be convinced that such initiatives will enhance quality without inappropriately jeopardizing their professional autonomy or individual patients' needs.[192]

Brent James, a physician, identified three general categories of work in HSOs: 1) support services, including admission/discharge, billing, medical records, and scheduling; 2) medical infrastructure, including services directly involved in patient care, such as blood bank, laboratory, radiology, and other ancillary services; and 3) clinical products—"the diagnostic and treatment processes that hospitals provide to patients. For example, normal obstetrical delivery, medical treatment of acute myocardial infarction (heart attack), and surgical treatment of appendicitis are all clinical products."[193]

James identified ways to increase physician involvement in CQI initiatives, which apply by extension to reengineering and strategic quality planning.[194] First, the principles of CQI are not new to physicians. They are trained in scientific, numbers-oriented investigation and reasoning. Management must educate physicians about the philosophy of CQI and train them to use CQI tools.

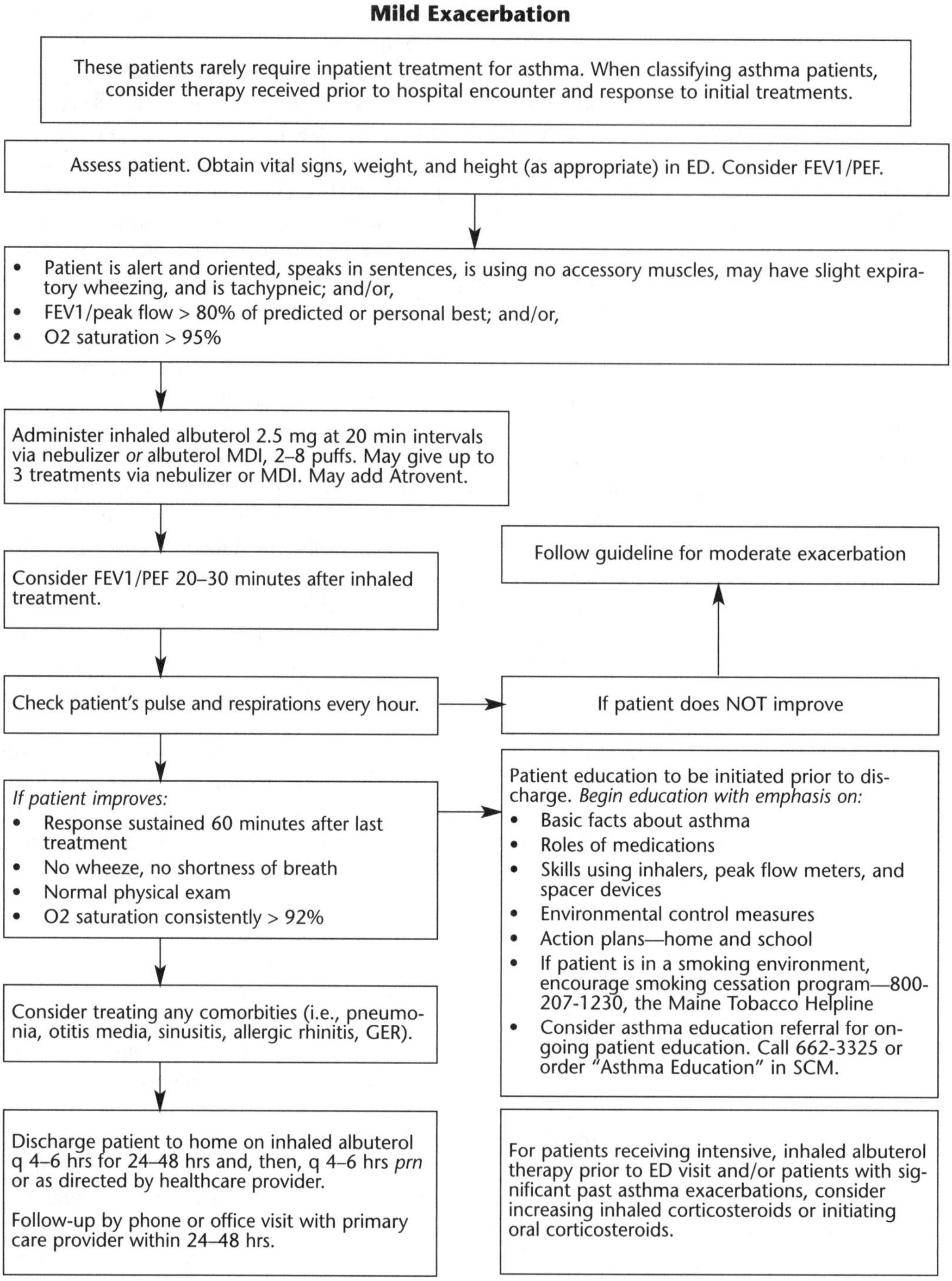

Mild Exacerbation

These patients rarely require inpatient treatment for asthma. When classifying asthma patients, consider therapy received prior to hospital encounter and response to initial treatments.

Assess patient. Obtain vital signs, weight, and height (as appropriate) in ED. Consider FEV1/PEF.

- Patient is alert and oriented, speaks in sentences, is using no accessory muscles, may have slight expiratory wheezing, and is tachypneic; and/or,
- FEV1/peak flow > 80% of predicted or personal best; and/or,
- O2 saturation > 95%

Administer inhaled albuterol 2.5 mg at 20 min intervals via nebulizer *or* albuterol MDI, 2–8 puffs. May give up to 3 treatments via nebulizer or MDI. May add Atrovent.

Consider FEV1/PEF 20–30 minutes after inhaled treatment.

Follow guideline for moderate exacerbation

Check patient's pulse and respirations every hour.

If patient does NOT improve

If patient improves:
- Response sustained 60 minutes after last treatment
- No wheeze, no shortness of breath
- Normal physical exam
- O2 saturation consistently > 92%

Patient education to be initiated prior to discharge. *Begin education with emphasis on:*
- Basic facts about asthma
- Roles of medications
- Skills using inhalers, peak flow meters, and spacer devices
- Environmental control measures
- Action plans—home and school
- If patient is in a smoking environment, encourage smoking cessation program—800-207-1230, the Maine Tobacco Helpline
- Consider asthma education referral for ongoing patient education. Call 662-3325 or order "Asthma Education" in SCM.

Consider treating any comorbities (i.e., pneumonia, otitis media, sinusitis, allergic rhinitis, GER).

Discharge patient to home on inhaled albuterol q 4–6 hrs for 24–48 hrs and, then, q 4–6 hrs *prn* or as directed by healthcare provider.

Follow-up by phone or office visit with primary care provider within 24–48 hrs.

For patients receiving intensive, inhaled albuterol therapy prior to ED visit and/or patients with significant past asthma exacerbations, consider increasing inhaled corticosteroids or initiating oral corticosteroids.

Figure 7.17. Asthma—ED Clinical Practice Guidelines, Mild Exacerbation. (From: Asthma—ED Clinical Practice Guidelines. www.mmc.org/workfiles/mmc_bush/AsthmaED.pdf. Retrieved August 13, 2007.)

"Quality improvement theory should be presented as a direct extension of the principles that the medical profession has always espoused."[195] Clinical quality initiatives seek improvement in medical outcomes; physicians should be comfortable with their data-driven scientific approaches and process orientation. These initiatives will result in better mobilization and utilization of resources to meet the needs of physicians and patients.[196]

Second, physicians are likely to distrust clinical measurement efforts unilaterally initiated by management.[197] Management must reassure clinicians and dispel any perception that quality projects are "thinly disguised efforts to reduce healthcare resource utilization, seemingly without regard for the potential impact of such actions on patients' health."[198] If trust is established, physicians and managers can work toward common goals in delivery of high-quality and cost-effective services.[199]

Third, quality teams already exist for clinical products, and they should be involved in other quality initiatives. Quality assurance (see Chapter 10) includes peer review "typically organized through sub-specialty medical staff groups and reports through an independent medical staff organization."[200] CQI techniques can be incorporated into this process. Because of physicians' independent self-interest in husbanding their time, James recommends structuring clinical improvement projects within staff meetings and allocating salaried physicians' use of work time.[201] Management "should consider physicians' self-perceived role as customers or providers as they plan physician involvement on quality improvement teams."[202]

Fourth, physicians should be encouraged to become involved in clinical product quality initiatives with other organization members and given administrative support in this effort.[203] This may include assigning staff to collect and analyze data and to support clinical QITs, as well as investing in real-time clinical/management information systems.[204]

Fifth, clinical CQI requires stable diagnostic and treatment processes. Physicians determine when these processes are used. This means management must ensure that physicians participate in Q/PI initiatives, that physicians understand they can be both customers and suppliers in a process, and that they are vitally interested in improving processes. As James observed, "It is more important how you [managers] implement than what you implement. The aim is to manage clinical processes, not to manage the physicians."[205]

Sixth, a 2-year study to identify and assess attributes of successful CQI initiatives in acute care hospitals concluded that physician involvement on clinical QITs early in the CQI program is essential for success.[206] Similarly, CQI will stimulate use of process measures by physicians.[207] Management must train a nucleus of physicians at the outset of a CQI initiative to stimulate a sense of physician ownership.[208]

Seventh, the focus should be strategically important clinical issues and procedures—those that are high cost and high volume and for which data are readily available and improvement opportunities are present.[209] It is suggested that management identification of these conditions will be an important motivating factor and reinforce the HSO's commitment to improving areas of concern to physicians.[210] Those involved should be physician leaders who have administrative appointments, as well as attending physicians who are highly respected by their peers.[211]

Eighth, management must be both patient and opportunistic[212] and be prepared to respond to the "neutral" majority of physicians who identify a clinical problem or concern.[213] When they do, management should be ready to show how CQI relates to them or their practices, orient them to CQI methods, and arrange for them to interact with physician champions who are committed to CQI.[214]

RESULTS OF INVOLVING PHYSICIANS

The rise of managed care has given impetus to improving the consistency of clinical practice and the development of evidence-based "best practice" guidelines. Data from implementing clinical guidelines and improving clinical performance in 25 integrated delivery systems and managed healthcare plans that provided healthcare to 40 million people are instructive. The most frequently cited method for improving clinical practice was feedback on clinical profiles of individual clinicians through audits of medical records and comparing their practice with peers or other benchmarks. The second most frequently cited method was clinician feedback from clinical department or administrative heads at regular department meetings. The third most frequent method was involvement of local physicians in developing practice guidelines; the same number of organizations also reported using or considering the use of financial incentives by "tying a small percentage of income to factors such as patient satisfaction, rates of preventative services, and efforts to improve quality."[215]

Failed approaches to achieving improvement in clinical performance reported were simply sending information to physicians or increasing their knowledge alone; feedback with group data alone; and development of practice guidelines outside of the managed care plan or practice unit without local physician involvement.[216] The success of clinical improvement was based on HSO/HS leadership's promoting a CQI culture, respect for physicians, involvement of physicians and other workers, a customer perspective, organizational support, and "viewing physicians as important participants but not necessarily the focus of a system whose performance is to be improved."[217] The latter point paraphrases Deming—blame problems with quality on the process, not the workers.

Regardless of their skills or professional eminence, contemporary physicians are as much a part of HSO processes as anyone and can be found as reifications of Juran's triple role. They are part of processes such as admitting, medication, therapeutic dietetics, laboratory, radiology, and discharge. They are "suppliers" by writing orders and providing information, they are "processors" by reviewing test results and judging the appropriateness of continued treatment, and they are "customers" by receiving information from various sources and using it in treatment decisions. Physicians, even surgeons, are part of processes in a variety of ways, and their work, regardless of their eminence, will be enhanced or diminished by the quality of the processes that support them and of which they are a part. If they ever existed in history, the days of the Lone Ranger are gone.[218] Modern medicine cannot be practiced in isolation.

▦ CQI—The Next Iteration

What is the future of CQI? The next iteration of CQI will be a quantum leap to involve multiple independent HSOs or HSs within a community. Acceptance of CQI by all health services providers in a community will be difficult to achieve, and the complexity of arrangements will be great.[219] Essential features will be 1) data sharing among participating provider organizations, which may be threatening to them and a possible barrier to cooperation; 2) accommodating different organizational cultures and answering questions of control; and 3) the shift in quality activities from independent providers to a collection within the community that represents "a transformation from hierarchies to markets."[220] CQI initiatives beyond the HSO or HS will likely use a public health model that relies on health status indicators, community satisfaction, and overall community benefit.[221] The Precede-Proceed model in Figure 1.2 reflects these elements.

CQI in the context of a communitywide model will require application of CQI principles, perhaps reengineering, and certainly strategic quality planning. However, it will be necessary to manage the changed leadership patterns among participating HSOs/HSs, lessen threats to them, and gain the cooperation of providers that have traditionally competed. Achieving this will be problematic. The following steps will facilitate the transformation from traditional organization-based to community-oriented quality initiatives:[222]

1. *Be cautious in implementing a conventional quality improvement infrastructure that may have worked in intraorganizational initiatives.* All organizations may not have the

same experience with quality initiatives; they may have different agendas and different priorities.

2. *Achieve the commitment of top management to community-based needs assessment.* Community-based indicators of need and quality must be developed, with HSO/HS leaders focusing on the needs of the community, not their individual organizations.

3. *Develop long-run objectives, but also set short-term measurable objectives.* Because of variability in commitment among different organizations, short-run objectives, perhaps involving modest initiatives, are necessary to demonstrate that communitywide quality initiatives can work.

4. *Select topics to utilize network participants who are ready for a common quality improvement approach to specific objectives, capitalizing on small wins.* Build consensus by selecting issues and areas for cooperation that the majority of key participants are ready to implement.

5. *Emphasize data feedback and improved insight.* Use feedback to lessen the concerns of HSOs/HSs, as well as autonomous professionals who may be conceding some sovereignty.

6. *Avoid "religious" wars.* One organization should not proselytize its concept of quality as the one and only.

7. *Build the network of organizations carefully.* Elicit the cooperation of community stakeholders who are critical to success.

8. *Recognize initial efforts as a coalition arrangement.* Indicate to potential participants how the community quality initiatives will benefit them and help to achieve their organization's objectives. Also, permit them to participate or not participate in initiatives; in a confederation, it is necessary to allow some freedom.

Efforts to improve the community's health will only be successful through interorganizational cooperation, a goal that all health services executives should strive to achieve.

DISCUSSION QUESTIONS

1. What important changes occurred in health services delivery in the 1980s and 1990s that stimulated HSOs/HSs to adopt the philosophy of CQI?

2. Define *CQI*. Why is it an organizational philosophy? What are its attributes? How can CQI lead to an enhanced HSO/HS competitive position?

3. Throughout history, a number of reformers have sought to improve the quality of medical care. What common thread connects them? Why did some fail?

4. Think about the nursing service in a hospital. Who or what are its customers? If the nursing service is the customer, who or what provides inputs (is the supplier)?

5. Identify several difficulties and several benefits of working with LIPs to improve quality. What considerations should managers bear in mind when working with them?

6. Identify the similarities and differences in the approaches to quality taken by Deming, Juran, and Crosby.

7. How does the PDSA cycle relate to the problem-solving model in Figure 6.4?

8. Define *reengineering*. What are its attributes? What is common to CQI and reengineering?

9. What are the four steps in strategic quality planning? How is it related to strategic planning as described in Chapter 8?

10. Why must physicians and other LIPs be involved in CQI? What steps are recommended to increase their involvement?

■ Case Study 1: Fed Up in Dallas[223]

Dear Ann Landers:

I've done at least $20,000 worth of business with a local printer. I've always paid my bills in installments, some as large as $1,000 a month.

My printer told me my payments were too small and she had to have all her money in one lump from then on. I paid her off and took my printing elsewhere.

I've patronized the same dry cleaner for 5 years. They know me on sight and have never asked for identification when they cash my checks. Suddenly, they are losing and damaging my clothes and acting as if it's not their fault.

This morning I drove into the service station where I've been a customer for 3 years. I asked the man to please check the pressure in a low tire. I was told that I'd have to buy gas in order to get full service. When I said, "OK," the attendant continued to gripe and then the owner got into the act. I told them to forget it, that I'd go elsewhere. The attendant replied, "You want me to take the air back out of your tire?" Needless to say, they won't see me again.

I've even had a run-in with a doctor I've been seeing for 6 years. I walked out of his office after being kept waiting for an hour and a half.

Ann, what's wrong with these people? Why don't they value those of us who keep them in business? In these times of economic hardship, you'd think they would do everything possible to please their customers. Am I wrong to expect a little service and courtesy in exchange for my business?

—Fed Up in Dallas

QUESTIONS

1. Obviously, Fed Up in Dallas is not a satisfied customer. In general, why do you think some organizations and their staffs are indifferent to customers who buy their products and services?
2. Describe an instance in which you or an acquaintance encountered a negative customer orientation by an HSO. What was your (or your acquaintance's) reaction?
3. Fed Up in Dallas describes negative experiences with four different businesses. Could she be the problem? What should organizations do when confronted with difficult customers?

■ Case Study 2: The Carbondale Clinic[224]

The Carbondale Clinic, located in Carbondale, Illinois, is a large group practice of about 30 physicians. The clinic employs about 100 people and serves a regional population of about 100,000. Specialties ranging from pediatrics to psychiatry are offered by the clinic, which also operates its own laboratory, basic imaging services, and outpatient surgical center.

For some years, the clinic has been receiving complaints from its patients that appointment times are not being met. For instance, a patient with an appointment for two o'clock might not get in to see the physician until four o'clock. However, the clinic has felt that such delays are unavoidable due to the uncertainty involved in the time it takes to adequately examine each patient and the possibility of emergency cases that must be inserted into the schedule.

Several criteria are used for scheduling. For instance, many patients are scheduled for annual physical exams. These are usually scheduled at least several weeks in advance because they require coordination of laboratory services and physicians' time. However, some physicians will begin examining a patient and decide that the patient needs a physical immediately. The physicians feel this does not really cause problems because they can send the patient down to the laboratory while they continue to see other patients.

Some patients also phone the clinic for an appointment when they have nonemergency, routine problems such as a mild fever or sore throat. Such patients are scheduled into available time slots as soon as possible—usually a day or two from the time they call. The objective here is to fit such patients in as quickly as possible without overloading the schedule with more patients than can reasonably be examined in a time period. Usually the plan is to schedule four patients per hour.

However, each day, various emergencies occur. These can range from a splinter in the eye to a heart attack, and these cases cannot wait. For an emergency that is not life threatening, the approach is to try to squeeze the person into a time slot that is not too heavily scheduled. However, a case of life or death—such as a heart attack—means that the schedule must be disrupted and the patient treated immediately.

Currently, all scheduling of appointments is done centrally. However, this frequently causes problems because the people making appointments often do not know how long it should take to examine a patient with a particular complaint. On the other hand, the nurses in each department are usually too busy to do the scheduling themselves. Generally, if there is a doubt about whether a patient can be fitted into a time slot, the preference is to go ahead and schedule the patient. This is because the physicians prefer not to have any empty times in their schedules. At times, if it looks as if there might be an available opening, the clinic even calls patients who were originally scheduled for a later time and asks them to come in early.

QUESTIONS

1. "For some years, the clinic has received complaints from its patients that appointment times are not being met." Why has no action been taken to correct the situation?
2. You are a member of a QIT that was asked to evaluate the appointment/scheduling process. Are there some "assumptions" in the narrative that you question? If data were sufficient for a Pareto diagram of problems with the appointment/scheduling process, what do you think the items would be? Please list them.
3. Draw a cause-and-effect (Ishikawa) diagram of causes for patient complaints.
4. What recommendations would you make to decrease patient waiting time?

■ Case Study 3: Noninvasive Cardiovascular Laboratory

The assistant vice president for operations at Barbarosa Hospital has identified a problem concerning the noninvasive cardiovascular laboratory (NCVL). First, patients have complained to their physicians about long waits and interruptions during tests. Second, the number of tests ordered increased when more LIPs joined the professional staff organization early this year, and the only NCVL technician, Loren Findley, has told his supervisor that he is overworked. Findley has threatened to resign if he does not get a full-time assistant. The hospital has no other employees who can perform the tests. The tests are not difficult; Findley could train someone to perform them in about 2 months.

Findley schedules all inpatient and outpatient tests ordered by house staff (residents) and attending physicians. Phone calls to schedule tests are received frequently during the day. On average, three of four of the tests Findley administers are interrupted by phone calls. It takes 10 minutes to return to the point in the test before the interruption (2 minutes talking on the phone and 8 minutes to restart the test).

Observing the technician and talking with him and his supervisor provided the following information. The NCVL is located on the third floor of the hospital. It is adjacent to the stress test laboratory, which has twice the space of the noninvasive laboratory but uses only half of it. The stress test technician is productive only 60% of the time. Findley's workspace is cramped and crowded with two patient beds, a very large desk, and supplies in boxes that are stacked floor to ceiling along two walls. The room's configuration does not permit easy movement, and some equipment must be placed in the hall. Consequently, Findley spends an average of 10 minutes moving equipment into or out of the room when setting up for a test that is different from the preceding one.

Findley is qualified to administer three tests:

1. Echocardiogram (ECHO): A graphic recording generated by ultrasound that is used to study the structures and motions of the heart
2. Ocular plethysmograph (OPG): A test to measure changes in size and volume of the eye
3. Pulse volume recording (PVR) plethysmograph: A test to measure changes in volume of a cross-section of a blood vessel over several heartbeats

Extensive observation showed the following standard times for each test (assume there is no difference for inpatients and outpatients):

Test	Standard time
ECHO	1 hour
OPG	½ hour
PVR	½ hour

Hospital records were used to compare the number of tests performed last year with the number performed in the first 3 months of the year:

		No. performed	
		This year	
Test	Previous year	First 3 months	Annualized
ECHO	800	300	1,200
OPG	200	75	300
PVR	200	75	300

The typical pattern for scheduled tests on any given day is ECHO, ECHO, OPG, ECHO, ECHO, PVR, ECHO, ECHO, OPG, and so forth.

QUESTIONS

1. Is Findley overworked? Why or why not? Should another technician be hired?
2. Assume that there is no budget to add a new technician. How should the current NCVL process be changed to improve quality and productivity?
3. Draw a cause-and-effect (fishbone) diagram of the reasons Findley's work is inefficient.
4. Draw a flow diagram showing the steps in the process(es) for Findley's work.

■ Case Study 4: Clinics

In the mid-1990s, Newland Hospital sought ways to increase the number of referrals to its inpatient services. The governing body approved a number of new initiatives, one of which was to purchase several primary care practices that were owned by family practice physicians who were in solo or two- or three-physician partnerships and who had clinical privileges on Newland's professional staff organization. Over a 2-year period, Newland purchased three practices with a total of eight physicians. In the purchase contract, Newland agreed to buy the practices, employ the physicians, and employ the clinical and clerical support staff who worked in the practices. These staff would report for administrative matters to Newland's vice president for ancillary services and would report to the physicians for clinical matters. The contract specified that the physicians would work 40 hours a week. The physicians would, however, control their hours of work and the patient schedule. The quality of care at the practices would be reviewed by Newland's chief medical officer.

It was assumed that the practices would benefit from the improved management that the hospital would provide. In addition, it was expected that there would be several efficiencies and economies of scale, especially in terms of staffing, logistics support, and the information technology provided by Newland. The practices were financially healthy when purchased, and allowing for the problems incident to the change in ownership, it was projected that the clinics would at least break even in the year following purchase and return to profitability no later than the 3rd year after purchase.

Now, the 5th year after purchase, all of the practices are losing money, with total annual loses in excess of $500,000. You are the vice president for ancillary services. The chief executive officer has asked you to prepare an analysis regarding the poor financial performance and to make recommendations regarding the actions to be taken.

QUESTIONS

1. Describe the system that Newland Hospital created by purchasing the primary care practices. How do the concepts of optimization and suboptimization of a system apply?
2. What reasons might explain why the practices are losing money?
3. Identify the economic value of the clinics to Newland Hospital. Identify the non-economic value.
4. Outline a plan that applies CQI principles and concepts to improve the healthcare delivery system composed of the primary care practices and Newland.

Notes

1. Laffel, Glenn, and David Blumenthal. "The Case for Using Industrial Management Science in Health Care Organizations." *Journal of the American Medical Association* 262 (November 24, 1989): 2,870; Merry, Martin D. "Total Quality Management for Physicians: Translating the New Paradigm." *Quality Review Bulletin* 16 (March 1990): 104; McLaughlin, Curtis P., and Arnold D. Kaluzny. "Total Quality Management in Health: Making It Work." *Health Care Management Review* 15 (Summer 1990): 7.
2. Kaluzny, Arnold D., and Curtis P. McLaughlin. "Managing Transitions: Assuring the Adoption and Impact of TQM." *Quality Review Bulletin* 37, 4 (November 1992): 380.
3. *Quality Management: A Management Advisory,* 1. Chicago: American Hospital Association, 1990; James, Brent C. *Quality Management for Health Care Delivery—Quality Measurement and Management Project,* 10. Chicago: Hospital Research and Educational Trust, 1989; Laffel and Blumenthal, "The Case for Using," 2,870; O'Connor, Stephen J. "Service Quality: Understanding and Implementing the Concept in the Clinical Laboratory." *Clinical Laboratory Management Review* 3 (November/December 1989): 330; Schumacher, Dale N. "Organizing for Quality Competition: The Coming Paradigm Shift." *Frontiers of Health Services Management* 5 (Summer 1989): 113. For a useful model of quality, see Lanning, Joyce A., and Stephen J. O'Connor. "The Health Care Quality Quagmire: Some Signposts." *Hospital & Health Services Administration* 35 (Spring 1990): 42.
4. Deming, W. Edwards. *Out of the Crisis,* 18. Boston: Massachusetts Institute of Technology, 1986.
5. Milakovich, Michael E. "Creating a Total Quality Health Care Environment." *Health Care Management Review* 16 (Spring 1991): 9.

6. Casurella, Joe. "Managing a 'Total Quality' Program." *Federation of American Health Systems Review* 22 (July/August 1989): 31.

7. James, *Quality Management,* 11.

8. *Glossary: Quality.* American Society for Quality. *http://www.asq.org/glossary/q.htm,* retrieved July 9, 2007.

9. James, *Quality Management,* 10.

10. McLaughlin, Curtis P., and Arnold D. Kaluzny. *Continuous Quality Improvement in Healthcare: Theory, Implementation, and Applications,* 12. Gaithersburg, MD: Aspen Publishers, 1994.

11. James, Brent. *Quality Management for Health Care Delivery.* HRET and the TRUST Award. July 25, 2005. *http://www.hret.org/hret/about/content/monograph.pdf,* retrieved January 9, 2007.

12. Re, Richard N., and Marie A. Krousel-Wood. "How to Use Continuous Quality Improvement Theory and Statistical Quality Control Tools in a Multispecialty Clinic." *Quality Review Bulletin* 16 (November 1990): 392.

13. Marszalek-Gaucher, Ellen, and Richard J. Coffey. *Transforming Healthcare Organizations: How to Achieve and Sustain Organizational Excellence,* 85. San Francisco: Jossey-Bass, 1990; Arndt, Margarete, and Barbara Bigelow. "The Implementation of Total Quality Management in Hospitals: How Good Is the Fit?" *Health Care Management Review* 20 (Fall 1995): 9.

14. Deming, W. Edwards. "Improvement of Quality and Productivity Through Action by Management." *National Productivity Review* 1 (Winter 1981–1982): 12–22; Deming, W. Edwards. *Quality, Productivity, and Competitive Position.* Boston: The MIT Press, 1982; Deming, W. Edwards. "Transformation of Western Style Management." *Interfaces* 15 (May/June 1985): 6–11; Deming, *Out of the Crisis.*

15. Juran, Joseph M. *Managerial Breakthrough: A New Concept of the Manager's Job.* New York: McGraw-Hill, 1964; Juran, Joseph M. "The Quality Trilogy." *Quality Progress* 19 (August 1986): 19–24; Juran, Joseph M. *Juran on Leadership for Quality.* New York: The Free Press, 1989; Juran, Joseph M. *Juran on Planning for Quality.* New York: The Free Press: 1988.

16. Crosby, Philip B. *Quality Is Free.* New York: McGraw-Hill, 1979; Crosby, Philip B. *Let's Talk Quality.* New York: McGraw-Hill, 1989; Crosby, Philip B. *Quality Without Tears.* New York: McGraw-Hill, 1984.

17. *Quality Management: A Management Advisory,* 2.

18. For ease of reading, when reference is made in this chapter to process improvement, it also includes input improvement.

19. The Joint Commission. *Specifications Manual for National Hospital Quality Measures, version 2.2.* December 1, 2006. *http://www.jointcommission.org/PerformanceMeasurement/WhatsNew/,* retrieved January 10, 2007.

20. The Joint Commission. *Specifications Manual.*

21. James, *Quality Management,* 1.

22. Anderson, Craig A., and Robin D. Daigh. "Quality Mind-Set Overcomes Barriers to Success." *Healthcare Financial Management* 45 (February 1991): 21; Kroenberg, Philip S., and Renee G. Loeffler. "Quality Management Theory: Historical Context and Future Prospect." *Journal of Management Science & Policy Analysis* 8 (Spring/Summer 1991): 204; McLaughlin and Kaluzny, "Total Quality Management," 7; Sahney, Vinod K., and Gail L. Warden. "The Quest for Quality and Productivity in Health Services." *Frontiers of Health Services Management* 7 (Summer 1991): 2.

23. Milakovich, "Creating a Total," 9.

24. McEachern, J. Edward, and Duncan Neuhauser. "The Continuous Improvement of Quality at the Hospital Corporation of America." *Health Matrix* 7 (Fall 1989): 7; Postal, Susan Nelson. "Using the Deming Quality Improvement Method to Manage Medical Records Department Product Lines." *Topics in Health Records Management* 10 (June 1990): 34.

25. *Quality Management: A Management Advisory,* 2; James, *Quality Management,* 1; Lynn, Monty L., and David P. Osborn. "Deming's Quality Principles: A Health Care Application." *Hospital & Health Services Administration* 36 (Spring 1991): 113.

26. Berwick, Donald M. "Managing Quality: The Next Five Years." *Quality Letter for Healthcare Leaders* 6, 6 (July/August 1994): 3.

27. Boerstler, Heidi, Richard W. Foster, Edward J. O'Connor, James L. O'Brien, Stephen M. Shortell, James

M. Carman, and Edward F.X. Hughes. "Implementation of Total Quality Management: Conventional Wisdom Versus Reality." *Hospital & Health Services Administration* 41 (Summer 1996): 143.

28. Taylor, Mark. "Quality as Gospel." *Modern Healthcare* 35, 18 (May 2, 2005): 32, 6 pages. *http://proquest .umi.com.proxygw.wrlc.org/pqdweb?index=3&did=8352241&SrchMode ...,* retrieved January 10, 2007. A good review of CQI, including barriers, can be found in Bigelow, Barbara, and Margarete Arndt. "Total Quality Management: Field of Dreams?" *Health Care Management Review* 20 (Fall 1995): 15–25 and in Gustafson, David H., and Ann Schoofs Hundt. "Findings of Innovation Research Applied to Quality Management Principles for Health Care." *Health Care Management Review* 20 (Spring 1995): 16–33.

29. Lynn and Osborn, "Deming's Quality Principles"; Taylor, Mark. "Quality as Gospel." *Modern Healthcare* 35, 18 (May 2, 2005): 32, 6 pages. *http://proquest.umi.com.proxygw.wrlc.org/pqdweb?index=3 &did=8352241&SrchMode ...,* retrieved January 10, 2007.

30. Towne, Jennifer. "Going 'Lean' Streamlines Processes, Empowers Staff and Enhances Care." *Hospitals & Health Networks Management* 80, 10 (October 2006): 34; Postal, "Using the Deming"; McEachern and Neuhauser, "The Continuous Improvement"; Sahney and Warden, "The Quest for Quality"; Walton, Mary. *Deming Management at Work.* New York: Putnam, 1990.

31. Ferguson, T. Bruce, Jr., Eric D. Peterson, Laura P. Coombs, Mary C. Eiken, Meghan L. Carey, Frederick L. Grover, and Elizabeth R. DeLong. "Use of Continuous Quality Improvement to Increase Use of Process Measures in Patients Undergoing Coronary Artery Bypass Graft Surgery: A Randomized Controlled Trial." *Journal of the Ameican Medical Association* 290, 1 (July 2, 2003): 49–56; James, Brent C. "TQM and Clinical Medicine." *Frontiers of Health Services Management* 7 (Summer 1991): 42–46.

32. Haugh, Richard. "The Demand for More Exacting Test Results—Fast!—Reformulates Hospital Labs." *Hospital & Health Networks* 80, 1 (January 2006): 46–48, 50, 52.

33. Benedetto, Anthony R. "Adapting Manufacturing-Based Six Sigma Methdology to the Service Environment of a Radiology Film Library." *Journal of Healthcare Management* 48, 4 (July/August 2003): 263–280;. Cascade, Philip N. "Quality Improvement in Diagnostic Radiology." *American Journal of Radiology* 154 (May 1990): 1,117–1,120.

34. Postal, "Using the Deming."

35. Zimmerman, Rosanne, Rhonda Smith, Christopher M.B. Fernandes, Teresa Smith, and Ayad Al darrab. "A Quest for Quality." *Quality Progress* 39, 3 (March 2006): 41–46.

36. Peterson, Charles D. "Quality Improvement in Pharmacy: A Prescription for Change." *Quality Review Bulletin* 16 (March 1990): 106–108.

37. Esimai, Grace. "Lean Six Sigma Reduces Medication Errors." *Quality Progress* 38, 4 (April 2005): 51–57.

38. Geboers, Harrie, Henk Mokkink, Pauline van Montfort, Henk van den Hoogen, Wil van den Bosch, and Richard Grol. "Continuous Quality Improvement in Small General Medical Practices: The Attitudes of General Practitioners and Other Practice Staff." *International Journal for Quality in Health Care* 13, 5 (October 1, 2001): 391–397.

39. Zimmerman, Rosanne, Rhonda Smith, Christopher M.B. Fernandes, Teresa Smith, and Ayad Al darrab. "A Quest for Quality." *Quality Progress* 39, 3 (March 2006): 41–46.

40. Chan, Yee-Ching Lilian, and Shih-Jen Kathy Ho. "Continuous Quality Improvement: A Survey of American and Canadian Healthcare Executives." *Hospital & Health Services Administration* 42 (Winter 1997): 529–534.

41. James, *Quality Management for Health Care Delivery*, p. 7.

42. O'Leary, Dennis S. "CQI—A Step Beyond QA." *Joint Commission Perspectives* 10 (March/April 1990): 2.

43. President of The Joint Commission, cited in Patterson, Pat. "JCAHO Shifts Its Emphasis to QI—Quality Improvement." *OR Manager* 6 (May 1990): 1.

44. Everett, Michael, and Brent C. James. "Continuous Quality Improvement in Healthcare: A Natural Fit." *Journal for Quality and Participation* (January/February 1991): 10.

45. Crosby, *Let's Talk Quality,* 63.

46. See also Berwick, Donald M., A. Blanton Godfrey, and Jane Roessner. *Curing Health Care: New Strategies for Quality Improvement,* 32–43. San Francisco: Jossey-Bass, 1990.

47. Darr, Kurt. "Applying the Deming Method in Hospitals: Part 1." *Hospital Topics* 67 (November/December 1989): 4.

48. Milakovich, "Creating a Total," 12.

49. Kaluzny, Arnold D., Curtis P. McLaughlin, and B. Jon Jaeger. "TQM as a Managerial Innovation: Research Issues and Implications." *Health Services Management Research* 6 (May 1993): 79.

50. Deming, *Out of the Crisis,* 3; Walton, Mary. *The Deming Management Method,* 25. New York: Perigee Books, 1986.

51. *Baldrige National Quality Program: Health Care Criteria for Performance Excellence,* p. 6. Washington, DC: U.S. Department of Commerce, Technology Administration, National Institute of Standards and Technology, 2007. (Pamphlet)

52. "Thomas Percival, 1740–1804." *http://www.thornber.net/cheshire/ideasmen/percival.html,* retrieved June 21, 2007.

53. "Ernest Amory Codman." *http://www.whonamedit.com/doctor.cfm/2558.html,* retrieved February 27, 2007.

54. "Ignaz Semmelweis." Wikipedia. *http://en.wikipedia.org/wiki/Ignaz_Semmelweis,* retrieved June 21, 2007.

55. Audain, Cynthia. "Biographies of Women Mathematicians: Florence Nightingale." *http://www.agnesscott.edu/lriddle/women/nitegale.ht,* retrieved June 22, 2007.

56. Riddle, Larry. "Biographies of Women Mathematicians: Polar-Area Diagram." *http://www.agnesscott.edu/lriddle/women/nightpiechart.htm,* retrieved June 22, 2007.

57. MacEachern, Malcolm T. *Hospital Organization and Management,* 17. Berwyn, IL: Physicians' Record Company, 1962.

58. Holleb, Arthur I. "Halsted Revisited." *American College of Surgeons Bulletin* 71, 9: 20–21.

59. The Joint Commission. "Ernest Amory Codman Award." *http://www.jointcommission.org/Codman/Ernest_Amory_Codman.htm,* retrieved February 14, 2007.

60. American College of Surgeons. "Public Information: What Is the American College of Surgeons?" *http://www.facs.org/about/corppro.html,* retrieved March 14, 2007.

61. "Ernest Amory Codman." *http://www.whonamedit.com/doctor.cfm/2558.html,* retrieved February 27, 2007.

62. Neuhauser, Duncan. "Heroes and Martyrs of Quality and Safety: Ernest Amory Codman, MD." *www.qualtyhealthcare.com,* retrieved February 27, 2007.

63. Neuhauser, Duncan. "Heroes and Martyrs of Quality and Safety.

64. Moen, Ron, and Cliff Norman. "Evolution of the PDSA Cycle." *deming.ces.clemson.edu/.../files/evolution_of_the_pdsa_cyclejul06.pdf,* retrieved January 12, 2007. This reference includes valuable background on the PDSA cycle and persons important in its evolution.

65. Moen, Ron, and Cliff Norman. "Evolution of the PDSA Cycle."

66. Lowe, Ted A., and Joseph M. Mazzeo. "Crosby, Deming, Juran: Three Preachers, One Religion." *Quality* 25 (September 1986): 22–25; Sahney and Warden, "The Quest for Quality," 4–7.

67. Lowe and Mazzeo, "Crosby, Deming, Juran," 22.

68. Deming, W. Edwards. "Walter A. Shewhart, 1891–1967." *The American Statistician* 21, 2 (April 1967): 39–40.

69. Darr, Kurt. "Eulogy to the Master: W. Edwards Deming." *Hospital Topics* 72 (Winter 1994): 4.

70. Deming, W. Edwards. *The New Economics for Industry, Government, Education,* 2nd ed., p. 2. Cambridge, MA: MIT-CAES, 2000.

71. Deming, *The New Economics for Industry, Government, Education,* 2nd ed., chap. 4, 92–115.

72. Deming, "Improvement of Quality"; Deming, *Quality, Productivity*; Deming, "Transformation of Western"; Deming, *Out of the Crisis.*

73. Darr, "Applying the Deming Method: Part 1"; Darr, Kurt. "Applying the Deming Method in Hospitals: Part 2." *Hospital Topics* 68 (Winter 1990): 4–6; Gabor, Andrea. *The Man Who Discovered Quality: How W. Edwards Deming Brought the Quality Revolution to America—The Stories of Ford, Xerox, and GM.* New York: Random House, 1990; Gitlow, Howard S., and Shelly J. Gitlow. *The Deming Guide to Quality and Competitive Position.* Englewood Cliffs, NJ: Prentice-Hall, 1987; Neuhauser, Duncan. "The Quality of Medical Care and the 14 Points of Edwards Deming." *Health Matrix* 6 (Summer 1986): 7–10; Scherkenbach, William W. *The Deming Route to Quality and Productivity.* Washington, DC: CEEP Press, 1986; Walton, *The Deming Management Method.*

74. Deming, *Out of the Crisis,* 199–203.
75. Darr, "Applying the Deming Method: Part 1," 4.
76. Deming's 14 points (in italics) are drawn from Deming, *Out of the Crisis,* 22–24.
77. Deming, *Out of the Crisis,* 200.
78. Deming, *Out of the Crisis,* 201.
79. Deming, *Out of the Crisis,* 202.
80. Deming, *Out of the Crisis,* 202.
81. Deming, *Out of the Crisis,* 202..
82. Deming, *Out of the Crisis,* 203.
83. Deming, "Improvement of Quality," 22.
84. Darr, "Applying the Deming Method: Part 1," 5.
85. Sahney and Warden, "The Quest for Quality," 4–5.
86. Personal communication, Juran Institute, January 1999.
87. "Joseph M. Juran." Wikipedia. *http://en.wikipedia.org/wiki/Dr._Joseph_Moses_Juran,* retrieved June 22, 2007.
88. Juran, *Managerial Breakthrough;* Juran, "Quality Trilogy"; Juran, *Juran on Planning;* Juran, *Juran on Leadership,* 361.
89. Sahney and Warden, "The Quest for Quality," 6–7.
90. Adapted with permission of The Free Press, a Division of Simon & Schuster Adult Publishing Group, from *Juran on Leadership for Quality: An Executive Handbook* by Joseph M. Juran. Copyright © 1989 by Juran Institute, Inc. All rights reserved.
91. Juran, *Juran on Planning,* 1.
92. Adapted with permission of The Free Press, a Division of Simon & Schuster Adult Publishing Group, from *Juran on Leadership for Quality: An Executive Handbook* by Joseph M. Juran. Copyright © 1989 by Juran Institute, Inc. All rights reserved.
93. Juran, *Managerial Breakthrough,* 7.
94. Juran, J.M., and Frank M. Gryna, eds. *Juran's Quality Control Handbook,* 4th ed., 6.19. New York: McGraw-Hill Book Company, 1988.
95. Crosby, *Quality Is Free,* 1.
96. Crosby, *Let's Talk Quality,* 104.
97. Sahney and Warden, "The Quest for Quality," 6.
98. The industrial concept of zero defects means conformance to standards or specifications. For example, size is allowed to vary by ±3 millimeters. *Zero defects* does not mean that the product is perfect, although *zero defects* has been used in industry as a slogan—an exhortation directed at workers. Deming opposes setting specifications except as general guides. He argues that efforts to seek perfection are thwarted if the goal is only to meet specifications. Point 10 of Deming's 14 points for improvement of management expresses his opposition to slogans. In his judgment, management has been unwilling to accept blame for poor processes and, instead, has blamed the workers, an attitude that has caused management to substitute slogans for process improvement. Deming believes slogans alone only cause worker anger and frustration.
99. Crosby, *Let's Talk Quality,* 9.
100. Crosby, *Quality Is Free,* 38–39.
101. Crosby, *Quality Is Free,* 132–138; Crosby, *Quality Without Tears,* 101–124; Crosby, *Let's Talk Quality,* 106–107. The quotation in Point 10 is from Crosby, *Quality Without Tears,* 117.
102. Crosby, *Quality Is Free,* 22.
103. Lowe and Mazzeo, "Crosby, Deming, Juran," 23.
104. Darr, "Applying the Deming Method: Part 2," 4.
105. Darr, "Applying the Deming Method: Part 2," 4.
106. James, *Quality Management,* iii.
107. Readers interested in HRET research projects can find information on the American Hospital Association web site at *http://www.aha.org/hret/R_ehm.html.*
108. James, *Quality Management,* 26–28, 32.
109. James, *Quality Management for Health Care Delivery.*

110. "Lean Six Sigma Training in Full Swing at USMA." U.S. Federal News Service, February 2, 2007. *http:// proquest.umi.com/pqdweb?index=3&did=1211124211&SrchMode=1&sid=1&Fmt= . . .* , retrieved February 26, 2007.

111. Strategos, Inc. "Just in Time, Toyota Production & Lean Manufacturing: Origins & History of Lean Manufacturing." Kansas City, MO. *www.strategosinc.com,* retrieved February 26, 2007.

112. Lean Manufacturing Guide. "Six Sigma Tools Used in Lean Manufacturing." *http://www.leanmanu facturingguide.com/tools.htm,* retrieved February 26, 2007.

113. Leslie, Marshall, Charles Hagood, Adam Royer, Charles P. Reece, Jr., and Sara Maloney. "Using Lean Methods to Improve OR Turnover Times." *AORN Journal* 84, 5 (2005): 849–855; Jennifer Town. "Going 'Lean' Streamlines Processes, Empowers Staff and Enhances Care." *Hospitals and Health Networks* 80, 10 (October 2006): 34–35.

114. Thilmany, Jean. "Thinking Lean." *Mechanical Engineering* 127, 7 (July 2005): 5.

115. Bukowski, Eugene R., Jr., and Mary Litteral. "Produce Perfect Products." *Quality* 45, 11 (November 2006): 40–43. Lean Synergy.pdf.

116. Laux, Daniel T. "Six Sigma Evolution Clarified—Letter to the Editor." *Six Sigma Healthcare. http:// healthcare.isixsigma.com/library/content/c020131a.asp?action=prin,* retrieved February 26, 2007.

117. "Statistical Six Sigma Definition." *iSix Sigma. http://www.isixsigma.com/library/content/c010101a.asp ?action=print,* retrieved February 26, 2007.

118. Brown, Lewis, and Denise Taylor. "Reducing Delayed Starts in Specials Lab with Six Sigma." *iSixSigma. http://healthcare.isixsigma.com/library/content/c070117b.asp?action=prin,* retrieved February 26, 2007.

119. International Organization for Standardization. "Overview of the ISO system." *http://www.iso.org/iso/ en/aboutiso/introduction/index.html?printable=true,* retrieved February 22, 2007.

120. "The Magical Demystifying Tour of ISO 9000 and 14000C." *http://www.iso.ch/iso/en/iso9000-14000/ understand/basics/general/basics_1.html,* retrieved January 12, 2007.

121. International Organization for Standardization. "ISO in Brief. 2006." *isoinbrief_2006-en.pdf.*

122. "Overview of the ISO system." *http://www.iso.org/iso/en/aboutiso/introduction/index.html#fourteen,* retrieved January 13, 2007.

123. International Organization for Standardization. "How Are ISO Standards Developed?" *http://www.iso .org/iso/en/stdsdevelopment/whowhenhow/how.html,* retrieved March 14, 2007.

124. Taylor, Mark. "Quality as Gospel." *Modern Healthcare* 35, 18 (May 2, 2005): 32, 6 pages. *http://proquest .umi.com.proxygw.wrlc.org/pqdweb?index=3&did=8352241&SrchMode ...,* retrieved January 10, 2007.

125. Conn, Joseph. "JCAHO Rival Has Setback." *Modern Healthcare* 36, 27 (July 3–10, 2006). *http://web .ebscohost.com/ehost/detail?vid=2&hid=6&sid=c4d9835c-c0de-4860-af93-f522...,* retrieved February 22, 2007.

126. Hammer, Michael. *Beyond Reengineering: How the Process-Centered Organization Is Changing Our Work and Our Lives,* 81–82. New York: HarperBusiness, 1996.

127. Kennedy, Maggie. "Reengineering in Healthcare." *Quality Letter for Healthcare Leaders* 6 (September 1994): 2–3.

128. Hammer, Michael, and James Champy. *Reengineering the Corporation: A Manifesto for Business Revolution,* 32. New York: HarperBusiness, 1993.

129. Stewart, Thomas A. "Reengineering: The Hot New Management Tool." *Fortune* 128 (August 1993): 41.

130. Bergman, Rhonda. "Reengineering Health Care." *Hospitals & Health Networks* 68 (February 5, 1994): 30.

131. Hammer, *Beyond Reengineering,* 80.

132. Hammer, *Beyond Reengineering,* 82.

133. Leatt, Peggy G., Ross Baker, Paul K. Halverson, and Catherine Aird. "Downsizing, Reengineering, and Restructuring: Long-Term Implications for Healthcare Organizations." *Frontiers of Health Services Management* 13 (June 1997): 17.

134. Hammer and Stanton, *The Reengineering Revolution,* 56.

135. Hammer and Stanton, *The Reengineering Revolution,* 57.

136. Hammer and Champy, *Reengineering the Corporation,* 102.

137. Leatt, Baker, Halverson, and Aird, "Downsizing, Reengineering," 5–6.

138. Hammer and Champy, *Reengineering the Corporation,* 49.

139. Johansson, McHugh, Pendlebury, and Wheeler, *Business Process Reengineering,* 15; Griffith, Sahney, and Mohr, *Reengineering Health Care,* 14.
140. Walston, Stephen L., and John R. Kimberly. "Reengineering Hospitals: Evidence from the Field." *Hospital & Health Services Administration* 42 (Summer 1997): 150.
141. Walston and Kimberly, "Reengineering Hospitals," 151.
142. Schweikhart, Sharon Bergman, and Vicki Smith-Daniels. "Reengineering the Work of Caregivers: Role Redefinition, Team Structures, and Organizational Redesign." *Hospital & Health Services Administration* 41 (Spring 1996): 22.
143. Walston and Kimberly, "Reengineering Hospitals," 151–152.
144. Walston and Kimberly, "Reengineering Hospitals," 151–152.
145. Arndt, Margarete, and Barbara Bigelow. "Reengineering: Déjà Vu All Over Again." *Health Care Management Review* 23 (Summer 1998): 63.
146. Hammer and Champy, *Reengineering the Corporation,* 128–133.
147. James, "Implementing Continuous Quality," 16.
148. Goldense, Robert A. "Attaining TQM Through Employee Involvement: Imperatives for Implementation." *Journal of Management Science & Policy Analysis* 8 (Spring/Summer 1991): 268.
149. Kazemek, Edward A., and Rosemary M. Charny. "Quality Enhancement Means Total Organizational Involvement." *Healthcare Financial Management* 45 (February 1991): 15; Kronenberg and Loeffler, "Quality Management Theory," 211–212.
150. "Joseph M. Juran." Wikipedia. *http://en.wikipedia.org/wiki/Dr._Joseph_Moses_Juran,* retrieved June 22, 2007.
151. McCain, Cecelia. "Using an FMEA in a Service Setting." *Quality Progress* 39, 9 (September 2006): 24–29.
152. "Most Airplane Crashes Caused by Human Error." *Quality Progress* 39, 11 (November 2006): 12.
153. Meyers, Susan. "Standardizing Safety: Borrowing Lessons Learned from the Airline Industry, Hospitals See the Results of Teamwork and Clear Communication." *Trustee* 59, 7 (July/August 2006): 12.
154. Meyers, Susan. "Standardizing Safety," 14
155. Meyers, Susan. "Standardizing Safety," 21.
156. Pizzi, Laura, Neil I. Goldfarb, and David B. Nash. "Chapter 44. Crew Resource Management and Its Applications in Medicine," 7. *http://www.ahrq.gov/clinic/ptsafety/chap44.htm,* retrieved June 11, 2007.
157. Harris, Karen T., Catharine M. Treanor, and Mary L. Salisbury. "Improving Patient Safety with Team Coordination: Challenges and Strategies of Implementation." *Journal of Obstetrics, Gynecology, and Neonatal Nursing* 35, 4 (July/August 2006): 557.
158. Dunn, Edward J. "Effects of Teamwork Training on Adverse Outcomes and Process of Care in Labor and Delivery: A Randomized Controlled Trial." Letter to the Editor. *Journal of Obstetrics and Gynecology* 109, 5 (June 2007): 1,457.
159. Anderson, Craig, and Peggy A. Rivenburgh. "Benchmarking." In *Total Quality Management: The Health Care Pioneers,* edited by Mara Minerva Melum and Marie Kuchuris Sinioris, 326. Chicago: American Hospital Publishing, 1992.
160. Anderson and Rivenburgh, "Benchmarking," 226.
161. Eastaugh, Steven R. *Financing Health Care: Economics, Efficiency, and Equity,* 258. Dover, MA: Auburn House, 1987.
162. Fogarty, Donald W., Thomas R. Hoffmann, and Peter W. Stonebraker. *Production and Operations Management,* 18. Cincinnati, OH: South-Western Publishing, 1989.
163. Selbst, Paul L. "A More Total Approach to Productivity Improvement." *Hospital & Health Services Administration* 30 (July/August 1985): 86.
164. James, Brent C. *Quality Management for Health Care Delivery—Quality Measurement and Management Project,* 10. Chicago: Hospital Research and Educational Trust, 1989.
165. In ABC inventory analysis, items are classified into A, B, or C groups based on volume, criticalness, or dollar value. A is high; C is low. The A group should have highest priority.
166. Laliberty, Rene, and W.I. Christopher. *Enhancing Productivity in Health Care Facilities,* chap. 5. Owings Mills, MD: National Health Publishing, 1984.
167. Mosard, Gil R. "A TQM Technical Skills Framework." *Journal of Management Science and Policy Analysis* 8 (Spring/Summer 1991): 237.

168. Anderson and Daigh, "Quality Mind-Set," 26.

169. The section on Hoshin planning is adapted and updated from Rakich, Jonathon S. "Strategic Quality Planning." *Hospital Topics* 78, 2 (Winter 2000): 5–11. Used with permission from Helen Dwight Reid Education Foundation. Published by Heldref Publications, 1319 18th St. NW, Washington, DC 20036-1802. Copyright © 2000.

170. See O'Brien, James L., Stephen M. Shortell, Edward F.X. Hughes, Richard W. Foster, James M. Carman, Heidi Boerstler, and Edward J. O'Connor. "An Integrative Model for Organization-wide Quality Improvement: Lessons from the Field." *Quality Management in Health Care* 3, 4 (1995): 21; Hyde, Rebecca S., and Joan M. Vermillion. "Driving Quality Through Hoshin Planning." *Joint Commission Journal on Quality Improvement* 22 (January 1996): 28; Horak, Bernard J. *Strategic Planning in Healthcare: Building a Quality-Based Plan Step by Step,* 2–4. New York: Quality Resources, 1997.

171. Demers, David M. "Tutorial: Implementing Hoshin Planning at the Vermont Academic Medical Center." *Quality Management in Health Care* 1 (Summer 1993): 64.

172. Shortell, Stephen M., Daniel Z. Levin, James L. O'Brien, and Edward F.X. Hughes. "Assessing the Evidence on CQI: Is the Glass Half Empty or Half Full?" *Hospital & Health Services Administration* 40 (Spring 1995): 6.

173. Kennedy, Maggie. "Using Hoshin Planning in Total Quality Management: An Interview with Gerry Kaminski and Casey Collett." *Journal on Quality Improvement* 20 (October 1994): 577.

174. Melum and Collett, *Breakthrough Leadership,* 4.

175. Melum and Collett, *Breakthrough Leadership,* 17.

176. Hyde and Vermillion, "Driving Quality," 30.

177. Plsek, Paul E. "Techniques for Managing Quality." *Hospital & Health Services Administration* 40 (Spring 1995, Special CQI Issue): 68–69.

178. Melum and Collett, *Breakthrough Leadership,* 21.

179. McLaughlin and Kaluzny, "Total Quality Management," 8.

180. Kelly, John T., and James E. Swartwout. "Development of Practice Parameters by Physician Organizations." *QRB* 16 (February 1990): 54. (Use of the term *practice parameters* is preferred by the American Medical Association, the American Academy of Neurology Quality Standards Subcommittee, and the American Academy of Pediatrics; Merritt, T. Allen, Donald Palmer, David A. Bergman, and Patricia H. Shiono. "Clinical Practice Guidelines in Pediatric and Newborn Medicine: Implications for Their Use in Practice." *Pediatrics* 99, 1 [January 1997]: 100–114.)

181. Kelly and Swartwout, "Development of Practice Parameters," 55.

182. Citrome, Leslie. "Practice Protocols, Parameters, Pathways, and Guidelines: A Review." *Administration and Policy in Mental Health* 25 (January 1998): 258.

183. Larsen-Denning, Lorie, Catherine Rommal, and Annie Stoekmann. "Clinical Practice Guidelines." In *Risk Management Handbook for Health Care Organizations,* 2nd ed., edited by Roberta Carroll, 575. Chicago: American Hospital Publishing, 1997.

184. Mendelson, Dan, and Tanisha V. Carino. "Evidence-Based Medicine in the United States—de Rigeur or Dream Deferred." *Health Affairs* 24, 1 (January/February 2005): 133–136.

185. Coffey, Richard J., Janet S. Richards, Carl S. Remmert, Sarah S. LeRoy, Rhonda R. Schoville, and Phyllis J. Baldwin. "An Introduction to Critical Paths." *Quality Management in Health Care* 1 (Fall 1992): 46.

186. Gillies, Robin P., Stephen M. Shortell, and Gary J. Young. "Best Practices in Managing Organized Delivery Systems." *Hospital & Health Services Administration* 42 (Fall 1997): 303.

187. "Good News on Guidelines." *Hospitals & Health Networks* 72 (January 5, 1998): 13.

188. Kelly and Swartwout, "Development of Practice," 55.

189. "Risk Management: Guideline Payoff." *Trustee* 51 (October 1998): 7.

190. Larsen-Denning, Rommal, and Stoekmann, "Clinical Practice Guidelines," 579.

191. Bigelow and Arndt, "Total Quality Management," 21.

192. Weiner, Shortell, and Alexander, "Promoting Clinical Involvement," 492.

193. James, Brent C. "How Do You Involve Physicians in TQM?" *Journal for Quality and Participation* (January/February 1991): 43.

194. See also Kaluzny, Arnold D., Curtis P. McLaughlin, and David C. Kibbe. "Continuous Quality Improvement in the Clinical Setting: Enhancing Adoption." *Quality Management in Health Care* 1 (Fall 1992):

37–44 and Berwick, Donald M. "The Clinical Process and Quality Process." *Quality Management in Health Care* 1 (Fall 1992): 1–8, for ways to enhance physician involvement in CQI.

195. James, "Implementing Practice Guidelines," 44.

196. Laffel and Blumenthal, "The Case for Using," 2,870.

197. Lagoe, Ronald J., and Deborah L. Aspling. "Enlisting Physician Support for Practice Guidelines in Hospitals." *Health Care Management Review* 21 (Fall 1996): 61–67.

198. James, "How Do You Involve," 44.

199. Succi, Melissa J., Shou-Yih Lee, and Jeffrey A. Alexander. "Trust Between Managers and Physicians in Community Hospitals: The Effects of Power Over Hospital Decisions." *Journal of Healthcare Management* 43 (September/October 1998): 398.

200. James, "How Do You Involve," 44.

201. James, "How Do You Involve," 44.

202. James, "How Do You Involve," 47.

203. James, "How Do You Involve," 47.

204. Shortell, Stephen M., James L. O'Brien, Edward F.X. Hughes, James M. Carman, Richard W. Foster, Heidi Boerstler, and Edward J. O'Connor. "Assessing the Progress of TQM in U.S. Hospitals: Findings from Two Studies." *Quality Letter for Healthcare Leaders* 6 (April 1994): 15–16.

205. James, "Implementing Practice Guidelines," 7.

206. Carman, James M., Stephen M. Shortell, Richard W. Foster, Edward F.X. Hughes, Heidi Boerstler, James L. O'Brien, and Edward J. O'Connor. "Keys for Successful Implementation of Total Quality Management in Hospitals." *Health Care Management Review* 21 (Winter 1996): 58.

207. Ferguson, T. Bruce, Eric D. Peterson, Laura P. Coombs, Mary C. Eiken, Meghan L. Carey, Frederick L. Grover, and Elizabeth R. DeLong. "Use of Continuous Quality Improvement to Increase Use of Process Measures in Patients Undergoing Coronary Artery Bypass Graft Surgery." *Journal of the American Medical Association* 290, 1 (July 2, 2003): 49–56.

208. Shortell, O'Brien, Hughes, Carman, Foster, Boerstler, and O'Connor, "Assessing the Progress," 15.

209. Lagoe and Aspling, "Enlisting Physician Support," 61.

210. Shortell, O'Brien, Hughes, Carman, Foster, Boerstler, and O'Connor, "Assessing the Progress," 15.

211. Berwick, "The Clinical Process," 3.

212. Kaluzny, McLaughlin, and Kibbe, "Continuous Quality Improvement," 40.

213. Shortell, O'Brien, Hughes, Carman, Foster, Boerstler, and O'Connor, "Assessing the Progress," 16.

214. Shortell, O'Brien, Hughes, Carman, Foster, Boerstler, and O'Connor, "Assessing the Progress," 16; Carman, Shortell, Foster, Hughes, Boerstler, O'Brien, and O'Connor, "Keys for Successful," 50.

215. Sisk, Jane. "How Are Health Care Organizations Using Clinical Guidelines?" *Health Affairs* 17 (September/October 1998): 97.

216. Sisk, "How Are Health Care," 99–100.

217. Sisk, "How Are Health Care," 106.

218. The Lone Ranger is a fictional comic book and movie character who fought evil and brought justice in the American West, aided only by his faithful Indian companion, Tonto. Characterizing someone as a "lone ranger" suggests that he or she alone, or with little assistance, will solve a problem.

219. Kaluzny, Arnold D., Curtis P. McLaughlin, and David C. Kibbe. "Quality Improvement: Beyond the Institution." *Hospital & Health Services Administration* 40 (Spring 1995, Special CQI Issue): 176.

220. Kaluzny, McLaughlin, and Kibbe, "Quality Improvement," 175.

221. Kaluzny, McLaughlin, and Kibbe, "Quality Improvement," 178–180.

222. Adapted from Kaluzny, McLaughlin, and Kibbe, "Quality Improvement," 181–185.

223. From the *Akron Beacon Journal,* July 12, 1991, C14; Ann Landers and Creators Syndicate, The Chicago Tribune, Chicago, IL. By permission of Esther P. Lederer Trust and Creators Syndicate, Inc.

224. From Vonderembse, Mark A., and Gregory P. White. *Operations Management: Concepts, Methods, and Strategies,* 2nd ed., 549–550. St. Paul, MN: West Publishing, 1991; reprinted by permission. Copyright © 1991 by West Publishing Company. All rights reserved.

8

Strategizing

One significant challenge for senior-level managers in health services organizations/health systems (HSOs/HSs) is establishing and maintaining sustainable relationships between these organizations and systems and their external environments. This requires continuous activity designed to assess internal and external environments and plan and carry out courses of action in response to what is seen there. These activities are referred to as strategic management, or strategizing. In this chapter, the term *strategizing* is used. Strategizing incorporates, but goes beyond, strategic planning, which is also examined.

Essentially, strategizing is achieving a "fit" or equilibrium between an organization and its external environment. The activities involved are future oriented and play a large role in how these entities establish and maintain sustainable relationships with their external environments. Of course, any equilibrium attained is at best temporary because of the constant flux (and growing complexity) of the environmental forces an organization must interact with and adapt to in order to survive and grow.

Strategizing can be viewed as providing the grand design and justification for the overall focus, direction, and operational management of HSOs/HSs. One useful perspective on strategic management, or strategizing, is that it requires managers who "understand the implications of external change, [have] the ability to develop strategies that account for change, and [have] the will as well as the ability to actively manage the momentum of the organization."[1]

Strategizing activities are better understood in the context of their relationship to systems theory and to planning in general. These two contextual aspects of strategizing are examined below to form a background for subsequent consideration of strategizing.

▬ Strategizing and Systems Theory ▬▬▬▬▬▬▬▬▬▬▬▬

Strategizing is consistent with, and presumes, a systems theory perspective. Morgan provides the image of the "organization as organism," building on the concept that organizations, like organisms, are open to and interact with their environment and must achieve an appropriate relation with that environment if the organization is to survive.[2] The organization seen as an open system continuously interacts with various forces and entities within its environment while these environmental factors are themselves dynamically interrelated. The management model presented in Figure 5.8 illustrates this for organizations.

CORE CONCEPTS OF SYSTEMS THEORY

Systems theory is built upon a set of core concepts. These are listed and briefly described below:

- *Input/conversion/output*—the system dynamic in which resources are imported into the organization from its environment as sources of energy to sustain its core technologies, which convert inputs into desired outputs (see Figure 5.7)
- *Feedback loops*—channels of information that allow the system to monitor its outputs, measure against standards, and adjust inputs and throughput as required
- *Homeostasis*—self-regulation using negative feedback
- *Entropy*—the tendency of systems to lose energy and become disorganized
- *Negative entropy*—the attempt to sustain the system (organism) and counteract entropy
- *Differentiation/integration*—the system dynamic that reflects the structural relationship of parts to the whole, in which units must be coordinated into subsystems and the latter into a unified whole for the system to be viable
- *Requisite variety*—the outcome of the organization's mapping of its environment to be able to respond to external forces and changes

The implication of the "requisite variety" attribute of general systems theory for HSOs/HSs is that their internal structures must map or correspond to the complexity of their relevant environments to achieve a good fit with the environment. For example, the rapid increase in regulations, and more recently in compliance processes, during the past four decades resulted in the hiring of in-house legal and risk management expertise to address compliance with the Employee Retirement Income Security Act (ERISA), Health Insurance Portability and Accountability Act (HIPAA), Americans with Disabilities Act (ADA), and Family and Medical Leave Act (FMLA), as well as changes in requirements and standards of The Joint Commission on Accreditation of Healthcare Organizations (The Joint Commission) and Centers for Medicare and Medicaid Services (CMS).

In anticipation of the application of Sarbanes–Oxley fiduciary requirements to the not-for-profit sector, governing bodies (GBs) and senior-level management must ensure that internal audit and compliance mechanisms are developed. Perhaps the most obvious adaptation of HSOs/HSs to environmental change is the pervasive impact of information technology/systems on both clinical and business operations, with the electronic health record becoming the gold standard in the industry. The development and implementation of health information systems and information technology have had implications for staffing, training, job design, process engineering, performance evaluation, incentives, and compensation, and more is anticipated.

An academic health center provides an example of the dynamics of an organization as an open system. Inputs include labor, expertise, supplies, cash, physical plant, and other resources. Throughput includes both core technologies, such as the medical, rehabilitative, diagnostic, and related clinical processes, and support technologies, such as food service, purchasing, financial management, legal counsel, and so forth. Outputs include

- Short-term process and activity measures, such as patient visits, physical therapy treatments, and intensive care unit nursing hours
- Clinical outcomes, such as lower cholesterol levels, increased range of motion, and decreased body mass index
- Impact/long-term effects on the health and well-being of the community, population, or "covered lives," such as lower prevalence of obesity, decreased teenage pregnancies, and decline in breast cancer mortality

Environmental Forces in an Open System

Organizations, as well as organisms, are affected by a wide variety of environmental forces, as shown in Figure 5.8. Organizations are influenced and constrained by these external forces, and organizations also may influence the forces. This depends upon the organization's size, asset base, financial health, reputation, and strategic direction. Using a large urban HSO as an example, the relevant environmental forces include but are not limited to the following:

- Demographic patterns and trends
- Economic conditions (local, regional, and national)
- Technological developments
- State of disciplinary knowledge/recommended practices
- Federal and state regulation and health policy
- Labor markets for providers, managers, and support staff
- Professional associations and organized labor
- Public officials and community leaders
- Organized interest groups and advocates
- Media representatives and opinion makers

HSOs/HSs engage in a continuous process of scanning their environments to address questions such as the following: How can we anticipate future demands and adapt to changes in our external environment? How is our mission established and reconsidered over time? How are objectives (desired outputs) established, and what influences their formulation? How do we develop and choose specific plans to accomplish objectives? Strategizing activities can help answer these and many other questions about how an organization establishes and maintains an effective relationship with its external environment, responding to both opportunities and threats emanating from that environment.

In addition to the sensing and responding mechanisms at work in its relationship to its external environment, an organization must also maintain effective feedback loops to ensure that it receives accurate, timely, and useful intelligence from its environment (see Chapter 13, Communication). The most useful feedback for the HSO would typically relate to its outputs and outcomes. A media report of a cluster of incidents of iatrogenic disease would serve as unwanted but nevertheless useful negative feedback as a sentinel indicator of problems in quality management and clinical processes. Similarly, an unusually high incidence of medical malpractice claims among one group of physicians within a preferred provider organizations (PPO) might occasion a review of physician recruitment and selection procedures as well as the clinical practices associated with this group. Alternatively, a highly favorable rating on quality indicators such as those in the Healthcare Effectiveness Data and Information Set (HEDIS) for a health maintenance organization (HMO) could be interpreted as an indication to "stay the course" in terms of its customer relationship management.

Strategizing and Planning

Before focusing on strategizing, it will be useful to establish some important definitions and concepts related to planning as background, because strategizing entails planning, especially strategic planning. *Planning,* in general, is defined as anticipating the future, assessing present conditions, and making decisions concerning organizational direction, programs, and resource deployment. The process of planning consists of a series of activities that include assessing present information about the organization and its environment; making assumptions about the future; evaluating present objectives, developing new ones, or both; and formulating organizational strategies and operational programs that will accomplish objectives when implemented.

Planning occurs at all levels of HSOs/HSs, which makes two distinct but related types of planning important: strategic and operational. *Strategic planning,* also known as strategizing, is performed at the GB and senior management levels with input from other organization members, including those of the professional staff organization (PSO) who hold leadership positions.[3] The GB exercises oversight to ensure that the strategic planning process is in place and accomplished appropriately.[4] Strategic planning, or strategizing, leads to the establishment of the intended outputs for an HSO/HS (see the Strategic Quality Planning: Hoshin Planning section in Chapter 7).

In turn, through operational planning, managers determine the means to accomplish the intended outputs. Operational planning is subservient to, is derived from, and must be in harmony with strategic planning. Operational planning involves establishing objectives along with operational programs, policies, and procedures in units of the organization that may encompass groups of departments, individual departments, and even smaller units and activities.

Strategic planning encompasses multiple years. Operational planning is usually short-term, with a time frame of 1 year or less. The GB and senior-level management are responsible for strategic planning. The GB is responsible for setting the HSO's/HS's direction—its mission and objectives. Senior-level management has significant input in formulating organization objectives and is charged with developing and implementing organizational strategies to accomplish them. The GB's role generally does not include originating strategy, although it is responsible for ensuring that strategic proposals brought to it by senior-level management are properly prepared and are consistent with the mission as well as responsibilities to stakeholders.

Middle-level managers are concerned with short-term operational planning and design and implementation of programs, policies, and procedures in their areas of responsibility. These most often occur at the level encompassing multiple departments. Finally, department managers and first-level managers also plan, usually in relation to specific operations or activities, such as in estimating workload, scheduling work activity, and allocating resources for which they have responsibility.

All planning has three distinctive attributes. First, planning can be considered futuristic because it anticipates what will be required of the HSO/HS and its component parts in the future and how this will be accomplished. When managers think systematically about the future and plan for contingencies, they greatly enhance their organization preparedness. Second, planning involves decision making because determining what is to be done and when, where, how, and for what purposes requires that alternatives be evaluated, decisions made, and resources allocated. All of this results in a clearer sense of organizational direction and enhanced effectiveness. Third, planning is dynamic and continuous—planned organizational activities are affected by future events and internal and external environmental forces. Consequently, continuous environmental surveillance and adaptive change are attributes of planning.

PLANNING AND THE MANAGEMENT MODEL

When related to the management model in Figure 5.8, the importance of planning in the management context is evident. Planning enables managers to deal with the external environment—the immediate healthcare environment and the larger general environment. Thus planning reduces uncertainty, ambiguity, and risk. By anticipating trends, and at times proactively influencing environmental variables, such as public policy, managers are more prepared for and able to respond to the myriad forces that affect them. Environmental forces that affect planning are more extensively discussed in Chapters 1 and 3.

Planning requires managers to focus on outputs. All organizational activity is directed toward accomplishing objectives, which are the ends, desired results, or outputs to be attained. From desired outputs, input needs are determined.

Planning enables managers to develop priorities and make better decisions about conversion design as well as allocation and use of resources. Integration of structure, tasks/technology, and people converts inputs to outputs. By identifying and focusing on objectives and formulating strategies and operational programs to achieve them, managers can design appropriate conversion processes and systems. These include some of the organizational arrangements that are presented in Chapter 2 and initiatives such as continuous quality improvement (CQI), work process design/redesign, and quality improvement described in Chapters 7 and 10. The function of decision making and its importance to the HSO's/HS's planned conversion of inputs to outputs are presented in Chapter 6.

As managers initiate organizational activity to accomplish predetermined objectives through chosen strategies and operational programs, they do so through people; Chapters 12 and 13 focus on leading and communicating with this important input resource.

Finally, planning is the foundation for resource allocation and control. It enables the HSO/HS to measure progress and determine whether expected results are being achieved. The control process described in Chapter 10 involves establishing standards for resource use and monitoring organizational activity against those standards. Criteria for measuring progress are based on objectives derived through planning.

HSO/HS PLANNING CONTEXT

All planning for HSOs/HSs, especially strategic planning, occurs in the context of external environments (see Figure 5.8). Managers are affected by the external environment, and they must anticipate, predict, or make assumptions about its future configuration and the effect on them. Several important environmental forces are noted above.

The general environment includes ethical/legal, political, cultural/sociological, economic, and ecological forces. The HSO's/HS's healthcare environment includes public policy (regulation, licensure, and accreditation), competition, healthcare financing (public and private), technology, health research and education, health status, and public health activities. For good or ill, these forces always affect what managers do and how they do it.

The post–World War II health services environment was highly supportive until the early 1980s. This was an era of expansion in capacity and growth in demand. The environment was relatively stable and predictable. Role clarity existed. Risk was low. Aggressive HSOs/HSs grew, those that were efficient thrived, and even many of the inefficient survived.

Since the mid-1980s, the healthcare environment has changed, becoming more turbulent, difficult, and even hostile. Most importantly, however, it is less certain. HSOs and HSs are less insulated. They are buffeted by fast-paced and changing external forces. The changes wrought by technology and new diagnostic and treatment procedures are breathtaking. Societal, consumer, and third-party payer assertiveness and demands for greater accountability are accelerating.[5] Power is shifting from providers to purchasers and consumers of care. Public and private sector initiatives to control costs are intensifying, and this heightens financial risk. These forces are contributing to intense competition among providers. Some of the results have been the formation of new financing and delivery arrangements, especially managed care organizations (MCOs) such as HMOs and PPOs; joint ventures; mergers and consolidations; and strategic alliances, especially the formation and growth of HSs.

As environmental turbulence gained momentum in the late 1980s, accelerated into the 1990s, and continues unabated in the 21st century, HSOs/HSs have been pursuing initiatives to contain the impact of external forces, decrease uncertainty, and lessen their risk. Recognizing that the rules of the game have changed, senior-level managers realize that their organizations and systems no longer have a guaranteed demand for their services from traditional constituencies, nor are they guaranteed a right to survive. Several proactive strategic responses to environmental forces are 1) embracing the philosophy of continuous improvement; 2) increasing recognition and prominence of marketing (see more in Chapter 9); and 3) undertaking formalized, systematic strategic planning, including strategic issues management, to enhance competitive position. Health services marketing is an environmental link to and integral part of strategic planning; strategic issues management is linked to strategic planning as a way of influencing public policy issues related to health services.

Environmental Planning Profile for the Early 21st Century

Even a cursory outline of key trends and characteristics of the most important forces in the environment in the late 20th and early 21st centuries suggests the complexity and turbulence of the external environment facing HSOs/HSs as they plan (strategically and operationally) for and in the years ahead. Selected characteristics of this environment include the following:

Demographics
- Graying of the population in the United States and Western Europe
  — "Old-old" (85+ years) as fastest growing age cohort
  — Baby boomer generation leaving the work force for retirement in this decade
- Increasingly diverse U.S. population (race, ethnicity, national origin, life style, religious practice, etc.)
  — Caucasian male now in the minority
  — Hispanic population with highest U.S. birth rate

Social Attitudes, Values, and Tensions
- A woman and an African American man as leading candidates for the Democratic Party nomination for the presidency in 2008
- Mainstream faith communities in conflict over sexuality, control of church property, and governance issues
- Partisan political conflict persisting over stem cell research, gay marriage, global warming, access to healthcare, American military interventions, and so forth

Health Policy, Legislation, and Regulation
- Part D amendments to Medicare providing partial prescription drug coverage for the elderly
- Managed care approaches to lower Medicaid costs
- HIPAA stipulations for ensuring confidentiality of health information and guarantees of health insurance portability
- Growth in state-initiated plans for universal health insurance coverage

- Cost shifting from employers to employees through increased deductibles, copays, and medical savings accounts
- Impact of Sarbanes–Oxley on corporate governance and fiduciary accountability

Scientific and Technological Developments

- Research and clinical applications of nanotechnology
- Developments in animal and human stem cell research
- New drugs to ameliorate memory recall in Alzheimer's patients
- Mapping the human genome
- Research and development of improved assistive technologies for individuals with physical and cognitive disabilities
- Intensive research efforts in structural and computational biology

Economic Trends

- Increasing globalization of the economy, including the interdependency of equities markets
- Growth in private capital funding of new businesses and technologies
- Outsourcing and off-shoring of U.S. manufacturing and service industries
- Privatization of traditionally public government functions, such as education, institutional corrections, and airline security
- Decline in numbers and influence of organized labor since the 1950s

Even such a highly selective list of environmental trends and influences suggests the persistence of the "turbulent white water" by which Vaill[6] characterizes the external environment facing all managers in the current era.

Products of Planning

In combination, strategic and operational planning yield tangible products, including statements of organizational missions, often including a vision and values for the HSO/HS; organization-level objectives, and subobjectives for its component parts; organization-level strategies, and substrategies for its component parts; and operational programs, policies, and procedures. Each of these products or outputs of planning is described below.

Mission, Vision, and Values

Virtually all planning efforts begin with and are grounded in mission statements. Mission statements "state the organization's purpose and reasons for existence" and "describe what the organization does and for whom."[7] In general, they include a specification of the organization's basic service, primary market, and technology or method of delivery.[8]

In short, the mission statement addresses these questions: What business(es) are we in and why? Who are our primary constituencies? How do we distinguish ourselves from our competitors (other organizations)? Although mission statements are typically broad and nonspecific, they should enable the organization to provide the public with a succinct (and preferably distinctive) statement of purpose.

Most HSOs/HSs link their mission statements to either vision statements or sets of core values or both. The vision statement, usually more condensed, less specific, and more philosophical than the mission statement, provides an articulation of how the organization's leadership wishes the organization to be perceived by its publics, along with a strategic view of its future direction and "a guiding concept of what the organization is trying to do and to become."[9] In addition, the organization often articulates its core values that serve as guiding principles for behavior of all members of the

TABLE 8.1.   SAMPLE OF MISSION, VISION, AND VALUES STATEMENTS OF HSOS/HSS

University of Pittsburgh Medical Center (UPMC) (www.upmc.com)

OUR MISSION AND VISION

The University of Pittsburgh Medical Center will redefine traditional models of healthcare delivery by becoming a truly integrated, self-regulating healthcare system, utilizing evidence-based medicine to produce superb clinical outcomes. The organization will be recognized nationally and internationally as a top tier academic center for research and clinical excellence, while remaining firmly rooted in the local community as a responsible corporate citizen and an integral part of western Pennsylvania.

OUR VALUES (EXCERPTS)

These values and principles guide the health system in achieving its mission and vision:

- We consider our people to be our greatest asset, and we seek to be responsive to the needs of individuals of all backgrounds.
- We strive for excellence in everything we do and believe that each member of the faculty and staff is responsible for the continuous improvement of quality in all aspects of the services we provide.
- We are committed to understanding and satisfying the expectations and requirements of our customers.
- We strive to provide an environment that supports and encourages the active leadership and participation of physicians throughout the system and fosters collaboration among healthcare professionals across programs and service lines.
- As stewards of the community's resources, we seek to operate in an efficient and effective manner in order to maintain financial strength and carry out the organization's mission, as well as to contribute to the economic stability and growth of the region.

Merck & Co., Inc. (www.merck.com)

OUR MISSION

The mission of Merck is to provide society with superior products and services by developing innovations and solutions that improve the quality of life and satisfy customer needs, and to provide employees with meaningful work and advancement opportunities, and investors with a superior rate of return.

OUR VALUES

- Our business is preserving and improving human life.
- We are committed to the highest standards of ethics and integrity.
- We are dedicated to the highest level of scientific excellence and commit our research to improving human and animal health and the quality of life.
- We expect profits, but only from work that satisfies customer needs and benefits humanity.
- We recognize that the ability to excel—to most competitively meet society's and customers' needs—depends on the integrity, knowledge, imagination, skill, diversity and teamwork of our employees, and we value these qualities most highly.

Miami–Dade County Health Department (www.dadehealth.org)

VISION

To Be a World-Class Public Health System.

MISSION

The mission of the MDCHD is to promote and protect the health of our community through prevention and preparedness today, for a healthier tomorrow.

VALUES

Integrity, Customer and Community Focus, Accountability; Teamwork, Excellence, Respect for People.

Presbyterian SeniorCare (www.srcare.org)

MISSION STATEMENT

For more than 70 years, Presbyterian SeniorCare has been improving the lives of older adults in southwestern Pennsylvania. A Christ-centered, non-profit organization, Presbyterian SeniorCare offers seniors a variety of living and care options, including assisted living, independent and supportive housing, nursing care, Alzheimer's care, home healthcare, CCRC living and more. Presbyterian SeniorCare assists and supports more than 5,000 older adults of all faiths and income levels annually at over 40 facilities throughout southwestern Pennsylvania.

organization. The value statements reflect the core operating values that form the infrastructure of the organizational culture and (in theory at least) provide criteria for the decision making of managers, professionals, and employees at all levels. Collectively, the mission, vision, and values statements should provide a coherent philosophy of management underlying the organization's behavior and its role in its environment and the broader society. The statements are "the foundation on which the rest of the strategic planning process is built,"[10] and the thoughtful consideration of these statements provides the first step for the strategic planning process.

Table 8.1 presents the mission, vision, and value statements of a sample of HSOs/HSs. Note the similarities and differences in these statements. Almost all such entities now display their statements of mission, vision, and values on their web sites.

Objectives and Subobjectives

Objectives are statements of the results to be accomplished. In the context of the management model in Figure 5.8, they also are HSO/HS outputs. They are the ends, targets, and desired results toward which all organization activity is directed. Most objectives are explicit, but some are implied. There are organization objectives—those to be accomplished by the organization or system as a whole— and subobjectives for particular differentiated units (i.e., divisions, departments, and programs).

Overall organization objectives are established by the GB, or in the case of HSs with differentiated subsidiary entities, entity objectives may be established by senior-level management with ratification by the GB. Often expressed in broad terms, organization objectives, when accomplished, result in mission fulfillment. Thus they are derived from and reflect the mission. Typical HSO/HS objectives are listed in Figure 5.8. Included are patient care and customer service; quality improvement; appropriate costs relative to quality; organizational survival and fiscal integrity; social responsibility and responsiveness to stakeholders; education, training, and research; and reputation. They are the outputs of the input-conversion process shown in Figure 5.7. Organization objectives seldom change in dramatic ways, but emphasis does change with circumstances. For example, survival becomes the foremost organization objective for an HSO/HS facing deteriorating market share, declining census and clinical staff, and insolvency.

Subobjectives are ends and results to be accomplished by various units of an organization or system. They provide direction for managers and other employees and are subsidiary to overall organization objectives. Figure 8.1 shows the hierarchical relationship between overall organization objectives and subobjectives for an HS and an HSO. In the case of the HS—which, for example, may be composed of a hospital, an MCO, and a nursing facility—each of these differentiated subsidiary entities that offer different services to different customers can have its own objectives set by the subsidiary's senior-level management. However, these objectives must be consistent with the system's overall objectives and mission. Subobjectives, in the case of the single HSO or subsidiary entities of an HS, are those that are pertinent to a specific unit or department. Typically, they are jointly formulated by middle- or first-level managers or both subject to senior-level management approval. They are derived from and must be consistent with subsidiary entity objectives, in the case of an HS, or overall organization objectives, in a single HSO.

Accomplishment of subobjectives at lower levels supports accomplishing overall organization objectives. At times, a conscious decision may be made to suboptimize subsidiary entity or unit objectives if doing so will enable the HSO/HS to accomplish overall organization objectives. For example, an HSO's chief medical officer may seek to accomplish a unit objective of providing the "best medical education in the world," to the detriment of HSO fiscal survival. In this instance, suboptimization (i.e., something less, such as achieving the "best medical education in its class of peer facility programs") would be appropriate.

Objectives that state realistic, attainable, and measurable results are critical to HSOs/HSs for the following reasons:

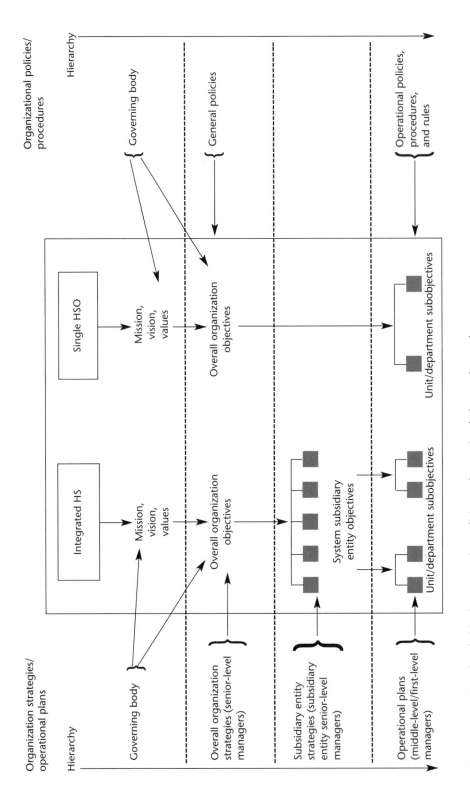

Figure 8.1. Hierarchy of objectives, strategies, policies, and operational plans and procedures.

1. They enable managers at various levels to focus attention on and initiate work toward specific ends.
2. They provide prioritizing criteria for decision making about services and programs.
3. They facilitate efficiency, particularly in allocating and using resources.
4. They give employees a uniform sense of direction that results in greater organization stability.
5. Knowledge of intended results is critical to formulating strategies to accomplish organization objectives and operational programs to achieve subobjectives.
6. They become criteria to be used in the control process when actual results (outputs) are compared with desired results (objectives).

Organizational Strategies and Operational Plans

Organization-level strategies are sets of activities that are selected and designed by GBs and senior-level managers to accomplish organization or system objectives. Strategies are long-term major patterns of activity requiring a substantial commitment of resources. *Strategy* is the term that is traditionally reserved to describe the means through which overall organization or system objectives can be accomplished. Examples of strategies include changing the scope of services, perhaps by specializing (e.g., adding a catheterization laboratory or an open-heart surgery unit); diversification (e.g., establishing a for-profit medical office building subsidiary); and forward or backward integration (e.g., expanding service area through a satellite family practice center or converting acute care beds to rehabilitation beds). Strategy formulation and implementation are the responsibility of senior-level management.

As presented in Figure 8.1, senior management, with oversight by the GB, formulates and implements overall organization or system strategies. In the case of an HS, senior-level managers in subsidiary entities formulate and implement strategies for their entities to accomplish entity objectives. However, they must support the system's objectives.

Conversely, operational plans are the specific sets of activities of individual units, departments, or programs. Their scope is less broad and global than that of organization strategies, and they are subsidiary to them. Just as all HSOs/HSs have a hierarchy of objectives, they also have a hierarchy of ways to accomplish them. As indicated in Figure 8.1, organization strategy is the means to accomplish overall organization/system objectives (and HS subsidiary entity objectives); operational plans are the subcomponents of strategies that accomplish HSO/HS unit (division, department, program) subobjectives.

Strategizing is overt, anticipatory, and long-term. In the case of a single HSO, its perspective embraces the whole organization rather than single departments or units; in the case of HSs, it embraces both the subsidiary (component) entities and the system as a whole. Strategizing is both externally and internally oriented and involves assessment of the HSO/HS vis-à-vis its external environment.[11] An integral part of effective strategizing is marketing, which is discussed in Chapter 9. Marketing facilitates environmental linkage.

Strategies are long-range, major patterns of activity requiring a substantial commitment of resources. It is appropriate to expand that definition here and add that strategies are the unified, comprehensive plans that capitalize on the HSO's/HS's strengths, take advantage of external opportunities, seek to reduce or overcome threats, and mitigate weaknesses. Strategies and the strategizing process are heavily influenced by a number of variables.

Organizational Culture

As discussed in Chapter 5, organizational culture is the ingrained pattern of shared beliefs, values, and assumptions that is acquired by organization members over time. Culture is the legacy—what the organization is and what it stands for. Culture shapes the acceptable behavior of members and depicts the desired nature of relationships between the HSO/HS and its stakeholders. Objectives must be consistent with mission and culture. Objectives that are inconsistent with the mission must be changed.

Stakeholders

Stakeholders are individuals, groups, or organizations affected by the HSO/HS who may seek to influence it and its objectives and strategies. Internal and external stakeholders, individually and in groups, seek to influence objectives and strategies.[12] It is the GB's responsibility to balance stakeholder demands and ensure that they are compatible with mission. Balancing requires maintaining ethical values and social responsibility and preventing inappropriate stakeholder demands from predominating.[13]

Values and Ethics

Establishing new objectives or modifying present objectives requires choice. The GB makes these choices. Just as culture and stakeholders influence objectives, so too do the values and ethics of those who make the choice. For example, new GB members with different values and preferences may influence an entity's direction.

General and Operational Policies and Procedures/Rules

Policies established by managers for HSOs/HSs (not to be confused with public policies) are officially expressed or implied guidelines and systems for guiding decisions and behaviors of organization members. Policies help organizations and systems attain objectives and thus must be consistent with those objectives and with the mission. Policies are classified as general or operational. The former apply to the entire organization or system and are formulated by senior-level management; the latter apply to a specific unit or department and are formulated by department managers to be consistent with general policy.

Familiar general policies governing human resources management are compensation, terms of employment, and on-the-job behavior. Examples are "we are an equal opportunity employer," "whenever possible, promotion will be from within," and "our compensation levels are competitive with those in the community." Other examples of general policies are "all patients will receive care regardless of ability to pay," "all employees are expected to ethically discharge their responsibility to patients/customers and each other," "capital equipment expenditures over \$50,000 must have prior senior-level management approval," and "life support for the terminally ill will be maintained unless the patient has an advance directive indicating otherwise."

Operational policies (sometimes called rules) for departments and other units are subsidiary to general policies and must be consistent with them. A human resources department operational policy might be to continuously update the compensation system's pay grades and rate ranges to remain competitive. A nursing department policy might be replacing licensed practical nurses with registered nurses to increase the intensity of nursing care as vacancies occur through attrition.

Procedures and rules guide actions for specific situations. Unlike policies, which are guidelines to decisions and behaviors, procedures are guides to action; rules prescribe specific actions. In general, they are expressed as a sequence of steps or tasks that are necessary to accomplish specific work. For example, there are procedures or rules for patient admission and discharge, requisition of supplies, ordering tests, sterilizing equipment, processing patient records, and reporting unsafe conditions or incident reporting of untoward events affecting patients.

Good policies and procedures are not easy to develop and implement. To be effective, a policy or procedure (or rule) must be clear and appropriate and must serve to guide the ways in which organizational activities are carried out. Good policies and procedures have several characteristics.[14] First, their impacts must be well thought out before they are formalized and must be in harmony with objectives. Policies or procedures whose negative effects have not been considered can be detrimental. For example, a PSO policy of ordering a full laboratory workup for every newly admitted patient may have a noble (or defensive) purpose but may be inconsistent with the HSO's/HS's objective of quality care at reasonable costs.

Second, policies and procedures must be flexible so they can be applied to typical as well as unique situations. Inflexible policies and procedures diverge from their intended purpose of providing guidelines for behavior and decision making. Situations may be encountered by managers or other employees that require judgment and atypical action. At times, managers appropriately deviate from policy and procedure—for example, not recording an employee's tardiness when delay was caused by an uncontrollable circumstance such as severe inclement weather.

Third, policies and procedures must be ethical and legal and reflect the values of the HSO/HS. A policy that permits employees to accept high-value gifts from suppliers may be legal, but it may be inconsistent with an integrity value.

Fourth, to be effective, a policy or procedure must be clear, communicated, understood, and accepted by those to whom it applies. A clear and communicated procedure on reporting sexual harassment informs employees how they must, and how they must not, perform in such a situation. Acceptability implies that employees consider the policy or procedure to be reasonable, legitimate, and fair. Policies and procedures that display unwarranted favoritism toward certain employee groups or those that appear to be arbitrary and with no sound purpose are more likely to be resisted or even ignored.

Fifth, to serve their purpose, policies and procedures/rules should be consistent with each other. They also should be consistent throughout the organization/system except when special and legitimate circumstances warrant differences. Unfounded inconsistency among policies and procedures and in application and enforcement of them is confusing and can cause employee dissatisfaction, frustration, and perhaps litigation, and it will detract from accomplishing objectives. Inconsistencies are most likely to occur among operational policies of various departments. Finally, to serve their intended purpose, policies and procedures must be continuously reevaluated and changed as necessary.

With the contextual background provided by the previous consideration of open system theory and planning, it is possible to construct a model of strategizing and to consider its interrelated components.

The Strategizing Process

The prevailing paradigm of strategizing, or as it is often called, strategic management, is that of a multi-level, iterative, and widely participatory process. It is an integrated set of planning, control, and decision-making processes looking outward to the HSO's/HS's environment; inward to its strengths, capabilities, and deficiencies; and forward to its future. Figure 8.2 illustrates the entire strategizing process, and each of its component activities is discussed in subsequent sections, beginning with situational analysis.

Situational Analysis

Situational analysis (see Figure 8.2) is the heart of strategizing. It essentially involves gathering and evaluating information about the past and present and making assumptions about the future. It is informed by external environmental analysis and internal environmental analysis. The results of assessment include identifying internal organizational strengths and weaknesses and external environmental opportunities and threats (hence the name *SWOT analysis:* strengths, weaknesses, opportunities, and threats), as well as risks, issues, and deficiencies.

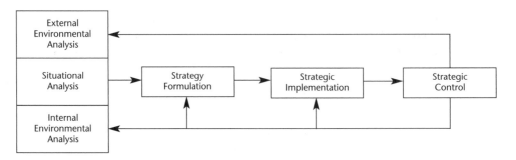

Figure 8.2. The strategizing process.

In essence, situational analysis is an ongoing review of strategic position as well as strategic alternatives. The senior-level managers are responsible for the assessment and for presenting its results to the GB for consideration, adjustment, and final approval.[15]

External Environmental Analysis

Environmental scanning to identify external threats and opportunities is critical to strategy formulation and choice among strategic alternatives. Threats in the environment are events that may adversely affect the HSO/HS. Examples include competition and new forms and places of service delivery; change in third-party reimbursement; change in target market demographics and health status; new technologies; changes in accreditation, regulation, and licensure; and economic conditions.

Opportunities are favorable or advantageous circumstances in the external environment that may be beneficial. Examples include change in demographics and service patterns, decline in primary care physicians in a rural area enabling a hospital to open a family practice center, and favorable alteration of a Medicare or Medicaid reimbursement policy.

A well-conducted external environmental analysis includes all the variables outside the boundaries of an HSO/HS that can influence the decisions and actions of its GB and managers. This may include complementary or competitive entities, patients/customers, suppliers, regulators, insurers, accrediting agencies, and so forth. It also includes other more general aspects of the external environment that can have a direct or indirect impact on the HSO/HS. Thus, for example, the general economy, the legal system, the physical environment, and community cultural norms and patterns are relevant.

The conduct of an external environmental analysis includes five interrelated steps: 1) scanning to identify relevant information (trends, developments, or possible events that represent opportunities or threats for the HSO/HS), 2) monitoring or tracking the relevant information identified through scanning, 3) forecasting or projecting the future directions of relevant information, 4) assessing the implications of the information, and 5) diffusing the information to those who can use it to guide decisions and actions.[16] Each step in the external environmental analysis process is described below.[17]

SCANNING

Scanning the external environment involves acquiring information that can affect an entity's future. Determination of what is important to scan—that is, what has strategic importance to an HSO/HS—has been described variously as being largely "judgmental," "speculative," or "conjectural."[18] Obviously, this makes the quality of the judgments, speculations, and conjectures about which of the vari-

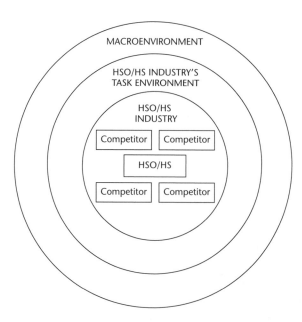

Figure 8.3. The external environment of a HSO/HS.

ables being scanned are of strategic significance quite important. For this reason, it is useful to have more than one person making these judgments.

One widely used approach to having multiple people involved in making these judgments is to rely upon a task force or ad hoc committee of people from within the HSO/HS to render a collective opinion. For example, a CEO might rely upon a group of senior- and middle-level managers for advice about what to scan. Another popular approach is to use outside consultants because managers can benefit from such expert opinions and judgments as to what is strategically important in their environments. It is also possible to utilize any of several more formal expert-based techniques.[19]

Although the determination of what is important to scan is specific to an HSO/HS, there are models designed to guide the conduct of situational analyses. For example, Figure 8.3 shows a focal HSO/HS at the center of a conceptualization of its external environment. The focal entity is shown along with the other similar organizations with which it directly competes. These form an industry; the hospital, nursing facility, and HMO industries are examples.

The focal organization and the other organizations in its industry exist in a task environment, which extends to clients or customers, suppliers, regulators, insurers, accrediting agencies, and so forth, with which the organization has direct interactions. Finally, the external environment of an HSO/HS includes its macroenvironment, or general environment, as it is also called. This is composed of everything outside the industry's task environment. In total, a focal entity's industry, task environment, and macroenvironment produce biological, cultural, demographic, ecological, economic, ethical, legal, policy, political, psychological, social, and technological information that the entity should include in its external environmental analysis. The external environments of HSOs/HSs are so extensive and complex that it is useful to have some means to organize the external environmental analysis. Sector analysis is one such device.

Sector Analysis

Sector analysis is one way to organize an environmental assessment: Threats and opportunities are identified and competitive position is assessed. Important sectors include the following:[20]

Macroenvironment: "includes major trends and events taking place outside the specific environment in which the organization operates, e.g., the global economy, industry trends, national economic indicators," business cycle, unemployment (loss of third-party health insurance).

Economic environment: "includes trends, events, and economic indicators that are specific to the marketplace in which the organization operates; also included in this area is an assessment of the growth, strength, and impact of managed care arrangements in the delivery of healthcare services in the marketplace."

Regulatory environment: "includes recent or expected changes in the myriad regulations that directly affect the organization," including those of local, state, and federal government.

Social environment/culture: "includes issues such as public health status of the marketplace, [and] health impacts of generalized social behaviors such as poor diet, sexually transmitted disease, smoking, [and] substance and alcohol abuse"; also includes cultural factors such as respect or disrespect for authority, attitudes of employees about work, sexual mores, personal ethics, and societal attitudes such as those regarding abortion.

Political environment: "includes factors such as recently enacted or pending legislation at the local, state, and federal levels"; healthcare as an actual or perceived right; public policy and federal responsibility for healthcare.

Demographics and market: includes demographic changes and trends in the marketplace, such as changes in service area composition or target market; age (Medicare), income (Medicaid), location, and patient–payer mix; demand for services.

Competitive environment: includes defining and assessing existing competitors who provide services similar to the HSO/HS; the extent of rivalry; and the HSO's/HS's competitive position in the marketplace, such as barriers to entry, threat of new entrants, potential for substitute services and products, and the strengths and weaknesses of other buyers/sellers and the organization's strength as a buyer/seller.

Technology environment: "includes assessment of advances in pharmaceuticals, genetics, and high-tech equipment, and the knowledge base, skills, and talents of the organization's workforce"; also includes medical education and research and the cost and pace of technology infusion.

Stakeholders: includes identifying and understanding stakeholder power and influence, their relative importance to the HSO/HS, and the demands they place on it.

Each of these sectors is a relevant component of an HSO's/HS's external environment.

MONITORING

Effectively scanning the external environment identifies specific information about trends, developments, and events that represent either opportunities or threats for continued attention through monitoring. Monitoring is more than scanning. It involves tracking or following important information over time.

Aspects of the external environment are monitored or tracked because they are thought to be of relevance. Monitoring these aspects of the environment, especially when there is ambiguity as to their importance to the future, permits more information to be assembled about trends, developments, and events to clarify their importance or determine the rate at which they may be becoming important.

Monitoring has a much narrower focus than scanning because the purpose in monitoring is to build a base of data and information around the set of important or potentially important aspects of the external environment that were identified through scanning or verified through earlier monitoring. Usually far fewer aspects of the external environment are monitored than are scanned.

Monitoring is extremely important because it is so often difficult to determine whether information about trends, developments, or events actually represents either real opportunities or threats for a program or project. Under conditions of certainty, managers would fully understand the information and all its consequences for their decisions and actions. However, uncertainty characterizes much about the external environments of HSOs/HSs, and it cannot be removed completely. Uncertainty can, however, be significantly reduced by the acquisition of more detailed and sustained information through effective monitoring. As with scanning, techniques that feature the acquisition of multiple perspectives and expert opinions can be helpful. Careful monitoring and tracking provides the background for the next step in analyzing an external environment—forecasting environmental changes.

FORECASTING

Scanning and monitoring cannot, in and of themselves, provide managers with all the information they need about the external environment. Often, if managers are to use this information effectively in strategizing, they need forecasts of future conditions or states. This may give them time to adjust desired results or formulate and implement successful operational plans in response to the new conditions.

Scanning and monitoring external environments involve searching for early signals that may be the harbingers of what will become strategically important information about trends, developments, and events. Forecasting involves extending information beyond its current state.

Forecasts of some types of information can be made by extending past trends or by applying a formula of some kind. In other situations, forecasting must rely upon conjecture, speculation, and judgment. Sometimes, sophisticated simulations can be conducted to forecast the future. However, uncertainty characterizes the results of all of these methods. It is especially difficult to include in any of these approaches the fact that few strategically important pieces of information exist in a vacuum. There are almost always many variables at work simultaneously, and no forecasting techniques or models that have been developed fully account for this fact.

Trend extrapolation is a widely used forecasting technique. When properly used, this technique can be remarkably effective and is relatively simple to use. Trend extrapolation is nothing more than tracking information and then using the tracking results to predict future states. It works best in the prediction of general trends, such as the number of patients/customers predicted to be served by an HSO/HS or reimbursement rates for certain services from Medicare or Medicaid. For example, if the number of patients/customers has increased by 5% for each of the past 5 years, it may be reasonable to assume a 5% increase in the next year.

Another useful forecasting technique is scenario development.[21] A scenario is a plausible prediction about the future. This technique is especially appropriate for analyzing environments that include many uncertainties and imponderables, conditions that often characterize the external environments of HSOs/HSs.

The essence of scenario development is to define several alternative future states. These possibilities can be used as the basis for developing contingency strategies from which a choice is made; alternatively, the set of scenarios can be used to select what managers consider the most likely future, the one upon which strategizing will be based.

Multiple scenarios permit several future possibilities to be explored. After a range of possibilities has been reflected in a set of scenarios, if managers wish to choose one as the most likely scenario, they can do so. However, a common mistake in using scenarios for strategizing is to envision too early in the process one particular scenario as the correct picture of the future. One example with four possible scenarios that a manager might imagine is this:

1. Our external environment will be mostly the same as today's only better.
2. Our external environment will be much better than today's.
3. Our external environment will be mostly the same as today's only worse.
4. Our external environment will be radically different from today's.

Each of these scenarios describes a different external environment that an entity might have to fit into. This effort would guide strategy choices. [22]

ASSESSING

Scanning and monitoring information that is relevant to strategizing comprise important steps in conducting an external environmental analysis. Another important step is making accurate forecasts of the future state reflected in the information. However, managers must also be concerned about the specific and relative strategic importance of the information they are analyzing. That is, they must assess the strategic importance and implications of the acquired information and forecasts for their HSOs/HSs.

Making these assessments is not an exact science. More than anything else, it relies upon the judgment of the people making the assessments. Even so, there are several bases upon which the strategic importance of information in an external environment can be considered. Prior experience with similar information is frequently a useful basis for assessing the importance of information. Other bases include intuition or best guesses about what particular information might mean, as well as advice and insight from others who are well informed and experienced. When possible, quantification, modeling, and simulation of the potential impacts can be useful.

Making accurate determinations of the relevance and importance of information to the future is rarely a simple task. Aside from the difficulties encountered in collecting and properly analyzing enough information to fully inform the assessment, there sometimes are problems that derive from the influence of the personal preferences and biases of those conducting the environmental analysis. Such problems can force assessments that fit preconceived notions about what is strategically important rather than reflect the realities of the impact of particular information. As with other steps in the external situational analysis, multiple judgments about the strategic importance of information can help avoid the bias problem.

USING AND DIFFUSING INFORMATION FROM ANALYSIS

The final step in assessing an HSO's/HS's external environment uses the acquired information and forecasts in strategizing, which may include diffusing or spreading the information to those whose decisions and actions may be affected by it. This step is frequently undervalued as part of the conduct of an external environmental assessment; it may even be overlooked. Unless information is diffused to and used by all who need it, however, it does not matter how well the other steps in the assessment are performed.

Managers must base their strategizing on valid information about the external environment if this core activity is to be properly performed. In many cases, they will need to share the information with others as well. For example, in a large HSO or an HS, there may be component units and other subdivisions with managers of their own who must engage in strategizing. There are three basic ways that managers can spread the strategically important information obtained through an environmental analysis:

1. Dictate use of the information. Use coercion or sanctions where necessary, to see that the information is used in all the appropriate places.
2. Persuade others to use the information by reasoning with them.
3. Educate others as to the importance and usefulness of the information in their strategizing activities.

In dictating use, managers simply rely on the power of their position to dictate that the information is to be used. Other participants are expected to carry out the dictates by using the information in their own strategizing. Such dictates have appropriate uses. For example, an abrupt change in a state's reimbursement policy for Medicaid services might require an immediate operational shift, leaving little time for anything but an edict to ensure the use of this information in strategizing.

Dictates have the advantage of speed, although a major drawback is their disruptiveness and the sense they give to those who receive them of nonparticipation in the environmental assessment. The more participative persuasion and education approaches work better when time permits their use. These approaches are greatly facilitated when those who will use the information from an external environmental assessment participate in its conduct. Participation can be achieved through such devices as membership on committees or teams charged to conduct the scanning, monitoring, forecasting, and assessing aspects of the assessment.

Using and diffusing the strategically important information about the external environment completes the process of assessing the external environment. The level of comfort those responsible for any HSO/HS feel about its external environment depends very heavily on the thoroughness and care with which the external environmental assessment is conducted.

Internal Environmental Analysis

An internal environmental analysis (see Figure 8.2) involves cataloging both the strengths and weaknesses inherent in an HSO/HS. This analysis provides managers with an inventory of capability and a resource base for use in strategizing. It permits managers to draw inferences about their entities' comparative advantages or distinctive competencies. The analysis focuses on the functional areas and results in an organization profile.

Examples of potential organizational strengths are referral patterns, reputation for quality, cost efficiency, technology, qualifications and stature of clinical staff and other professionals, financial and other resources, range and types of services and products provided, a cohesive organizational culture, and proactive management. In addition, as summarized in Chapter 5, management skills (technical, human, and conceptual), roles (interpersonal, informational, and decisional as well as those of designer, strategist, and leader), and competencies (conceptual, technical managerial/clinical, interpersonal/collaborative, political, commercial, and governance) or, using the National Center for Healthcare Leadership's framework, transformation, execution, and people can be strengths. Weaknesses may include deficiencies in any of these elements; shortage of capital; outdated physical plant and equipment; hostile labor environment; poor quality/reputation; aging or decreasing numbers of physicians; or reactive management.

FUNCTIONAL AREA ANALYSIS

Functional area analysis is one method by which systematic internal environmental analysis can be performed to identify strengths and weaknesses and to provide a comprehensive organization profile. Among the functional areas typically analyzed are[23]

> *Marketing and service:* "includes analysis of the characteristics of current patients, such as payer source, acuity, demographics, origin and destination; referral sources; review of the current level of usage of services or product lines offered; channels or mechanisms for service delivery; promotional techniques; and success rate with each"; also includes target markets, reputation, specialization, image, barriers to market entry, breadth and depth of service, market share, access, and quality of clinical staff
>
> *Clinical systems:* "includes evaluation of output measures of volume and quality; level of technology available; level of technology needed; and skills and

knowledge base of clinicians"; also includes patient management control; skills, age and composition of medical staff; and status of clinical delivery CQI initiatives

Production: includes design of work processes and methods; cost of production; quality of outcomes; tasks–technology–people relationships; work scheduling and idle capacity; and equipment and facility size, capacity, and age

Financial: "includes evaluation of the availability and use of capital funds; use of operating revenues; ratio analysis; budget variances, and internal control mechanisms"; also includes patient–payer mix, leverage, financial reserves, accounting and billing systems, and earnings or residuals

Human resources: "includes evaluation of the skill levels in technical areas; availability of appropriately prepared personnel; recruitment and retention track record"; also includes quality of personnel skills, attitudes, compensation, stability of employment, productivity, commitment to CQI, and labor relations

Management: "includes evaluation of the number of levels; strength of each level as a whole and the individuals in that level"; also includes organizational structure and linkages; assessment of skills, roles, competencies, leadership and effectiveness of managers; and managers' perspectives, experience, values, ethics, and philosophies

Governing body: includes the composition, strength, skills knowledge, cohesiveness, commitment, oversight, and support to the HSO/HS and to the fulfillment of its mission

Culture: (not a functional area but important because it affects the functional areas) includes the organization's values and ethics; cohesiveness of the culture; philosophy about CQI, customers, and employees; and compatibility of culture with mission

Awareness of strengths in all functional areas and culture permits conclusions to be drawn about comparative advantage and the ability to implement strategies chosen. Some of these conclusions identify the organization's or system's particular competences, where it excels compared with other organizations, and how it can be differentiated. Is the HSO/HS the lowest cost provider? Does it provide the highest quality service? Does it have the best reputation? Is it committed to CQI and customer satisfaction? Is it on the cutting edge of technology application? Comparative advantage is a barrier to entry that others must overcome to compete with an entity. Information about comparative advantage, strengths, and weaknesses allows consideration of organizational strategies that capitalize on the first two and mitigate the last.

The systematic assessment and appraisal through external and internal environmental analysis identifies external threats and opportunities facing the HSO/HS as well as internal organizational strengths and weaknesses. Conclusions can be drawn about the HSO's/HS's comparative advantage and competitive position. This is often referred to as SWOT analysis (strengths, weaknesses, opportunities, and threats).[24] It enables managers to identify risks, issues, organizational deficiencies, and gaps in objectives that are the difference or discrepancy between actual and desired results.

Strategy Formulation

Figure 8.2 indicates that strategizing includes formulation of strategies based on information and insight provided by situational analysis. This part of the overall process includes identifying strategic options and selecting from among the options strategies for implementation.

At any time, an array of strategies can be identified, evaluated, chosen, and implemented to achieve objectives. Alternative strategies are extensively discussed in the literature, and several are discussed in this section. Those more specifically related to marketing are discussed in Chapter 9. To categorize or classify organizational strategies, two important points must be made. First, the categorization is always relative to the frame of reference of the HSO/HS—that is, its core services and products. For example, an acute care hospital's adding a full-line family practice center would be categorized as related diversification (i.e., not part of a core service); if the center were freestanding in a different geographic or market area, it also would be categorized as vertical integration (i.e., closer to the consumer—forward, or downstream). However, in the case of a physician group practice, adding a related service such as a laboratory or dietary counseling to its family practice center to provide a full line of services would be horizontal integration (i.e., related to its core service and at the same point in production). The second point is that managers rarely choose and implement only one strategy; it is common for multiple strategies to be implemented concurrently.

COMMON STRATEGIES

A catalog of many of the strategies available to an HSO/HS is shown in Table 8.2. As is done in this table, the numerous strategic alternatives can be classified into several different types.[25]

Directional strategies are developed and articulated in an HSO's/HS's mission, vision, values, and objectives (see Table 8.2, which contains examples). Directional strategies help guide the strategic choices in the adaptive, market entry, competitive, and implementation categories of strategies.

Adaptive strategies delineate how the HSO/HS will expand, contract, or stabilize operations, whether through diversification, vertical integration, market development, or product development. Contraction strategies include divestiture, liquidation, and retrenchment.

Market entry strategies are formulated to provide the means by which strategies to expand or

TABLE 8.2. SCOPE AND ROLE OF STRATEGY TYPES

Strategy	Scope and Role
Directional Strategies	The broadest strategies set the fundamental direction of the organization by establishing a mission for the organization (Who are we?) and providing a vision for the future (What should we be?). In addition, directional strategies specify the organization's values and the broad goals it wants to accomplish.
Adaptive Strategies	These strategies are more specific than directional strategies and provide the primary methods for achieving the vision of the organization—adapting to the environment. These strategies determine the scope of the organization and specify how the organization will expand scope, contract scope, or maintain scope.
Market Entry Strategies	These strategies carry out the expansion of scope and the maintenance of scope strategies through purchase, cooperation, or internal development. These strategies provide methods for access or entry to the market. They are not used for contraction of scope strategies.
Competitive Strategies	Two types of strategies, one that determines an organization's strategic posture and one that positions the organization vis-à-vis other organizations within the market, are market oriented and best articulate the competitive advantage within the market.
Implementation Strategies	These strategies are the most specific strategies and are directed toward value added service delivery and the value added support areas such as the culture, structure, and strategic resources. In addition, individual organizational units develop action plans that carry out the value added service delivery and value added support strategies.

Source: Swayne, Linda E., W. Jack Duncan, and Peter M. Ginter. 229. Strategic Management of Healthcare Organizations, 5th ed. Malden, MA: Blackwell Publishing, 2006. Used by permission.

maintain the scope of an organization are carried out in the marketplace. These strategies include acquisitions and mergers, internal development, alliances, and joint ventures, among others. These market entry strategies may be used to carry out an adaptive strategy.

Competitive strategies, sometimes called positioning strategies, relate to how consumers view an HSO's/HS's services and products in the context of products and services available from competitors. Often called generic strategies, the competitive strategies include cost leadership, differentiation, and focus strategies.

Implementation strategies are developed to implement directional, adaptive, market entry, and competitive strategies. Implementation strategies can apply to the entire HSO/HS, as do changing organizational culture or reorganizing, or they can be specific to one or more of its functional departments, such as marketing, finance and, human resources.[26]

A number of adaptive, market entry, and competitive or positioning strategies in addition to those shown in Table 8.2 are extensively used in HSOs/HSs. Several of these are described below.

SPECIALIZATION/NICHE STRATEGIES

Specialization is a strategy in which HSOs/HSs emphasize selected services or products, often based on disease or acuity of illness. Some hospitals, for example, are known for their specialization in oncology, organ transplantation, and cardiac surgery; nursing facilities specialize in long-term care; hospices specialize in the care of those who are terminally ill. A niche strategy involves focusing on a service area, such as the inner city, or a target market, such as outpatients. An HS specialization strategy might involve the HS's component organizations' focusing on rehabilitation or acute care services. Both strategies are essentially the same as the Porter focus strategy (see Chapter 9) and usually are implemented in tandem—as in the case of a pediatric hospital that specializes by type of care (e.g., neonatal) and has a niche in a specific target market (children)—and may involve differentiation based on low-cost, high-technology leadership.

VERTICAL INTEGRATION AS A STRATEGY

The vertical integration strategy occurs when an HS operates at more than one point on a chain of production, distribution, or both. Vertical integration results in a "broad range of patient care and support services operated in a functionally unified manner."[27] It adds upstream or downstream services.[28] Vertical integration is generally based on patients' acuity of illness, which can range from acute to chronic. Examples of forward (i.e., downstream) integration for an acute care hospital include involvement in an HS featuring ambulatory care, satellite family practice clinics, or wellness promotion. Backward (i.e., upstream) integration includes long-term care and rehabilitation, as well as acquired home health agency services.[29]

Vertical integration also may occur in nonservice areas—that is, in factors of production that involve make/buy decisions. Examples are the development or acquisition of businesses that provide contracted housekeeping or information system services for the HSO/HS or that supply or manufacture generic pharmaceuticals, prosthetic devices, or intravenous solutions.

HORIZONTAL INTEGRATION AS A STRATEGY

In contrast to the strategy of vertical integration, horizontal integration occurs when an HSO expands its core services or products at the same point in the production process and in the same part of the industry. In the case of an HS, it would be "lateral relationships among like entities."[30] Horizontal integration usually is done to round out core service/product lines and to enter new markets with existing types of services.

Horizontal integration may be achieved through internal development, acquisition, or merger. An acute care hospital that adds coronary bypass surgery to its existing core surgical services or that builds a suburban acute inpatient hospital is horizontally integrating. Hospital systems or nursing facility chains in which member facilities offer the same core services are horizontally integrated, and they most often use this strategy to reach new markets and to achieve economies of scale for support and management services, enhance access to capital, and lower overall organization risk.

Horizontally linked HSOs/HSs may be closely coupled through ownership or loosely coupled through affiliations or alliances. Examples of geographically dispersed, horizontally integrated, for-profit HSs include Beverly Enterprises (*www.beverlycares.com/BeverlyHealthcare*) and HCA, Inc. (*www.hcahealthcare.com/CPM/CurrentFactSheet1.pdf*). Beverly operates about 82 nursing facilities across the United States. HCA operates about 173 general acute hospitals across the United States.

DIVERSIFICATION AS A STRATEGY

Diversification strategies permit HSOs/HSs to add new services/products, enter new markets, or both where neither is directly related to their core services/products. Diversification usually is defined relative to 1) the traditional main line of business, core services, or both and 2) whether the activity is related or unrelated. For acute care hospitals, diversification includes adding new non-inpatient care services/products, such as industrial medicine or women's medicine, or such nonacute care services as rehabilitation or substance abuse.

There are two types of diversification: concentric and conglomerate. Concentric diversification occurs when different but related healthcare services/products are added to the existing core of services. This may be done to increase revenues or to enhance competitive position and reach new target markets. Concentric diversification also may constitute forward or backward integration. For example, an acute care hospital that diversifies into long-term care by converting acute care beds is also engaging in vertical integration.[31] One way of classifying strategy as vertical integration or diversification is by intent relative to patient flow. If the purpose is to control patient flow, such as by an acute care hospital's acquiring physician practices, then this strategy can be classified as vertical integration. If the purpose of acquiring a nursing facility is entering a growth market and not controlling patient flow from the hospital, this strategy can be classified as concentric diversification.

The second form of diversification is conglomerate diversification. Here an HSO/HS produces non–health-related products/services that are unrelated to its principal business or core services. An example is a hospital's providing laundry or computer services to other organizations; investing in real estate, such as shopping centers, homes, or apartments; or providing catering services. Although concentric diversification is the most common form for HSOs/HSs, some do engage in conglomerate diversification.

RETRENCHMENT/DIVESTITURE AS A STRATEGY

A strategy of retrenchment, or downsizing, involves reducing the scope or intensity of products/services, partial withdrawal from a market area, or decreasing capacity in terms of facilities, equipment, or staff. A divestiture is eliminating a group of services or products, complete withdrawal from a market area, or closing facilities. In highly competitive markets in which the HSO/HS has no comparative advantage or in instances in which demand has decreased, it may implement a strategy of retrenchment—in extreme cases, divestiture.

The more commonly implemented strategy is retrenchment. This reduces losses, permits reallocation of resources to more promising services, and in extreme cases, enables an entity to survive. Declining birth rates in a service area may cause a hospital to downsize obstetrics; high levels of uncompensated care may cause an HSO to close (retrench/divest) its trauma centers; and low inpatient occupancy rates may cause another HSO to reduce the number of acute care beds (retrench) while converting those beds to long-term or rehabilitative care (both vertical integration and concentric diversification).

STRATEGIC ALLIANCES AS A STRATEGY

Joint ventures, mergers, and consolidations are strategic alliances (SAs) that represent prevalent strategic arrangements in health services delivery. SAs as a strategy grew in the 1990s and continue to be popular today. Frequently, the strategy is coupled with one or more other strategies. For example, joint ventures can be coupled with vertical and horizontal integration. SAs arise from mutual need and a willingness among the participating HSOs/HSs to share knowledge, capabilities, risks, and costs; to leverage innovation; and to take advantage of complementary strengths and capabilities. "Such alliances are designed to achieve strategic purposes not attainable by a single organization, providing flexibility and responsiveness while retaining the basic fabric of participating organizations."[32]

SELECTING STRATEGIES

The range of alternative strategies considered, and of those eventually selected, is greatly influenced by the context in which the choice of strategies is made. Although there are other aspects of the context in which strategic choices are made, key ones include

- Type of organization
- Strategic decision style
- Managerial philosophy
- Organizational culture and choice-maker values
- Portfolio analysis
- Organization life cycle
- Competitive position

Each of these elements is discussed below.

Type of Organization

Type of organization refers to self-image and how the HSO/HS adapts to its external environment, competitors, and customers. A useful typology is that developed by Miles and Snow:[33] prospector, analyzer, defender, and reactor. This typology has been applied to studies of HSOs/HSs[34] and is discussed further in Chapter 9.

    Prospectors might occasionally redefine markets, routinely seek new target markets, seize the initiative, and capitalize on opportunities; they are proactive, tending to be innovative and at the forefront of applying new technologies. Analyzers also are proactive but not as much so as prospector organizations. They seek to maintain stability in selected areas of operation, although, following and guided by the experience of prospectors, they seek new opportunities. A defender seeks to maintain the status quo and stability; it is not innovative. In general, such HSOs/HSs vigorously protect what they have, such as a niche or specialized service/product domain. Reactors are passive and usually stir to action only in a crisis or when external environmental forces cannot be ignored.

Strategic Decision Style

Strategic decision style describes the process by which strategic alternatives are formulated and evaluated and decisions are made. It can be classified as systematic, entrepreneurial, or incremental.[35] A systematic strategic decision style is proactive. It involves comprehensive external and internal analysis; understanding interrelationships of threats, opportunities, strengths, and weaknesses; considering all strategic alternatives; and selecting an organizational strategy on the basis of rational criteria.

Entrepreneurial strategic decision style reflects decisions made on "gut feelings," hunches, or intuition. It in general does not include full and comprehensive strategic assessment, only selected review; thus it is a style in which strategic decisions are made quickly. In mature HSOs/HSs, entrepreneurial decision style is, in general, inappropriate. However, it may be appropriate for emerging or even mature HSOs/HSs in a turbulent, fast-changing environment, especially if windows of opportunity close rapidly, thus making quick decisions imperative.

Incremental strategic decision style is generally reactive and usually involves change at the margin. Sometimes it means simply muddling through.[36] Incremental decision styles are piecemeal approaches to strategy choice and do not include comprehensive, systematic strategic assessment or reviewing and evaluating a full range of potential strategies.

Managerial Philosophy

Managerial philosophy in the context of choosing strategies is best described as a continuum that ranges from opportunity maximization to cost minimization. The former is a proactive, prospector, systematic/entrepreneurial perspective. It implies that organizational strategies are chosen to take advantage of opportunities and capitalize on strengths.

Cost minimization as a philosophy implies conservatism. It may be seen in a defender but is certainly found in a reactor. It focuses on how to "save a buck" without considering opportunity costs. Organizations are never entirely at one end of the continuum but usually are closer to one end or the other. Other similar descriptive terms are *aggressive-innovative* versus *lethargic-conservative* or *risk taking* versus *risk averse*. HSOs/HSs that are opportunity maximizers, aggressors-innovators, and risk takers usually consider and choose different strategies than those at the other end of the continuum.

Organizational Culture and Choice-Maker Values

Organizational culture and the values of decision makers who formulate strategies are contextual variables that often affect the selection of strategies from among options. Organizational culture is a continuum from harmonious to divisive, and the values of those formulating strategy can be consistent or inconsistent with culture. Cultural disarray—perhaps caused by splintered factions, internal hostility, and a lack of cohesion, mutual support, and shared beliefs—leads to divisiveness. Under such circumstances, it may be impossible to gain the commitment of participants to implement complex strategies and weather the resulting changes required by the strategy. Mismatching culture and strategy causes implementation difficulties. This restricts the range of realistic strategies.

HSOs/HSs with strong, cohesive cultures and values shared by GB members and senior-level managers can prospect, be more opportunistic, and successfully implement a wider range of organization strategies than those with a divisive culture and managerial values at variance with the culture. As has been observed, "what a business is able to accomplish may be determined as much, if not more, by its culture than its strategic plan. Strategies are only as good as the culture that exists to encourage and support them."[37]

Portfolio Analysis

Portfolio analysis is borrowed from marketing and describes and categorizes resource-producing or resource-consuming services and products. The typical nomenclature is *cows, hogs, and stars*.[38] Cows are services or product lines that yield more than they consume; hogs consume more than they yield; and stars, if nurtured, will evolve from embryonic resource consumers into cows.

Portfolio analysis of services or product lines in an HSO, for example, might determine that pharmacy and radiology are cows, obstetrics is a hog, and sports medicine is a star. Organizations with a preponderance of cows and stars are in a better position to prosper and have greater latitude in strategy formulation than those with a preponderance of hogs. Portfolio analysis is important to strategy formulation because it allows strategic managers and GBs to recognize the cows, hogs, and stars of their organizations and how alternative strategies may change the ratio of these three categories.[39]

Another variable that affects the context of strategy formulation is strategic business unit analysis, or as applied in HSOs/HSs, strategic service unit (SSU) analysis. This type of segmentation is like portfolio analysis except that *SSU* generally refers to identifiable, relatively autonomous organizational units with distinct services and product lines that are offered to distinct target markets. SSUs have reasonable control over their activities, are separate from other SSUs, compete with external groups for market share, and have their own revenues and costs.[40] Each differentiated subsidiary unit in a vertically integrated HS is a separate SSU. For example, a vertically integrated HS that owns two hospitals, an HMO, and a nursing facility could segment them into four SSUs. SSUs are important to the context of strategizing because a distinct and even different strategy may be chosen and implemented for each.

Organization Life Cycle

Organization life cycle refers to the stage of development of an HSO/HS. Conceptually, organization life cycle borrows from theories of aging in human beings and product life cycle in marketing. All organizations, including all HSOs/HSs, go through stages of emergence, growth, maturity, decline, and perhaps regeneration, although time spans vary. Figure 8.4 presents this concept graphically.

It is important to note that external or internal events (changing technology, competition) can increase or decrease the slope of the life cycle curve, lengthen or shorten it, and enable the HSO/HS to regenerate from one stage (maturity) to another (growth) or accelerate from one stage (maturity) to another (decline). Where an HSO/HS is in its life cycle helps determine the strategic alternatives available as well as the best choices. In the growth stage, HSOs/HSs may choose aggressive, expansionary-type strategies such as forward and horizontal integration and concentric diversification. They are likely to be prospectors and opportunity maximizers. Those in decline likely will be forced to retrench, minimize cost, and perhaps pursue niche strategies.

A variation on the organization life cycle concept is the service, product, or market life cycle. This is a life cycle concept especially appropriate to marketing (see Chapter 9). This concept applies the paradigm of biological development to the marketing of a product or service. As the biological

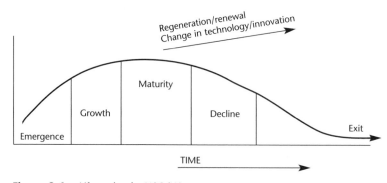

Figure 8.4.   Life cycle of a HSO/HS.

organism follows a cycle of birth to death, so do most services, products, and markets. The service, product, or market life cycle is usually presented as having at least five stages: birth (entry), growth, maturity, decline, and death. A sixth phase, of rebirth or renewal, may also be considered. The life cycles of services, products, or markets can be presented as curves plotted against time on the *x*-axis and growth (sales or revenues) on the *y*-axis. The curves look much like the one in Figure 8.4, which shows the life cycle of an organization.

The market entry phase shows a slow growth in revenues, usually accompanied by negative profits due to the high start-up costs. Assuming that the new service/product survives its infancy, it enters a phase of usually rapid growth in revenues and in profitability, which typically lags behind. Upon the organization's maturity, the life cycle curve peaks and flattens, suggesting stagnant growth. The life cycle curve then slants downward, reflecting decline in sales and profits, heading toward death (market exit and/or product termination). However, by an infusion of resources, product modifications, and creative promotion, the decline may be reversed and the life cycle continued.

Competitive Position

The feasible set of strategies that can be considered is partially predicated on an entity's competitive position. Barriers to market entry, threat of new entrants (competitors), availability of substitute products or services, and the HSO's/HS's strength as a seller or buyer are attributes of competitive position. Table 8.3 presents a matrix of strength of competitive position and product (or service) life cycle that suggests strategic behavior for each condition. Competitive position ranges from dominant to weak; life cycle ranges from embryonic to aging. The behaviors suggested in the table cells are determined by the strength of the HSO's/HS's competitive position and the position of its services in the product life cycle. An HSO/HS with a mature service, such as acute inpatient care, in a dominant position would seek to hold its market share and grow with the industry. One in a weak competitive position but with a growth service, such as cardiac surgery, could choose to make a substantial resource commitment (turnaround) to strengthen competitive position or could choose to abandon that service and redirect resources.

TABLE 8.3. COMPETITIVE POSITION/PRODUCT LIFE CYCLE MATRIX

Strength of competitive position	Life-cycle stage			
	Embryonic	Growth	Maturity	Aging
Dominant	Hold position All-out push for share	Hold position Hold share	Hold position Grow with industry	Hold position
Strong	Attempt to improve position All-out push for share	Attempt to improve position Push for share	Hold position Grow with industry	Hold position or harvest
Favorable	Selectively attempt to improve position Selective or all-out push for share	Attempt to improve position Selective push for share	Custodial or maintenance Find niche and attempt to protect it	Harvest Phased withdrawal
Tentative	Selectively push for position	Find niche and protect it	Find niche and hang on Phased withdrawal	Phased withdrawal or abandon
Weak	Up or out	Turnaround or abandon	Turnaround or phased withdrawal	Abandon

From Digman, Lester A. *Strategic Management: Competing in the Global Information Age,* 8th ed., 326. Mason, OH: Thomson Custom Publishing, 2006; reprinted by permission from Elsevier.

STRATEGY CHOICE

In strategy formulation (see Figure 8.2), a critical activity is choosing organizational strategies from among the strategies potentially available. The major context variables that influence these choices were examined above, including type of organization, strategic decision style, managerial philosophy, organizational culture and choice-maker values, portfolio analysis, organization life cycle, and competitive position. Heavily influenced by these context variables, choices from among strategic alternatives are also guided by a set of criteria used by specific entities in selecting strategies.

These criteria can provide answers to such questions as: Will the organizational strategy accomplish objectives? Will the strategy address risks, issues, deficiencies, and gaps? Will the strategy take advantage of opportunities in the environment and capitalize on strengths and comparative advantage? Will the strategy lessen threats and overcome weaknesses? In addition, attention must be given to the relationship between potential organizational strategies and the internal functional areas. That is, considering strengths and weaknesses, is the strategy feasible? Does the organization have the capacity—financial resources, managerial systems and human resources, and productivity and conversion processes—necessary to implement the strategy successfully? If so, implementation is the next step in strategizing, as depicted in Figure 8.2.

▪ Strategic Implementation

Once organizational strategies are selected, operational plans, policies, procedures, and rules are developed for the entire HSO/HS and/or for units or segments of the organization. As depicted in Figure 8.1, the plans, programs, and activities are derived from the strategies and must be consistent with them. It is necessary to gather and allocate resources and make organizational design arrangements that will support implementation of strategies. Challenges involved in carrying out strategies can be very significant. Strategies, no matter how carefully crafted, do not implement themselves.

A cardinal rule of good strategizing is that the process cannot ignore the fact that strategies must be implemented. Inherent in the consideration of culture, strengths, and weaknesses, as part of the situational analysis that provides background for selecting strategies, is the fact that there is a direct connection between an HSO's/HS's capabilities to implement particular strategies and the appropriateness of such strategies for the organization or system. This connection is very important. Entities that are designed for implementing particular strategies are more likely to implement them well than organizations and systems that have been designed for different strategies.[41] Strategic managers who have designed for stability and centralized decision making can have great difficulty implementing a corporate growth strategy of unrelated diversification, for example. Similarly, people who are experienced only in implementing growth strategies will have difficulty shifting to divestiture or retrenchment strategies.

Ideally, strategic managers recognize the connection between strategy and implementation capability in the strategy formulation stage, and they factor this into strategy choices. Sometimes, however, they do not. Divestiture, retrenchment, and other degenerative strategies are often forced on HSOs/HSs by the realities of their external environments. In such cases, it does not matter that the GB and senior-level managers prefer growth strategies. Consider what strategies have been forced on HSOs/HSs by public policies initiated to slow the rates of growth in the Medicare and Medicaid programs, for example. In other cases, the preference of strategic managers for particular strategies overrides the fact that implementation capabilities are not well matched to the preferred strategies.

When mismatches occur between strategies and implementation capabilities, whether imposed by external policy or market changes or the result simply of poor judgment by strategic managers, problems invariably arise in implementation. Such mismatches can be overcome in two ways: 1) strategies can be changed or 2) capabilities to implement a strategy can be changed. In the latter case, resources can be redirected, people can be provided with additional training and education, and new people can be brought into the situation to support strategy implementation.

Even when there is a close match between strategies and implementation capabilities, strategy implementation requires that those responsible for strategic implementation establish appropriate organizational structures, assemble a workforce with the skills and abilities to carry out the implementation of strategies, and build and maintain well-coordinated relationships among organizational units, as crucial factors in successful implementation. Similarly, the ability of strategic managers to motivate the necessary levels of effort on the part of many different organizational participants is vital to successful strategic implementation.

Strategic Control

As managers are implementing strategies, it is necessary to control. Control is very important in strategizing and, as is discussed in Chapter 10, controlling is an important activity in general in managing. The discussion here is limited to control as an element in effective strategizing.

In this context, results of strategies must be monitored and evaluated to determine whether objectives are being accomplished and whether resource allocation and utilization are effective. If not, adaptation must occur, including going back to the beginning of the strategic management process depicted in Figure 8.2. In fact, strategic management is a cyclical process. Even though present strategies may result in achieving objectives, strategic assessment must monitor internal and external environments with respect to whether and how they are changing and what the response should be.

The strategizing process (Figure 8.2) is brought full circle through strategic control and subsequent adaptations and changes. In the control stage, implementation is monitored and the resulting information is used to control ongoing decisions, actions, and behaviors affected by the organization's strategies. Figure 10.2 models the basic control process, in which actual results are monitored and compared with previously established objectives and standards, and deviations are corrected. In effective strategic control, senior-level managers, who have overall responsibility for their entities' performance, evaluate that performance and make changes when they are indicated.

STRATEGIC CONTROL SYSTEMS

Strategic managers must develop effective strategic control systems to achieve the successful implementation of their strategies by detecting discrepancies between desired and actual performance, which trigger corrective actions when necessary.[42] HSOs/HSs typically employ a number of strategic control systems or devices, including budgets, routine activity reports, exception reports, employee performance appraisal systems, and consumer or patient satisfaction surveys. Effective strategic control systems

- Facilitate coordination in organizations and systems
- Motivate effort toward achievement of organizational objectives
- Provide an early detection system to warn that the assumptions and conditions underlying strategies are wrong or have changed
- Provide a means through which strategic managers can intervene to correct an ineffective or inappropriate strategy

MECHANISMS OF STRATEGIC CONTROL

Assuming that missions and objectives have been established as part of the strategy formulation and strategic implementation stages of strategizing, then strategic control entails monitoring actual organizational strategic performance, comparing actual results with desired results, and correcting deviations or adapting to new strategic realities.

Monitoring Performance

In monitoring and comparing, strategic managers monitor actual performance in their domains and compare this to the desired states of performance they seek. Where clear, concrete objectives and standards exist, monitoring outcomes and then comparing them to the standards is a straightforward process. But to carry out this step effectively, strategic managers must observe more than mere operating results, although such bottom-line outcomes are always important in judging the success or failure of strategies. One very serious problem with relying on outcomes is that they often occur too late to permit the effective corrective actions necessary to fully meet objectives. In addition to this problem, final results may not point to why deviations occurred. To overcome such problems, effective strategic managers design their monitoring systems and techniques very carefully.

Management information systems (MISs) can be designed so that information relevant to strategic control can be collected, formatted, stored, and retrieved to support monitoring and comparing activities. These systems can be tailored to provide information that is useful in the strategic control of quality assessment and in improvement as well as cost control activities, for example. If MISs are to be useful in support of monitoring and comparing actual performance with desired standards of performance activities, they should possess certain characteristics, including the following:

- The MIS should match the elements of information it covers to the strategies being managed. The closer the match between the information and the specific nature and structure of strategies, the more effectively the control stage in the strategic management process can be carried out.
- The elements of information should point out exceptions at critical points. Effective strategic control requires attention to those factors most critical to organizational performance. Generally, the more strategic managers concentrate on critical points, the more effective will be the results of their control efforts. Related to this characteristic, the elements of information in an MIS should be economically selected and worth their cost.
- The elements of information should be understandable to those who will use them. Some strategic control systems are supported by MISs—especially those based upon mathematical formulas, complex statistical analyses, and computer simulations—that include information elements that are not always understandable to the people who must use them. The inclusion of such elements in an MIS can be dysfunctional.
- The MIS should report deviations promptly. The ideal MIS for strategic control purposes detects deviations soon after they actually occur. Only if information about difficulties with their strategies reaches strategic managers in a timely manner can they take effective corrective action.
- The MIS should be forward looking. Although perfect control would be instantaneous, the facts of organizational life include a time lag between deviations and corrective actions in strategic management. Nevertheless, a crucial precursor to effective strategic control is the ability to detect potential or actual deviations from established strategies early enough to permit effective corrective action. Thus, strategic managers usually prefer a forecast of what will probably happen next month, next quarter, or next year—even though this contains a margin of error—to information that is accurate to several decimal points but about which nothing can be done.
- Finally, the MIS should point to corrective action. A strategic control system that detects deviations from the desired results established for strategies will be little more

than an interesting exercise if it does not show the way to corrective action. An adequate system will disclose where failures are occurring, who is responsible for them, and what corrective action can be undertaken.

Taking Corrective Actions and Adapting to New Strategic Realities

Based on monitoring and comparing with desired results, corrective actions are taken to bring performance deviations back into line with performance objectives. This step often presents difficult problems for strategic managers, even if they are guided by good information from their strategic control systems. It is often difficult to determine why strategies fail or why their implementation falters, because so many underlying factors can be involved. The strategic management model shown in Figure 8.2 implies, as discussed on page 373, that the effort to trace the source or sources of deviations and to decide where to intervene goes back to each stage of the process where questions such as these can be answered: Is the information produced in the situational analysis still accurate, complete, and relevant? Are the strategies still appropriate? Are the steps being taken to implement the strategies the correct ones? And so on.

Armed with a determination of the causes of deviations, strategic managers can undertake corrective actions with some hope for successful results. In doing this, managers become change agents. They must adapt and adjust prior decisions and activities within the overall strategizing process in Figure 8.2. Strategic control, and the adaptation and change that it triggers, brings the strategic management processes full circle. These important steps in the processes are where strategic managers determine the continuing relevance of their strategies and make adaptations and changes.

One of the most important contributions that senior-level managers, with involvement of GBs, make to the ability of their HSOs/HSs to fulfill their missions, attain their organizational objectives, and achieve their desired levels of overall organizational performance is to know when adaptations in strategies and other organizational changes are needed and how to smoothly and effectively make them. Adaptations occur because managers perceive performance gaps—discrepancies between desired and actual states—in their areas of responsibility and take actions to address the gaps. In effect, managers must know how to act as change agents. Strategic adaptation can be defined as a discernible, measurable modification in form, quality, or state over time in an HSO's/HS's mission, objectives, and strategies.[43] Such modifications occur so ubiquitously that adaptation can be considered a constant responsibility of managers.

Pressures to add or delete strategies or to adapt existing strategies to new realities come from internal and external sources. Internally, for example, a new technology may provide an opportunity to diversify into new services. The dynamic external environments of HSOs/HSs provide another set of forces for adaptation and change. For example, growing, declining, or aging populations in their market areas or the plans and actions of competitors have significant implications for the strategies of HSOs/HSs, usually requiring them to adapt in a variety of ways in response. Public policies and regulations also exert strong and direct external pressures for strategic adaptation.[44] Changes in reimbursement policy for the Medicare and Medicaid programs routinely drive strategic adaptation in HSOs/HSs. [45]

Mechanisms of Strategic Adaptation

One of the facts of organizational life in organizational settings is the tendency of many people to resist things that are new and different. Thus, strategic managers invariably must deal with resistance to strategic adaptations. A crucial step in smoothing adaptation and change is devising a suitable overall approach to making the adaptation or change. Many possible approaches fit into one of two broad categories. One is based on the use of power, in which managers use coercion or sanctions to bring about change. Such approaches are also called force-coercion approaches and are top-down in nature.[46] Alternatively, approaches can rely on reason and rational persuasion. In these approaches, managers make strategic adaptation and organizational changes more easily because, by convincing those involved of the need for change and explaining the rationale for it, they improve the chances that adaptations and changes will be accepted.

In the power (force-coercion) approaches, managers determine and announce the adaptations and changes that they wish to make; other participants are expected to accept them. Changes in strategic direction of HSOs/HSs often require top-down power approaches, as do quick responses to important environmental changes. For example, a change in the reimbursement policy of a major insurance carrier may require an immediate adaptation or change that leaves little time for anything but a top-down edict.

Approaches that rely on reason and persuasion to implement adaptation and changes come in many forms, although they share the common element of being participative. In these approaches, participation in making adaptations and changes increases, although the degree of participation can vary widely. In general, increasing the level of participation or involvement of others in decisions about adaptation and change can allow managers to reap substantial rewards, including better decision making, which can lead to higher-quality and other desired performance results. Approaches that rely on participation are very different from top-down approaches. Participation suggests the opposite of top-down edicts from senior-level managers who direct what and how change will be made.

When information, rewards, knowledge, and power are concentrated at the top of an HSO/HS, little opportunity exists elsewhere for meaningful involvement or participation in adaptation and change. In contrast, when these factors are decentralized, opportunities to participate in managing adaptation and change are greatly increased.

When permitted higher levels of participation, more people can decide about adaptations and changes in their work and also have meaningful input into changes in mission or objectives, culture, strategies, tasks, technologies, people, and structures. Such high involvement, which is sometimes called a bottom-up approach, works best when senior-level managers encourage and facilitate its use. An important advantage of a high-participation, bottom-up approach to strategic adaptation and organizational change is that it stimulates creativity in the HSO/HS. It also fosters commitment to making adaptations and changes in those who participate. HSOs/HSs frequently use high-involvement, bottom-up approaches when adaptations and changes involve small parts of the organization or system, such as single departments, or when changes are modest and operational.

Strategic managers cannot ensure that a strategic adaptation will be successfully implemented, although certain actions increase the likelihood of success. Perhaps the most important action is that those involved in or affected by an adaptation understand the necessity for it. Managers should provide information as far in advance as possible—including details concerning reasons for the change, its nature and timing, and the expected impact.

It may be useful for a substantial adaptation or change to be introduced on a trial basis. Familiarity gained through experience with an adaptation or change, as well as assurances that it is not irrevocable, can reduce initial insecurity and increase the likelihood of acceptance. Allowing time for a change to be digested by those involved almost always increases their acceptance of it.

Another useful action for managers when adjusting or changing is to minimize the disruption of customs and informal relationships. The HSO/HS culture has value because it helps people adjust to the workplace and to their roles in it. Change almost invariably disrupts the culture, but such disturbances can be reduced by facilitating widespread participation in making the adaptations and changes.

In considering how to minimize resistance to strategic adjustment and organizational changes, strategic managers should remember that people respond to change in predictable, often negative, ways. Some people may view change negatively and resist it because of their background and experience. They also may react negatively to change because of the work environment. For example, when an HSO/HS has been stable for a long time, it may be especially difficult to introduce strategic adaptations without strong resistance. When people become part of the status quo and believe it is permanent, even minor changes can be disruptive. Conversely, when change is part of the culture, it is expected and more readily accepted.

Being a change agent is never easy. It is most difficult when it involves major strategic adaptations or complex organizational changes. The successful management of a complex adaptation requires that strategic managers have a purpose for the adaptation or change, the skills that are necessary to make the change, incentives and resources to make the adaptation possible, and a plan for making the change. If any of the necessary ingredients are missing, the adaptation may not succeed, or it may be more difficult and limited than it would be if all necessary ingredients were present.

Strategic Issues Management

To conclude, following the outline of Figure 8.2, the discussion to this point has focused on strategizing as creating a more favorable match between the HSO/HS and its external environment. The emphasis traditionally has been on changing/adapting the organization and its strategies to meet the threats and opportunities emanating from the external environment to enhance its competitive position. Strategic issues management (SIM), which is a logical extension of strategizing, is a systematic process that focuses on influencing the external environment so that it is more favorable to the organization.[47] That is, SIM involves proactively influencing and affecting strategic issues versus simply reacting and adapting to them. Public policy and its impact on HSOs/HSs provide a good example of strategic issues.

Longest defines policy competency as having "the dual capabilities to successfully *analyze* and *influence* the public policymaking process."[48] Others characterize SIM as "political strategy."[49] Whatever it is called, senior-level managers must proactively seek to influence public policy issues related to their organizations—otherwise they would not be fulfilling their responsibilities to defend and further the interests of their organizations. For HSOs/HSs, "survival depends as much on an ability to anticipate and influence the public policy issues that arise in the sociopolitical environment as the competitive issues that arise in the economic environment."[50]

In the management model in Figure 5.8, HSOs/HSs interface with the external environment, which includes the healthcare environment as well as the general environment. In both, public policy issues take on significance because managers must respond to them reactively (adapt) when regulations/legislation are imposed or proactively (influence) in helping frame the debate about issues and playing a role in shaping the outcomes. With the latter response, managers strategically seek to affect the external environment to be more favorable or less unfavorable to their entities by influencing the course and pace of externally imposed change. Trade associations such as the American Hospital Association or American Association of Homes and Services for the Aging can be very effective allies in these efforts. Identifying and acting on policy issues requiring political action are essential for success.[51]

DISCUSSION QUESTIONS

1. Define *strategizing*.
2. How does systems theory relate to strategizing?
3. All planning, whether strategic or operational, has three distinctive attributes no matter where it occurs. Briefly describe each attribute.

4. Figure 8.2 illustrates the entire strategizing process and each of its component activities. Briefly describe the components of the strategizing process.
5. Compare adaptive, market entry, and positioning strategies in HSOs/HSs.
6. Discuss the influence of the context in which the choice of strategies is made.
7. Discuss the internal and external strategic assessment components identified in Figure 8.2.
8. Discuss strategic control.
9. Resistance is often the human response to strategic changes. What can managers do to overcome resistance?

Case Study 1: No Time for Strategizing

Downstate Medical Center is a 400-bed teaching hospital with a board composed of business and community leaders. Downstate is considered by most in the region it serves to be the key hospital. The board is devoted to the hospital and meets quarterly. Its executive committee meets monthly and follows financial, quality, and other operational activities at the hospital closely in exercising its oversight duties. The executive committee and the entire board scrutinize the key aspects of the hospital's operation closely and regularly.

It is the custom of Clare Lipton, who chairs the Downstate board, and Nathan Robertson, president and CEO of the hospital, to have lunch together in the hospital's boardroom on a weekly basis. Recently, the conversation has focused on how to get the board more engaged in strategizing.

Lipton has made the point that she feels the board is happy about how things are going at the hospital, and with Robertson's performance, but has added, "We are sailing along nicely, but we don't know what the future holds for the hospital and where it fits into that future."

QUESTIONS

1. What are the appropriate roles of the CEO and the board in strategizing the future of Downstate Medical Center?
2. If things are going well at Downstate, why should its leaders give more attention to strategizing?
3. What do you recommend to Nathan Robertson and to Clare Lipton as a way to begin strategizing for Downstate Medical Center?

Case Study 2: A Response to Change

As business office manager of Group HMO, Inc., Dana Smith was responsible for the work of approximately 45 employees, of whom 26 were classified as secretarial or clerical. At the direction of the HMO president, a team of outside systems analysis consultants was contracted to make a time study and work-method analysis of Smith's area to improve the efficiency and output of the business office.

The consultants began by observing and recording each detail of the work of the secretarial and clerical staff. After 2 days of preliminary observation, the consultants indicated that they were prepared to begin their time study on the following day.

The next morning, 5 of the business office employees participating in the study were absent. On the following day, 10 employees were absent. Concerned, Smith sought to find reasons for the absenteeism by calling her absent employees. Each related basically the same story. Each was nervous, tense, and physically tired after being a "guinea pig" during the 2 days of preliminary observation. One told Smith that his physician had advised him to ask for a leave of absence if working conditions were not improved.

Shortly after the telephone calls, the head of the study team told Smith that if there were as many absences on the next day, then his team would have to delay the study. He stated that a scientific analysis would be impossible with 10 employees absent. Realizing that she would be held responsible for the failure of the study, Smith was very concerned.

QUESTIONS

1. What caused the reactions to the study?
2. Could these reactions have been predicted? How?
3. What steps should Smith take to get the study back on track?

■ Case Study 3: Free Clinic Woes[52]

As the director of Franklin Creek District Health Department, Jane Potterfield was proud of herself. She had gotten a small grant from a local corporation for a part-time receptionist and had received free use of an old store in one of her counties—the county that was most rural. She also had gotten two big-city physicians who were willing to travel to that store twice a week. She had all she needed to start a free clinic.

This primary care clinic would be available for those in the rural county who were working but unable to afford health insurance. In other words, they were too poor to afford an individual health plan but probably too rich to be eligible for Medicaid. Because all services were to be free, the state would furnish special help, such as free malpractice insurance coverage for the doctors.

Furthermore, the state health department had given Jane's health department approval to hold a childhood vaccine program in the same rural building twice a month. This would make it possible to increase the number of rural children who got immunized according to the state timetables.

Jane was at her desk preparing an agenda for the next board of health meeting, with all this good news on it. She felt that she was really making a difference in her region.

Suddenly, there was a knock at her office door.

Jane looked up to see a member of the board of health, Dr. Karen Matthewsen. Jane felt Karen was the best board member they had. Karen was a country doctor who worked in the rural county where Jane's concerns were the strongest, and Karen was a champion of the medically indigent throughout the whole region.

"Come in, Karen," Jane said with enthusiasm. "You can perhaps give me some help drawing up the agenda item about the wonderful new free clinic and vaccine program."

"Well, that is why I wanted to come see you, Jane—I am worried about those new developments." Karen said these words as she sat down in the guest chair by Jane's desk. Karen was clearly upset.

"But you are the biggest champion for the dispossessed on our board. I thought you would be tickled pink to see more services opening where the need is so great." Jane was also getting a little upset. This reaction from her old friend was not expected.

"As you know, Jane, I see more poor patients than any other doctor in the area, and I must say that it is tough enough to make a living in a rural county without having neighboring doctors come in and give free care. I know they are not supposed to take my Medicaid patients, but I operate on a close margin—closer than you might expect—and the loss of even underpaying private-pay patients and maybe some Medicaid ones, too, is problematic. Some patients might even prefer your services to going on Medicaid, while I work to get my uninsured patients covered by Medicaid and never turn a Medicaid patient down.

"Furthermore, lots of residents of our rural county could use the new childhood vaccine program you are offering, and those vaccines represent 20% of my practice net income every summer in the month before school opens."

Jane countered by noting that the free clinic would be encouraging eligible individuals to sign up for Medicaid and to see local doctors, but Karen noted that the free clinic would not be operating but two half days a week, and with volunteer labor, it would be unlikely to do a lot of follow-up and paperwork.

"No," Karen said, looking Jane straight in the eye, "I must say that, for the first time, I am against a new health department program aimed at the indigent. I believe country doctors like me need to be free of well-meaning government initiatives that are redundant, with private enterprises already struggling financially. I plan to vote against the clinic."

QUESTIONS:

1. How do you feel about Karen's position? What are its strengths and weaknesses?
2. Organizational staff people like to avoid having many split votes on crucial issues. What can Jane do to meet the needs of her community and maintain the board's unity. Is there an effective compromise position that can be championed?
3. If you were a working but poor person needing care in that rural county, what would you recommend the board do?

■ Case Study 4: Closing Pediatrics

City Hospital has a pediatrics department with 35 beds. For the past several years, the occupancy has varied between 40% and 60%. There is a definite downward trend, but it appears to be stabilizing at about 45% occupancy. The low occupancy has caused a financial strain. Other area hospitals are experiencing similar situations. As a result, several hospitals have proposed forming a community task force to study the situation and determine whether one or more pediatric departments should be closed, thereby increasing occupancy for those remaining. It is hoped that this will reduce costs and increase quality.

Although this proposal may benefit the community as a whole, it raises questions for City Hospital. Among them is the effect on two objectives: to provide a full range of quality services and to offer a full range of graduate medical education, including residencies in pediatrics.

QUESTIONS

1. What effect would the retrenchment strategy have on City Hospital's objectives?
2. Identify the stakeholders that influence the decision.
3. Are there other strategies that can be considered by City Hospital?
4. Argue against the closure. What reasons support your position?

Notes

1. Swayne, Linda E., W. Jack Duncan, and Peter M. Ginter. *Strategic Management of Healthcare Organizations,* 5th ed., 7. Malden, MA: Blackwell Publishing, 2006.
2. Morgan, Gareth. *Images of Organization,* 39. Thousand Oaks, CA: SAGE Publications, 2006.
3. Zuckerman, Alan M. "Hospital and Medical Staff Strategic Planning: Developing an Integrated Approach." *Physician Executive* 20 (August 1994): 15–17; Zuckerman, Alan M. *Healthcare Strategic Planning: Approaches for the 21st Century,* 37. Chicago: Health Administration Press, 1998.

4. Orlikoff, James E., and Mary Totten. "Strategic Planning by the Board." *Trustee* 48 (July/August 1995): SS1–SS4.

5. Labovitz, George H. "Customer Expectations in the New Millennium." *Healthcare Executive* 13 (January/February 1998): 47.

6. Vaill, Peter B. *Managing as a Performing Art: New Ideas for a World of Chaotic Change*. San Francisco: Jossey-Bass, 1991.

7. Zuckerman, Alan M. *Healthcare Strategic Planning: Approaches for the 21st Century,* 37. Chicago: Health Administration Press, 1998.

8. Pearce, John A., II, and Richard B. Robinson, Jr. *Strategic Management: Formulation, Implementation, and Control,* 5th ed., 33. Burr Ridge, IL: Irwin, 1994.

9. Thompson, Arthur A., Jr., and A.J. Strickland, III. *Strategic Management: Concepts and Cases,* 10th ed. Boston: Irwin/McGraw-Hill, 1998.

10. Whyte, E. Gordon, and John D. Blair. "Strategic Planning for Healthcare Providers." In *Healthcare Administration: Principles, Practices, Structure, and Delivery,* 2nd ed., edited by Lawrence F. Wolper, 289–326. Gaithersburg, MD: Aspen Publishers, 1995.

11. Bruton, Garry D., Benjamin M. Oviatt, and Luanne Kallas-Burton. "Strategic Planning in Hospitals: A Review and Proposal." *Healthcare Management Review* 20 (Summer 1995): 16–25.

12. Whyte, E. Gordon, and John D. Blair. "Strategic Planning for Healthcare Providers." In *Healthcare Administration: Principles, Practices, Structure, and Delivery,* 2nd ed., edited by Lawrence F. Wolper, 289–326. Gaithersburg, MD: Aspen Publishers, 1995.

13. For an extensive treatment of stakeholder analysis, see Blair, John D., and Myron D. Fottler. *Challenges in Healthcare Management: Strategic Perspectives for Managing Key Stakeholders*. San Francisco: Jossey-Bass, 1990.

14. Donnelly, James H., Jr., James L. Gibson, and John M. Ivancevich. *Fundamentals of Management*. New York: The McGraw-Hill Companies, 2000.

15. Begun, James, and Kathleen B. Heatwole. "Strategic Cycling: Shaking Complacency in Healthcare Strategic Planning." *Journal of Healthcare Management* 44 (September/October 1999): 339–351.

16. The first four steps are adapted from Swayne, Linda E., W. Jack Duncan, and Peter M. Ginter. *Strategic Management of Healthcare Organizations*, 5th ed., 70. Malden, MA: Blackwell Publishing, 2006. The fifth step is adapted from Longest, Beaufort B., Jr. *Managing Health Programs and Projects*. San Francisco: Jossey-Bass, 2004.

17. These steps are also discussed in Longest, Beaufort B., Jr. *Managing Health Programs and Projects,* 42–47. San Francisco: Jossey-Bass, 2004 and Longest, Beaufort B., Jr. *Seeking Strategic Advantage Through Health Policy Analysis,* 55–82. Chicago: Health Administration Press, 1997.

18. Klein, Harold E., and Robert E. Linneman. "Environmental Assessment: An International Study of Corporate Practices." *Journal of Business Strategy* 5 (Summer 1984): 66–77.

19. Swayne, Linda E., W. Jack Duncan, and Peter M. Ginter. *Strategic Management of Healthcare Organizations,* 5th ed., 75–86. Malden, MA: Blackwell Publishing, 2006.

20. Adapted from Whyte, E. Gordon, and John D. Blair. "Strategic Planning for Healthcare Providers." In *Healthcare Administration: Principles, Practices, Structure, and Delivery,* 2nd ed., edited by Lawrence F. Wolper, 295. Gaithersburg, MD: Aspen Publishers, 1995; reprinted with permission of Jones and Bartlett Publishers, Sudbury, MA (www.jbpub.com).

21. Luke, Roice D., Stephen L. Walston, and Patrick M. Plummer. *Healthcare Strategy: In Pursuit of Competitive Advantage,* 54–57. Chicago: Health Administration Press, 2004.

22. Luke, Roice D., Stephen L. Walston, and Patrick Michael Plummer. *Healthcare Strategy: In Pursuit of Competitive Advantage,* 55–56.

23. Adapted from Whyte and Blair, "Strategic Planning," 296–297; reprinted by permission.

24. Luke, Roice D., Stephen L. Walston, and Patrick Michael Plummer. *Healthcare Strategy: In Pursuit of Competitive Advantage,* 49–53.

25. Swayne, Duncan, and Ginter, *Strategic Management of Healthcare Organizations,* 228.

26. Swayne, Duncan, and Ginter, *Strategic Management of Healthcare Organizations,* 228–230.

27. Conrad, Douglas A., and William L. Dowling. "Vertical Integration in Health Services: Theory and Managerial Implications." *Healthcare Management Review* 15 (Fall 1990): 9–22, p. 9.

28. Brown, Montague, and Barbara P. McCool. "Vertical Integration: Exploration of a Popular Strategic Concept." *Healthcare Management Review* 11 (Fall 1986): 7–19.

29. Campbell, Sandy. "Using Wellness and Prevention as a Strategic Platform for a Hospital System." *Healthcare Strategic Management* 16 (May 1998): 15.

30. Satinsky, Marjorie A. *The Foundations of Integrated Care: Facing the Challenges of Change.* Chicago: American Hospital Publishing, 1998.

31. For a good discussion of hospital diversification into long-term care, see Giardina, Carole W., Myron D. Fottler, Richard M. Shewchuk, and Daniel B. Hill. "The Case for Diversification into Long Term Care." *Healthcare Management Review* 15 (Winter 1990): 71–82.

32. Zuckerman, Howard S., Arnold D. Kaluzny, and Thomas C. Ricketts, III. "Alliances in Healthcare: What We Know, What We Think We Know, and What We Should Know." *Healthcare Management Review* 20 (Winter 1995): 54–64, p. 54.

33. Miles, Raymond E., and Charles C. Snow. *Organizational Strategy, Structure and Process.* New York: McGraw-Hill, 1978; reissued in 2003 by Stanford University Press.

34. Ginn, Gregory O., and Gary J. Young. "Organizational and Environmental Determinants of Hospital Strategy." *Hospital & Health Services Administration* 37 (Fall 1992): 291–302.

35. Hunger, J. David, and Thomas L. Wheelen. *Essentials of Strategic Management.* Reading, MA: Addison-Wesley, 1997.

36. Whyte and Blair, "Strategic Planning," 293.

37. Digman, Lester A. *Strategic Management: Concepts, Decisions, Cases,* 2nd ed., 335. Homewood, IL: BPI/Irwin, 1990.

38. Hunger, J. David, and Thomas L. Wheelen. *Essentials of Strategic Management,* 90–91. Reading, MA: Addison-Wesley, 1997.

39. Rutsohn, Phil, and Nabil A. Ibrahim. "Strategically Positioning Tomorrow's Hospital Today: Current Indications for Strategic Marketing." *Journal of Hospital Marketing* 9 (1995): 13–23.

40. Swayne, Linda E., W. Jack Duncan, and Peter M. Ginter. *Strategic Management of Healthcare Organizations,* 5th ed., 34. Malden, MA: Blackwell Publishing, 2006.

41. Galbraith, Jay R., and Robert K. Kazanjian. *Strategy Implementation: Structure, Systems, and Process.* St. Paul, MN: West Publishing Company, 1986.

42. Camillus, John C. *Strategic Planning and Management Control.* New York: Lexington Press, 1986.

43. Van de Ven, Andrew H., and Marshall S. Poole. "Explaining Development and Change in Organizations." *Academy of Management Review* 20 (July 1995): 510–540, p. 512.

44. Longest, Beaufort B., Jr. *Health Policymaking in the United States,* 4th ed. Chicago: Health Administration Press, 2006.

45. Longest, Beaufort B., Jr. *Seeking Strategic Advantage Through Health Policy Analysis.* Chicago: Health Administration Press, 1997.

46. Chinn, Robert, and Kenneth D. Benne. "General Strategies for Effecting Changes in Human Systems." In *The Planning of Change,* 4th ed., edited by Warren G. Bennis, Kenneth D. Benne, and Robert Chinn, 22–45. New York: Harcourt Brace, 1985.

47. Reeves, Phillip N. "Issues Management: The Other Side of Strategic Planning." *Hospital & Health Services Administration* 38 (Summer 1993): 229–241.

48. Longest, Beaufort B., Jr. *Health Policymaking in the United States,* 4th ed., 125. Chicago: Health Administration Press, 2006.

49. Bigelow, Barbara, Margarete Arndt, and Melissa Middleton Stone. "Corporate Political Strategy: Incorporating the Management of Public Policy Issues into Hospital Strategy." *Healthcare Management Review* 22 (Summer 1997): 53–63.

50. Bigelow, Arndt, and Stone, "Corporate Political Strategy," 53.

51. Reeves, Phillip N. "Strategic Planning Revisited." *Clinical Laboratory Management Review* 20 (November/December 1994): 549–554.

52. Written by Gary E. Crum, Ph.D, M.P.H., Executive Director, Graduate Medical Education Consortium, The University of Virginia at Wise (Past Director, Northern Kentucky Health Department). Used with permission.

9

Marketing

Marketing closely aligns with strategizing, as discussed in Chapter 8. Marketing is critical to success in strategizing, whether in helping identify strategic alternatives, selecting from among them, or implementing and evaluating the strategies selected. Effective marketing is essential to implementation of virtually any strategy and ultimately to fulfillment of the mission. From this perspective, the objectives of marketing must be congruent with and complement several aspects of health services organizations/health systems (HSOs/HSs):

- Mission, vision, values, objectives, and organizational strategies
- Priorities, preferences, and commitments of governing bodies (GBs) and senior-level managers
- Financial targets and constraints
- Potential for growth and diversification in relevant markets
- Technological developments and requirements of the core business
- Corporate citizenship and accountability to society as a whole, the community, covered lives, and individual patients

The importance of effective marketing activities to the strategic success of HSOs/HSs cannot be overstated.

This chapter was cowritten by Wesley M. Rohrer, III, Assistant Professor of Health Policy and Management, Graduate School of Public Health, University of Pittsburgh.

▬ Marketing Defined ▬▬▬▬▬▬▬▬▬▬▬▬▬▬▬▬▬▬▬▬

The central concept of marketing is that of a voluntary *exchange* of things of *value*. The buyer receives something of value (a product or service) from the seller in exchange for something of value. This concept holds that achieving organizational objectives depends on "determining the needs and wants of target markets and delivering the desired satisfactions more effectively than competitors do."[1] Consummation of such exchange requires that sellers/providers create and make available, and that buyers/consumers locate and choose, services and products. Applying this basic concept, marketing can be defined broadly as "the analysis, planning, implementation, and control of carefully formulated programs designed to promote voluntary exchanges of values with target markets with the purpose of achieving organizational objectives."[2] Another widely used definition was provided by the American Marketing Association in 2008: "Marketing is the activity, set of institutions and processes for creating, communicating, delivering and exchanging offerings that have value for customers, clients, partners, and for society at large."[3] This is considerably broader than the original definition of marketing given by the American Marketing Association in 1935: "Marketing is the performance of business activities that direct the flow of goods and services from the producer to the consumer."[4]

The financial or commercial success of organizations is affected by the use of traditional marketing. In addition, the ability of organizations and systems to develop and implement certain kinds of clinical programs and activities in their markets may depend upon their use of *social marketing*. Both types of marketing are useful in HSOs/HSs, although the two types differ and are distinguished from each other in this chapter. Most of the discussion in this chapter pertains to the traditional type of marketing, but an extension of traditional marketing into social marketing will also be discussed.

Adapting the definition by Kotler and Clarke[5] to the healthcare context, marketing is defined as planning, implementing, and evaluating activities designed to bring about voluntary exchanges with people and other organizations in target markets for the purpose of achieving the mission and objectives established for an organization or system.

Obvious markets for organizations and systems include current patients/customers who utilize their products or services and potential new patients/customers, as well as others who can influence existing or potential patients/customers, such as referring physicians and health plans that may permit or limit use of the services by their subscribers or members. Other important target markets are potential employees and staff, donors, and volunteers. Commercial marketing focuses on facilitating exchanges between organizations and their target markets, including identifying and quantifying the target markets.

Although these definitions of marketing differ in emphasis and precision, common elements can be identified, including the essential nature of marketing as an exchange process in which the exchanges involve things of value to the parties. These definitions collectively address

- The perception and expression of an unfulfilled need or want (e.g., Maslow's hierarchy of physiological, safety/comfort, social, ego/achievement, and self-actualization needs, as shown in Figure 12.4)
- An entity (supplier) willing and capable of satisfying that need or want with a product or service
- Goods and services that can be valued or priced and made available to exchange now or in the future
- Channels (means or media) for communicating about the terms and conditions of the exchange
- A location, distribution network, or other mechanism to facilitate the transaction (including delivery of the physical product or service and the payment)

Any activity that includes these components can be considered a marketing transaction regardless of the industry, organizational ownership, private or public sector, or for-profit or not-for-profit nature of the business, including healthcare.

SOCIAL MARKETING DEFINED

Although this chapter focuses on traditional marketing concepts in healthcare settings, social marketing will be discussed in later sections. Adapting a widely accepted definition,[6] social marketing is defined as the application of commercial (or traditional) marketing technologies to planning, implementing, and evaluating services that are designed to influence the voluntary behavior of target audiences in order to improve their personal welfare and that of society. Another useful way to define social marketing is to view it as "a process for influencing human behavior on a large scale, using marketing principles for the purpose of societal benefit rather than commercial profit."[7] Social marketing has been defined by Kotler and Zaltman as the "design, implementation, and control of programs calculated to influence the acceptability of social ideas."[8] In essence, social marketing can be viewed as a relatively new way of thinking about some very old human endeavors. Since social systems first formed, attempts have been made to inform, persuade, influence, and motivate individuals and groups in order to gain their acceptance of certain ideas. Social marketing has become an important mechanism in these efforts.

In the United States, social marketing has been used widely in areas such as energy conservation and recycling and especially in addressing health issues. The health issues that have been addressed through social marketing include such issues as obesity, antismoking, safety, drug abuse, drinking and driving, HIV/AIDS, nutrition, physical activity, immunization, breast cancer screening, mental health, and family planning. Canada, especially, has made significant use of social marketing in seeking to improve the health of Canadians through widespread social marketing campaigns.

Health Canada, which is the federal department responsible for helping the people of Canada maintain and improve their health, has created a wide range of social marketing programs and campaigns. Their web site[9] contains descriptions of many of these, along with extensive educational materials about social marketing in health, including a seven-step tutorial on developing a social marketing plan.

WHAT MARKETING IS NOT

In clarifying what marketing is, it may be instructive to distinguish between marketing and associated activities that are often regarded as being equivalent to marketing. Marketing, according to the prevailing paradigm, is not (primarily or exclusively)

- Selling
- Advertising
- Promoting
- Generating revenues

Although these activities are relevant to marketing, they must be managed carefully and applied in the context of the HSO's/HS's mission, values, and objectives. Marketing from a quality management perspective entails building long-term relationships based on trust, mutual respect, and enduring values. Consequently, relationship building, service excellence, and commitment to quality must be given priority over "closing the sale" and inventory turnover.

A distinction should also be made between commercial marketing and *public relations*. Public relations entails the management of communications between the organization and its stakeholders using public media channels to create, enhance, protect, and/or maintain the desired public image of the organization overall or a perception of an event or activity. While related to and supportive of marketing, public relations is not marketing.

Health promotion involves the dissemination of knowledge and expert judgment using the media and other targeted communication channels to prevent disease, illness, and injury and to advocate for improved health and wellness. It is similar to, and may be used in, social marketing efforts. It could be argued that public relations, health promotion, and health communications are all subsumed within *health communications*, "the study and use of methods to inform and influence individual and community decisions that enhance health."[10] Certainly, the core idea of influencing health-related behavior is relevant to all these concepts, directly or indirectly.

HSOs/HSs have engaged in marketing-like activities for decades.[11] Examples include

- Engaging in public relations to influence public perceptions of the organization's overall image and specific events
- Providing health education/health promotion messages to patients and community groups
- Distributing annual reports to key stakeholders and the wider community
- Investing in donor development and fund-raising
- Developing new products and services to respond to patient needs
- Pursuing aggressive recruitment and retention of physicians and other key staff
- Implementing patient demographic origin studies and patient satisfaction surveys[12]

WHAT MARKETING IS

Marketing in HSOs/HSs has changed significantly in the past few decades. It is no longer viewed as a segregated, stand-alone activity consisting of disseminating information about types of services and products and their quality or as gathering information about patient/customer satisfaction. Informed individuals do not construe marketing only as advertising and selling, with the implication that physicians and patients will use the HSO's/HS's facilities only when there is a substantial promotional effort. It is not the artificial creation of demand for services that is discussed in Chapter 4. Marketing is properly consumer focused.[13] Market-oriented HSOs/HSs "are characterized by a concerted effort to collect, share, and respond to consumer information."[14]

The contemporary perspective of marketing is that it is a designed process, integrated with other activities, in which the organization identifies and satisfies the needs and wants of stakeholders—especially patients/customers and clinical staff, as well as the community at large—so that mission and objectives can be accomplished. Kotler and Clarke, for example, observe that marketing is "a central activity of modern organizations. To survive and succeed, organizations must know their markets, attract sufficient resources, convert these resources into appropriate products, services, and ideas, and effectively distribute them to various consuming publics."[15]

While marketing in the past was viewed primarily as a set of periodic and loosely coupled advertising and promotional activities of limited relevance to, and outside, the core business of the HSO/HS, the consensus today is that marketing is an essential component of strategizing as well as contributing to the achievement of more short-term financial, clinical, and other operational objectives. Specifically, it is generally recognized that marketing extends well beyond advertising and other promotional efforts to generate "artificial" demand for services.[16]

Like most service industries in the 21st century, healthcare marketing has become assertively consumer focused. Consequently, market-oriented organizations are characterized by a concerted effort to collect, share, and react and respond to consumer information.[17] "To survive and succeed, organizations must know their markets, attract sufficient resources, convert these resources into appropriate products, services, and ideas, and effectively distribute them to various consuming publics."[18] For this characterization to be consistent with the current marketing paradigm, emphasis must be added to developing long-term relationships with stakeholders and to doing so from the environmental analysis stage through product/service design and forward to outcome measures and stakeholder satisfaction feedback.

Strategic Marketing Management and Analysis

Marketing requires careful management. In many respects, marketing management parallels the strategizing process illustrated in Figure 8.2, especially the analysis of the external and internal environments. The focus in marketing management is on analysis of factors associated with an organization's competitive situation. Effective marketing managers perform four interrelated forms of analysis as key parts of marketing management:

- *Market analysis,* which includes the structure, maturity, geographical scope, core technology, prevailing marketing mix, elasticity of demand for products/services, barriers to entry and exit, and other factors necessary to define and address a specific product/market
- *Competitor analysis,* which emphasizes competitors, including their number and size, market concentration and intensity, market share distribution, and distinctive advantages of the major competitors
- *Customer analysis,* which includes assessment of both the articulated needs and wants of potential customers (needs assessment) and the demographics of the community (as potential customer base) and current customers, including ethnicity, life style, age distribution, educational level, occupation, and family income, among other variables
- *Capabilities analysis,* which includes internal strengths and capacities such as the expertise and skill set of the human resources, leadership and management development, financial health and resources, technological development, institutional accreditation, and certification or other recognition of quality and performance

The information derived from these focused assessment processes must be integrated with the broader assessment of the internal and external environment associated with overall strategizing, as discussed in Chapter 8. These processes may occur independently but may be incorporated in a comprehensive *marketing audit,* which is the systematic evaluation of the effectiveness of the overall marketing function in an organization or system. This formal evaluation is consistent with the specific analyses just discussed and typically includes

- Identifying target markets, customer needs, and external opportunities and threats
- Scanning and assessing the competitive environment
- Assessing the current service mix or product line,[19] using the benchmark of customers' needs and preferences
- Enhancing all aspects of the marketing experience, consistent with internal strengths and weaknesses

The Marketing Mix:
Core Concepts in Marketing Management

One of the key concepts in marketing management is termed the *marketing mix*. The marketing mix provides a framework and the logic for marketing management and practice by defining the essen-

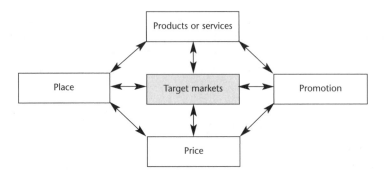

Figure 9.1. Elements of marketing. (From Longest, Beaufort B., Jr. *Managing Health Programs and Projects,* 250. San Francisco: Jossey-Bass, 2004. Used with permission.)

tial components of a marketing initiative. These components are known famously as the "4 *P*s of marketing"—product, place, price and promotion.[20] Although an alternative scheme has been used (SCAP: service, consideration, access, and promotion),[21] the traditional 4 *P*s typology is useful and fits health services marketing well. Decisions about the marketing mix and the associated resource commitments define a marketing strategy. Figure 9.1 presents these elements of marketing that are necessary to achieve the exchange between consumer and seller. Each element is described below.

PRODUCT/SERVICE

A large variety of products and services is offered by HSOs/HSs to address real or perceived needs in their markets. From a marketing management standpoint, this marketing component incorporates product development and design as well as the specific attributes of the product/service. This component includes direct healthcare rendered, as well as the amenities associated with a healing environment or experience, including aesthetics and comfort of the facilities, the interpersonal encounters with providers and support staff, and the availability and quality of support services, such as food service, chaplaincy, and hours of visitation. In the context of continuous quality improvement (CQI), all aspects of the customer's experience with the organization are included in the assessment of product and service quality.

Relational marketing entails potential customer participation in ongoing product development through focus groups, customer satisfaction surveys, customer complaints, and unsolicited feedback. This marketing component addresses the question, What products with what characteristics do we offer to whom?

Based upon marketing managers' identification of target markets and their evaluations of these markets' attributes, the needs of specific target markets, the satisfaction of present customers,[22] and the extent of competition, managers can continue ensuring that suitable services and products are developed. Such information allows the service mix (scope and intensity) and product lines to be expanded, reduced, realigned, or focused. Target markets can be large or small and are defined geographically. A general acute care hospital may have a target market (also called a service area) encompassing the community and its environs; a tertiary hospital target market may encompass a large region.

Target markets can be classified by type of care (preventive, acute/short-term, chronic/longterm, rehabilitative), service (medical and surgical, obstetrics and gynecology, oncology), age (gerontology, pediatrics), income level, or type of payer (self-pay, commercial, managed care, public). Assessment information may reveal gaps in the service mix or product line, as well as potential target markets, competitive and other marketplace threats, and whether special opportunities exist.

As target markets change, as competition and technology intensify, and as needs, preferences, and attitudes shift and change, HSOs/HSs need to evaluate and realign their mix of services, products, and programs. Such realignment must be consistent with the organization's mission, capabilities, and strengths and may include expansion or elimination of services under conditions of downsizing. For example, a competitor's introduction of an urgent care center or the formation of a health maintenance organization (HMO) in the service area may require reassessment of the target market, plans for how to reach that market, and changes in services. Decline in birth rate may mean reevaluating obstetrics with the possible aim of redirecting resources to other services. New technology may suggest the need to introduce new or expanded services. Identified opportunities may lead to a hospital offering wellness and employee assistance programs to large corporations, pharmacy services to nursing facilities, and home health services to discharged patients or residents.

PLACE

The place component of marketing refers to the sites or loci of obtaining the products/services offered by an organization or system. It also takes into consideration the channels for distributing the product/services to consumers. With the expansion of online marketing technologies, the issue of "place" becomes more complex. The nature of health services entails that timely access, such as affordable transport to the site, convenient hours of operation, and bilingual staff, is important and sometimes critical.

Establishing satellite ambulatory care and family practice centers and mobile screening units enhances access to services and expands the potential market area. Increasingly, family medicine and therapist group practices have extended evening and weekend hours to accommodate working adults and to enhance their competitive position. This component of the marketing mix responds to the question: Where do we locate our facilities to ensure effective distribution and convenient access by our customers?

PRICE

Price considerations refer to the charges or rates assigned as the perceived values of products/services to customers. Pricing is complex because it must be based on considerations of actual costs of production and delivery, prices for equivalent and substitute goods in the market, the elasticity of demand, the number and concentration of competitors, and the service or product life cycle. In competitive markets, HSOs/HSs recognize and must respond to the price sensitivity of large self-insured employers and insurers that are bundling and pricing services nontraditionally and negotiating aggressively.

To the extent that the responsibility for payment rests directly on consumers, it is more likely to act as a barrier to access. However, when the costs of the health services consumed are paid by third-party payers rather than the ultimate consumers, the consumers may be indifferent to price. Beyond out-of-pocket expenditures, the pricing decision should also reflect intangibles such as patient anxiety, inconvenience, and opportunity cost of time spent in waiting for and receiving treatment. Certainly these considerations may influence the consumer's decision making. In addition, the image and reputation of premier HSOs/HSs might affect the purchase/exchange decision.[23]

The trend toward shifting costs to the consumer, through higher deductibles and copayments for third-party coverage and medical savings accounts, has likely made many consumers more price conscious. The fundamental question relevant to pricing is What price should we charge consumers, relative to our costs and competitive position in the market?

PROMOTION

The promotion component of marketing relies heavily on advertising, defined as "any paid form of non-personal presentation and promotion of ideas, goods or services by an identifiable sponsor that is transmitted via mass media."[24] Consumer awareness is an especially important and challenging component in health services marketing. Customers or their intermediaries must be informed about services (type, scope, quality) that are offered, where and when, and at what cost. Through effective promotion, such information can be conveyed, and organizations can build a reputation or protect an image, analogous to brand identification for products.

Advertising efforts may be addressed to a broad public or focused on a segment of the market. Promotion includes various incentives to encourage trial use, purchase, and acceptance of the service or product, including point-of-sale samples, discount coupons, rebates, and so on. Although promotion should not be seen as synonymous with marketing (especially not in health and human services), nonetheless, effective advertising and promotion can be critical for the success of a marketing strategy.

Most of the criticism about healthcare marketing has been directed at promotion, especially advertising, which some would argue artificially generates demand for services. However, this argument is weak, given the psychology associated with healthcare decision making. For example, few would choose a colonoscopy unless it was deemed necessary to maintain good health and prevent illness. Furthermore, such criticism is inconsistent with the marketing concept[25] if promotion is properly regarded as the beneficial and necessary dissemination of information about heathcare options, risks, pricing, and access so that consumers can make more-informed purchase decisions.

THE MARKETING MIX IS NOT CARVED IN STONE

The marketing mix is an evolving concept in healthcare marketing. As noted above, an alternative, although very similar, scheme to the 4 *P*s model exists in the form of SCAP (service, consideration, access, and promotion).[26] English has gone so far as to challenge the relevance of the 4 *P*s as applied to health services marketing by noting that "this model has never been a comfortable fit for healthcare."[27] Instead, English proposes an alternative paradigm, the 4 *R*s:

- *Relevance,* reflecting the HSO's/HS's commitment to be a listening organization by practicing customer-focused marketing
- *Response,* by which English means "the creation of brand expectations and delivering on them"[28]
- *Relationships,* reflecting the need for providers to build long-term relationships with customers that "ultimately involve a paradigm shift" for managers from "episode management to relationship building"[29]
- *Results,* representing the need for measures of both the hard and soft benefits of effective marketing

Macstravic[30] rejects English's "premature obituary" of the 4 *P*s, claiming that they are not only relevant to healthcare marketing but essential. Macstravic concedes the usefulness of the 4 *R*s but as distinct and (for the most part) complementary factors to the 4 *P*s. Furthermore, he offers two new factors to consider, a fifth *P* and a fifth *R*:

- *Prompting,* by which Macstravic means encouraging consumers to adopt and maintain healthy, beneficial behaviors
- *Reminding,* by which he means communicating with consumers to increase their awareness of the health and wellness benefits that they receive from their HSOs/HSs

Macstravic claims that the last factor has considerable untapped potential "to reinforce lasting relationships [with consumers]."[31] Although the value of the 4 *P*s is attested by their persistence in marketing literature and practice, the 4 *R*s do provide a useful parallel perspective on the current paradigm of relational marketing.

Challenges in Identifying the Customer and Target (Desirable) Markets

External environmental analysis in the strategizing process (see Figure 8.2) may partially identify present and potential target customers and target markets. This includes the ultimate consumers of services but also those who may influence purchase decisions on behalf of patients/customers such as some third-party payers. Traditionally in health services, the common view has been that the consumer in the marketing exchange is the patient or other direct recipient of services. However, others who may intervene and influence the consumer's choices—which services, for what price, when and where—must be considered as potential partners in marketing transactions, as the agents for direct care recipients.[32] For example, physicians serve as moral agents by representing the patient's interests, structuring the array of healthcare options offered to the patient, and controlling access to inpatient healthcare facilities and, sometimes, nursing facilities. Physicians not only influence the demand for services in these ways but also may participate in utilization review of other health services providers.

Third-party payers, including government agencies such as the Centers for Medicare and Medicaid Services (CMS) and the Department of Veterans Affairs (DVA), large employers, and managed care organizations (MCOs), influence access to, duration of, and price of services to the ultimate consumer. Federal and state regulation influences directly or indirectly the type and intensity of services provided, through licensure, quality assessment, sanctions, and reimbursement mechanisms. Professional and industry associations, such as The Joint Commission on Accreditation of Healthcare Organizations (The Joint Commission), the AMA and its local counterparts, and the American College of Healthcare Executives (ACHE), influence the quality of care and behavior of practitioners by establishing clinical and management standards and benchmarks and codes of ethics for professionals.

HMOs, health plans, and other MCOs have been especially important in influencing access to and pricing of healthcare services for healthcare consumers. Furthermore, the pervasive availability and growing use of accessible online technology to support healthcare decision making has also complicated the marketing process. In summary, it is clear that determining Who is my customer? and What is my target market? is a complex and challenging task.

SEGMENTING MARKETS

Berkowitz defines market segmentation as "the process of grouping into clusters consumers who have similar wants or needs to which an organization can respond by tailoring one or more elements of the marketing mix."[33] Market segmentation is best understood in contrast to mass marketing, which is based on the assumption that all actual and potential consumers in a given market need and want essentially the same thing, that is, the same service/product attributes. Mass marketing assumes that all customers are willing to pay the same price for the product/service in the same place (or means of distribution) and will respond to the same promotional messages. Prior to the advent of sophisticated marketing tools, advances in service and product production processes, information technology, and the rising expectations associated with the post-WWII consumerism trends, mass marketing was the primary tool and was partially effective. Generic products like baker's flour, concrete, trash bags, and perhaps even computer chips may be appropriate for mass marketing in their respective markets.

However, increasingly, consumer marketing, including the marketing of health services, relies upon segmentation of the population or customer base. Berkowitz distinguishes these two marketing approaches by noting that "while mass marketing can be described as bending demand to the will of supply, market segmentation . . . [is] the bending of supply to the will of demand."[34] Underlying this distinction is a critical difference in envisioning the relationship with the customer and the implications for quality of product or service. Mass marketing assumes a pliable pool of consumers whose needs and wants may be easily manipulated to gain the acceptance and stimulate purchases of the products/services being marketed. The organization's marketing approach might be characterized as primarily that of sales management. Alternatively, segmentation suggests a more nuanced and customer-focused marketing philosophy that emphasizes relationship management, which is clearly the case in HSOs/HSs.

Thomas[35] identifies the conditions necessary for useful identification of a cluster or cohort of consumers as constituting a marker segment. An important attribute is that the segment possesses characteristics that can be cost-effectively identified, measured, and analyzed. The segment must be potentially accessible to promotional and other communication activities. Finally, the segment must be sufficiently large to justify product/service and market development to address its perceived needs and wants.

Although various factors or criteria for market segmentation are potentially useful, the following set of categories is commonly cited and applied:

- *Demographic:* Useful factors include age, gender, socioeconomic status (SES), race/ethnicity, income/wealth, and other quantifiable (objectively measurable) variables. This approach to segmentation is especially relevant to identifying markets for health services.
- *Geographic:* Geographical distribution of existing and potential customers may be defined for markets at the national, regional, or state and local levels. For services, ZIP code distribution has become increasingly important for assessing needs, patient satisfaction, and potential market segmentation.
- *Psychographic:* This refers to the psychological attitudes, values, and other traits that predispose an individual to adopt one lifestyle (or stable pattern of social behaviors) rather than another. Individual lifestyle may also be closely related to, or expressed in terms of, the person's social class or other referent group. For example, the term *yuppie,* popular in the 1990s, combined age cohort and SES to characterize a lifestyle of social and economic upward mobility.

    In response to what Yankelovich and Meer[36] regard as a current overreliance on this basis for segmentation, these authors contend that "the psychographic profiling that passes for market segmentation these days is a mostly wasteful diversion from its original and true purpose—discovering customers whose behavior can be changed or whose needs are not being met."[37]
- *Usage Pattern:* This criterion targets segments on the basis of actual or projected level of consumption or use of products/services, ranging from nonusers (refusers) to heavy users. The pattern of access to healthcare services is especially important in health services marketing and has implications for the health status and well-being of the patient, e.g., compliance with therapy. Brand loyalty is a closely related marketing concept based on measures of purchase and consumption patterns that has become a popular criterion of marketing effectiveness in healthcare.
- *Cohort membership:* Berkowitz defines the cohort as "a group of people bound together in history by a set of [major] events . . . [that] form and shape attitudes."[38] The shared attitudes, values, and beliefs of a cohort based on their shared history and life experiences provide the glue that constitutes the cohort as a meaningful market

segment. It can be argued that cohort segmentation is especially relevant to healthcare organizations and services. A number of classification schemes for identifying and classifying cohorts have been proposed.[39]

- *Benefit to Users:* The benefit sought by the consumer or the need to be satisfied by use of the product/service is another potentially useful basis for market segmentation. Although in some consumer markets, such as retail groceries, the link from products offered to benefits sought seems to be quite clear and direct, in others the links may be more complex because of multiple benefits being sought and needs to be satisfied. For example, the purchaser of a Gucci handbag is likely seeking benefits beyond convenient storage and portability of personal items. The consumers of health services may be seeking relief from pain, peace of mind, increased longevity, sense of well-being, and accountability to loved ones. The application of this segmentation criterion should encourage a more in-depth analysis of consumer needs and wants.

QUANTIFYING PATIENT/CUSTOMER TARGET MARKETS

Managers in HSOs/HSs seek to identify and quantify target markets, as well as understand the needs and wants of people in these markets, so that they can tailor effective marketing strategies to facilitate exchanges. To facilitate marketing focused on patient/customer target markets, it may be useful to segment them along several dimensions. As discussed earlier, common dimensions for segmenting markets include demographic segments such as age, gender, race, income, occupation, and health insurance status; psychographic segments such as lifestyle preferences (e.g., urban/suburban/rural residence, preference for alternative medicine, and willingness to utilize new products or services); use-based segments such as frequency of usage of medical and dental services, health clubs, or fitness centers; benefit segments such as desire to obtain certain product/service benefits (e.g., luxury, thriftiness, scheduling convenience, or ease of access); and geographic segments such as those based on location (e.g., ZIP code, community, region, or state).

Of course, the identification and quantification of target markets and segments within them are only the beginnings of understanding the potential of the target markets and segments to produce actual demand for the HSO's/HS's services/products. Such determinations require additional analysis, which can be aided by use of techniques such as the epidemiological planning model.[40] An example of the application of this model follows.

Epidemiological Planning Model

Suppose an HSO/HS wishes to initiate a medically monitored fitness center for people at risk for heart disease. Such programs typify those in which the level of normative need for services in a target market—which is often one or more demographic categories (e.g., adult men and women) in a geographic community (e.g., a cluster of ZIP codes)—can be estimated using the epidemiological planning model (EPM).[41]

The EPM is an equation in the following general form through which an estimate of the demand for a particular service can be made:

$$\left\{\begin{array}{c}\text{Demand for}\\\text{a service}\end{array}\right\} = \left\{\begin{array}{c}\text{Population}\\\text{at risk}\end{array}\right\} \times \left\{\begin{array}{c}\text{Incidence}\\\text{rate}\end{array}\right\} \times \left\{\begin{array}{c}\text{Average use}\\\text{per incidence}\end{array}\right\} \times \left\{\begin{array}{c}\text{Market}\\\text{share}\end{array}\right\}$$

This program's managers may be interested in estimating the demand for such services as counseling, exercise programs, and relaxation therapies. An estimate of demand for services will be useful in taking the steps necessary to ensure that the program can provide them in an effective and timely manner. Effective marketing strategies require that the needs and wants—which translate into demand for services—of those in target markets are known *and* that programs can satisfy the demands.

The estimate of the demand for counseling services for adults at risk for heart disease, for example, would be based on current information for the terms in the EPM equation, or on projections if managers were interested in projecting future demand. In this example, where the service area is a particular set of ZIP codes around the entity that is considering adding the service, the demand calculation for annual counseling services is made as follows:

- *Population at risk* is determined from information on the county's population, available from the U.S. Census Bureau (*www.census.gov*). Assume that such data show that there are about 200,000 adult men and women in the ZIP codes under consideration and that this group can be broken down into cohorts based on gender and other demographic segments.
- *Incidence rate* is determined by using national data on at-risk populations, available through the National Center for Health Statistics (*www.cdc.gov/nchs*). Overall, the rate of risk for heart disease in adult populations may be 6 in 10. This means that as many as 120,000 of the 220,000 adults in the targeted ZIP codes could be at risk for heart disease (200,000 × 0.6 = 120,000).
- *Average use* of counseling sessions *per incidence* is determined by the number of counseling sessions that managers plan to provide to each program client; assume four sessions per client per year. This can be based on the operation of similar programs and on clinical judgments.
- *Market share* in this situation is based on the fraction of the population at risk that the program's managers think they will serve; this number can be guided by actual experience in other ongoing programs and perhaps by market surveys. It will obviously be affected by the presence of competitors and their strength in the market under consideration. In this instance, assume that 15% of the population at risk will be served.

  Thus, demand for counseling services can be *estimated,* by the following calculation, at 72,000 counseling sessions per year:

$$\begin{Bmatrix} \text{Demand for} \\ \text{counseling} \\ \text{sessions} \end{Bmatrix} = \begin{Bmatrix} \text{Population} \\ = \\ 200{,}000 \end{Bmatrix} \times \begin{Bmatrix} \text{Incidence} \\ \text{rate} = \\ 600/1{,}000 \end{Bmatrix} \times \begin{Bmatrix} \text{Average use} \\ \text{per incidence} = \\ 4 \end{Bmatrix} \times \begin{Bmatrix} \text{Market} \\ \text{share} = \\ 15\% \end{Bmatrix}$$

Once target markets and segments within them are identified and quantified, however, managers still must develop effective marketing strategies if they are to achieve productive exchanges with the people in target markets and segments. As seen in the next section, there are several well-established types of marketing strategies.

Examples of Marketing Strategies

Two important sets of typologies of marketing strategies are those developed by Miles and Snow[42] and Porter's competitive strategies.[43] These are discussed in the next two sections, followed by discussion of other well-known prototypical strategies.

MILES AND SNOW TYPOLOGY

Miles and Snow constructed a typology of strategies three decades ago that remains popular today.[44] "Specifically, they identified four strategic patterns that differ from one another by the degree to which an organization's leaders are willing to assume risk or take aggressive action in the pursuit of competitive advantage."[45] Applying the Miles and Snow typology to HSOs/HSs yields four models of the patterns that might be pursued in marketing strategies:

- *Prospectors:* HSOs/HSs that aggressively search for new market opportunities and frequently engage in experimentation and innovation
- *Analyzers:* HSOs/HSs that maintain stability in selected areas of operation but seek new opportunities in other areas (often following the lead of prospector HSOs/HSs)
- *Defenders:* HSOs/HSs that rely on previously successful strategies and rarely make changes in strategies, or even small adjustments in existing strategies
- *Reactors:* HSOs/HSs that perceive threats and opportunities from their external environments but are unable to adapt on a consistent and effective basis

PORTER'S COMPETITIVE STRATEGIES

Another important typology of strategic alternatives was developed by Michael Porter. As discussed in Chapter 8, positioning strategies relate an HSO/HS to its competitors. In fact, Porter's classic analysis of such strategies labels the positioning strategies as competitive strategies. He identified three categories of competitive strategies: low-cost leadership strategy, differentiation strategy, and focused strategy.[46] Each is described below.

Low-Cost Leadership

The HSO/HS that pursues a low-cost leadership strategy seeks to reach a broad market of buyers with services or products that are perceived to be of at least equal value/quality as those of competitors but at lower prices. To sustain this strategy, the HSO must continuously seek to drive down costs while maintaining or enhancing quality. As discussed in Chapter 7, continuous quality improvement (CQI), reengineering, and strategic quality planning—in which quality enhancement is central to the strategizing process—are initiatives that can lead to increased quality, productivity improvement (i.e., cost effectiveness relative to quality), and enhanced competitive position. It should be noted that even if ultimate consumers are less sensitive to pricing strategies because they are buffered from the impact of full charges, the payer/insurer will almost certainly be responsive to price differentials. Furthermore, focus on cost control has the potential benefit of increasing gross margins, independent of short-term competitive effects.

Product Differentiation

Product differentiation refers to a strategy in which the HSO/HS attempts to distinguish its products and services from those of its competitors on some product attributes (other than price) considered to be important to the consumer. In healthcare, differentiation can take the form of providing more comfort or amenities (e.g., private rooms in acute care and birthing suites), emphasizing state-of-the-art technology (e.g., electronic health records and "green facilities"), emphasizing prevention and well-being (e.g., offering "silver sneakers" fitness classes at a community hospital), or increasing visibility of the HSO's reputation and image (e.g., banners announcing the HSO's national rankings for quality of care). An effective promotional campaign is almost always necessary for a product differentiation strategy to have a competitive effect.

Focused (Niche)

A focused strategy entails the identification of a specific and narrow market segment, or niche, in which the HSO can focus its entire marketing effort to attract a customer base with unique needs and wants. In niche markets, the customer base is smaller, but competitors are also fewer. Once established in a niche market, a successful competitor is likely to experience a high level of brand loyalty and relatively price-inelastic levels of demand. Given the uniqueness of niche market segments, focused strategies often entail product differentiation and may be compatible with low-cost leadership.[47] Health services examples include elective cosmetic surgery and antiaging creams for affluent consumers, and various alternative health regimens, such as acupuncture and natural pharmaceuticals.

As may be evident from the discussion above, these strategies are not mutually exclusive, are potentially complementary, and may be implemented in combination or sequentially. A low-cost strategy may yield a clearly differentiated set of service/product offerings and may be attractive in a narrowly segmented market. An urban medical center may use multiple strategies for different market segments, such as bariatric surgery for a more affluent niche market, a low-cost strategy for community hospital services and outreach in an economically distressed community, and a range of tertiary clinical services differentiated on the basis of world-class quality.

OTHER PROTOTYPICAL MARKETING STRATEGIES

Marketing strategies must (as discussed above) be consistent with the HSO's/HS's mission and vision, core values, strategic direction, goals, and access to resources. Although there are various schemes for classifying marketing strategies, the following discussion represents a typical set of categories of market *growth* and *contraction*. It could be argued that virtually every HSO/HS will adopt one of these strategies at some point in the organization's history and life cycle.

Growth strategies include market entry, expansion, and adaptation and are almost certainly the most commonly pursued strategies. Growth of staff, assets, facilities, revenues, and profits is such a common indicator of the enterprise's success that anything other than a growth strategy seems to require special justification.

Expansion includes market penetration, market/product development, and diversification.[48] Market penetration entails increasing revenues and market share of current products and services within established markets. In a market in which the demand for services is flat or declining, market penetration by one HSO results in a "zero sum" game where growth in market share for one competitor can only result from loss of business by another. Assertive advertising, expanding access to services, and negotiated pricing can be used to support this strategic choice. Market development (entry) requires introducing the current product line and services into new markets or to additional market segments. This may be achieved through geographical expansion, such as establishing a satellite clinic for an urban academic health center in a rapidly growing suburban community, or by attracting new market segments. An example of the latter might be a long-term care facility opening a wellness center onsite targeted to active, independent-living elderly in the community. Product development refers to the design and introduction of new or improved products and services in existing markets. Adding a managed care health plan to an academic health center would be an example of product development, closely related to the core business of the HSO.

Contraction strategies reflect a declining position in the target market and/or changes in the perceived attractiveness of the market. Contraction can take several forms, including divestment, harvesting (or starving), and exit. In divestment, the organization sells the assets or otherwise eliminates a product, product line, or service that is considered to be underperforming or no longer a good strategic fit with the core business. This may be necessary to increase liquidity and decrease debt when the organization faces severe fiscal and related crises. *Harvesting* is used somewhat euphemistically to refer to a strategy of milking a product/service for its cash flow but starving it of sustaining resources beyond the short term. It might serve as a precursor to an eventual market exit strategy. Market exit, or retrenchment, entails the departure of an organization from an entire market. Although such a move may seem wise, even inevitable for strategic reasons, as long as there is some demand for the withdrawn services, the exit costs must be considered in terms of adverse impact on the community and the HSO's/HS's image. Such closings of facilities and programs are associated with reorganizations, mergers, and consolidations and often are justified on grounds of optimal resource allocation within the larger system.

▬ Industry Structure and Competitive Position: Porter's Model ▬

A seminal contribution by Porter to understanding the variety and suitability of marketing strategies is his Five Forces Model.[49] This classical methodology for evaluating an industry's structure and an organization's competitive position within it was developed by Porter some years ago. It consists of the following five elements, or forces:

1.   Existing intensity of the competition among providers within the target market
2.   Potential for new entrants in the marketplace
3.   Availability of substitute products and services
4.   Bargaining power of buyers
5.   Bargaining power of sellers/suppliers

Figure 9.2, which shows the relationship of these five forces driving industry competition, is particularly appropriate to consider in analyzing the competitive position of organizations and systems.

INTENSITY OF COMPETITION (RIVALRY)

Rivalry among competing sellers/suppliers characterizes their efforts to gain favorable position in the market by managing the marketing mix and perhaps an associated strategy, such as price competition. This means the seller will utilize such variables as service and product attributes (including quality), image or brand identification, and promotion to achieve an advantageous competitive position. "Rivalry can range from friendly to cutthroat, depending on how frequently and how aggres-

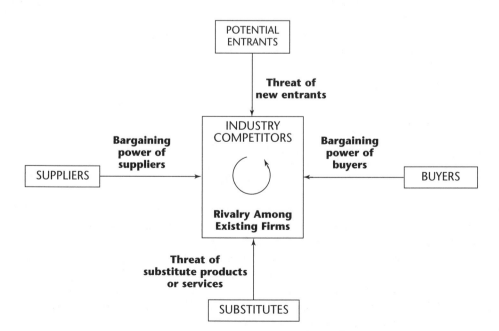

Figure 9.2.   Forces driving industry competition. Reprinted with permission of The Free Press, a Division of Simon & Schuster Adult Publishing Group, from *Competitive Strategy: Techniques for Analyzing Industries and Competitors* by Michael E. Porter. Copyright © 1980, 1998 by The Free Press. All rights reserved.

sively companies undertake fresh moves that threaten a rival's profitability,"[50] and can result in both offensive and defensive responses by the rival. The characteristics of competitive relationships in health services markets are discussed below:[51]

1. Competitive intensity is greatest when competitors are numerous and evenly balanced in size of staff, assets, and so forth. Most urban areas in the United States are characterized by intense competition among a decreasing number of large, integrated healthcare systems. Stand-alone community hospitals in small towns or rural areas are likely to be insulated from competition if they are not the targets of merger and acquisition strategies of larger HSOs/HSs.
2. Rivalry intensifies with sudden changes in demand for services within a market as competitors attempt to increase their market share. Similarly, competition intensifies whenever significant excess capacity is present, such as an oversupply of hospital beds in an area.
3. Competition is strong when the services and products offered are relatively undifferentiated and/or there are negligible costs to the consumer in switching to another provider. The more effectively an organization or system differentiates its services by brand identification, quality, convenience, and/or price, the stronger its market position in the face of competition. An organization can also affect the switching costs and incentives faced by its customers by contracting to provide its health services through an independent managed care insurer or a captive (i.e., subsidiary) MCO.
4. Competitive rivalry increases when fixed costs are high and there is overcapacity in the market. For example, if trauma centers are not used to capacity, the fixed costs remain without offsetting revenue. This same logic holds for excess hospital beds.
5. Rivalry increases when exit barriers are so high that it might cost more to discontinue the service and exit the market than to continue to operate at some reduced level. Acute care hospitals, for example, face high exit barriers. Their relatively high fixed plant and equipment costs can discourage them from leaving the market, as can other nonfiscal factors such as the ethical issues associated with their commitment to mission.
6. Competition may also intensify due to acquisitions, mergers, or consolidations of HSOs/HSs in a market. For example, when a weak HSO is acquired by or merged into another HSO outside the market, the acquiring HSO will likely initiate an aggressive promotional and public relations campaign to increase its visibility and public awareness and the market share of the acquired entity. These efforts are likely to stimulate defensive responses from other competitors in the same market.

SUBSTITUTE PRODUCTS[52]

The existence of or potential for substitute services/products can increase competitive pressures for organizations by posing a threat to their competitive position. The threat "is strong when substitutes are readily available and attractively priced, buyers believe substitutes have comparable or better features, and buyers' switching costs are low."[53] Potato chips and pretzels, Coke and AriZona Green Tea, and XBox and Monopoly can be considered substitute products. In health services, however, providers delivering lower-quality care and/or services that are difficult to access are no substitute for those that are delivering high-quality, accessible care.

Substitute products and services in health services include such products and services as pharmaceuticals versus psychoanalysis for depression, open heart surgery versus percutaneous transluminal angioplasty (PCTA) to prevent heart attacks, and diet and exercise regimen versus bariatric surgery. An HSO/HS offering only one of an array of alternative services is exposed to competition from those offering substitutes. When the substitutes are perceived to be of similar quality and efficacy but also offered at lower cost, the competitive threat of substitutes will increase. Examples are influenza shots provided by the county health department versus through a physician's office, and purchasing a generic equivalent to a brand-name drug.

POTENTIAL FOR NEW ENTRANTS

New entrants increase capacity to meet demand for services or products in a given market, which increases the intensity of competition and may drive marginal providers out of the market. In healthcare, new entry urgi-care centers compete with hospital-based emergency departments for non–life-threatening care, and freestanding ambulatory care imaging and surgery centers compete with acute care hospitals. Barriers to market entry influence the likelihood and ease of entry of new competitors, and the level of competition is decreased when barriers are high. Barriers to entry include the following:[54]

1. *Capital requirements* represent the costs of physical plant, other fixed assets, technology, and equipment required to sustain operations. High capital requirements and the associated fixed costs drive the need for *economies of scale,* that is, the need to achieve high volume to "spread the overhead" and lower the average cost of services. The inability to obtain sufficient capital, to achieve economies of scale, and to break even within a reasonable time will raise the costs and decrease the likelihood of new entry. An example is a new competitor building a new medical complex in an overbedded urban area. In comparison, the opening of a family practice clinic using leased space in an urban mall has relatively low capital requirements and has different implications for the economics of production and profitability.
2. *Product/service differentiation* forces potential competitors to allocate substantial resources to overcome the competitive advantage of an established provider relative to quality, stature, reputation, and image. It would be difficult for a potential new entrant to succeed in matching or exceeding the high quality and stature of the internationally renowned Mayo Clinic, Cleveland Clinic, Memorial Sloan-Kettering Cancer Center, or University of Pittsburgh Medical Center's organ transplantation program.
3. *High switching costs* lock in buyers/patients and are a barrier to new entrants. The lower the switching costs are, the easier it is for competitors to enter markets. In a geographical area with a large commercial insurance plan, there may be lower switching costs for insured people and thus a lower barrier for a new service provider/entrant than when a larger percentage of the population is enrolled in managed care. To succeed under the latter condition, the new entrant would need to convince the managed care insurer to contract with it to eliminate patient switching costs.
4. *Government policy and regulation* can be a barrier to entry. In the past, certificate-of-need legislation tended to preclude competitors from entering markets and offering certain healthcare services. Regulation and licensure, such as that for skilled nursing facility beds, restricts entry.

BARGAINING POWER OF BUYERS[55]

The competitive strength of buyers in an industry also is a major influence on the level of competition. Buyers have strength if the goods they purchase are undifferentiated, switching costs are low, they purchase in large volume, and many suppliers are available. Bargaining power is enhanced when the buyer has the potential to backward integrate and avoid the seller altogether. Integrated healthcare delivery systems, multi-institutional systems, strategic alliances, and networks have greater bargaining power than stand-alone HSOs because of the greater volume of purchases of the former.[56] Similarly, an MCO has greater bargaining power than independent HSOs when contracting services, due to the number of insured enrollees it represents. Consequently, an MCO can negotiate discounts in price and other favorable terms with the suppliers of its services.

"Health plans and providers coexist in a complex, reciprocal buyer–seller relationship."[57] When the bargaining power of one party weakens, the market power of the other is strengthened. Brown indicates that "sellers of service are bundling products [to enhance their supplier bargaining power] while buyers, including managed care firms, seek to unbundle. That tug of war will continue for the near term."[58]

An example of the application of buying power to gain competitive advantage is an HS's developing its own subsidiary health plan to market health insurance products to the public and especially to large employers. By directing its enrollees (covered lives) to the HS's health services facilities and network of licensed independent practitioners (LIPs), the HS increases its bargaining power relative to other competitors.

BARGAINING POWER OF SUPPLIERS[59]

The bargaining power of suppliers also has potential influence on the intensity of competition within a healthcare market. Suppliers' bargaining power is strong when competitors are few, products and services are differentiated, buyers' switching costs are high, few if any substitute products are available, and the supplier's costs are low relative to other competitors. The supplier has enhanced market power if it has the capacity to integrate backward to produce the products and services it offers to the market. Also, "vertical integration augments the firm's market [supplier/selling] power."[60] Vertically integrated HSs have enhanced bargaining power both backward and forward: as buyers with their suppliers and as suppliers with buyers of their services, such as MCOs and employers.

The reverse market conditions will result in reduced bargaining power for the supplier. As in the earlier example, an independent acute care hospital in a competitive market likely has weak supplier power relative to an established MCO. Conversely, its bargaining power may be greater if its services are appreciably differentiated from those of other suppliers based on attributes such as quality, good will, technology, and expertise and reputation of the clinical staff.

An alliance between a hospital and a physician–hospital organization (PHO) provides another example of how the buyer–supplier power relationship may be influenced.[61] PHOs often are structured as joint ventures with shared hospital–physician ownership, an arrangement by which the hospital and physicians can contract with MCOs to provide services to the health plan's subscribers. Consequently, PHOs "may increase the negotiating clout of their individual members with managed care organizations"[62] and provide a vehicle for risk sharing among providers and encourage collaborative efforts in utilization management and quality improvement.[63]

▬ Market Position Analysis ▬▬▬▬▬▬▬▬▬▬▬▬▬▬▬▬▬▬▬▬

Several tools have been developed to facilitate analysis of the position of organizations in their current market(s) relative to their competition. One of the earliest and still utilized is the Boston Consulting Group Matrix (BCG Matrix) developed by Bruce Henderson.[64] Another more sophisticated and widely used tool is the GE/McKinsey Matrix. This tool was developed by McKinsey & Company as a means of screening General Electric's extensive portfolio of strategic business units (SBUs). Both tools are described below.

BCG MATRIX

The BCG Matrix is a graphic approach allowing the organization or system to position its products within a 2×2 matrix based on two variables, current market share and projected market growth. The market share measure is calculated as the ratio of the organization's market share to that of its most

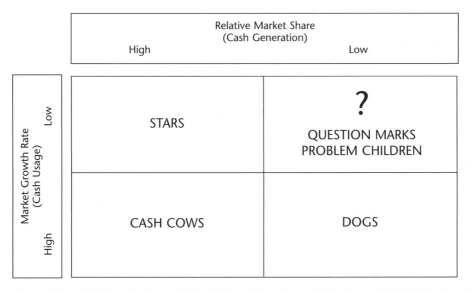

Figure 9.3. BCG Growth–Share Matrix. (Adapted from Bruce D. Henderson (1973). "The Experience Curve—Reviewed IV, The Growth–Share Matrix or The Product Portfolio." Boston: The Boston Consulting Group, page 1. http://www.bcg.com/publications/files/Experience_Curve_IV_Growth_Share_Matrix_1973. Used by permission of the Boston Consulting Group.)

dominant competitor. One assumption underlying the model is that high market share of revenues produces high profits as well, an assumption that may not be warranted. The market growth variable is measured as the rate of growth in total revenues in the target market. The resulting matrix provides a means to indicate an organization's current array of products and services and to project their likely or desired position at some future time.

The four cells in the matrix have been traditionally labeled "stars" (high market share, high growth), "cash cows" (high share, low growth), "question marks" or "problem children" (low share, high growth), and "dogs" (low share, low growth). Figure 9.3 is an adaptation of the BCG Matrix.

Each of the cells in the matrix reflects a prototypical market position with strategic implications. The stars are successful and profitable high-revenue-producing products in a market experiencing a high rate of revenue growth. The optimal strategic choice may be to continue to support this product at current or higher levels of resources, assuming that its growth and profitability will continue.

The cash cows represent mature products continuing to generate revenues in a slow-growing or stagnant market. The optimal strategy in this position is to "milk" the product for revenues, even if profitability is declining, while reallocating resources to other promising products.

The question marks, or problem children, identify services/products with a low share in high-growth markets. As such, they represent classic underachievers. The strategic choices with question marks seem clear: Feed and discipline these problem children so that they are able to compete to increase their market share, or starve (divest) them and reallocate the resources to more deserving siblings.

Finally, the dogs are low-share products in low/no-growth markets. In this case "let sleeping dogs lie" is usually not a wise strategy, because continuing to invest in such products is unlikely to yield adequate returns and is likely to depress potential earnings for the entire product/service mix. In this case, a mercy killing (liquidation and market exit) may be a better strategy than slow starvation.

GE (GENERAL ELECTRIC)/MCKINSEY MATRIX

The GE/McKinsey Matrix (see Figure 9.4) is a more sophisticated, multidimensional alternative to the BCG model. It uses a similar approach by positioning services/products and service/product lines

		Business Unit Strength		
		Strong	Average	Weak
Market Attractiveness	High			
	Medium			
	Low			

Figure 9.4. GE/McKinsey Matrix. (Adapted from Charles W. Hofer and Dan Schendel, 1978. *Strategy Formulation Analytical Concepts.* St. Paul, MN: West Publishing, page 32. Used by permission of South-Western, a division of Thomson Learning (www.thomsonrights.com). Fax 800-730-2215.)

against two variables—in this case, competitive strength and market attractiveness. The variables are derived as weighted, multifactor indices that provide a richer measure of the underlying variables. Market attractiveness is a composite of 9 variables, including market size (revenues), growth rate, profit margin, competitive intensity, and inflation sensitivity. Business, or competitive, strength is composed of 12 variables, including current market share, rate of share growth, brand strength, product quality, distribution network, and cost and managerial factors.

The GE/McKinsey Matrix provides a 3 × 3 field with market attractiveness ranging from low to high and with business strength from weak to strong. Each of the nine cells is associated with a proscriptive strategic option; for example, a product positioned with weak business strength with average (medium) market favorability is associated with "harvest or divest" options. Although the GE/McKinsey Matrix is logically equivalent to the BCG model, it does encourage more thorough analysis and more precise positioning.

Strategic Marketing Postures

Organizations differ in their behavior in confronting competitive markets and market opportunities. Typical styles (postures) have been identified to distinguish how organizations respond to their environments, competitors, and customers. Thomas characterizes five distinct strategies and corresponding marketing roles: dominant leaders, market followers ("second fiddle"), challengers ("frontal attack"), niche players, and flankers.[65]

Dominant leaders have attained the greatest market share and base their strategy on maintaining or increasing their market control. Typically, the market behavior and performance of these players serve as the norms and benchmarks, respectively, for competitors in the same market.

Market followers pursue a "wait-and-see" or copycat strategy that is essentially cautious and risk avoiding. This posture may be considered especially prudent when a variant of the dominant player, the *market pioneer,* has heavy investments in a new technology, radically differentiated products and services, or innovative distribution channels. The follower avoids the risks the pioneer accepts but also will forego the initial returns of successful market entry. Once the follower senses that it's safe to enter the water (with evidence of the market's acceptance of the new product), the "second fiddle" competitor makes its entry into a calmer, lower-risk environment with a copycat or marginally differentiated product or service.

In contrast, the *challenger* mounts an aggressive response to the market leader in the attempt to erode the leader's market share and competitive advantage. With the increasing consolidation and growth of healthcare systems, a typical pattern has emerged in many large metropolitan areas: that of a few large systems competing for market dominance with smaller systems and a few stand-alone hospitals on the fringe, struggling to survive. As the smaller and less well resourced HSOs lose market share, they face acquisition by larger HSOs/HSs, divestiture of unprofitable product lines, or liquidation.

Niche players focus their resources and attention on some narrowly defined market segment with the goal of attaining dominance in that segment. This focused strategy allows the organization to concentrate resources on the development and marketing of one product/service or product/service line for a well-defined and easily identified population. Once the niche player establishes a strong position in its narrow market, it may play a role equivalent to the dominant leader in the broader market. Its knowledge of the niche market and brand loyalty, as well as the limited potential for market growth, will likely serve as barriers to entry for other competitors. Examples of a niche strategy in health services include elective, cosmetic surgeries; Botox treatments; eye (ophthalmologic) hospitals; and acupuncture clinics.

Flankers, or fringe players, may be seen as pursuing a variation on the niche strategy by avoiding direct competition with the dominant leaders and challengers while not achieving market strength in a well-defined niche. This can be considered a defensive or reactive marketing strategy, in which flankers react to the moves of dominant players by competing on the fringes of markets by pursuing low-cost, low-quality (bare bones) strategies. One example of this approach is that of the initial market entry of Jet Blue and other "no frills" air carriers. In health services, a stand-alone community hospital providing limited inpatient and ER services may be seen as playing a flanker role relative to the major healthcare providers.

As one example of the typical pattern of market roles in U.S. healthcare in the 21st century, the University of Pittsburgh Medical Center (UPMC) has established market dominance in southwestern Pennsylvania by acquiring many of the formerly independent community hospitals in the region and several prestigious specialty providers, such as Magee-Womens Hospital and Children's Hospital of Pittsburgh, and has most recently pursued a "white knight" acquisition of a financially distressed member of a faith-based network, Mercy Hospital of Pittsburgh. The remaining major market challenger, West Penn Allegheny Health System, was formed by West Penn's takeover of the flagship hospital of another system upon its financial collapse and by its acquiring other fiscally challenged community hospitals. In such a concentrated market, the remaining independent hospitals have very few choices other than adopting a niche or flanker strategy or ultimately agreeing to be acquired.

Market Research

Market research may be defined as the application of quantitative and qualitative methods of data collection and analysis to better understand consumer needs, wants, attitudes, and behaviors relevant to managing all aspects of the marketing mix and developing effective marketing strategies. Market research relies on both primary and secondary data sources for a wide range of objectives, including assessing the needs and preferences of a target market segment, designing new and enhanced products, predicting customer acceptance and use, evaluating and comparing the efficacy of alternative promotional channels, obtaining data on obstacles to access for subgroups of consumers, and analyzing the impact of alternate pricing strategies.

All the tools of the social and behavioral sciences are available, in principle, to the marketing researcher in health services. Statistical analysis of patient demographics and psychographics, geographic information system (GIS) and ZIP code analyses of customer residency and access patterns, advertising yields, and trends in pricing of services represent applications of market research in healthcare. However, given the focus on relationship and customer-focused marketing, qualitative methods such as customer satisfaction surveys, in-depth interviews, focus groups, and "mystery shopping" are increasingly used. Almquist and Wyner[66] call for greater use of experimental designs and methods in marketing to take advantage of their predictive power, precision, and cost-effectiveness relative to more traditional techniques. Certainly the efficacy of any marketing strategy will depend in large part on the validity and reliability of the data collected; they are the basis for understanding and making predictions about consumer needs, preferences, and behaviors as well as consumers' and competitors' responses to variations in the components of the marketing mix and strategic marketing initiatives of contemporary HSOs/HSs.

MARKETING AUDITS

Because organizations and systems are so consumer focused, they "are characterized by a concerted effort to collect, share, and respond to consumer information."[67] These efforts often take the form of marketing audits, which are systematic evaluations of the entity's marketing situation. They include 1) identifying target markets and their needs, identifying opportunities, and assessing competition through environmental surveillance and 2) evaluating present service mix or product lines relative to identified target market needs.

A marketing audit identifies present and potential target markets for the HSO/HS—potential purchasers of services as well as those who may influence purchase decisions on behalf of patients/customers. Central to this assessment is identification of consumers' present and future needs, wants, and desires.

In healthcare, the traditional view is that the consumer in the exchange process is the patient. However, there are others who may intervene and influence who buys what service, for what price, and where, thus functioning as customers. For example, physicians not only control admission to hospitals and, sometimes, nursing facilities but also review the services that are provided. Third-party payers, in particular government, large corporations, and MCOs, influence the prices of services. Directly or indirectly, regulation influences the type and intensity of services provided through such mechanisms as accreditation, quality assessment, and reimbursement mechanisms. Self-insured corporations influence where customers receive service by advocating alternatives such as HMOs and PPOs and, through purchasing power, also can influence type of, scope of, and price charged for services. Consequently, HSO/HS marketing must seek to satisfy wants and needs of patients as well as to identify, recognize, address, and satisfy the wants and needs of others who influence the purchasing decision.

HSOs/HSs must effectively audit their markets and use the information to reconsider and realign their service and product mixes and make many associated changes. Information from the marketing audit can reveal potential new target markets and other opportunities, as well as marketplace threats from competitors and other threats, such as demographic shifts.

For example, a competitor's introduction of an urgent care center or an ambulatory surgery center could require significant reassessment of a target market's threats or opportunities. Similarly, declining population in a market or an increasing number of elderly in the target market could stimulate changes in service. The addition of living arrangements and health services for the elderly is an example. This means not only new services for a new market, but also new strategies and plans designed to help reach the new market.

Conceptually, the list of potential new opportunities and threats arising in target markets can mean significant and ongoing changes in services. The likelihood of such changes, many of which are listed in the earlier section on Product/Service, illustrates how vitally important effective marketing audits are to HSOs/HSs.

Ethics in Marketing

Ethics in marketing receives more attention in Chapter 4. Suffice it to say here that because marketing is largely a human endeavor involving exchanges of value, it is subject to a variety of ethical considerations. Ethics has been applied to health services managers as representing "a special charge and a responsibility to patients, organization and staff, to themselves and the profession, and ultimately, but less directly, to society."[69] Certainly this mandate and accountability apply to those responsible for the marketing function in HSOs/HSs. The core values at the root of ethical decision making in health services and healthcare that have achieved general consensus include respect for persons, beneficence, nonmaleficence, and justice.[70]

Respect for persons includes autonomy, truth telling, confidentiality, and fidelity, not only in interactions with patients but with all stakeholders. Perhaps the foundation of this value commitment is the willingness to treat others as independent decision makers worthy of trust and respect. *Beneficence* refers to doing good acts, including those motivated by altruism and professional standards of practice. *Nonmaleficence* refers to avoiding evil or harmful acts. This value is captured in the Code of Hammurabi, in which physicians face harsh sanctions if their treatments result in injury or death, and is consistent with "above all, do no harm!" *Justice* requires fairness and due process to all, entailing, for example, that all patients who present with the same medical circumstances be treated in a similar fashion. *Fidelity* provides the ethical underpinning for the healthcare providers' fiduciary responsibility to their patients, acting as agents for the patients both morally and legally. Veracity, or *truth telling,* is the foundation upon which all other values are based. Without truth telling in ongoing relationships among people, there is no basis for trust that the other values will be honored, nor any solid ground for meaningful, enduring relationships.

The application of these values to marketing processes is straightforward. If an HSO/HS or its agents (managers, staff, and care providers) are not seen as honest in business transactions, trust will be eroded along with public image and credibility. If the organization or its agents demonstrate lack of respect to stakeholders, such as by violating confidentiality or exhibiting patronizing attitudes, again trust and good will be impaired if not destroyed.

Marketing management has a special responsibility for honesty and fidelity in communication to promote and advertise with current and potential customers. In fact, marketing may face the challenge of restoring the public image of an HSO/HS and maintaining market position in the face of some significant ethical breach by management or affiliated healthcare providers.

All HSOs/HSs must be responsive to their stakeholders, especially patients, payers, and employees; for-profits are also accountable to owners and stockholders. Not only is the organization or system obligated to engage in prudent fiscal stewardship, but it can carry out its mission only by remaining solvent. These organizations and systems must balance their responsibility for the health and well-being of the communities they serve with the business case for maintaining, expanding, or contracting their market positions. Decisions about product/service mix, price, access to services, and the channels for and content of marketing messages all have ethical as well as business implications. For example, if an affluent market segment is targeted for cosmetic surgery and fitness club services, will "profit" be used to subsidize charitable care or medical education? What actions should an HSO/HS take to ameliorate the impact on a medically underserved community if it decides to exit the market? Effective marketing management requires that ethical concerns be considered when strategic choices are made.

▨ DISCUSSION QUESTIONS

1. Discuss variation in the definition of *marketing,* and state the preferred definition used in this chapter.
2. Discuss what marketing is and is not, as described in this chapter.
3. What is social marketing?
4. Discuss the 4 *P*s of the marketing mix.
5. Briefly describe Porter's ideas on competitive strategies.
6. Discuss some of the key challenges in identifying target markets for HSOs/HSs.
7. Identify and describe each of the five forces in Porter's model of competition.
8. Compare and contrast the BCG Matrix developed by the Boston Consulting Group and the GE/McKinsey Matrix developed by McKinsey for General Electric.
9. Discuss ethics in marketing, including its importance.
10. Discuss the role of marketing audits.

▨ Case Study 1: Lactation Services at Women's Wellness Hospital[71]

Women's Wellness Hospital (WWH), one of the oldest and most prestigious hospitals for obstetrics and gynecology (OB-GYN) and other women's health services in the United States, is part of a large, rapidly growing urban academic health center located in the Middle Atlantic states. Due to a declining base of women of childbearing age in this urban region and an increasingly older population, WWH has diversified its patient base and is considering an array of new products and services to increase its market dominance beyond the 52% share it currently has. While searching to expand its product line beyond its core OB-GYN and maternal health services, WWH's governing body and senior-level managers also want to ensure that it retains its focus on the high-quality, high-touch women's services it has traditionally offered.

WWH offers a cluster of services associated with lactation (breast feeding) but without having incorporated these services into a coherent marketing strategy. These services and resources include

- Inpatient access to seven board-certified lactation consultants on a fee-for-service basis
- Outpatient scheduling for lactation consults
- General breast-feeding inpatient information from nursing staff
- Lactation education for medical and nursing staffs
- Breast-feeding aids and accessories for rental or purchase, such as breast pumps, nursing bras, and parenting books

Among the considerations that must be addressed in developing a marketing strategy for lactation services are the following:

- Such services are not covered under any Medicaid or any other federal or state-funded health program, and it is not clear that the current fees cover the costs of providing the consulting services.
- Some of the lactation specialists have expressed the opinion that they are over-scheduled with inpatient consults.
- Corporations have expressed interest in accommodating their employees who choose to breast-feed.

- Currently the lactation consultants share a crowded office in the basement adjacent to the environmental services area.
- The other major healthcare system in the county also offers board-certified lactation services within its OB-GYN and pediatric units.
- The national Women, Infants, and Children Program administered by the U.S. Department of Agriculture assertively promotes breast feeding to its primary constituency (mothers of lower socioeconomic status) as well as to the broader public.

QUESTIONS

1. Assuming that you are an external marketing consultant contracted to help WWH develop a marketing strategy for lactation services, what additional information would you need to gather as part of your marketing research? Identify at least two questions you might ask for each of the 4 *P*s of the marketing mix.
2. What specific issues must be considered in order for you to price the lactation services that are to be offered?
3. Is place (location) of these services an important concern for an effective marketing strategy in this situation? Why or why not?
4. What would be the likely implications of deciding to eliminate the board-certified lactation specialists and shift responsibility to the nursing staff exclusively?

■ Case Study 2: What Is Marketing?

Marketing has been defined in numerous ways (review the Marketing Defined section in this chapter). For example, in 1935, the American Marketing Association defined marketing as the "performance of business activities that direct the flow of goods and services from the producer to the consumer."[72] In 1985, the association redefined marketing as "the process of planning and executing conception, pricing, promotion and distribution of goods, ideas and services to create exchanges that satisfy individual and organizational goals."[73]

By 2004, this definition had morphed into "marketing is an organizational function and a set of processes for creating, communicating and delivering value to customers and for managing customer relationships in ways that benefit the organization and its stakeholders."[74] By 2008, the American Marketing Association's official definition had become "marketing is the activity, set of institutions and processes for creating, communicating, delivering and exchanging offerings that have value for customers, clients, partners, and for society at large."[75] So, what is marketing?

QUESTIONS

1. What are primary differences in these definitions?
2. Why has the American Marketing Association's official definition of *marketing* evolved in this way?
3. Does the 2008 definition fit well with contemporary marketing in HSOs/HSs?

■ Case Study 3: Marketing Turmoil—Pharmaceuticals[76]

George Hinton was a local pharmacist in rural Alabama. He had served his community of 900-plus people for more than 40 years. He was also an officer in the local Rotary Club, and his business cosponsored several community events such as the annual Girl Scout picnic. In addition to drugs, his little shop sold cosmetics and nostrums, and it had a restaurant counter where a waitress would bring you the latest blue plate special each weekday noon, if you had $5.

It was Monday (meatloaf day) when Mrs. Olive Murden, age 63, entered the establishment and, using her cane, shuffled back to the pharmaceutical area in the rear. She called to George as he counted pills in the side room.

"How do you do, Mrs. Murden?" George amiably inquired as he walked over to speak with her.

"I am still fighting my arthritis," she offered with a half smile.

"What brings you in today—you still have some of your prescriptions don't you?" George asked.

"Yes, I do, and I really appreciate your driving in and opening up your store for me last Sunday at midnight when I found myself out of the expensive pill. I was really hurting."

"Well, we've been doing business together for a long time, and you still are my number one customer for Brinklie's Magnolia Blossom Perfume," he said with a smile.

Mrs. Murden's face grew darker as she told George what she had come to say. "I will be needing my prescriptions transferred, I am afraid."

George was disturbed but not surprised. "Moving to that special discount drug program the big chain department store is offering, are you, Mrs. Murden?"

"No, though I considered it until I learned my expensive pill was not on their list." Mrs. Murden shifted her feet, plainly uncomfortable with the news she was giving her old friend. "The local Chamber of Commerce is offering a no-cost drug discount card, and by using it, I can save a lot of money on my expensive pill."

"Well, I can fill that for you here with that card and get you the same discount," George said, though he knew what she was going to say next.

"Well, yes . . . but they say I can save even more if I use the card and order my pills by mail from someplace in Delaware."

"I see—many people are buying their pills by mail nowadays—the drug companies can reduce overhead and middlemen, and you can get more for the dollar, but it of course is hurting us local pharmacies." George was plainly upset. Mrs. Murden was the 10th customer that month he had lost to the marketing initiatives of his huge competitors, and the expensive pills that she and other customers needed were major sources of his income. His bottom line was getting thinner every day.

In the months that followed, Mrs. Murden came to George's store once for some of her special perfume but then stopped coming altogether.

QUESTIONS

1. The largest company doing business in Alabama during 2007 was a company offering discount cards for pharmaceuticals. It is clear that the money Mrs. Murden is saving is only a fraction of what these discount mail houses—and the manufacturers who work with them—save when they bypass people like George. Is there some way we could share those funds with local pharmacies to help keep them in business? Should we?

2. George came down and opened his store at midnight for his longtime client—but the big chain stores have pharmacies that are open 24 hours, 7 days a week, and if you mail your orders on time, you will never even need to drive to the pharmacy again. Would you stay with your old friend George if you were on a pension and it cost you 5% of your disposable income in increased drug costs to do so?

3. How could you market George's products and services to maintain/increase his market share and keep him in business?

■ **Case Study 4: Hospital Marketing Effectiveness Rating Instrument**[77]

Complete the following instrument. Choose a hospital, another HSO, or an HS with which you are familiar. Circle the one most appropriate answer (A, B, or C) for each question below.

Customer Philosophy

1. How does the HSO/HS view its markets?
    A. Management thinks in terms of serving patient needs based on the facilities and clinical staff currently available.
    B. Management attempts to offer a broad range of health services, performing all of them well.
    C. Management thinks in terms of serving the needs of well-defined patient and physician segments that offer to the HSO/HS the best prospect for long-term growth and financial return.

2. What is the status of the HSO's/HS's publicity, promotion, and community education programs?
    A   There is limited activity in this area.
    B. The HSO/HS has a number of programs in this area, but coordination among them is limited.
    C. The HSO/HS has a well-coordinated program of information and community outreach efforts, all under the guidance of one staff member.

3. How does the HSO/HS attract and retain the clinical staff?
    A. Primary responsibility for selection and attraction of staff resides with current staff members.
    B. The HSO/HS relies on specific incentives such as high salaries or special equipment to attract new members.
    C. As part of the planning and coordination process, the HSO/HS has developed a comprehensive system to determine and influence the factors affecting the professional staff organization affiliation decision.

Integrated Marketing Organization

4. Is there a vice president or director of marketing responsible for planning, executing, and coordinating the marketing functions?
    A. No such individual exists.
    B. Yes, but there is little integration of this individual within the planning/decision-making process. This individual primarily provides marketing services.
    C. Yes, and the individual participates in HSO/HS policy making as well as providing marketing services.

5. To what extent are marketing-oriented functions (e.g., planning, public relations, marketing research, advertising, promotion, and fund-raising) coordinated in the HSO/HS?
    A. Not very well. There is sometimes unproductive conflict among these functions.
    B. Somewhat. There is some formal integration, but less than satisfactory coordination and control.
    C. Very well. There is effective coordination and control of these functions.

6. Is there a formal systematic procedure for evaluating potential new services and technologies?
    A. There is no formal procedure.
    B. A procedure exists, but it does not include major input from marketing.
    C. The procedure is well developed and includes major input from marketing.

Marketing Information System

7. Does the HSO/HS conduct patient exit interviews and other surveys of patient satisfaction and suggestions?
    A. Rarely or never
    B. Occasionally, but not on a formal basis
    C. Yes, systematically, on a formal basis

8. Does the HSO/HS collect information regarding trends in demand for various types of treatments and the availability in the market of competitive services?
    A. Rarely or never
    B. Occasionally
    C. Yes, on a systematic, continuous basis

9. Does the HSO/HS have an information system containing relevant and up-to-date marketing data?
    A. Such information is limited and is not maintained on an ongoing basis.
    B. Adequate records are maintained and updated on a routine basis, essentially in hard copy form.
    C. An extensive, computer-based information system is provided for systematic storage, maintenance, update, and analysis of marketing data.

Strategic Orientation

10. Does the HSO/HS regularly monitor and evaluate patient services, to identify potential new services to offer and current services to curtail or drop?
    A. The HSO/HS does not evaluate the marketing viability of its various services.
    B. The HSO/HS occasionally evaluates its current services and studies potential new services.
    C. The HSO/HS regularly evaluates its current services and systematically studies potential new services.

11. Does the HSO/HS carry out strategic market planning as well as annual marketing planning?
    A. Strategic market planning is only initiated under special circumstances, such as when facility expansion or debt financing is being considered.
    B. Strategic market planning is carried out regularly but is not done very well.
    C. Strategic market planning is carried out regularly and is done very well.

12. Does the HSO/HS prepare contingency plans?
    A. No.
    B. Contingency plans are occasionally developed to meet major threats.
    C. Contingency plans are routinely developed as part of the normal planning process.

13. Does HSO/HS management know the costs and profitability of its various services?
    A. Such information is not available.
    B. Limited information is available.
    C. HSO/HS management knows the costs and profitability of its various services.

14. Are marketing resources used effectively on a day-to-day basis?
    A. Such resources either are not available or are inadequately used.
    B. The resources are adequate and used to a significant extent but not in an optimal manner.
    C. Yes. Such resources are employed adequately and effectively.

15. Does management examine the results of its marketing expenditures to know what it is accomplishing for its money?
    A. No
    B. To a limited extent
    C. Yes

Scoring

For all of the 15 questions, indicate the number of

A responses	_____ × 0 = _____
B responses	_____ × 1 = _____
C responses	_____ × 2 = _____
Total score	_____

The following scale shows the HSO's/HS's level of marketing effectiveness:

0–5	=	None
6–10	=	Poor
11–15	=	Fair
16–20	=	Good
21–25	=	Very good
26–30	=	Superior

QUESTION

How does the HSO/HS that you evaluated score on the marketing effectiveness rating instrument? If it was low, explain why.

Notes

1. Kotler, Philip, and Gary Armstrong. *Marketing: An Introduction,* 4th ed., 10. Upper Saddle River, NJ: Prentice-Hall, 1997.
2. Kotler, Philip, and Roberta N. Clarke. *Marketing for Healthcare Organizations,* 2nd ed., 5. Englewood Cliffs, NJ: Prentice-Hall, 1987. For similar definitions of marketing, see Cooper, Philip D. "What Is Healthcare Marketing?" In *Healthcare Marketing: Issues and Trends,* 2nd ed., edited by Philip D. Cooper, 3. Rockville, MD: Aspen Publishers, 1985; Keith, Jon G. "Marketing Healthcare: What the Recent Literature Is Telling Us." In *Healthcare Marketing: Issues and Trends,* 2nd ed., edited by Philip

D. Cooper, 15–16. Rockville, MD: Aspen Publishers, 1985; MacStravic, Robin E. *Marketing Religious Healthcare,* 1. St. Louis: The Catholic Health Association of the United States, 1987; and Winston, William J. *How to Write a Marketing Plan for Healthcare Organizations,* 3. New York: Haworth, 1985.

3.   American Marketing Association. "Dictionary of Marketing Terms." *www.marketingpower.com,* retrieved February 25, 2008.

4.   Bennett, Paul D. *Dictionary of Marketing Terms,* 2nd ed. Chicago: American Marketing Association, 1995.

5.   Kotler, Philip, and Roberta N. Clarke. *Marketing for Healthcare Organizations,* 2nd ed., 5. Englewood Cliffs, NJ: Prentice-Hall, 1987.

6.   Andreasen, Alan R. *Marketing Social Change: Changing Behavior to Promote Health, Social Development, and the Environment,* 7. San Francisco: Jossey-Bass, 1995; Andreasen, Alan R. *Social Marketing in the 21st Century.* Thousand Oaks, CA: Sage, 2005.

7.   Smith, William A. "Social Marketing: An Evolving Definition." *American Journal of Health Behavior* 24, 1 (January/February 2000): 11–17, p. 11.

8.   Kotler, Philip, and Gerald Zaltman. "Social Marketing: An Approach to Planned Social Change." *Journal of Marketing* 35 (1971): 3–12, p. 4.

9.   Health Canada. *http://www.hc-sc.gc.ca/index_e.html.*

10. Freimuch, Vickie, Galen Cole, Susan D. Kirby. "Issues in Evaluating Mass Mediated Health Communication Campaigns." In *Evaluation in Health Promotion: Principles and Perspectives,* edited by Irving Rootman, Michael Goodstadt, Brian Hyndman, David V. McQueen, Louise Potvin, Jane Springet, and Erio Ziglio. Geneva: WHO Regional Publications, 2001. European Series, No. 92.

11. MacStravic, Robin E. "The End of Healthcare Marketing." *Health Marketing Quarterly* 7 (1990): 3.

12. See Sturm, Arthur C., Jr. *The New Rules of Marketing: Strategies for Success,* 23. Chicago: Health Administration Press, 1998.

13. Cooper, Philip D. "Managed Care Positives and Negatives for Healthcare Marketing." *Health Marketing Quarterly* 12 (1995): 59.

14. Proenca, E. Jose. "Market Orientation and Organizational Culture in Hospitals." *Journal of Hospital Marketing* 11 (1996): 6.

15. Kotler, Philip, and Roberta N. Clarke. *Marketing for Healthcare Organizations,* 2nd ed., 4. Englewood Cliffs, NJ: Prentice-Hall, 1987.

16. Fisk, Trevor A. "Strategic Planning and Marketing." In *The AUPHA Manual of Health Services Management,* edited by Robert J. Taylor and Susan B. Taylor, 311. Gaithersburg, MD: Aspen Publishers, 1994.

17. Proenca, E. Jose. "Market Orientation and Organizational Culture in Hospitals." *Journal of Hospital Marketing* 11 (1996): 3–18.

18. Kotler, Philip, and Roberta N. Clarke. *Marketing for Healthcare Organizations,* 2nd ed., 4. Englewood Cliffs, NJ: Prentice-Hall, 1987.

19. Zelman, William N., and Deborah L. Parham. "Strategic, Operational, and Marketing Concerns of Product-Line Management in Healthcare." *Healthcare Management Review* 15 (Winter 1990): 29.

20. Kotler, Philip, and Gary Armstrong. *Marketing: An Introduction,* 4th ed., 13. Upper Saddle River, NJ: Prentice-Hall, 1997.

21. Keith, Jon G. "Marketing Healthcare: What the Recent Literature Is Telling Us." In *Healthcare Marketing: Issues and Trends,* 2nd ed., edited by Philip D. Cooper, 15–16. Rockville, MD: Aspen Publishers, 1985.

22. A good review of methods to measure customer satisfaction can be found in Ford, Robert C., Susan A. Bach, and Myron D. Fottler. "Methods of Measuring Patient Satisfaction in Healthcare Organizations." *Healthcare Management Review* 22 (Spring 1997): 74–89.

23. MacStravic, Robin E. "Price of Services." In *Healthcare Marketing: Issues and Trends,* 2nd ed., edited by Philip D. Cooper, 232–234. Rockville, MD: Aspen Publishers, 1985.

24. Thomas, Richard K. *Marketing Health Services,* 83. Chicago: Health Administration Press, 2005.

25. Kotler, Philip, and Roberta N. Clarke. *Marketing for Healthcare Organizations,* 2nd ed., 25. Englewood Cliffs, NJ: Prentice-Hall, 1987.

26. Keith, Jon G. "Marketing Healthcare: What the Recent Literature Is Telling Us." In *Healthcare Market-*

ing: Issues and Trends, 2nd ed., edited by Philip D. Cooper, 15–16. Rockville, MD: Aspen Publishers, 1985.

27. English, Joel. "The Four 'P's of Marketing Are Dead." *Marketing Health Services* 22, 2 (Summer 2000); 20–23, p. 20.

28. English, Joel. "The Four 'P's of Marketing Are Dead." *Marketing Health Services* 22, 2 (Summer 2000): 20–23, p. 21.

29. English, Joel. "The Four 'P's of Marketing Are Dead." *Marketing Health Services* 22, 2 (Summer 2000): 20–23, p. 22.

30. Macstravic, Scott. "The Death of the Four 'P's: A Premature Obituary." *Marketing Health Services* 22, 4 (Winter 2000): 16–20.

31. Macstravic, Scott. "The Death of the Four 'P's: A Premature Obituary." *Marketing Health Services* 22, 4 (Winter 2000): 16–20, p. 19.

32. Bigelow, Barbara, and John F. Mahon. "Strategic Behavior of Hospitals: A Framework for Analysis." *Medical Care Review* 46 (Fall 1989): 298.

33. Berkowitz, Eric N. *Essentials of Healthcare Marketing,* 164. Sudbury, MA: Jones and Bartlett Publishers, 2006.

34. Berkowitz, Eric N. *Essentials of Healthcare Marketing,* 164. Sudbury, MA: Jones and Bartlett Publishers, 2006.

35. Thomas, Richard K., and Michael Calhoun. *Marketing Matters: A Guide for Executives,* 185. Chicago: Health Administration Press, 2007.

36. Yankelovich, Daniel, and David Meer. "Rediscovering Market Segmentation." *Harvard Business Review* (June 2006). (Reprint R0602G.)

37. Yankelovich, Daniel, and David Meer. "Rediscovering Market Segmentation." *Harvard Business Review* (June 2006). (Reprint R0602G, p.1.)

38. Berkowitz, Eric N. *Essentials of Healthcare Marketing,* 183. Sudbury, MA: Jones and Bartlett Publishers, 2006.

39. Berkowitz, Eric N. *Essentials of Healthcare Marketing,* 183–184. Sudbury, MA: Jones and Bartlett Publishers, 2006.

40. Griffith, John R., and Kenneth R. White. *The Well-Managed Organization,* 6th ed., 121–123. Chicago: Health Administration Press, 2007.

41. Griffith, John R., and Kenneth R. White. *The Well-Managed Organization,* 6th ed., 121–123. Chicago: Health Administration Press, 2007.

42. Miles, Raymond E., and Charles C. Snow. *Organizational Strategy, Structure and Process.* New York: McGraw-Hill, 1978. Reissued in 2003 by Stanford University Press.

43. Porter, Michael E. *Competitive Strategy: Techniques for Analyzing Industries and Competitors.* New York: The Free Press, 1980.

44. Miles, Raymond E., and Charles C. Snow. *Organizational Strategy, Structure and Process.* New York: McGraw-Hill, 1978. Reissued in 2003 by Stanford University Press.

45. Luke, Roice D., Stephen L. Walston, and Patrick Michael Plummer. *Strategy: In Pursuit of Competitive Advantage,* 139. Chicago: Health Administration Press, 2004.

46. Porter, Michael E. *Competitive Strategy: Techniques for Analyzing Industries and Competitors,* 35. New York: The Free Press, 1980.

47. McIlwain, Thomas F., and Melody J. McCracken. "Essential Dimensions of a Marketing Strategy in the Hospital Industry." *Journal of Hospital Marketing* 11 (1997): 42.

48. Berkowitz, Eric N. *Essentials of Healthcare Marketing,* 47–50. Sudbury, MA: Jones and Bartlett Publishers, 2006.

49. Porter, Michael E. *Competitive Strategy: Techniques for Analyzing Industries and Competitors.* New York: The Free Press, 1980.

50. Thompson, Arthur A., Jr., and A.J. Strickland, III. *Strategic Management: Concepts and Cases,* 10th ed., 74. Boston: Irwin/McGraw-Hill, 1998.

51. Porter, Michael E. *Competitive Strategy: Techniques for Analyzing Industries and Competitors,* 17–23. New York: The Free Press, 1980.

52. Porter, Michael E. *Competitive Strategy: Techniques for Analyzing Industries and Competitors,* 23–24. New York: The Free Press, 1980.

53. Thompson, Arthur A., Jr., and A.J. Strickland, III. *Strategic Management: Concepts and Cases,* 10th ed., 81. Boston: Irwin/McGraw-Hill, 1998.

54. Porter, Michael E. *Competitive Strategy: Techniques for Analyzing Industries and Competitors,* 7–17. New York: The Free Press, 1980.

55. Porter, Michael E. *Competitive Strategy: Techniques for Analyzing Industries and Competitors,* 24–27. New York: The Free Press, 1980.

56. Brown, Montague. "Mergers, Networking, and Vertical Integration: Managed Care and Investor-Owned Hospitals." *Healthcare Management Review* 21 (Winter 1996): 29–37.

57. *Mapping Your Competitive Position: Medicare PSOs and Health Plans,* 12. Washington, DC: Ernst & Young, 1997. (Score Retrieval File No. 000168.)

58. Brown, Montague. "Mergers, Networking, and Vertical Integration: Managed Care and Investor-Owned Hospitals." *Healthcare Management Review* 21 (Winter 1996): 36.

59. Porter, Michael E. *Competitive Strategy: Techniques for Analyzing Industries and Competitors,* 27–29. New York: The Free Press, 1980.

60. Walston, Stephen L., John R. Kimberly, and Lawton R. Burns. "Owned Vertical Integration and Healthcare: Promise and Performance." *Healthcare Management Review* 21 (Winter 1996): 83–92, p. 84.

61. Burns, Lawton R., and Darrell P. Thorpe. "Trends and Models in Physician-Hospital Organization." *Healthcare Management Review* 18 (Fall 1993): 7–20.

62. Kongstvedt, Peter R. *Essentials of Managed Care,* 2nd ed., 42. Gaithersburg, MD: Aspen Publishers, 1997.

63. Kongstvedt, Peter R. *Essentials of Managed Care,* 2nd ed., 42–43. Gaithersburg, MD: Aspen Publishers, 1997.

64. Henderson, Bruce D. "The Experience Curve—Reviewed. IV. The Growth Share Matrix or the Product Portfolio." Boston: The Boston Consulting Group, 1973. (Reprint: available at *http://www.bcg.com/publications/files/Experience_Curve_IV_Growth_Share_Matrix_1973.pdf.*)

65. Thomas, Richard K. *Marketing Health Services,* 261. Chicago: Health Administration Press, 2005.

66. Almquist, Eric, and Gordon Wyner. "Boost Your Marketing ROI with Experimental Design." *Harvard Business Review* (October 2001). (Reprint R0109K.)

67. Proenca, E. Jose. "Market Orientation and Organizational Culture in Hospitals." *Journal of Hospital Marketing* 11 (1996): 3–18.

68. A good review of methods to measure customer satisfaction can be found in Ford, Robert C., Susan A. Bach, and Myron D. Fottler. "Methods of Measuring Patient Satisfaction in Healthcare Organizations." *Healthcare Management Review* 22 (Spring 1997): 74–89.

69. Darr, Kurt. *Ethics in Health Services Management,* 1. Baltimore: Health Professions Press, 2005.

70. Darr, Kurt. *Ethics in Health Services Management,* 23–29. Baltimore: Health Professions Press, 2005.

71. Written by Wesley M. Rohrer, III, and used with his permission.

72. American Marketing Association. *www.marketingpower.com,* retrieved February 25, 2008.

73. American Marketing Association, February 25, 2008.

74. American Marketing Association, February 25, 2008.

75. American Marketing Association, February 25, 2008.

76. Written by Gary E. Crum, Ph.D, M.P.H., Executive Director, Graduate Medical Education Consortium, The University of Virginia at Wise (Past Director, Northern Kentucky Health Department). Used with permission.

77. Adapted from Kotler, Philip, and Roberta Clarke. *Marketing for Health Care Organizations,* 2nd ed., 32–35. Englewood Cliffs, NJ: Prentice-Hall, 1987; reprinted by permission. This instrument was prepared by Rick Heidtman under the supervision of Professor Philip Kotler.

10

Controlling and Allocating Resources

Control is typically last in the list of management functions and follows planning, organizing, staffing, and directing. In many ways, controlling is the most important, but it cannot occur until the results of the first four have been implemented. Managers control to ensure that the expected results actually occur after a structure or task is integrated with technology or people. Control depends on information conveyed to managers who continuously monitor sensors to ensure that individual work results are effective and desirable and that organization objectives are accomplished within resource constraints. The management model in Figure 5.8 reflects these relationships.

Control allows managers to know if an HSO's or HS's services are high quality. Control enables managers to determine the effectiveness of processes. Control measures the quality of input resources, whether they are properly allocated, and whether resource use is appropriate. Control enables a determination that organization objectives are being achieved. Quality control, infection control, performance improvement, risk management, cost control, utilization review, narcotics control, budgets, position control for staffing levels, and credentials review are all control or control-like activities.

Chapter 5 describes the controlling function as gathering information about and monitoring activities and performance, comparing actual results with expected results and, as appropriate, taking corrective action by changing inputs or processes. Control and planning are closely linked; the standards and desired results used in control are derived from the HSO's/HS's strategic and operational plans.

Monitoring (Control) and Intervention Points

Control systems are information based. The generic control system in Figure 10.1 identifies monitoring (control) and intervention points. Control collects and monitors information at three points: input utilization, functioning of conversion processes, and outputs. Results inconsistent with expectations or standards cause intervention and change, which can occur at either the input point [A] or process point [B] or both.

OUTPUT CONTROL

Feedback control is the best-known type of output control.[1] It is retrospective and measures the quantitative and qualitative output of individuals, departments, and organizations. Whether measured qualitatively or quantitatively, output or results are usually expressed numerically.

Job performance is a type of individual measure. Quantitative department measures include the numbers or units of outputs such as laboratory tests performed, radiographs taken, surgical procedures done, meals served, patients admitted, medication orders filled, and pounds of laundry processed. Qualitative department measures can include accuracy, timeliness, and customer satisfaction. Organizationwide quantitative measures can include average length of stay (ALOS), occupancy rate, market share, and financial integrity. Qualitative measures include quality of care, range of services, and stakeholder satisfaction. Output standards and expectations are derived from, and reflect, unit and departmental subobjectives and overall organization objectives.

PROCESS CONTROL

Converting inputs into outputs requires processes. The quality of outputs is determined by the effectiveness of processes that produce them and the amount and appropriateness of inputs. Usually, controlling directs attention at outputs (quantity and quality of service), but it is equally important to monitor the myriad integrative conversion processes whose total effort generates outputs. The foundation principle of continuous quality improvement (CQI) is that processes can be improved. This can occur only if there is a monitoring system to identify how well they are functioning. Examples of integrative conversion processes in HSOs/HSs include

- Work systems such as patient admitting and discharge, transportation, materials handling and distribution, direct patient care, and ancillary services
- Specific job design and staff, and machine, technology, and facility interrelationships
- Financial record keeping and information collection, storage, retrieval, and dissemination systems
- Decision and resource allocation and planning processes
- Managerial methods, practices, and styles, along with organizational structuring, coordination, and communication methods and flows

Because process (in combination with inputs) yields outputs, concurrent process control is important. Also known as screening control,[2] process control "focuses on activities that occur as inputs are being converted [into] outputs."[3] Furthermore, process is one of two points at which intervention can occur if outputs are inconsistent with expectations (see Point B in Figure 10.1). Standards and expectations are easier to develop for processes that produce tangibles, are consistent, and are simple to document and understand. Developing standards and expectations is more difficult for less tangible processes. For example, what are the effects on conversion (and, ultimately, on output) of different managerial methods of problem solving and decision making, leadership and supervisory

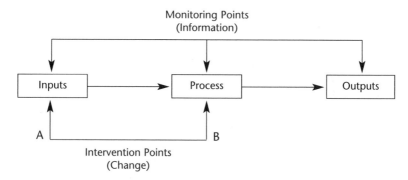

Figure 10.1. Generic control system.

styles, approaches to motivation, or methods of communication? This may help explain why control has historically focused on outputs generated and inputs consumed rather than on processes. CQI directs the control function at a process.

INPUT CONTROL

As noted, resource consumption in creating outputs is a major focus of control. Effective HSOs/HSs control inputs by developing standards and expectations about resource consumption. Examples include nursing hours per patient day, materials and supplies consumed, and the ratio of various types of staff to beds. Often called feedforward control, "it is an approach to control that uses inputs to a system of organizational activities as a means of controlling the accomplishment of organizational objectives [outputs]."[4] The philosophy of CQI suggests that choosing the best inputs before conversion will diminish the potential for problems with outputs. For example, the quality of human resources inputs can be controlled by credentialing and licensure, which help ensure that clinical staff have certain levels of training and skills. Input control, however, cannot substitute for process and output control.

▬ Control Model ▬▬▬▬▬▬▬▬▬▬▬▬▬▬▬▬▬▬▬▬▬▬▬

Thus far, control has been described as a process to collect information about results and performance at the monitoring (control) points of inputs, process, and outputs. Comparing actual results with standards and expectations, appraising comparisons, and making changes at either the input or process points or both are the remaining components of control. Figure 10.2 incorporates these components in an expanded control process model to show actual results measured and compared with standards and expectations. Depending on results, the control process follows one of four loops, each of which may indicate the necessity of intervention.

IN CONTROL LOOP

The "in control loop" in Figure 10.2 is the simplest. When evaluation of information from the three monitoring points—inputs, process, and outputs—indicates that standards and expectations are being met, intervention is unnecessary, and activity continues.

ACCEPTANCE CONTROL LOOP

When monitoring indicates that performance does not meet expectations, managers investigate to determine the cause(s) of deviation. If deviation is desirable or acceptable, or its cause is uncontrol-

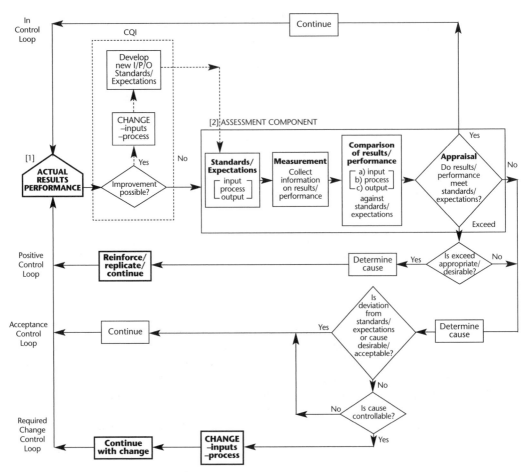

Figure 10.2. Expanded control model.

lable, there is no intervention. For example, overtime higher than that budgeted (standard) may be acceptable if the census is proportionately higher.

If the deviation is undesirable but the cause is uncontrollable, actual performance must be accepted. For example, a number of registered nurse hours per patient that is less than that desired but more than the minimum needed for good patient care may result from an inadequate pool of registered nurses.

REQUIRED CHANGE CONTROL LOOP

Intervention should occur when information indicates that deviation is unacceptable and the cause is controllable. For example, if the average length of stay (ALOS) is substantially longer than the standard, intervention is required. This deviation may occur if physicians (input point) do not write orders to discharge patients in a timely manner or if ineffective work systems (process point) cause delays in reporting test results. Another example is higher than normal staff turnover that results from a negative organizational climate, inadequate compensation, or poor supervision. Here, too, input or process point intervention is required.

POSITIVE CONTROL LOOP

Control isn't only negative, however. For example, the cause of performance that exceeds standards should be identified, reinforced, integrated into the process, and replicated elsewhere whenever possible. A work unit consistently under budget with superior individual work results and high quality and customer satisfaction may be a function of effective managerial style, positive employee attitude and commitment, and well-designed processes. Improvement control that recognizes and emphasizes the positive should not be forgotten.

There are instances when it is undesirable for actual performance to be better than standards. For example, it may seem desirable that nursing service hours per patient be below budget (i.e., standard), but evaluation may show this to be unacceptable if quality of care is at risk. The expenditures for physical plant maintenance may be less than budget, but this is undesirable if preventive maintenance is postponed. If actual results and performance are better than standards and expectations but are undesirable or inappropriate, the cause should be determined, and either the "acceptance" or "required change" control loops should be used to intervene.

Levels of Control

Managers use three basic levels of control: strategic, operational, and functional. *Strategic* control focuses on attaining overall HSO/HS objectives, including financial performance. Senior-level managers monitor organizational performance to determine whether the strategies that have been implemented are accomplishing strategic objectives and whether a changed external environment requires reevaluation. Figures 8.2 and 8.3 depict the role of the external environment in the strategizing process. *Operational* control monitors operational plans and day-to-day unit or department activities. This level of control is largely the responsibility of middle- and first-level managers who are concerned with their unit or department work schedules, budgets, and use of resources. *Functional* control focuses on logically grouped functional areas such as clinical services, finance, information systems, and marketing. Senior functional-area managers, as well as middle- and first-level managers, are responsible for control in these areas.[5]

Control and CQI

Meeting standards is not the end of the control process in HSOs. The philosophy of CQI uses continuous inquiry to improve processes and inputs so that outputs can be improved. Figure 10.2 shows CQI in the rectangle outlined by dashes. If no improvement of processes or inputs is possible, the control loop flows from actual results/performance [1] through to the assessment component [2]. If improvement is possible, change is made to either inputs or processes or both, and new standards and expectations are developed to replace those used previously in the assessment component [2].

Control and Problem Solving

As noted in Chapter 6, problem solving is largely based on information produced through the control function. The four conditions that initiate problem solving are opportunity/threat, crisis, deviation, and improvement. *Opportunity* is prospective and anticipatory and results from favorable internal or external circumstances that enable the HSO/HS to achieve or enhance desired results. *Threat* is also prospective and anticipatory, but it is the converse of opportunity, and problem solving seeks to minimize potential internal and external threats to achieving its goals. *Crisis* problem solving occurs when not acting promptly will cause untoward results. *Deviation* problem solving is the most common and occurs when individual and organizational work results are inconsistent with those desired. Problem solving under the condition of *improvement* improves processes or inputs to affect outputs positively.

Control Considerations

Several managerial and design considerations are important in managing control systems.

MANAGERIAL CONSIDERATIONS

Managerial questions to be answered when a control system is established or modified are the following:

- *Where is control focused?* Control may focus on input (resource use), process or conversion (efficiency of work systems that convert inputs to outputs), or output (individual process, aggregations of processes, or organizationwide results).
- *What types of measures are used for standards and monitoring results?* Measures used in control depend on focus, quantifiability of results, and the extent to which measures convey accurate, usable, and meaningful information.
- *Who has the authority to establish standards?* A principle of control is that those whose activities are monitored have input but not sole authority to establish standards and monitor results. Checks and balances are universal in accounting systems; for example, cashiers who handle cash do no final audits or reconciliations. Similarly, utilization review is not performed by those providing the services.
- *How flexible should standards be?* Blind and inflexible use of numerical measures for control purposes can cause distortions. Changes and unforeseen circumstances require that judgment, common sense, and flexibility be used in control systems.
- *Who has access to control system information?* Controlling requires dissemination of information, but some information is appropriately restricted to certain levels of management or specific managers.
- *Who is responsible for intervention?* Just as organizations have a defined authority–responsibility hierarchy, managerial considerations in control include who is responsible and who intervenes.

DESIGN CONSIDERATIONS

Sometimes, control systems cause unintended or undesirable consequences, cost more than they save, measure the wrong things correctly, or measure the right things incorrectly. Control systems should include the following to decrease the potential for dysfunctional outcomes:

- *When possible, control should be prospective.* Control cannot always be forward looking or predictive. Usually, data flow or organizational constraints limit information to that which is concurrent or retrospective. If available, however, feedforward control provides information to managers that enables them to anticipate deviation and makes them more effective.
- *Control should be organizationally realistic and understandable to users.* Control systems must be harmonious with the organization, fit realistically, and be understandable. A system that creates barriers or artificial constraints is dysfunctional. For

example, inventory data are best controlled by materials management. Centralizing access to and control of photocopiers in one location may be unrealistic and inefficient.

- *Control should be accurate, timely, and reliable.* When control systems are designed, the standards and measurements need to be accurate and reliable. Corrections that use inaccurate or unreliable information defeat the purpose of control, as does using data unreflective of the current situation.
- *Control should be significant, have economic benefit, or both. Significant* refers to the importance of what is being controlled. *Economic benefit* refers to the cost of control relative to the value of what is controlled. There is little economic benefit to disposal (destruction) control of used syringes. Its benefits result from preventing use by drug addicts and protecting those who handle medical waste. Narcotics control has significant clinical and economic benefits and is required by law. Conversely, control of disposable surgical gowns has little economic value—control costs will exceed benefits.
- *Control should be information appropriate.* Too much or too little information is undesirable. Important indicators are lost when information is excessive. Too little information prevents managers from focusing on critical elements. Control systems should give managers sufficient, discriminating information in a timely, usable manner.

Information Systems and Control

Managers require information. Effective planning, problem solving, and control occur only when managers receive appropriate, accurate, and timely information that is based on reliable data and presented in a usable format. "The organization that can successfully and efficiently manage information will produce better quality healthcare because it will be able to measure, monitor, and improve the care it delivers."[6] Information systems (IS) improve access to information and facilitate communication among providers and team members, contribute to reduced costs, and enhance competitive position.[7] Chapter 3 considers the applications of IS technology to the clinical aspects of health services delivery.

Management IS is a generic concept that refers to computer systems that gather, format, process, store, and report data that are converted to information retrievable by managers for use in planning, executing, and controlling organizational activities. Traditional IS is applications driven; data are retrieved from discrete files created for specific purposes by organization units. In IS design, users specify the type and extent of data. IS applications in HSOs began in the 1960s with systems developed by in-house systems analysts and programmers. In the 1980s, an increasing number of commercial vendors began providing software for administrative and clinical support functions.[8]

IS in HSOs/HSs generally falls into two broad categories. First, administrative and financial systems provide information supporting administrative operations and managerial planning, resource allocation, and control activities. Second, clinical and medical systems provide information to support patient care activities. Other uses include cost accounting, resource utilization and productivity analysis, and market intelligence. Table 10.1 shows associated IS applications by core functions for a managed care organization (MCO).

The senior-level manager responsible for IS is the chief information officer (CIO). The CIO should be 1) technically competent, including in managing internal systems and being aware of technology used by competitors and developments in IS; 2) compatible with organization objectives,

TABLE 10.1. MANAGED CARE ORGANIZATION FUNCTIONS AND ASSOCIATED INFORMATION REQUIREMENTS

Core functions	Examples of applications
Financial monitoring	Balance sheets Income statements Financial statements General accounting Cost accounting Premium billing and accounts receivable Payment tracking for contracts, subcontracts
Preparation of standard analytical reports and decision models	Performance statistics Utilization management Provider reporting: inpatient and outpatient Referral patterns Inpatient and outpatient out-of-network use Case-mix analysis Provider profiling Actuarial analysis
Management control and reporting	Membership analysis Eligibility/verifications tracking Utilization rates by groups, age, gender Quality indicators Financial reporting Regulatory reporting Budgeting models Forecasting models Contract modeling and projections
Claims payment and prospective/capitation payment processing	Capitation payments Claims payment, network and out-of-network Claims adjudication Encounter statistics Claims grouping by episodes of care
Management of multiple lines of business	Government accounts (Medicare, Medicaid, etc.) Individual coverage Group billing, benefits management, eligibility
Marketing and sales support	Enrollment and disenrollment trends Geographic distribution of members and providers Contract negotiation and management Rate management/actuarial services Account management and analysis Forecasting models Provider databases and credentials
Profitability	Per member per month costs and premiums Medical loss ratios
Member/customer services	Customer service inquiry Internet access to MCO Member health/wellness education and promotion Epidemiological analysis
Employer information needs	HEDIS reporting Outcomes measurement Employer group enrollment tracking and reporting Utilization history and claims experience of covered population

From Austin, Charles J., and Stuart B. Boxerman. *Information Systems for Health Services Administration*, 5th ed., pp. 350–351. Chicago: Health Administration Press, 1998; reprinted by permission.

stage of evolution of information technology, and clientele; 3) business savvy, to understand information's importance in a competitive market and the technology's high cost; and 4) a leader, especially as a change agent, team builder, and communicator.[9]

INFORMATION SYSTEMS: LANs AND WANs

The sophistication of IS ranges from applications reporting systems to database management systems to decision support systems. Applications reporting is the most familiar to HSO/HS managers and consists of tailored reports about organizational operations or areas of activity such as payroll, inventory, budgets, admissions, census, and scheduling.

Advances in computer hardware and software make database IS ubiquitous in HSOs/HSs. Data from throughout the organization are integrated and consolidated in a single database or multiple databases that are accessible by authorized users, rather than segregated for specific applications reporting. Often, these systems are inquiry based.

Local area networks (LANs) allow communication among computers and peripherals within an organization or among organizations in a limited area.[10] Extended into large geographic areas, LANs become wide area networks (WANs), which allow long-distance input and inquiry information access. WANs enable geographically distant operating units to "interchange information, create computer-based patient records, and develop integrated outcome measures and statistics."[11] Chapter 3 notes the initial use of WANs in community health information networks (CHINs). CHINs have been superseded by regional health information organizations (RHIOs). Figure 3.7 shows how RHIOs can be linked to entities such as HSOs, payers, physicians, and pharmacies.

MANAGEMENT AND CLINICAL IS

MDSS. Management decision support systems (MDSSs) are a type of specialized IS application in HSOs/HSs. The MDSS merges external databases, financial databases, clinical systems, and other data sources into a decision support systems database from which users obtain data that can become the information needed for decision making.[12] MDSSs are model based, and they can perform statistical analyses and simulations. An interactive capability allows managers to make hypothetical queries such as What would be the effect on net margins if Medicare days were to increase 20%? Or a bed assignment model might be used to determine the implications for resource allocation and utilization.[13]

Management Expert Systems. Management expert systems go beyond the data storage, retrieval, modeling, and reporting capabilities of a decision support system. They seek to replicate the reasoning process a human being uses to make a decision.

> An expert system consists of a *knowledge base* containing the system expertise, a *database* that the knowledge base is matched against, an *inference engine* that generates suggested conclusions, a *user interface* that links the user to the system, and *workspace* that serves as a "scratchpad."[14]

CSS. Patient care applications of IS are widely used in HSO clinical support systems (CSSs). Use of IS in CSSs is generally of two types: managing internal processes and communicating with other departments or processes. For example, the laboratory uses IS to automate and control processes and to report results of laboratory testing. Medical imaging and radiology services' use of IS is also of two types—clinical and management. Medical imaging systems use computer technology to process and enhance digital images, and radiology IS schedules procedures, records and reports test results, reports charges, and prepares management reports. A clinical application is computer-aided detection (CAD) used in diagnosing mammograms. CAD is effective in finding microcalcifications in breast tissue. Its sensitivity results in many false positives, and overreliance by radiologists may cause a false sense of confidence.[15] IS applications can be found in the pharmacy, physical and respiratory therapy, nursing service, critical care units, and emergency services.[16]

CDSS. Like MDSS, the clinical decision support system (CDSS) is a leap in technology application. CDSSs are another type of expert system, and they assist physicians in diagnosis and treatment planning. CDSSs "generally consist of static and dynamic modeling routines, driven by normative data bases and vast stores of 'automated' clinical knowledge; their outputs consist of quantitative comparisons of clinical outcomes associated with alternative medical decisions."[17] The Acute Physiology and Chronic Health Evaluation (APACHE), whose development began at the George Washington University in the early 1980s, is an example. APACHE uses physiological variables, age, and chronic health status to predict probable outcomes of treatment. It is especially useful to support decision making in intensive care units.[18]

ELECTRONIC HEALTH RECORDS

The electronic health record (EHR) allows easy access to the entire medical record and, if accessible throughout an HSO/HS and from remote locations, offers a significant technological advantage. Chapter 3 details EHR's advantages and disadvantages. For purposes of context, several benefits are summarized here:[19]

1. Immediate caregiver access to patient information from provider sites
2. More timely and complete medical records
3. Legible entries
4. Eliminating "lost" information in the record
5. Improved turnaround time for scheduling patient appointments
6. Improved timeliness and access to billing information
7. Improved capability for abstracting research data
8. Improved access to quality management data
9. Elimination of faxing, copying, and mailing patient information among provider sites
10. Reduced clerical staff involved in moving and retrieving records
11. Reduced storage costs

IS ISSUES

Advances in IS technology in the past 2 decades have been profound. They have enhanced resource utilization through better managerial control and improved patient care outcomes through better clinical decision making. However, the advances have been costly. Hardware and software are expensive, as is IS support staff. Many issues have been raised in regard to patient care and clinical IS use. For example, applications such as CDSS typically build on IS originally designed for administrative and claims/transactions processing,[20] and thus they may be working from contaminated databases or may lack standardization when different databases are accessed. Incompatible system architectures create problems relative to compatibility.

"Patient and financial tracking across the network requires integrated information systems that operate on multiple vendor hardware and software. Standardization of databases and coding mechanisms are imperative."[21]

IS USES

Given that quality and control depend on information, Austin and Boxerman delineate several areas, with examples, in which IS can support managers and clinicians:[22]

Applications	Examples
Patient care	• Computer-based patient records • Order entry and results reporting
Clinical support	• Laboratory automation and laboratory ISs • Pharmacy ISs • Nursing ISs • Other service department ISs—PT, OT, pulmonary, ED • Clinical decision support systems • Computer-assisted medical instrumentation • Quality of care applications
Other clinical	• Telemedicine, teleradiology, telehealth • Long-term care ISs • Home health ISs • Medical research and education ISs
Management & administration	• Financial ISs • Human resources ISs • Resource utilization and scheduling systems • Materials management ISs • Facilities and project management ISs • Quality of care applications
Managed care	• Applications to link MCOs with purchasers, consumers, providers • Quality of care applications • Claims processing and adjudication ISs

The uses of IS in telemedicine are discussed in Chapter 3.

In terms of control, IS should provide information that meets the managers' specific needs. It should allow them to 1) monitor input, process, and output; 2) provide, for each level of management and its area of responsibility, reports that contain accurate, relevant, and timely information that will improve their decisions on control (intervention); and 3) extract and pinpoint critical and high-priority items requiring management analysis and, perhaps, intervention. Clinical IS that incorporates practice parameters for use by physicians and other licensed independent practitioners (LIPs) improves quality and achieves a level of control. Also known as clinical guidelines, practice guidelines, and critical paths, practice parameters guide clinical decision making. Clinical IS allows comparisons of clinical outcomes and resource use over time, against other HSOs and benchmarks, and can be used to profile physician practice patterns. Practice parameters are discussed in Chapter 7.

▬ Control and Human Resources ▬▬▬▬▬▬▬▬▬▬▬▬▬▬▬▬▬

In 2006, 15.6 million persons were employed in the healthcare industry.[23] HSOs are labor intensive; the costs of staff are about two thirds of total expenses. This makes human resources the most significant input component in delivery of health services. Health professions occupations are highly fragmented by skills area. About 200 different types of positions are required to staff a general acute care community hospital; more than 300 for a large teaching facility. The number of types is growing. Acquiring and retaining a qualified work force are among the most significant tasks facing HSO/HS management. Artificial scarcity of various health occupations has been created by professional associations that accredit educational programs, as well as those who certify practitioners. This has added greatly to salaries and healthcare costs.

To implement strategies, accomplish objectives, and fulfill their missions, HSOs must be properly staffed. When managers integrate technology and people into formal structures (organizational arrangements), meaningful work occurs. The human element is the catalyst in the organizational equation that causes other inputs (material, supplies, technology, information, and capital) to be converted into outputs in the form of individual and organizational work results (see the management model in Figure 5.8).

Standards of The Joint Commission on Accreditation of Healthcare Organizations (The Joint Commission) in the *Comprehensive Accreditation Manual for Hospitals* address the human resources function:

> The goal of the human resources function is to ensure that the hospital determines the qualifications and competencies of staff positions based on its mission, population(s), and care, treatment, and services. Hospitals must also provide the number of competent staff needed to meet patients' needs.

This goal is met by the following:

- *Planning:* The planning process defines the qualifications, competencies, and staffing necessary to provide for the organization's care, treatment, and services.
- *Providing competent staff:* The hospital provides for competent staff through traditional employer–employee arrangements or through contractual arrangements with other entities or persons.
- *Orienting, training, and educating staff:* The hospital provides ongoing in-service and other education and training to increase staff knowledge of specific work-related issues.
- *Assessing, maintaining, and improving staff competence:* Ongoing, periodic competence assessment evaluates staff members' continuing abilities to perform throughout their association with the organization.
- *Promoting self-development and learning:* Staff is encouraged to pursue ongoing professional development goals and provide feedback about the work environment.[24]

Human resource standards for other types of HSOs accredited by The Joint Commission are similar.

HUMAN RESOURCES MANAGEMENT

Personnel administration is the historic term that described the staffing activities, programs, and policies related to acquisition, retention and maintenance, and separation of human resources. As Chapter 5 notes, the contemporary concept is human resources management (HRM). All managers have some responsibility for HRM activities such as selection, performance appraisal, promotion, training and development, discipline and corrective counseling, and compensation of employees. However, most HRM is centralized and coordinated by a human resources (HR) manager in the HR department that establishes organizationwide or systemwide policies and procedures and provides support for HR acquisition, retention, and separation services, and for labor relations when there is a bargaining unit.

The HR department recruits and screens potential new staff (acquisition), enhances competencies of current staff and keeps those who are effective in the organization (maintenance and retention), facilitates the exit (separation) of those who leave, and develops policies for staff in the organization (coordinating). HR is a staff department (as opposed to a line department) that assists various HSO units and managers with expertise and programs. The centralized role of the HR department and the importance of staff as an asset mean the HR manager is included in senior-level management. This manager integrates all HRM activities with the HSO's/HS's strategic plans.[25]

Even though the staffing function is centralized in the HR department, managers must have a working knowledge of its role and activities. First, HRM policies provide structure and define interactions among managers, who are ultimately accountable for the quality and productivity of their operations and employees. Second, HRM policies reflect societal norms as expressed in legislative enactments and judicial decisions regarding nondiscriminatory hiring, discipline, promotion, and compensation. Better-informed managers will be more effective in using human resources and less likely to act unethically or illegally.

Staffing Activities

Staffing activities can be viewed as a time flow of distinct phases, as shown in Figure 10.3. Acquisition includes HR planning, recruitment, screening, and orientation after selection by the relevant manager. Retention and maintenance include performance appraisal, placement, training and development, discipline and corrective counseling, compensation and benefits administration, employee assistance and career counseling, and safety and health. Separation is the third phase.

ACQUIRING HUMAN RESOURCES

HR Planning

Human resources planning occurs when the HR department interacts with HSO managers to forecast staffing needs. The result is a plan to meet those needs through recruiting and hiring, transferring, and/or enhancing the skills of current staff through training and development. Acquisition, the first activity in the process model in Figure 10.3, highlights the need for HR planning. HSOs are dynamic, staffing needs change, and the work force must be considered in this context. Staff mix and staffing levels are functions of organizational growth, services offered, employee turnover, and changes in technology. HR planning ensures that the organization has the right number of staff with needed qualifications and skills to deliver appropriate levels and quality of services.[26] It involves profiling, estimating, inventorying, forecasting, and planning.

Step 1: Profiling

Profiling the HSO/HS at a future point and estimating the numbers and types of jobs (skills) required has an element of subjectivity. The strategic plan, anticipated demand for services, changes in professional practice or labor supply, and staffing for new technologies are considered in making projections.

Step 2: Estimating

Once a profile is developed, human resource estimates are made. If the determining variables can be identified and quantified, this step is straightforward because the health services industry has estab-

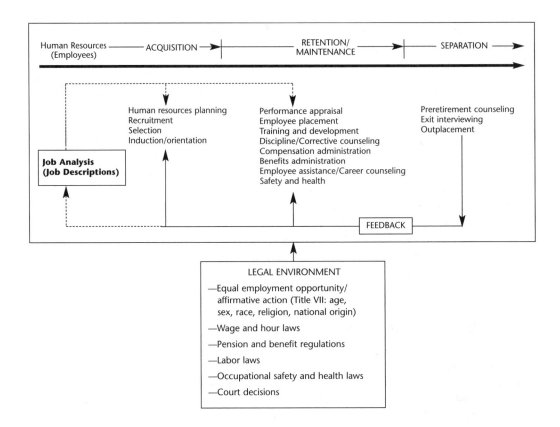

Figure 10.3.   Personnel/human resource management activities time flow.

lished staffing ratios for most major functions. Knowing the square feet in a new facility allows projections of environmental services staff needed. Similarly, nurse staffing ratios can be applied if new patient beds are added.

Step 3: Inventorying

Sometimes called a talent inventory, assessing the skills, abilities, and potential of human resources and how they are being used is vital.[27] The HR audit involves compiling data about each staff member's job title, experience, length of service, performance, education, special skills, and placement.

Step 4: Forecasting

Planners forecast changes in the HSO's/HS's work force that result from entry, transfer, and exit due to retirement, death, voluntary separation, or discharge. Historical data are often used to forecast future staffing.

HSOs differ greatly from other types of organizations because the clinical work force is credentialed and/or licensed for specific work. This greatly diminishes upward or lateral movement to unrelated positions. States may require continuing education for health services occupations, and professional associations that certify their members are likely to have similar requirements. Succession planning for senior management positions should be performed. All such aspects must be considered when making work force forecasts.

Step 5: Planning

The assumptions and information from Steps 1 through 4 support the action plan that ensures that the appropriate number of staff with requisite skills is available as needed. HR needs identified through organizationwide or systemwide CQI efforts are factored into the plan as well.

Sources of Staff

Staff can be obtained internally and externally.[28] Filling vacancies by internal transfer or promotion is cost-effective, is usually faster, has lower recruiting and relocation costs, and enhances employee morale. Effective use of current employees requires that the skills inventory includes career path planning, as appropriate, and that training is provided to upgrade employees with potential for promotion or transfer.

Staff are also recruited externally. Advertising vacancies or relying on present employees to "pass the word" will generate applications. Some HSOs pay financial incentives to staff who recruit certain categories of employees. Visits to training programs and schools and colleges, contacts with public and private employment agencies, and recruitment through professional organizations are also useful. Other external sources of workers are those who inquire about employment, temporary staffing agencies, and contract employees.[29]

The source used depends on the qualifications required, supply in the labor market, geographic area, employer's reputation, and teaching affiliations. Recruiting is complicated by job fragmentation and specialization, uneven work force distribution, increasing demand for health services, career alternatives for women, and differences in public support for education.

Job Analysis and Job Descriptions

A fundamental responsibility of the HR department and an example of control is developing and maintaining job descriptions for all positions. It is in the HSO's financial interests to staff at a level, and with the minimum qualifications, that ensures quality at the lowest cost. Monitoring this component of HR management is especially important, given the proliferation of job classifications in health services and the propensity of health services workers and their professional associations to limit market entry through accreditation and licensing and to enhance credentials and certifications.

HRM staffing activities such as work force planning, recruitment, selection, performance appraisal, and compensation administration depend on job descriptions.[30] In addition, much of equal employment opportunity law uses the job description as a basic document. This makes developing and maintaining job descriptions a good investment.

Job Analysis

New staff can be recruited only when training, skills, and experience are known. This information is commonly obtained from job analysis.[31] The job analysis conducted by the HR department uses questionnaires and interviews directed at incumbents, observes and studies the job to determine its content (duties and responsibilities), describes conditions under which the job is performed, and identifies relationships to other jobs. This analysis identifies the skills, training, and abilities needed to do the work.[32] Information from job analysis is the source for a job description.

Job Descriptions

Generally, job descriptions include job title, location, job summary, five to nine general duties and responsibilities, supervision given or received, special working conditions (including equipment or systems used), hazards, and qualifications. The statement of qualifications includes the minimum education, training, experience, and demonstrated skills required.[33] Job descriptions should be concise to ease understanding and worded to permit maximum flexibility in work design.

Job descriptions should be updated as job content, performance requirements, or qualifications change. They are used for most HRM functions—recruitment, selection, training, performance appraisal, career counseling, and compensation,[34] and they are fundamental documents in legal disputes. The information simplifies communication among managers, employees, applicants, and the HR department. When a vacancy occurs, HR is notified that the position must be filled. The job description provides vital information as the recruitment process is begun.

Recruitment

As noted, recruiting involves attracting internal or external applicants. Recruiting staff is largely a function of the labor market. If no special skills or training are required for a job and supply is ample, recruitment may be little more than reviewing applications from those who inquire about employment. Health professions in short supply require the organization to compete for staff. Internally, job posting, promotion, and transfer of existing staff are sources. External sources are recruiting at schools, job fairs, employment agencies, and professional associations.[35]

Selection

The essence of selection is to determine an applicant's suitability for the job in terms of training, experience, and ability.[36] Three basic sources of information are used: application forms, preemployment interviews, and testing.

As Figure 10.3 suggests, HSO/HS managers work in a complex legal environment, especially in terms of equal employment opportunity and nondiscriminatory practices. HR managers take the lead to ensure that the organizationwide staffing function and HRM policies comply with federal, state, and local laws, but all managers must have a basic understanding of employment law. The content of application forms, preemployment interviews, and preemployment testing are subject to state and federal law, regulations, and court decisions. This complexity necessitates that managers consult with the HR manager and legal counsel, as needed.

Selection—A Joint Responsibility

Despite myriad techniques, selection is an inexact science. Ideally, the decision is made by the manager to whom the new employee will report, with the advice and counsel of HR. This approach has the advantages that credentials are appropriate, employment laws are followed, organizational policies are met, and those selected meet quality standards and conform to the HSO's/HS's values and culture. Hiring only those who have a good fit with the organization's value system is critical in minimizing turnover, enhancing morale and job satisfaction (Deming's "joy in work"), and maximizing delivery of high-quality care.

Orientation

Induction and orientation follow selection. Induction activities are typically performed by the HR department and include enrolling the new employee in benefit plans, issuing an identification badge, and creating an individual database. HSOs require a physical examination before new employees begin their duties to screen for communicable diseases, ensure that the individual can perform the job without danger to self or others, determine workers' compensation risk, and detect and document preexisting health conditions.

Orientation should include information about the physical facility, organizational structure, universal precautions, fire and safety programs, the employee health service, the employee assistance program (EAP), and other HR department services. Organization policies and benefits should be explained in detail. In some departments, orientation may include an extended period of training and orienting the employee to department-specific work methods. This is done through techniques such as on-the-job training, use of preceptors, and formal classroom instruction.

An important part of inducting new employees into the HSO/HS is informing them about its mission, vision, and values. Successful orientation builds employees' sense of identification with the organization, helps them gain acceptance by fellow workers, and gives them a clear understanding of what they need to know. Ideally, the orientation program enables new employees to become familiar with the entire organization as well as their own work area and department. This can be accomplished by a tour of the facilities, using media such as videos or DVDs, and/or a reception for new employees.

RETAINING EMPLOYEES

HRM maintenance and retention activities begin after placement. These include appraising job performance; moving employees within the organization through promotion, demotion, and transfer; disciplinary counseling and separation; compensation and benefits management; employee assistance and career counseling; and ensuring a healthful workplace and personal safety (see Figure 10.3).

Performance Appraisal

The HR department establishes and maintains an organizationwide employee performance appraisal system that is used by all managers.[37] Appraisal systems evaluate an employee's work by comparing actual with expected performance. It is essential that managers understand the limited role that staff have in affecting the outcomes of their individual work effort. Deming's conclusion that 85%–94% of work results occur because of the process must be borne in mind. Beyond the emphasis on process improvement, the primary purpose of employee appraisal should be to focus on the training or other needs of employees, rather than to assume that they are the cause of poor outcomes. In this regard, managers should act as mentors and coaches to their staff and do all they can to facilitate workers' ability to do their jobs well and achieve "joy in work."

Uses of Performance Appraisal

Performance appraisal has many uses.

- *Determining if individual work results are consistent with expectations:* Performance appraisal systematically collects information to determine whether results are those expected and, if not, to determine the reason. A focus on the process must be maintained.
- *Providing feedback to employee and supervisor:* The performance appraisal interview is a formal opportunity for two-way communication. Positive performance can be reinforced. Less-than-satisfactory performance can be discussed, reasons for it identified, interventions formulated, and future expectations established.
- *Identifying high, marginal, and unsatisfactory performers:* Depending on an assessment of performance, various interventions can be used. Less-than-satisfactory performance most often results from employee variables, such as lack of technical job skills or experience, or from poor process or job design. Based on this information, interventions such as developmental education, skills training, or job redesign may be warranted. If performance is unsatisfactory for reasons of attitude and behavior, then counseling, discipline, or separation may be warranted. The purpose of performance appraisal is to monitor and, if possible, improve each employee's ability to do the job well.
- *Identifying potential and desirable employee movement within the organization:* Results of performance appraisal can influence an employee's candidacy for promo-

tion, as well as transfer and demotion. High performers may be promoted with or without further skill building; low performers may be transferred to more suitable jobs.

- *Providing information for compensation:* Organizations with wage and salary systems that incorporate merit increases should be cautious in using appraisals to determine adjustments in pay. Here, too, the overriding importance of the process in determining how well employees perform must be understood.
- *Providing information for employee assistance and counseling:* If an employee's performance is unsatisfactory because of substance abuse or off-the-job personal problems, performance appraisal may reveal a need to recommend assistance.

Most HRM retention activities are linked to performance appraisal. As a result, it is a control and information-gathering system of great importance to managers and the HSO/HS.

Benefits of Systematic Appraisal

Formal written appraisals of all employees are normally required on an annual basis; however, good management practice and maintenance of high productivity require more frequent feedback on an informal basis. If an employee has just started a new or more responsible position, then an appraisal within 3 months is advisable. In some organizations, appraisals are made according to hire dates; in others, all appraisals are made once or twice a year on fixed dates. As an employee achieves longevity, periodic appraisals have an important influence on morale. They reaffirm the manager's interest in the employee's continuous development and improvement.

Appraisals done in the traditional manner are roundly disliked by staff *and* managers. Often, they are seen as arbitrary; a popularity contest among staff; and a distasteful, subjective exercise by managers. The addition of ranking, rating, and forced distributions only compounds the problems with appraisals. In addition, they stimulate competition among staff when, in fact, every effort should be made to encourage cooperation and team work. Organizations will do well to reconsider their traditional appraisal methods or, better yet, abandon them entirely.

Continuous Quality Improvement

Peter Drucker noted that "quantity without quality is the worst thing and will result in total failure."[38] Performance appraisals are useful in monitoring quality because they provide data to help managers make several measurements: success of current job design and work flow (processes); progress in achieving objectives; and individual performance, to the extent that it affects quality because, for example, an employee is inadequately trained. Real-time performance feedback is required for the achievement of CQI. Cascio identified criteria for evaluation, including using customer expectations to drive expectations for quality improvement teams and/or individual performance, or both; pre-identifying results/expectations and whether they are met or exceeded; and identifying and measuring behavior skills that make a difference in improving quality results and customer satisfaction (see the discussion of CQI in Chapter 7).[39]

Training and Development

Training is another basic HRM activity in maintaining and retaining human resources. Training changes behavior, and it expands employee knowledge and skills through an organized process by which employees learn the skills, abilities, and attitudes needed for successful job performance.[40] Training may be provided by the HR department or by a separate unit. Large HSOs have training departments to educate staff about CQI, develop managerial skills, and facilitate departmental (line) training. Other approaches include training shared among several independent HSOs; or HSs may centralize and provide training for system members.

Line training is department specific and is usually the responsibility of functional or service line managers. Special mention should be made of supervisory and management development as a type of training. HSOs/HSs have special needs in preparing supervisors and managers because so many are drawn from staff with technical education. Management development increases the capabilities of managers beyond their technical base.[41] The focus is on general managerial skills such as leadership, motivation, communication, and problem solving. Specific skills training in report writing and budgeting may be included.

Developing and enhancing employees' skills or cross-training them to do more than one job are investments in the HSO/HS.[42] It is value-added activity that is important to quality and productivity improvement and ensures staff competence.

Discipline (Corrective Counseling)

Disciplinary actions should be rare. Given that qualified, carefully selected staff are correctly placed within the organization, there is every reason to believe that they come to work to do a good job and will do their work as well as the process allows. Management must look first to the processes in which they and their staff work for answers to performance problems. This means assessing all connected processes: the HR recruitment process may have failed to secure someone well prepared for the job; the orientation or training processes may have been deficient; staff members may not understand their role(s) in a process and how what they are doing affects the process; the staff member may be in the wrong job or wrong part of the process. Everyone involved in processes must understand Juran's description of the triple role as customer, processor, and supplier. Managers must first be mentors and coaches to their staff and do all they can to facilitate workers' ability to do their jobs well.

Despite managers' best efforts, however, there may be instances when "corrective counseling" is necessary. If corrective counseling is to be positive, policies and practices must be reasonable, and employees must understand what is expected of them. It must be understood that the employer has a right to a well-disciplined, cooperative work force and, if necessary, has authority to take whatever action the situation requires.

Compensation Administration

Effective compensation administration is essential to maintaining and retaining a suitable work force. *Compensation* is a generic term for wages, salaries, and fringe benefits and directly affects an organization's ability to attract and retain qualified employees. HR departments in HSOs/HSs are responsible for developing, implementing, and administering an organizationwide compensation program.[43]

Equity is key in compensation programs. Depending on size and clinical activities, an HSO may have more than 200 different types of jobs. Determining the pay for each type involves using three factors: internal equity, external equity, and philosophy of the HSO.

- *Internal equity*—How does the pay of various jobs compare? What should a nurse earn compared with a social worker or dietitian? There are various ways to achieve internal equity. At a minimum, job requirements must be identified and their complexity evaluated. Evaluation is usually reduced to a numerical factor (rating) so that jobs can be more easily compared.

- *External equity*—How does the organization's pay for jobs compare with those in competing organizations? External equity became more important as market forces increasingly affected HSOs/HSs. Shortages of staff such as medical technologists, sonographers, and pharmacists caused wage wars, and union pressures prompted an analysis of the market in terms of pay competitiveness.
- *Philosophy*—How does the HSO/HS pay relative to the market? A mature pay philosophy will succinctly describe how the HSO/HS will use data obtained by answering the questions about internal and external equity to compete for staff in the labor market. For example, the philosophy might be "our pay range midpoints will be 10% above the projected median of our market for professional (higher level) jobs and equal to the projected median of our market for service (lower level, entry) jobs." There is no "right" pay philosophy, because factors such as labor supply, market definition, projected human resources needs, type of organization, and fiscal constraints must be considered.

Establishing and Administering a Compensation System

Job evaluation is a formal system to determine the relative value of jobs in an organization and is the heart of a wage-and-salary administration program.[44] Jobs are analyzed using job descriptions. Each job is rated according to an evaluation plan with the purpose of establishing specific rates of pay or specific wage ranges (salary grades).

Job evaluation can be performed using ranking, job classification, and point and factor comparison systems. Regardless, the outcome is a scheme of hourly rates and wage ranges that relate logically to one another; a procedure that permits changes in compensation within grades, using criteria such as performance and experience; a means to move employees to new grades or classifications, based on changes such as job enrichment; and a way to maintain internal equity.

Executive and Incentive Compensation

In the 1990s, the need to recruit and retain well-qualified senior-level managers prompted HSOs/HSs to join industry in using bonuses that link compensation incentives to organization performance.[45] Incentive compensation programs attract talented managers, encourage development of multiple skills, increase tolerance for risk taking, motivate innovative behavior, and reward cost reductions.

Benefits Administration

Fringe benefits are an increasing part of total employee compensation and are typically one fourth to one third of payroll costs. Typical fringe benefits are health insurance (hospital, professional service, and perhaps dental and vision), pension plan contributions, life insurance, disability insurance, and paid vacation, holidays, and sick leave. Federal- and state-mandated payments include Social Security, workers' compensation for on-the-job injuries, and unemployment insurance.

HSOs/HSs have sought to control benefits costs by using methods such as self-insuring. Employers self-insure to cover the costs of certain benefits (other than mandated programs) by establishing a trust fund to pay claims directly without using an insurance carrier. Premium expense savings fund the trust and cover claims. Excess liability coverage (stop loss insurance) with a high deductible is used to limit employer risk and losses.

Another way to control benefits costs while maximizing employee satisfaction is the cafeteria, or full flexible, benefit plan.[46] In this arrangement, the employer allocates a specific dollar amount to each employee, who then designs a benefits package from a menu of items. Choosing a set of benefits that fits individual needs increases employee satisfaction. An added advantage to employers is that costs are more predictable.

Flexible spending accounts for health and child care expenses are key parts of cafeteria plans and are frequently offered as freestanding benefits. Employees place pretax dollars in accounts reserved for their use during the year. Unused dollars may be lost. Employers do not pay Social Security or income taxes on funds in the flexible spending accounts, which further reduces cost and increases employee take-home pay. The high proportion of female and single-parent employees has caused HSOs/HSs to increasingly provide on-site child care services, which reduce employee absenteeism, enhance recruitment, increase morale and retention, and reduce parental stress.

Employee Assistance Programs

Beginning with a narrow focus—assisting employees with alcoholism—EAPs have broadened their mission to help employees solve problems that negatively affect their work, including substance abuse and legal, financial, and emotional problems, and to assist with general health issues and in personal development. In terms only of chemical abuse, EAPs have significant potential, given the estimates that 15%–20% of the general work force use illicit drugs or abuse alcohol. These employees are three to four times more likely to be injured on the job than nonusers, have 47% of serious workplace accidents, file close to 50% of workers' compensation claims, and are 33% less productive.[47] EAPs have the potential for significant savings through decreased turnover rates, lower insurance costs, decreased use of sick time, improved employee job performance, enhanced quality and productivity,[48] and salvaged human resources. HSOs also provide EAP services to industry through their outpatient services. They are an ideal source for industry because a separate, effective EAP incorporates confidentiality, and self-referred employees get help without fear of retribution or a record of counseling that might affect their employment.

Career counseling is a second area in which HR departments provide employee assistance. Shortages have caused HSOs to develop the skills of current employees. Expenditures for direct skills training, subsidized professional education, and management development have become a large part of the HSO's investment in its staff. Career counseling and needs assessment by the HR department can reduce the costs of mismatching people and jobs and enhance the organization's return on its employee investment.

Health education and health promotion are a third and increasingly vital area of employee assistance. By educating the work force to manage its health better and assist efforts in areas such as stress management and weight and smoking reduction, employers can improve employee morale and productivity, reduce health insurance costs, and contribute to the positive climate required for employee retention. These initiatives invest in the HSO's/HS's human resources.

Workplace Health and Safety

HSOs are dangerous places. Caustic and toxic chemicals in the laboratory and pharmacy, food processing equipment in dietary, radiation in radiology, chemicals and gases used for sterilization, and infections in patient care areas are but a few of many hazards. Attention is also being given to reducing workplace violence.[49]

Enactment of the Occupational Safety and Health Act of 1970 (PL 91-596), also known as the Williams-Steiger Act, affected organizations of all types.[50] The law covered nongovernmental HSOs and was enacted to address safety and health problems associated with machines, chemicals, pollutants, and environmental threats in the workplace. The Occupational Safety and Health Administration (OSHA) implements the law and requires organizations to perform three major activities: 1) promulgation and enforcement of safety standards to eliminate or lessen hazards, 2) record keeping, and 3) training and education.

Acquired immunodeficiency syndrome (AIDS) poses unique problems for HSOs. Protecting healthcare workers from patients is compounded by the need to protect patients from healthcare workers. Use of universal precautions assumes that every patient is human immunodeficiency virus (HIV) positive; the precautions are designed to protect healthcare workers and other patients by reducing the risk of cross-infection. Mandatory testing of healthcare workers, especially physicians and dentists, is unresolved.

SEPARATION FROM EMPLOYMENT (EXIT)

Employees leave HSOs/HSs for various reasons; HR departments assist and monitor separation. Activities include facilitating the individual's exit; collecting employer-provided equipment, keys, and records; completing personnel records; processing final pay; and conducting an exit interview. Other activities include preretirement planning and outplacement:

- *Preretirement Planning:* Preretirement counseling prepares employees for the psychological, emotional, and financial changes at retirement. Experts are used to help employees understand lifestyle changes, emotional and physical needs, financial planning, Social Security benefits, pensions, and legal affairs such as estate planning.
- *Outplacement*: Outplacement occurs most often when jobs are eliminated because services are retrenched or abandoned or facilities close or merge. Outplacement recognizes the employer's social and financial commitment to assist employees in securing employment. It may include making contacts with other employers, advertising on employees' behalf, counseling, retraining, and providing the services of outplacement firms.
- *Exit Interviews*: The HR department conducts confidential exit interviews to try to gain candid feedback about the work environment. Goals include confirming the reason for separation and learning job likes and dislikes and opinions of supervisors, the facility, the benefits package, and compensation. Efforts are made to resolve problems so the employee leaves on a positive note. Information from the exit interview is used to help develop a profile of programmatic strengths and weaknesses and identify a possible need for intervention.[51] Despite being retrospective, exit interviews provide important information to management.

HUMAN RESOURCES DEPARTMENT AND CLINICAL STAFF

The functions and scope of the HR department have grown significantly, but professional staff organization (PSO) relations remain the exclusive domain of the HSO/HS governing body and senior management. This is understandable when LIPs typically are not employees. Salaried LIPs have most characteristics of typical employees, including participating in the employee benefits program. Even here, however, the HR department is rarely involved in salary administration or personnel file maintenance. HSOs/HSs simply do not consider LIPs to be typical employees.

HUMAN RESOURCES IN HSs

HRM activities apply to HSs, but in a more centralized way. The role of HSs includes setting overall human resources policy, coordinating HRM activities among affiliated organizations, and providing support for their programs. Corporate efforts include establishing systemwide guidelines ranging from compensation and benefits, regional training and development, and recruitment and selection to intraorganizational behaviors such as workplace romances and sexual harassment. Corporate assistance can be provided to components relative to specific programs, such as succession planning and regional training. Corporate support ranges from informal consultation on compensation plan design to benefit plan administration. Well-directed corporate HR functions save time and money for individual components and expand the capabilities of their HR services.

RM and Quality Improvement

Historically, safety programs and efforts to measure the quality of clinical services were separate control activities that were usually limited to acute care hospitals. In the early 1970s, safety programs began evolving into the broader concept of risk management (RM) and included proactively managing risk.

> Risk management functions encompass activities in health [services] organizations that are intended to conserve financial resources from loss. Those functions include a broad range of administrative activities intended to reduce losses associated with patient, employee, or visitor injuries; property loss or damages; and other sources of potential organizational liability.[52]

A comprehensive RM program includes identifying, controlling, and financing risks of all types. Inherent in RM is preventing risk and minimizing the effects of untoward events, should they occur. RM programs are common in HSOs/HSs and are required in a number of states.[53]

Internal and external factors caused these changes. Internally, HSO/HS managers increasingly recognized their ethical duty to provide a safe environment for patients, staff, and visitors and to deliver high-quality clinical services. External stimuli included 1) an increasingly litigious society and court decisions that put greater legal liability on HSOs/HSs; 2) state laws mandating RM programs, as indicated above; 3) federal laws such as the Occupational Safety and Health Act of 1970,[54] which mandated the study of hazards in acute care hospitals so that national standards could be set; and 4) the requirements of private organizations such as The Joint Commission and public bodies such as the Department of Health and Human Services (DHHS) and their state counterparts, which increasingly emphasized the quality of services and managing risk. Better RM programs followed as it became apparent that HSOs/HSs had to effectively manage the economic costs of risk.

In the 1990s, improving clinical quality (quality assessment and improvement, or QA/I) for patients was an important part of this expanded concept of RM. In 1992, The Joint Commission moved away from the terms and methodology of quality assurance and mandated QA/I as a better, more proactive and effective focus to evaluate and improve quality. Those standards linked, but did not integrate, QA/I and RM activities. The evolution continued, and by the late 1990s, QA/I and RM were fully integrated into performance improvement.* In 2008, RM activities are a source of "relevant information" and integrated into performance improvement.[55] Integrating QI and RM is prudent and enhances the effectiveness of both. HSOs/HSs must never suggest, however, that they are more concerned with reducing economic risk than with providing high-quality clinical services, despite their clear connection.

RM and efforts to improve clinical quality are similar. The Venn diagram in Figure 10.4 shows the overlap between RM and QI, most of which is found in performance improvement. Risk financing, employee benefits, and general liability issues have been unique to RM and are likely to remain so. Patient satisfaction, employee empowerment, and performance improvement are largely linked to QI, even though they may affect risk. The evolution of quality assessment (QA) to performance improvement expands the historical focus of QA beyond clinical activities to include improvement of the processes that support them. This change further diminishes the distinctions between RM and

---

*Productivity improvement and performance improvement are similar concepts, although not synonymous. The quality improvement literature uses the former, The Joint Commission the latter.

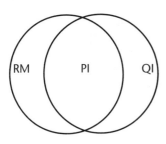

- Patient/customer focus
- Data-driven, complementary databases
- Includes clinical *and* administrative areas
- Process improvement orientation
- Staff involvement at all levels
- Loss(es) viewed as process failure
- Leadership from the top
- Ongoing education of staff
- QI viewed as step to managing risk
- Problem identification
- Culturally embedded

Figure 10.4.   Relationship and integration of RM and QI.

clinical activities and increases their linkages and the need for integration. Opportunities to benefit from cooperation will increase. In the meantime,

> for some professionals on both sides, integration means that one function envelops and subsumes the other—a circumstance that would not be in the best interests of either function. . . . Operational linkages is a term that is vague enough to allow for a variety of organizational models, reporting relationships, and data flow.[56]

RISK MANAGEMENT

As late as the 1970s, it was common even for larger HSOs and HSs to assign the director of maintenance collateral duties in facility safety. Directors of maintenance were unlikely to have formal preparation in RM and patient safety. RM was underdeveloped, and various risks facing the HSO were neither integrated nor handled comprehensively. Insurance was the typical means of protecting HSOs from monetary loss; proactive RM likely came from insurance companies wanting to decrease their exposure. Figure 10.5 shows a risk control (management) system with four quadrants: consequential loss, property loss, liability loss, and bodily injury. It illustrates the relationships that arise among governance, senior-level management, and the HSO's/HS's organization, staff, and activities.

Link to Senior Management

Regardless of the integration between RM and QI, encouragement and commitment by senior management are necessary for a successful RM program. Governing body support is shown by allocating adequate resources to the chief executive officer (CEO) for RM activities, support that should be readily available given the economics of prevention. RM has a staff, rather than a line, relationship to the CEO. A RM committee develops policy and provides general oversight. To the extent that RM and QI are integrated, this committee includes members of professional staff organization committees and is more clinically oriented.

The Risk Manager

Common preparation for health services risk managers includes an understanding of RM, nursing, management of HSOs, insurance, and law.[57] Larger HSOs and HSs need a full-time risk manager. Integrating RM and QI suggests the need for more academic preparation, perhaps as an adjunct to a clinical background. RM in an HS is likely to be managed by someone with significant operational experience, perhaps supplemented by legal and clinical preparation. A master of health services administration degree is good preparation for either the HSO or HS risk manager.

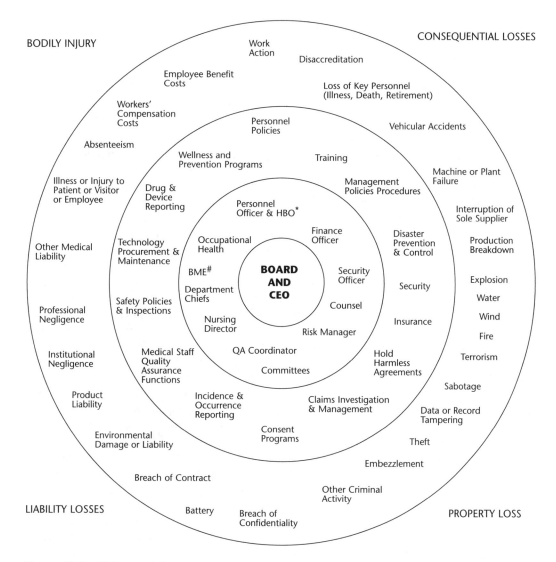

Figure 10.5. Risk control (management) system (*HBO, health benefits officer; #BME, biomedical equipment). (From Kavaler, Florence, and Allen D. Spiegel. *Risk Management in Health Care Institutions: A Strategic Approach*, 6. Sudbury, MA: Jones & Bartlett, 1997. www.jbpub.com. Reprinted by permission.)

Risk managers have become increasingly important in HSOs/HSs. As the risk managers' role matured, their duties came to include identifying and evaluating risks, loss prevention and reduction, managing the insurance program, safety and security administration, litigation management and claims handling, assisting in adjusting losses, RM consultation, and QI and related activities.[58] Reviewing business relationships (including contracts) is a necessary function for risk managers; examples include clinical and educational affiliations, vendor relationships, interorganizational relationships (in an HS and among HSOs), contracts with clinicians, management services, employment contracts, equipment purchase and lease agreements, and joint ventures.[59]

Risk managers depend on various HSO/HS units and constituent departments. Working effectively with persons over whom the risk manager has no line authority requires good interpersonal skills and an ability to coordinate and integrate various resources and sources of information. The risk manager may have the effect of exerting *de facto* line authority by providing information that is the basis for senior management decision making, as well as by persuading senior management to take action. Nevertheless, the risk manager's influence is indirect.

Principles of Managing Risk

The steps in managing risk include identifying, evaluating, eliminating, reducing, and transferring risk. Risk to the HSO is identified in several ways. The most common is to collect and aggregate data about problems or potential problems. Examples are workers' compensation claims, patient infections, injuries to staff from "sharps," unexpected patient deaths, patient falls, and injuries to visitors. Contributing to these data are the written occurrence, or incidence, reports completed by staff with knowledge of the circumstances of the event.

Finding patterns in these data is especially important. Safety inspections and audits of various activities and functions, ranging from financial (e.g., contracts) to fire protection, are ways to identify potential problem areas. Managing risk must be more than reactive, however. It should concentrate on evaluating, eliminating, reducing, and transferring risk.

Evaluating risk means reviewing and categorizing information about problems over time, which allows the risk manager to focus where problems are greatest. Evaluating risk should be prospective, too, because it can be predicted actuarially that certain types of problems will occur or have a probability of occurring. Prospective, retrospective, and concurrent efforts can use evaluative techniques such as cost–benefit and cost-effectiveness analyses to select the best course of action. Evaluation assists in identifying strategies to eliminate, reduce, or transfer risk.

Eliminating or reducing risk (or both) can be achieved in many ways. Examples include sponsoring education and awareness programs for staff, modifying physical plant and structure, enhancing the credentialing process and review of clinical staff activities, improving processes and procedures, initiating material management systems, improving patient and staff relations, and hiring qualified personnel in appropriate categories. It is preferable to eliminate risk, but this may be impossible for many types. Here, the emphasis must be on minimizing risk.

Corporate reorganization (restructuring) can eliminate certain economic risks. For example, assets of a separately incorporated operating HSO may be leased from the HS, which may make the HSO immune from recovery by successful plaintiffs. Establishing trusts and foundations in the corporate reorganization, which is common when HSs are established or when restructuring occurs, has the same effect. Putting HSO assets beyond the legal reach of successful plaintiffs has its place and is a legitimate business strategy. Failing to provide a means to fairly compensate persons who have been clinically or financially injured because of interacting with an HSO or HS, however, is socially irresponsible and unethical.

Some risks can be transferred to others. A common method of doing this is with the "hold harmless" agreement. It requires that a party doing business with an HSO/HS indemnify it for any liability incurred because of that party's negligence. Equipment purchase contracts commonly include such clauses. As permitted by law, transfer of risk clauses should be used in all agreements with subcontractors. Insurance may be the most common way to transfer risk.[60] Entering a risk pool—joining those with similar exposure to risk—allows risk to be shared and spread among others. Actuarial methods can determine the potential for loss, a premium can be assigned, and this allows individual exposure to loss to be minimized.

Financing Risk

Some risks, such as casualty (e.g., damage from fire, water, or wind storm), general liability (e.g., for injury to visitors or suppliers), business interruption (e.g., from equipment failure, strike, vandalism, or acts of nature), theft (e.g., embezzlement), and medical malpractice can be minimized but cannot be eliminated or transferred. The financial viability of the HSO/HS must be protected from them. Insurance is the most common means of doing so. Commercial insurance requires that insureds pay a premium. Coverage under the contract of insurance provides specified protection against certain losses for a fixed period. This contract between the HSO/HS (the insured) and the insurer (carrier) puts obligations on the insured, as well. Examples include staff training, providing inspection reports to insurance carriers, promptly reporting circumstances that might cause liability, and cooperating in the carrier's investigation and defense of claims. In addition to commercial insurance, HSOs/HSs may participate in insurance programs through captive insurance companies that have been established by the state, a trade association, a consortium of HSOs/HSs, or a large HSO/HS. "Off-shore" insurance companies are an example. Recurring malpractice "crises" resulting from rapid increases in malpractice insurance premiums made these variations popular. Some commercial insurance carriers stopped writing medical malpractice liability insurance, which made availability a factor, as well.

Prior to the 1980s, medical malpractice liability insurance was written on an "occurrence" basis—the insured had coverage if a policy was in effect at the time of the event (occurrence). Occurrence coverage protected the insured from a claim if the claim was filed within the statute of limitations, regardless of how long that was after the injury. This resulted in a "long tail," meaning that claims could be brought years or even decades after the event that caused a claim to be filed. The statute of limitations begins to run only after the event is, or should have been, discovered, and this adds more length to the "tail." For example, a newborn infant can bring suit for 21 years plus the statute of limitations for negligent medical treatment. Insurance carriers argued that this made it virtually impossible to actuarially predict their risk (exposure), which made it impossible to calculate an appropriate premium. To avoid this problem, they began to write policies with "claims-made" coverage, that "eliminated the 'long tail' of occurrence coverage because the insurer knows at the expiration of a given policy all of the claims that will be reported against that policy. The insurer need not be concerned with unknown claims that may be made in future years at inflated costs."[61] This change means that the insured must have a policy in effect when the claim is brought rather than when the insured event occurs, as with occurrence coverage. This shift seems to have reduced the rate of increase in medical malpractice liability insurance premiums.

Larger HSOs/HSs are more able to self-insure. Self-insurance programs are usually broader than medical malpractice liability and may include financial protection against risks such as business interruption, fire, and other casualty losses and bonding for employees with financial responsibilities. Establishing a self-insurance program involves much more than simply stating that the HSO/HS is self-insured. Actuarial studies must be done to determine the potential for various types of losses, including special attention to the specific risk from clinical services offered or contemplated. Based on these data, the HSO/HS must establish dedicated financial reserves to meet expected claims. Usually several years are needed to accumulate the reserves needed for a self-insurance program to be financially viable. In the interim, commercial coverage is necessary. In addition, after the program is fully established, vigilance is necessary so that the fund is both adequate to meet expected claims and not raided for other purposes. Underfunding or stripping reserves for self-insurance protection can have disastrous consequences for the organization's economic viability.

Even when the self-insurance program is mature, HSOs/HSs will carry excess liability and casualty coverage against large claims. For example, an HSO/HS might self-insure for all losses up to $3 million; beyond that it may have a policy with a commercial carrier to a total coverage of $20 million. It is important to note that even if an HSO/HS has only commercial insurance, the policy is likely to have a deductible, which is a form of self-insurance. Deductibles must be met from reserves.

Good business practice demands that HSOs/HSs protect themselves against the full range of financial risks. In addition, it is socially responsible and ethical that they do so. "Going bare" in terms of medical malpractice claims means that the HSO/HS neither self-insures nor carries commercial insurance. This practice is not uncommon among LIPs with poor medical malpractice liability records. Their assets are in spouses' names or otherwise beyond the reach of plaintiffs. This, too, is socially irresponsible. It is prudent for HSOs/HSs to require that LIPs on their professional staffs provide evidence of insurance coverage as a condition of having clinical privileges. This is standard practice in acute care hospitals.

Non-LIP caregivers and managers should carry personal liability insurance to protect themselves as individuals from legal actions for alleged negligence. Individual malpractice policies have become common among registered nurses, and there are significant legal and professional reasons to purchase such coverage, even if the employer has an umbrella policy that covers employees.[62] Managers should remember that they, too, are liable for errors and omissions (malpractice) committed in their professional activities. The HSO's/HS's umbrella liability policy will cover employees. Nonetheless, the effects of litigation have many nuances for employers and employees. Soon after litigation begins, it becomes apparent that the various parties have substantially different interests. Umbrella policies of the type commonly found in HSOs/HSs typically do not include employees as named insureds. This means that, legally, an individual employee has no voice in a decision to settle a lawsuit. Although not a legal determination, settling may suggest admission of fault. This may be adverse to employees' interests from the standpoints of professional reputation, licensure, certification, and references. Conversely, a personal policy gives one a much more powerful position. The Health Care Quality Improvement Act of 1986[63] requires that payments made for the benefit of physicians and LIPs be reported to a national data bank. This greatly increases the effects of settling a malpractice claim and makes it important for affected parties to have maximum control.

Members of the HSO's/HS's governing body are not employees. They should be protected against legal actions for errors and omissions under a directors' and officers' liability policy, a policy that should be provided by the HSO/HS. They, too, should consider a personal errors and omissions liability insurance policy.

Process of RM

It is crucial that a RM program systematically report circumstances that put HSOs/HSs at risk. These can be fire and safety problems, accidents, or any type of negligence. Data collection for analysis of actual and potential loss may be done with a sophisticated RM software program or a simple manual entry system. "Establishing databases for incident reports, claims, insurance coverages, hazardous materials, and other sources of information may be accomplished through the use of both internal and external sources. One of the richest internal sources is quality data."[64]

Common to internal control systems is a written statement, usually called an incident, or occurrence, report. Incident reports alert risk managers to specific problems, and aggregating the data will show problem areas and patterns. Because incidence reporting and associated activities are used to improve the quality of care as part of peer review, laws in most states prevent plaintiffs' attorneys from obtaining (discovering) them. The laws were passed in the belief that access to such information would have a chilling effect on physicians' willingness to engage in peer review. A collateral result of limiting access to documents is that the plaintiff (injured party) is less likely to prevail. On balance, however, society's interests are served by promoting activities whose purpose is to improve the quality of care, even given the potential for abuses by overuse of the shield.

Analysis of data from reporting systems is used in the feedback loop—it informs the risk manager about problems and suggests steps to correct them. For example, data about falls resulting from patients' excessive waits for assistance with toileting could be used to support a nursing service request for more staff. Data about postsurgical wound infections could be used to improve staff training in sterile processing, or it could be used to teach correct hand washing techniques to clinical staff. Data about injuries to staff who move bariatric patients could justify a training program about proper lifting techniques and purchase of specialized equipment.

Legal counsel review of the RM program is indispensable. If counsel are available on-site (in-house counsel), it is likely they will be more involved in RM than would be external or retainer counsel. Some HSOs/HSs use in-house counsel as risk managers. Regardless, legal counsel must participate to provide the legal perspectives for RM.

After injury to a patient has occurred, the risk manager can minimize loss by immediately taking four steps. First, if the patient has been discharged, the medical record (including radiographs) should be obtained, and absolute custody of it should be retained by the risk manager. Second, if the patient continues under treatment and the record is active, it should be photocopied (with new entries photocopied on a regular basis) and the copies retained by the risk manager. This standard operating procedure should be known throughout the HSO/HS. Third, meetings should be held with the patient, the family, or both to determine their interest in settling any potential claim. Once an injured patient retains legal counsel, the case is almost certain to become more complex and costly. Fourth, the HSO/HS should do whatever it can to retain the patient's goodwill; above all, insult should not be added to injury. An injured patient who needs additional services should never be billed for them. Angry patients are much more likely to sue than are those who believe the HSO/HS did the best it could under the circumstances and acted responsibly. To reduce anger, the HSO's staff must communicate honestly with the patient and family. Injured parties who believe they are being misled or kept from the truth will react with anger and a strong desire to learn what happened. Expressing concern, providing information, and, perhaps, apologizing diminish the likelihood that an injured party will take legal action.[65]

Efforts at early settlement raise a duality of interests that can cause a conflict of interest. Patients and their relatives should clearly understand that the risk manager is an employee of the HSO/HS. Risk managers must never allow patients or family members to believe that they are advocates for the patient or acting as legal counsel on the patient's behalf. Honesty and forthrightness succeed far better than other tactics. At a minimum, fraud or misrepresentation by the risk manager are unethical. Further, it will cause a court to set aside any agreement and may result in criminal charges or punitive damages against the HSO/HS.

IMPROVING QUALITY AND PERFORMANCE

Early concerns about the quality of clinical practice in HSOs focused on hospitals and were addressed through peer review, which is defined as physician review of the care that is provided by physicians and other types of caregivers. In 1912, the American College of Surgeons began developing the concept of peer review. By 1918, it published *The Minimum Standard,* part of which addressed peer review of medical practice: "The [medical] staff [shall] review and analyze at regular intervals their clinical experience in the various departments of the hospital."[66] Chapter 7 discussed Ernest A. Codman's contribution in developing the standard and establishing the American College of Surgeon's hospital survey program, whose work, Chapter 1 noted, was continued by The Joint Commission upon its establishment in 1951.

The process of peer review was called *medical audit,* terminology that continued into the 1960s. Enactment of Medicare codified utilization review (UR), which focused on appropriate use of services. UR did not directly affect the quality of care in hospitals, except that reviewing appropriateness of admission, use of ancillary services, and length of stay minimized nosocomial (institution-caused) and iatrogenic (physician-caused) problems. The focus of UR in Medicare is discussed in Chapter 1. Medical audit and UR placed little emphasis on solving the problems identified, however.

Efforts to measure quality continued to evolve. In the early 1970s, The Joint Commission required quality assessment activities, a variation on medical audit. In the middle 1970s, the words were changed to *medical care evaluation,* but it remained essentially medical audit. By 1980, the concept of quality assurance had become a Joint Commission standard. Quality assurance meant that The Joint Commission standards had evolved from finding and describing problems (medical audit) to be more proactive and dynamic by stressing problem solving to improve clinical quality. As noted earlier, performance improvement is now the umbrella concept for all quality-related Joint Commission standards.

Historically, quality has been defined as the degree of adherence to standards or criteria. As applied in health services, ensuring quality meant using prospectively determined criteria to measure performance, with the measurement being done retrospectively. Newer definitions of quality are discussed in Chapter 7 in the context of CQI. These include conformance to requirements and fitness for use or fitness for need and are customer driven because they focus on customer expectations and do not exclusively reflect criteria or standards developed using professional expertise. It is suggested that *quality* should be defined as meeting latent needs—identifying "needs" customers may not even know they have but will be pleased to have identified and met by the provider. CQI defines *customer* broadly to include all who receive goods or services.

Measuring quality using the concepts of quality assurance required that the HSO/HS establish standards (criteria), typically through peer judgments. Developing criteria was but the first step. Two other elements were necessary: a means of surveillance to identify deviations requiring action, and stopping the deviation or minimizing its recurrence—the corrective action. These steps are simple in theory and may be in practice as well, depending on what is being measured. Much of the conceptual framework used to measure quality was developed by Avedis Donabedian, a physician, whose nomenclature of *structure, process,* and *outcome* became standard in health services. Structure and process were the major foci of The Joint Commission's QA standards in the 1980s.

Donabedian noted the difficulties in defining the quality of medical care and measuring the quality of the interpersonal relationship between physician and patient—a relationship essential to the process of care, as reflected in the outcome of care. Technical aspects of care are more definable and measurable than are interpersonal relationships.[67] Regardless, measuring quality under traditional QA began with criteria developed internally and/or externally imposed.

Structure, Process, and Outcome in Quality Theory

Donabedian defined *structure* as the tools and resources that providers of care have at their disposal and the physical and organizational settings where they work.[68] *Process* is the set of activities that occur within HSOs and between practitioners and patients. Here, judgments of quality may be made either by direct observation or by reviewing recorded information. Donabedian considered this means of measuring quality to be largely normative, in that the norms come either from the science of medicine or from the ethics and values of society.[69] *Outcome* is a change in a patient's current and future health status that can be attributed to antecedent healthcare.[70] Donabedian defined *outcome* broadly to include improvement of social and psychological function, in addition to physical and physiological aspects. Also included are patient attitudes, health-related knowledge acquired by the patient, and health-related behavioral change.[71]

Donabedian concluded that "good structure, that is, a sufficiency of resources and proper system design, is probably the most important means of protecting and promoting the quality of care."[72] He added that assessing structure is a good deal less important than assessing process and outcome. Comparing process and outcome, Donabedian concluded that neither is clearly preferable. Either may be superior, depending on the situation and what is being measured. He emphasized that it is critical, however, to know the link between the content of the process and the resulting outcome. Only by knowing this link (preferably at the level of a causal relationship) can what is done or not done in the process be modified to improve the outcome. Not knowing how a desirable outcome was achieved means replication is only a matter of chance. Table 10.2 shows the advantages and disadvantages of

TABLE 10.2.   ADVANTAGES AND DISADVANTAGES OF PROCESS AND OUTCOME MEASURES OF QUALITY

Process		Outcome	
Advantages	Disadvantages	Advantages	Disadvantages
Practitioners have no great difficulty specifying technical criteria for standards of care. Even not fully validated standards and criteria can serve as interim measures of acceptable practice. Information about technical aspects of care is documented in the medical record and usually is accessible as well as timely—it can be used for prevention and intervention. Use of this information permits specific attribution of responsibility so that credit or blame can be more easily ascertained and specific corrective action can be taken.	Great weakness in the scientific basis for much of accepted practice and use of prevalent norms as the basis for judging quality may encourage dogmatism and perpetuate error. Because practitioners prefer to err on the side of doing more than is necessary, there is a tendency toward overly elaborate and costly care; this is reflected in the norms. Although technical aspects are overemphasized, the management of the interpersonal process tends to be ignored, partly because the usual sources of data give little information about the physician–patient relationship.	When the scientific basis for accepted practice is in doubt, emphasis on outcome tends to discourage dogmatism and helps maintain a more open and flexible approach to management. An open and flexible approach may help in the development of less costly but no less effective strategies of care. Outcomes reflect all of the contributions of all of the practitioners to the care of the patient and thus provide an inclusive, integrative measure of the quality of care. Also reflected in the outcome is the patient's contribution to the care that may have been influenced by the relationship between patient and practitioners; a more direct assessment of the patient–physician relationship can be obtained by including aspects of patient satisfaction among measures of care.	Even expert practitioners are unable to specify the outcomes of optimal care, as to their magnitude, timing, and duration. When indicators of health status are obtained, it is difficult to know how much of the observed effect can be attributed to medical care. Choosing outcomes that have marginal relevance to the objectives of prior care is an ever-present pitfall; even when relevant outcomes are selected, information about many outcomes often is not available in time to make it useful for certain types of monitoring. Waiting for a pattern of adverse outcomes can be questioned on ethical grounds. Examining outcomes without examining means of attaining them may result in a lack of attention to the presence of redundant or overly costly care.

Adapted from Donabedian, Avedis. *Explorations in Quality Assessment and Monitoring. Vol. 1, The Definition of Quality and Approaches to its Assessment*, 119–122. Chicago: Health Administration Press, 1980.

focusing on process and outcome to measure quality. Outcome indicators in Donabedian's taxonomy focus on the overall outcomes of medical care, such as health status and disability.

Development and application of QA peaked in the late 1980s with adoption of a 10-step QA process. From then to the present, The Joint Commission began its evolution to use of outcome indicators (measures). In 1987, its Agenda for Change initiated a major shift to adopting CQI. These activities were subsumed into what became known as the ORYX® initiative.[73] It was generally conceded that the QA implemented in the 1980s did little to improve the quality of care. "On the whole, to the extent that quality measurement tools have been developed at all, they tend to unveil the fact of flaw, not its cause."[74]

The first clinical indicators developed were hospitalwide care and obstetrical and anesthesia care.[75] In early 1989, 12 key principles of organizational and management effectiveness were announced by The Joint Commission, and pilot testing was undertaken. The purpose was to characterize an acute care hospital's commitment to continuously improve its quality of care. A central tenet was that identifying and monitoring outcome indicators were necessary for a hospital to focus its QI activities. By 1991, indicators had been developed for anesthesia, obstetrics, cardiovascular medicine, oncology, and trauma care.[76] These indicators focused on high-risk, high-volume, and problem-prone aspects of care. Hospitals could choose from among hundreds of performance measurement systems and thousands of performance measures. A major goal of ORYX® is to develop standardized, evidence-based measures.[77] As of 2007, five core performance measure sets have been identified for hospitals: those for acute myocardial infarction, heart failure, pneumonia, pregnancy and related conditions, and surgical infection prevention.[78] The number and range of evidence-based performance measures by which hospital outcomes can be compared will increase and is strongly supported by the Centers for Medicare and Medicaid Services (CMS).

Importance of QI

The importance of evaluating and improving quality was suggested in Chapter 1 and is expanded here. The Joint Commission and other accreditors such as the Community Health Accreditation Program and the American Osteopathic Association require organized, effective QI activities. Unaccredited HSOs/HSs are not in "deemed" status and can be reimbursed for services to federal beneficiaries only by meeting the conditions of participation established by the DHHS. Accreditors of medical education programs require the HSO to be Joint Commission accredited. Insurers expect HSOs/HSs to be accredited. Lending institutions and organizations that rate bond offerings consider accreditation in their decisions. Chapter 2 details the importance of credentialing clinical staff, an activity indispensable to QI. In addition, failing to effectively assess quality increases the likelihood of adverse malpractice judgments because the HSO has not met the legal standard of care.

QI is considered important by managerial, clinical, and support staff who want to do their best. They strive to do so because they have internalized the motivation to provide high-quality care and achieve excellence in their HSO/HS. This necessitates learning what is being done well, what is not, and how to close the gap.

QI and QA Compared

HSOs/HSs that immerse themselves in the philosophy and techniques of CQI have achieved a paradigm shift away from the traditional approaches to quality. As described in Chapter 7, QI uses powerful tools that result from a radically different philosophy about relationships between managers and staff. Table 10.3 suggests the differences between QI and QA; several should be highlighted.

QA is a negative process. It focuses on the "who" and seeks to identify those who seem to cause the problems. QI seeks the "why." Workers are not the focus. QI implements the philosophy of W. Edwards Deming, whose theories are detailed in Chapter 7, that 85%–94% of problems result from the process; few are caused by the workers.

Commonly, QA measures only the quality of clinical practice, The Joint Commission's focus until the 1990s. QI measures clinical outcomes but is more concerned with the myriad processes and systems that support delivery of clinical services, as well as those that are administrative, such as admitting and patient accounts. The clinical and administrative aspects of many processes cannot be separated easily, and QI seeks to improve integrated or cross-functional processes as well as those that are intradepartmental. Improving quality in support and administrative processes positively affects clinical processes and, thus, delivery of care, because there is greater organizationwide quality consciousness and because, without exception, these areas affect clinical services. For example,

TABLE 10.3. CHARACTERISTICS OF QI VERSUS QA

QI	QA
"Why" focused (positive)	"Who" focused (negative)
Prospective	Retrospective
Internally directed	Externally directed
Follows patients	Follows organizational structure
Involves the many	Delegated to the few
Integrated analysis	Divided analysis
Bottom up	Top down
Proactive	Reactive
Employee focused	Management focused (directing)
Full staff involvement	Limited staff involvement
Process based	Event based
Process approach	Inspection approach
Quality is integral activity	Quality is separate activity
Focus on all processes to improve fitness for use	Focus on meeting clinical criteria
Focus on improving processes	Focus on solving problems
Makes no assumption about irreducibility of problems	Assumes problems/numbers of problems reach irreducible number

inefficient intradepartmental or interdepartmental admitting processes directly and indirectly affect patient care. It is certain they affect patient satisfaction.

Another important difference is that QI focuses on improving processes, whereas QA focuses on solving the problems that result from a faulty process. QA addresses the unusual or unique—what Deming called special causes—and investigates indicators that exceed thresholds. Similarly, the QA philosophy means that managers spend much of their time "fighting fires." Putting out fires is necessary, but doing so neither improves processes nor increases efficiency or effectiveness. Putting out a fire only returns the process, more or less, to the state it was in before the fire. QI asserts that unique and unusual results or outcomes should be ignored unless they pose a significant risk or danger; attention should focus on improving the process(es). HSO/HS managers cannot ignore unusual or unique events that affect patients, but the effort spent on them should be minimized because the real gain comes from improving processes to reduce variation, error rates, and other inefficiencies.

Finally, assumptions that were made about the irreducibility of problems were the most insidious aspect of the philosophy of QA and were probably responsible for delaying improvement in the quality of care. Psychologically, it is crucial that "good enough" is no longer acceptable; the QI philosophy rejects it. An element of "good enough" is suggested when HSOs/HSs compare outcome indicators or other performance measures with their own criteria or with external criteria. Criteria and indicators are important starting points and provide a macro-level understanding of outcomes produced by an HSO/HS, generally, or from a specific process. The fact is that organizations in which CQI has been implemented improve quality by reducing waste, rework, and redundancy, not by accepting a place within the herd. Until a systematic search for the root causes of medication errors has been done using the tools of QI, for example, no one knows what the irreducible level of medication errors in an HSO is.

In the final analysis, improving clinical (and managerial) quality requires change. If Deming is correct that only 6%–15% of problems result from causes within workers' control, management must work with staff to improve quality. Managers must shed the traditional view that poor quality occurs because employees choose to perform suboptimally. What must be remembered, especially with the increased emphasis on outcome indicators, is that the link between process and outcome must be understood. Unless it is known how the outcome was produced, desired outcomes cannot be purposefully replicated, nor can a process be changed to prevent undesired outcomes.

SUMMARY

Readers should have a clear sense of the importance of managing risk and assessing and improving the quality of clinical and managerial performance. These processes have an important place in the control function of managers in HSOs/HSs. Making changes is difficult in HSOs/HSs, where much that is done is a personal service rendered by clinical staff who are often independent contractors and have no employment relationship with the organization. For the manager, this requires attention to interpersonal skills and an ability to work with and through people. Maintaining and improving the quality of care for patients and protecting employees and visitors depend largely on these skills.

Improving quality (and minimizing risk) is part of the manager's control function that is shown in the control model in Figure 10.2. It is platitudinous, but true nevertheless, to say that managers must be part of the solution or they will remain part of the problem. Managers should be unwilling to accept an attitude anywhere in the HSO/HS that what is being done is "good enough."

■ Control Methods

Managers use numerous methods and techniques to monitor and control inputs, processes, and/or outputs. RM and performance improvement are examples of structured, programmatic control methods. Others are budgeting, activity-based costing, and operational activity and financial ratio analyses.

BUDGETING

Budgets are among the most common methods of control. They serve a dual purpose. First, they are numerical expressions of plans,[79] and second, they become control standards against which results are compared.[80] Types of budgets and time frames vary. Most are made for 1 year, such as operating expense and revenue budgets. Capital budgets are likely to be multiyear.

Budgeting depends on planning and forecasting. Individual cost centers or departments forecast the volume of services that they expect to deliver, the workload demand, and the resources that are needed in the next budget period. Cost centers are organizational units in which there is a well-defined relationship between inputs and outputs. Examples are surgical services, nursing service, clinics, laboratories, pharmacy, diagnostic testing, dietary, patient billing, medical records, and maintenance. Based on projected workloads, revenue budgets can be derived for those units with which revenues can be associated; examples are the emergency department, clinics, diagnostic testing, pharmacy, and surgery. For all departments, including those in which revenues typically cannot be directly associated, such as nursing service, social services, maintenance, and administration, operating expense budgets are derived that reflect the amount and types of resources that are necessary to perform the projected workload. Managers who insist that all departments and functional areas must "pay their own way" are thinking in boxes—they do not see the organization as a system in which all parts must work to achieve the aim of the system. Managers should understand that some units may have to suboptimize their performance if the performance of the entire system is to be optimized.

Operating expense budgets include two types of expenses: direct and indirect. Direct expenses are those incurred by a cost center or a department and that can be specifically attributed to it. They include labor and nonlabor components. Human resources requirements must be converted to dollars paid for salary, wages, and fringe benefits. Nonlabor expenses are supplies and equipment. From a cost perspective, indirect expenses can be allocated to the various units, including overhead costs, such as general facility maintenance, building depreciation, utilities, and management staff not identified with specific cost centers. Indirect costs are usually allocated among cost centers on bases such as space occupied, number of employees, or volume of output.[81] Usually, cost centers have control over only their direct expenses.

Operating budgets can be fixed, variable, or fixed-variable. Fixed budgets represent a resource commitment to a cost center or department for the budget period. They are based on planned workload. Variable budgets recognize that as volume, workload, or service demands change, so will resource needs.[82] Hybrid fixed-variable operating budgets separate fixed and variable components, with the latter changing as workload increases or decreases.

Budgets force managers to be aware of inputs used and the associated costs of staff, materials, equipment, or supplies. Preparing a budget requires a manager to project the cost and amount of resources that will be consumed and used in achieving outputs (conversion). Budgets are standards against which results can be compared. Typically, monthly reports compare actual expenditures for the month, and the year to date, with the amount budgeted. Variances that indicate deviations of actual from budgeted amounts can be identified and used for control.

A sample emergency department (ED) budget for a 100-bed hospital is shown in Table 10.4. It reports operating revenue and direct operating expenses, but it does not include allocated indirect costs such as overhead. The array of data allows several types of comparisons of ED performance with budget. This type of report enables managers to exercise greater control over resource use and allows them to determine whether revenue and costs are lower than, are equal to, or exceed expectations.

COST ALLOCATION

HSOs/HSs typically control resource consumption and conversion through the budget process at the level of cost center or department. This form of budgeting, in which direct and indirect costs are identified and monitored, has limitations, however. Prior to implementing prospective pricing by use of diagnosis-related groups (DRGs) in the early 1980s, the Health Care Financing Administration (HCFA, predecessor to the CMS) required providers to use step-down costing for Medicare payments. Subsequently, this costing system was used by HSOs to develop base rates that became the basis for DRG reimbursement. Step-down cost allocation allocates direct costs and pools of indirect costs to specific services and or departments. For example, pooled indirect costs such as those for maintenance, housekeeping, utilities, administration, information services, and marketing would be allocated to cost centers on some logical basis such as labor hours, space occupied, number of employees, or units of service, and the direct and indirect costs of a department would be stepped down to specific services. The goal of step-down cost allocation is to present a more complete financial picture of the costs of treating individual patients and providing specific services. By analyzing input—labor, materials, and equipment—and indirect and overhead costs throughout the organization and associating them with different products or services, standard costs by type of output can be determined. Control is exercised by comparing actual costs of final output with prospectively determined standard costs. Analysis of variance allows inferences to be drawn about the appropriateness of input consumption and efficiency of conversion.

Before cost allocation procedures were widely adopted by HSOs/HSs, managers had difficulty defining end products (services) and the costs associated with producing them, and there were few incentives to do so. A unit of service such as "patient day" is a poor output measure because it fails to reflect variations in resource use resulting from factors such as admission type or severity of medical problems (e.g., acuity level). For example, providing care for a high-risk premature infant requires very different resources from various cost centers than does care for a full-term infant not at risk. Also, the nursing service resources necessary to care for severely ill rather than convalescing patients differ, although the intermediate output measure—patient day—is the same.

TABLE 10.4. COMMUNITY HOSPITAL EMERGENCY DEPARTMENT REVENUES AND EXPENSES[a]

	A Current month this year	B Current month budget	C[b] Current month variance	D Year-to-date this year	E Year-to-date budget	F[b] Year-to-date variance	G Year-to-date last year
Operating revenue							
Inpatient	76,858	49,072	27,786	654,580	629,564	25,016	593,286
Outpatient	190,505	181,667	8,838	1,681,516	1,737,482	-55,966	1,675,505
Total net revenue	267,363	230,739	36,624	2,336,096	2,367,046	-30,950	2,268,791
Operating expenses							
Salaries & wages	72,044	61,319	10,725	598,818	586,746	12,072	547,616
Purchased services	0	116	-116	5,797	1,044	4,753	925
Repair, maintenance, rent, lease	987	2,115	-1,128	6,806	19,035	-12,229	18,819
Supplies, pharmacy, food	9,336	7,626	1,710	75,524	73,402	2,122	69,932
Other	196	282	-86	2,769	2,538	231	3,041
Total operating expenses	82,563	71,458	11,105	689,714	682,766	6,948	640,333
Department profit (loss)	184,800	159,281	25,519	1,646,382	1,684,280	-37,898	1,628,458

[a]All amounts in U.S. dollars.

[b]Minus denotes the revenue and/or expenses were under the budget amount for the period.

ACTIVITY-BASED COSTING

Activity-based costing (ABC) differs from conventional approaches to cost allocation.[83] ABC is a bottom-up method of allocating costs "because it finds the costs of each service at the lowest level, the point where resources are used, and aggregates them upward into products. ABC is based on the paradigm that activities consume resources and processes consume activities."[84] This contrasts with the top-down method of step-down allocation, which begins with all costs and allocates them downward to various services.[85] These differences are depicted in Figure 10.6.

ABC is a more precise way of allocating all direct and indirect costs to activities that produce patient services. It provides managers with more precise measures of the costs of services, or residuals in the case of revenue centers (revenues minus costs), and it is useful in identifying non–value-added activities. ABC has two dimensions: 1) process assessment and 2) identification of activities involved in patient services—"cost drivers"—and cost assignment for resources used in each activity. Thus, ABC focuses on both expenses and the processes that generate expenses. It enhances con-

Traditional Costing

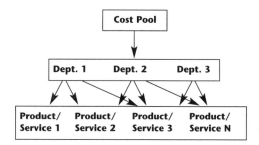

- Costs (labor, supplies, facilities) of various kinds of functions (purchasing, setup, monitoring, service delivery)

- Organizational units that deliver or support the delivery of service

- Various services (lab tests, CBC, physical exam)

Activity-Based Costing

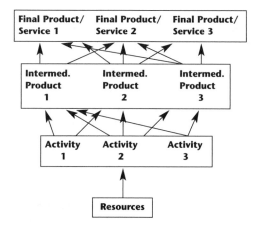

- Normal delivery, bypass surgery, etc.

- Physical, well-baby visits, meals, lab tests, radiology procedures, etc.

- Patient history, writing orders, chest X-ray, urinalysis, test setups, purchasing, billing, 15-min outpatient visits, echocardiogram, telemetry, etc.

- Labor, supplies, materials

Figure 10.6. Comparison of traditional and activity-based costing. (From Zelman, William N., Michael J. McCue, and Alan R. Millikan. *Financial Management of Health Care Organizations: An Introduction to Fundamental Tools, Concepts, and Applications,* 465. Malden, MA: Blackwell, 1998; reprinted by permission.)

trol of resource consumption and is a logical adjunct to CQI because it facilitates an understanding of processes and activities that do or do not add value.[86] By focusing on process, Peter Drucker observed, "activity-based costing asks, 'Does it have to be done?'"[87]

Evaluating the flow of a patient's receipt of services makes it possible to identify all activities (elements) of work. These activities are called cost drivers because they result in resource use. ABC allocates both indirect and direct costs to each specific activity. Tracing costs across cost centers and departments to the final product or service gives a more accurate understanding of work processes and the costs to provide service.[88] For example, for a service such as a surgical procedure, ABC will "develop cost information on all different activities along the critical path from preadmission to discharge."[89] The costs of admission, billing, and accounts receivable can be assigned to the final product (surgery), as can other costs such as nursing service, operating suite, and recovery costs associated with the particular surgical procedure. For costs to be identified, the specific resources consumed for any patient encounter must be identified. To do so requires process analysis of required activities. ABC offers management a more precise way of matching the costs of resources consumed to services provided.[90] This allows evaluation of processes to identify activities that can be improved, substituted, or eliminated. Furthermore, understanding the true cost of a service enables HSOs/HSs and their LIPs to make better strategic and tactical pricing decisions, determine if a service is profitable, and know more precisely the resources needed to provide it.[91] In addition, providers are better able to evaluate services, programs, and managed care contracts. These data contribute to CQI because process input costs are more easily recognized. Again, some units may need to suboptimize their financial performance if the performance of the entire system is to be optimized.

FINANCIAL STATEMENTS

Eventually, all HSO/HS activity is reflected in its financial statements. The two most important are the income statement and the balance sheet. Both are indispensable for management control. Table 10.5 shows a sample income statement and balance sheet for a hypothetical hospital. The organization's income statement shows revenue and expenditures for a 1-year period, including profit, which is described as the excess of income over expense for not-for-profit HSOs/HSs. Gross revenue is usually defined as inpatient, outpatient, premium, and other revenue, such as that from grants, investments, and auxiliary operations. Premium revenue is that earned from capitated contracts. Gross revenue is what the HSO/HS would have received if everyone paid charges, or full price. Most third-party payers negotiate rates (prices) that are less than 100% of charges, however. The difference between charges and negotiated rates plus the value of charity care make up the total discounts and contractual allowances, which are deducted from gross revenue. Net patient revenue is what the HSO/HS received for the services it provided.[92] The balance sheet shows the organization's current and fixed assets and its liabilities and equity.

The profit and loss statement and the balance sheet enhance management's ability to monitor and control the organization's financial situation by showing profitability (e.g., profit margin, return on investment, and return on equity), capital structure risk (e.g., debt to assets), and efficiency of asset utilization (e.g., fixed and total asset turnover, accounts receivable collection period, and inventory turnover). These measures are discussed in the Financial Analysis section below.

RATIO ANALYSIS

A language common to all organizations is numerically expressed data. For example, HSOs/HSs are described by number and types of beds, number and types of employees, and size and specialty mix of their PSOs. HSOs/HSs are partly evaluated by numbers of patients admitted, procedures performed, and expenditures.

TABLE 10.5.   EXAMPLE OF COMPOSITE AVERAGE INCOME STATEMENT AND BALANCE SHEET (,000)

		2000	2006	Compound Annual Growth Rate (%)
Income Statement				
Revenues		$70,646	$75,636	1.37
	Premium revenue	$0	$1,265	N/A
	Other revenue	$6,982	$9,435	6.21
	Total revenues	$77,628	$86,336	2.15
Expenses				
	Interest expense	$1,509	$1,726	2.72
	Depreciation & amortization	$4,699	$6,015	5.06
	Bad debt expense	$2,569	$3,167	4.27
	Other expense	$63,584	$69,318	1.74
	Total expenses	$72,361	$80,226	2.09
Excess of Revenues over Expenses (profit)		$5,267	$6,110	3.01
	Other equity changes	$367	($125)	−180.62
Increase in Equity		$5,634	$5,985	1.22
Balance Sheet				
Assets				
	Cash & short-term investments	$7,012	$12,413	12.10
	Accounts receivable	$9,238	$10,692	2.97
	Inventory	$769	$1,036	6.14
	Other current assets	$2,973	$3,763	4.83
	Total current assets	$19,992	$27,904	6.90
Net Fixed Assets		$35,617	$40,357	2.53
	Replacement funds	$13,089	$21,397	10.33
	Other assets	$5,601	$8,516	8.74
	Total assets	$54,307	$70,270	5.29
Liabilities & Equity				
	Current liabilities	$9,349	$15,267	10.31
	Long-term debt	$19,367	$23,089	3.58
	Other liabilities	$3,108	$4,670	8.48
	Equity	$40,384	$61,048	8.62
	Total liabilities and equity	$72,208	$104,074	7.58

Managers use similar data to monitor and control the HSO's/HS's functioning and how well it is accomplished. This may be done by comparing an activity to predetermined standards or by ratio analysis, which involves evaluating a relationship expressed as an index or percentage. These analyses are simple measures and typically are expressed in two modes: point specific and longitudinal. These analyses are applied to operational activity and financial status.[93]

OPERATIONAL ACTIVITY ANALYSIS

Operational activity analysis is control by evaluating input, process, or output variables. Control charts are one type of analysis. Run charts record performance over time and are the basis for control charts. Run chart data are used in calculating upper and lower control limits, which changes the run chart into a control chart. Control charts allow managers to distinguish common cause variation from special cause variation, which they must do before undertaking process improvement. Figure 7.10 is a control chart that shows the performance of process between the time noon meal food trays leave the kitchen and the time the first patient receives a tray on a nursing unit. Control charts can be developed for the performance of any process.

Another method for operational activity analysis is using and evaluating nonfinancial indices expressed in ratios or percentages. Managers can design operational activity ratios (or percentage indices) to meet specific control needs if they can be expressed numerically. Ratios are flexible and can be used as point-specific input, conversion, and output standards, as well as indicators of improvement. They can be tracked and compared longitudinally to show trends. Three broad categories are performance-to-utilization ratios, input-to-output ratios, and key indicator ratios.

Performance-to-utilization ratios provide index information about activities such as inventory turnover by area (dietary services, pharmacy, supply, laboratory), inventory dollar value per occupied bed, percentage of readmissions, and staff turnover and absenteeism by unit or type of employee. Ratios also yield information about capacity utilization, such as average length of stay, percentage occupancy, and efficient use of space and time (in surgical suites, clinics, emergency department, radiology). Finally, ratios provide indices of specific process outputs, usually expressed in patient days or other denominators, such as radiographs per admission, laboratory tests per patient day, clinic visits per day, pounds of laundry processed per occupied bed, and full-time equivalent employees (FTEs) per occupied bed.

Input-to-output ratios compare resource consumption by type to units of output. Examples are the hours by various types of staff per unit of service, such as nursing hours per patient day, radiographs per radiology technologist hour, and square feet cleaned per environmental services employee hour. Others are total revenue to FTEs, cost per discharge, and cost per patient day.

Key indicator ratios differ from the previous two groups. Ratios about patients and staff allow inferences to be drawn about quality. Examples include patient incidents and injuries per 100 patient days, percentage of incomplete medical records 30 days after patient discharge, gross and net death rates, anesthesia deaths per 10,000 surgical procedures, infection rates, and percentage of normal tissue removed in operative procedures. Other key indicator ratios include patient mix by type of payer, clinical staff mix by age or specialty, and patient origin mix by service area segment.

This discussion of performance-to-utilization, input-to-output, and key indicator ratio groupings is not exhaustive, but it illustrates that ratios can be derived by comparing any two numbers. When used in control, ratio analysis should address two issues. First, does the ratio provide meaningful information? Some do not; for example, the ratio of maintenance expenditures per Medicare patient day is meaningless. Managers must evaluate the underlying derivation of the ratio, what it measures, and its meaning. Second, judgment must be used in interpreting results. Particularly important is assessing the many causes of single-point deviation (i.e., deviation occurring at one point) or longitudinal deviation (i.e., change over time). Ratios are only one type of many indicators that show how actual results deviate from desired results. The cause of the deviation must be investigated, understood, and corrected, if necessary. Blindly using ratios will result in inappropriate conclusions and intervention, and almost certain undesirable consequences.

DATA ANALYSIS SERVICES

Data analysis services that provide comparative performance-to-utilization, input-to-output, key indicator, financial, and productivity and efficiency analyses for HSOs are available from vendors. The Center for Healthcare Industry Performance Studies (CHIPS) and Solucient are two examples.[94] Both provide industry data for performance indicators. Reports can be generated for individual hospitals to show indicators over time, provide benchmarks with similar hospitals, and present comparative results for virtually any hospital department. Furthermore, vendors can provide industry indicators by classifications such as bed size, urban/rural, region, state, teaching/nonteaching, system affiliation, and national averages.

BENCHMARKING

Benchmarking compares the organization's performance in various operational and clinical measures to reference standards and industry "best practices."[95] The comparison is with HSOs/HSs of similar type. CHIPS and Solucient provide benchmark data and "best practices" reference information. Benchmarking can also occur internally, as in the case of a horizontally integrated HS that compares system hospitals' performance. For control purposes, benchmarking provides standards against which comparisons can be made. Benchmarking is also discussed in Chapter 7.

FINANCIAL ANALYSIS

If numeric data are the common language of organizations, their lifeblood is finance. Financial ratio analysis calculates and evaluates various indices that measure the HSO's/HS's risk exposure, activity, and profitability. The accepted conventions for these measures are usually grouped into four categories, as summarized in Table 10.6:[96]

1. *Liquidity ratios* are risk measures that refer to the organization's ability to meet short-term obligations. Included are current ratio, acid test (also called quick) ratio, and collection period (or accounts receivable) ratio.
2. *Capital structure ratios* are also risk measures. They reflect the ratio of debt (borrowed funds) to total capital structure and, in the case of investor-owned HSOs/HSs, the proportion of debt to owners' investment (equity). In general, higher debt ratio(s) mean greater leverage and higher risk. Other risk-measuring ratios include cash flow to debt, and times interest earned.
3. *Activity ratios* are turnover measures that reflect asset utilization. In a sense, this is the degree to which various categories of assets generate revenue. Those presented in Table 10.6 compare operating revenue to total, net fixed, and current assets as well as to inventory.
4. *Profitability ratios* are indicators of the HSO's/HS's performance expressed in financial terms. Particularly critical measures are deductions (allowances for contractual adjustments and uncollectible accounts), operating margin, nonoperating revenue contribution, and return on assets. A measure that is important to investor-owned organizations is return on equity (operating income plus interest divided by stockholders' equity).

Financial and other data analyses, such as profitability, liquidity, capital structure, asset efficiency, and other financial ratios for comparison purposes, are available from vendors. Data are available by classifications such as hospital bed size, urban/rural, region, state, teaching/nonteaching, system affiliation, and national averages.

Use of Analytical Techniques in Resource Allocation

Converting inputs to outputs requires allocating and using resources. One dimension of control is determining if the allocation and use are appropriate and meet expectations. One dimension of CQI is improving processes to more efficiently use resources. Managers must understand the range of

TABLE 10.6. COMMON FINANCIAL RATIOS USED FOR CONTROL

Liquidity

1. Current $= \dfrac{\text{Current Assets}}{\text{Current Liabilities}}$

2. Acid Test $= \dfrac{\text{Cash + Marketable Securities}}{\text{Current Liabilities}}$

3. Collection Period $= \dfrac{\text{Net Accounts Receivable}}{\text{Average Daily Operating Revenue}}$

4. Average Payment Period $= \dfrac{\text{Current Liabilities}}{(\text{Total Operating Expenses} - \text{Depreciation}) \div 365}$

Capital Structure

5. Long-Term Debt to Fixed Assets $= \dfrac{\text{Long-Term Debt}}{\text{Net Fixed Assets}}$

6. Long-Term Debt to Liquidity $= \dfrac{\text{Long-Term Debt}}{\text{Unrestricted Fund Balance}}$

7. Times Interest Earned $= \dfrac{\text{Net Income + Interest}}{\text{Interest}}$

8. Debt Service Coverage $= \dfrac{\text{Net Income + Depreciation + Interest}}{\text{Principal Payment + Interest}}$

9. Cash Flow to Debt $= \dfrac{\text{Net Income + Depreciation}}{\text{Total Liabilities}}$

Activity

10. Total Asset Turnover $= \dfrac{\text{Total Operating Revenue}}{\text{Total Assets}}$

11. Fixed Asset Turnover $= \dfrac{\text{Total Operating Revenue}}{\text{Net Fixed Assets}}$

12. Current Asset Turnover $= \dfrac{\text{Total Operating Revenue}}{\text{Current Assets}}$

13. Inventory Turnover $= \dfrac{\text{Total Operating Revenue}}{\text{Inventory}}$

Profitability

14. Mark-Up $= \dfrac{\text{Gross Patient Revenue}}{\text{Operating Expenses}}$

15. Deductible $= \dfrac{\text{Allowances for Contractual Adjustments and Uncollectible Accounts}}{\text{Gross Patient Revenue}}$

16. Operating Margin $= \dfrac{\text{Operating Income}}{\text{Operating Revenue}}$

17. Nonoperating Revenue Contribution $= \dfrac{\text{Nonoperating Revenue}}{\text{Net Income}}$

18. Return on Assets $= \dfrac{\text{Operating Income + Interest}}{\text{Total Assets}}$

Composite

19. Viability Index $= \dfrac{[\text{Total Liabilities}]}{[\text{Total Assets}]} \times \dfrac{[\text{Operating Expense}]}{\text{Operating Revenue}} \times \dfrac{1}{\text{Current Ratio}} \times 4.0$

From Cleverley, William O. "Financial Ratios: Summary Indicators for Management Decision-Making." *Hospital & Health Services Administration* 26 (Special Issue, 1981): 30–31. Reprinted by permission. Chicago: Health Administration Press.

analytical techniques available as they make decisions about allocating resources, using resources, and improving processes.

Analytical techniques are methods or procedures that systematically arrange and evaluate information. They help managers focus on important aspects and compare them against criteria. Results are expressed in objective terms. The problem-solving process model in Figure 6.4 shows that analytical techniques help evaluate and select alternatives, especially those concerning resource allocation. It should be remembered that nonquantitative considerations are important when evaluating alternatives and that only when both nonquantitative and quantitative measures are included do effective problem solving and decision making occur. Analytical techniques are the predominant means for deriving objective information.

Analytical techniques are used to evaluate allocation and utilization of resources for new projects and improvement of current processes. Techniques described below are volume analysis (with and without revenue as a variable), capital budgeting, cost–benefit analysis, and simulation. Volume analysis with revenue as a variable is used to evaluate the economic viability of an alternative, such as adding a service or buying equipment. When revenue is not a variable, volume analysis can be used to evaluate alternatives with different fixed and variable cost characteristics and to evaluate the resource implications of improving an existing process. Capital budgeting is a ranking method used to compare several proposed alternatives. Cost–benefit analysis identifies and compares the resource consequences of two or more proposed alternatives, one of which can be the current situation. Finally, simulation yields "what if" information about the resource consequences of changes in existing situations—such as adding staff to decrease patient waiting time or modifying the flow of a process—without actually making the changes. Analytical techniques that are not included but that can be used are critical path analysis using Gantt charts; PERT charts; force field analysis; decision matrix analysis; decision trees; inventory analysis; linear programming; network analysis; plus/minus/interesting analysis; queuing; statistical techniques such as forecasting, hypothesis testing, and regression; and strengths/weaknesses/opportunities/threats (SWOT) analysis.[97] Table 10.7 briefly describes several of these techniques.

VOLUME ANALYSIS WITH REVENUE

Volume analysis with revenue as a variable is often called *break-even analysis.* It is one of the simplest analytical techniques available to evaluate the economic viability of a proposed alternative involving resource allocation. Figure 10.7 depicts volume analysis for an urgent care center. For such an analysis to be used, identifiable costs and identifiable revenue must be available. Important components of volume analysis with revenue as a variable are

- Identifiable revenues measured by price or charge (P) per unit of output or service (x) (e.g., charge per emergency department, outpatient, or office visit; per laboratory test, electrocardiogram, or radiograph; or per day of hospital or nursing facility stay)
- Identifiable fixed costs (FC)—costs that do not vary with output or volume (e.g., associated capital costs for facility and equipment lease or depreciation, and pay for minimum staffing levels)
- Identifiable variable costs (VC)—costs that vary with output or volume (e.g., for supplies, materials, medications, staff beyond minimum levels, and overtime)

Three variants of volume analysis yield different results depending on which variables are known. The break-even model determines the economic viability of an alternative. If fixed and variable costs and price/charge per unit of output/service are known, the break-even model determines

TABLE 10.7. QUANTITATIVE TECHNIQUES FOR DECISION ANALYSIS

Technique	Linear programming	Queuing theory	Network analysis	Regression analysis
Description	This technique attempts to optimize the distribution of scarce resources among competing activities. This is accomplished by the maximization or minimization of a dependent variable, which is a function of several independent variables that are subject to a set of restraints, i.e., limited resources. This method is capable of being executed manually, but is very adaptable to solution by a computer.	Queuing theory is the study of the probabilities associated with the length of a waiting line and the time an individual must wait in the queuing system. This information is used to achieve a balance between the cost of waiting for a service and the cost associated with providing this service. "Cost in a medical setting invariably includes elements defined by 'good medical care' which are, at best, difficult to quantify but must be included with monetary cost to obtain the proper solution." In queuing theory, the waiting line may be organized on a first-in–first-out basis, a random basis, or by some other priority technique. The waiting line can have a finite or infinite calling population, and it is assumed that the average service rate is greater than the average arrival rate for a single-channel–single-server queuing model.	Network analysis is characterized by a network of events and activities. Activities are defined as the actual performance of tasks, whereas events represent the start or completion of an activity. Events do not consume time. This technique allows the determination of probabilities of meeting specified deadlines; identifies bottlenecks in the project; evaluates the effect of shifting resources from a noncritical activity to a critical activity and vice versa, and enables the manager to evaluate the effect of a deviation of the actual time requirement for an activity from what had been predicted. Specific network analysis models include critical path methods (CPM), program evaluation and review techniques (PERT), and graphical evaluation and review techniques (GERT). The difference between these systems lies in their different abilities to analyze complex network systems.	This is a technique that derives a mathematical equation to describe or express the relationship between the data of two or more variables over a period of time. The variable to predict in this equation is referred to as the dependent variable. The other variables in the equation are called independent variables or predicting variables. The basic measure of the relationship between the dependent variable and the independent variable(s) is depicted by a regression line, which is computed by the method of least squares. This will result in an equation, based on historical data, that will predict the future behavior of the dependent variable. This technique is used primarily for the purpose of forecasting and control.
Hospital applications	Physician, nurse, and patient scheduling problems; purchasing problems associated with hospital supplies and equipment; hospital transportation problems and assignment problems	Determination of the most effective serving system for food service operations, outpatient clinic operations, admission operations, telephone switchboard operations, etc. In each of these situations, queuing theory balances the cost of an individual waiting with the cost of additional facilities that would be incurred to prevent the individual from waiting.	Hospital planning and control efforts associated with building or research and development projects or the determination of flow allocations through a health care system, such as a mass screening facility	Used to forecast dependent variables such as a number of hospital admissions, inpatient days, outpatient visits, outpatient days, average daily census, cost per patient day, etc., and to control deviations from the planned costs associated with each of these variables

Data required	Manager must express desires in a unidimensional objective function; data that pertain to an objective function expressed in terms of maximization of benefits or minimization of costs, set of constraints, variables, and alternative courses of action	Average number of arrivals per a unit of time; specified unit of time; average service time per arrival; number of waiting lines, number of waiting line phases, and number of people in the waiting line	Data that pertain to the determination of project activities and events; determination of optimistic, pessimistic, and most likely time estimates with associated mean activity times and time required for an activity in terms of probability distribution and associated parameters	Historical data compiled daily, monthly, quarterly, or annually with respect to the dependent and independent variables of the problem
Advantages	Optimum use of productive factors; potential to increase decision quality; highlights problem bottlenecks; forces objectivity and quantification	Description of probabilities that a waiting line will contain a certain number of individuals; expected length of the waiting line and the expected waiting time for the individual	Determination of longest time paths through a network; identification of the relative frequency of occurrence of different paths; evaluation of program changes	Provides accurate forecasts of dependent variables in a three-month to two-year time frame. Allows management to analyze deviations from the planned cost of an activity or event.
Disadvantages	Inability to represent several goals/objectives in a unidimensional objective function; costs associated with data upkeep; homogeneous values in constraints; assumption of linearity	Assumption that both arrival and service completion lines follow a Poisson distribution; upkeep of data	Accurate time forecasts for activities	Cost of data upkeep; assumption of linearity; the assumption that no causal relationship exists between the variables

Excerpted from Helmer, F. Theodore, William H. Kucheman, Edward B. Oppermann, and James D. Suver. "Basic Management Science Techniques for Decision Analysis." *Hospital & Health Service Administration* 27 (March/April 1982): 68–69. Reprinted by permission. Chicago: Health Administration Press.

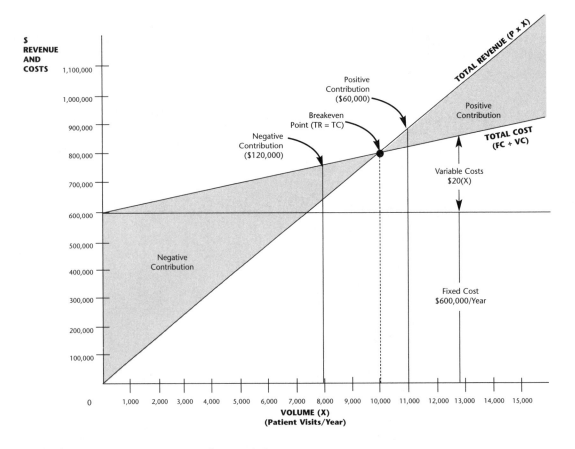

Figure 10.7. Urgent care center volume analysis.

the volume of output/service (x) needed to break even. It should be noted that type of provider reimbursement (fixed, such as DRG; capitated; cost-based; or charges) and payer mix significantly complicate the use of volume analysis.[98] Breaking even occurs when total revenue (price per unit of service times volume) equals total costs (fixed plus variable). The general formula is (solve for x)

$$\text{Breakeven point} = \frac{FC + VC(x)}{P(x)}$$

or

$$(P)(x) + VC(x) = FC$$

$$(P - VC)x = FC$$

$$x = \frac{FC}{P - VC}$$

A second variant of volume analysis is determining the net (positive or negative) contribution (*NC*) that results from an alternative when price or charge, total volume, and fixed and variable costs are known. Positive net contribution occurs when total revenue (volume times price) exceeds total costs (fixed plus variable); net contribution is negative when total costs exceed total revenue. The general formula is (solve for *NC*)

$$P(x) = FC + VC(x) + NC$$

or

$$NC = P(x) - [FC + VC(x)]$$

The third variant of volume analysis is to use it as a price- or charge-setting model. If fixed and variable costs and volume are known, the technique yields the price or charge per unit of output/service required to meet end-result criteria ranging from breaking even (where total revenue equals total costs) to attaining a specific net positive contribution. When *NC* is set at the value desired—which may be zero—the general formula is (solve for *P*)

$$P(x) = FC + VC(x) + NC$$

or

$$P = \frac{FC + VC(x) + NC}{x}$$

HSOs/HSs encounter many situations with identifiable cost and revenue attributes in which volume analysis can be applied. Examples are acquiring new equipment (magnetic resonance imager, laboratory diagnostic equipment), expanding facilities (new beds, parking deck), adding new services (neonatology, open-heart surgery), and embarking on new ventures (emergency care center, ambulatory surgery center, physicians' office building). Depending on known variables or assumptions made about them, volume analysis can determine economic viability. Will the project break even? Will it have a net positive or negative contribution? Volume analysis can be used, too, as a price-setting model to meet specific criteria, that is, break even or yield a net positive contribution. Figure 10.7 shows these relationships. An acute care hospital proposes to open a freestanding satellite urgent care center. Fixed costs (building and equipment depreciation, minimum staffing levels) are $600,000/year. Variable costs (supplies and materials) per patient visit are assumed to be $20. The average price/charge per patient visit is $80. Volume analysis can be used to determine what number of patient visits per year (or per day) will be necessary to break even. This is determined as follows (solve for *x*):

$$P(x) = FC + VC(x)$$

$$\$80(x) = \$600,000 + \$20(x)$$

$$\$60(x) = \$600,000$$

$$x = \frac{\$600,000}{\$60}$$

$$x = 10,000$$

Thus, for the project to break even, 10,000 patient visits per year (28/day) will be necessary.

If other information (knowledge about competition, population in the service area) is available, the decision maker can judge whether it is reasonable to expect 10,000 patient visits per year (28/day) and determine the economic viability of the project. If only 8,000 patient visits can be expected each year, the net (negative) contribution would be –$120,000, as indicated in Figure 10.7. Algebraically, this is determined as follows (solve for NC):

$$P(x) = FC + VC(x) + NC$$
$$\$80 \,(8{,}000) = \$600{,}000 + \$20 \,(8{,}000) + NC$$
$$\$60 \,(8{,}000) = \$600{,}000 + NC$$
$$\$480{,}000 = \$600{,}000 + NC$$
$$NC = \$480{,}000 + (-\$600{,}000)$$
$$NC = -\$120{,}000$$

Similarly, if volume were 11,000 patient visits per year, net (positive) revenue would be $60,000. Freestanding satellite urgent care centers often see patients whose needs are greater than they can meet. Estimates must be made as to the income (or loss) that might result from referral of these cases to the acute care hospital's emergency department or other services. Hospital management must see the system (hospital and urgent care center) as a whole. It may be necessary (or desirable) for the urgent care center to suboptimize its financial performance so that performance of the entire system is optimized, whether in terms of community service or referrals and/or revenue.

VOLUME ANALYSIS WITHOUT REVENUE

Often, HSOs/HSs have alternative situations that do not have identifiable revenue attributes but do have volume and fixed and variable cost attributes. Volume analysis without revenue evaluates and compares the cost consequences of alternatives. It may be used in situations in which there is no revenue or when revenue is indeterminate. Because revenue is not a variable, the analysis focuses on fixed and variable cost trade-offs among volume alternatives.

Figure 10.8 illustrates the concept. Leasing one of two photocopying machines is being considered. Machine A is slow (10 copies per minute) and leases for $200/month (fixed cost). Machine B is faster (30 copies per minute) and leases for $600/month. Machine A has a lower fixed cost than Machine B ($FC_a < FC_b$); however, the variable cost of staff waiting at the machine while photocopying is higher ($VC_a > VC_b$). Given the different fixed and variable cost attributes, the preferred alternative is different at various volume levels. If volume is x_1, then Machine A is preferred because total costs are lower ($TC_{a1} < TC_{b1}$). If volume is x_2, then Machine B is preferred ($TC_{b2} < TC_{a2}$). Alternative preference is thus dependent on the extent to which there are fixed and variable cost trade-offs relative to volume.

Volume analysis without revenue is powerful because it focuses on the relationship of cost components to volume alternatives. Applications include equipment replacement and machine/technology–people substitution. As larger percentages of HSO/HS revenues are prospectively determined by case (i.e., DRGs) or capitated, alternative evaluation from a cost trade-off perspective becomes more important.

CAPITAL BUDGETING

Capital budgeting refers to techniques that evaluate, compare, and rank multiple capital investment alternatives or compare single alternatives to a given criterion such as rate of return. The degree of sophistication ranges from simply determining payback period to complex evaluations of revenue and cost streams that are discounted to net present value.[99]

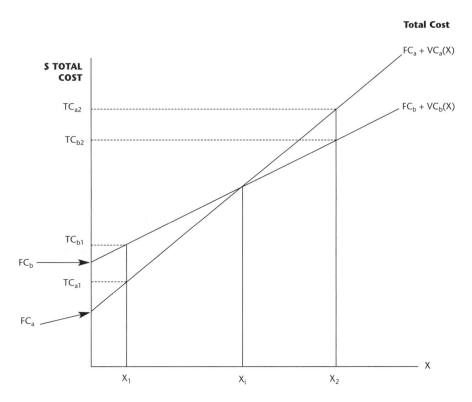

Figure 10.8. Volume analysis without revenue.

Payback is an uncomplicated capital budgeting technique because it does not consider the net present value of revenue and cost streams for investment alternatives under consideration. It simply determines the number of years needed to recoup an initial investment and yields a gross index of the desirability of investment alternatives. In any comparison of multiple investment alternatives, the one with the shortest payback period (lowest index) is preferred. Results are distorted, however, if revenue and cost streams are dissimilar and the useful lives of alternatives differ appreciably. Type of provider payment and payer mix also affect the analysis. A more precise ranking index is the net present value of alternatives.

In payback analysis, necessary components for each alternative are

- Identifiable annual revenue generated
- Identifiable annual costs
- Identifiable investment and salvage value

The payback technique has two elements. The first is net investment, which is initial cost minus salvage value. The second is annual net benefit from the investment, if selected. Net benefit is determined by revenue generated minus operating expenses. Dividing net investment by net benefit determines the number of years to return the cost of the investment. The general formula for the payback period is

$$\text{Payback period} = \frac{(\text{Cost of the proposed investment}) - (\text{Salvage value})}{(\text{Revenue generated from investment}) - (\text{Operating expenses})}$$

It should be noted that payback is used predominantly to rank and compare multiple capital investment alternatives (e.g., whether to acquire personal computers for managers or fetal monitoring equipment) or alternatives for the same use (e.g., which vendor's personal computers to acquire). If investment, cost, and revenue streams are discounted to present value (and assuming a given rate of interest), a new present value index similar to the payback index can be used to rank alternatives. Applications usually involve equipment addition or replacement or facility expansion or alternatives such as building a parking deck or office building.

COST–BENEFIT ANALYSIS

Conceptually, cost–benefit analysis is similar to payback analysis and is "the analysis of healthcare resource expenditures relative to possible medical benefit."[100] Unlike payback analysis (a capital budgeting technique), cost–benefit analysis may be used whether or not there is an identifiable revenue stream. Cost–benefit analysis is often used to evaluate government programs.

Cost–benefit analysis is widely applicable in most areas of an HSO's/HS's operations and can be used readily in process improvement decisions. It involves comparing two or more alternatives, one of which may be an existing situation. Cost components are required; a revenue component can be incorporated if present, although revenue is not required for the analysis.

Important components in cost–benefit analysis are

- Identifiable imputed or actual costs associated with the proposed alternatives (one of which may be the current situation)
- Identifiable changes in productivity (and imputed value of the productivity) that represent cost savings associated with the proposed alternatives (one of which may be the current situation)
- Identifiable changes in revenue associated with the proposed alternatives (though not required for the analysis)
- Other considerations that may not be quantifiable

Actual or imputed costs associated with an alternative can include capital expenditures for equipment, space, employees, and materials and supplies. Net benefit is the marginal difference between the components listed previously for each of the proposed alternatives. That is, net benefit equals Alternative A minus Alternative B for the previous components. A positive net benefit suggests that the proposed alternative is better. However, nonquantifiable considerations, such as effect on customer satisfaction or organizational control, may argue for acceptance of a particular alternative even though it may have higher costs and/or fewer benefits. In this instance, the decision maker evaluates the importance of nonquantifiable considerations and whether they outweigh the quantifiable effects.

Cost–benefit analysis has wide applicability in HSOs/HSs. Examples include evaluating the cost–benefit of using disposable versus nondisposable tableware in the cafeteria, computer system upgrades, owning or leasing a phone system, and outsourcing in-house services such as IS, environmental services, and food service. Applications can occur in all situations that have identified or imputed costs and benefits (which may be revenue based but more often are cost-savings based) associated with alternatives, one of which may be the existing situation.

Table 10.8 is an application of cost–benefit analysis. Community Memorial Medical Center, a 211-bed facility, is considering two alternatives. Alternative A involves upgrading its existing information system to include more-sophisticated cost accounting and decision support capability. Alternative B is to outsource this application. Table 10.8 indicates that Alternative A would require Community Memorial Medical Center to make a one-time expenditure for additional hardware of $4,000; pay software purchasing/licensing fees of $75,865 in the first year and $15,173/year there-

TABLE 10.8. COMMUNITY MEMORIAL MEDICAL CENTER, ANYTOWN, USA (211 ADJUSTED OCCUPIED BEDS)[a]

	Year 1	Year 2	Year 3	Year 4	Year 5	Year 6	Year 7
Alternative A: medical center–related costs							
Annual costs							
Computer hardware	4,000						
Software license	75,865	15,173	15,173	15,173	15,173	15,173	15,173
Annual cost standards maintenance							
(starts in second year)		15,628	16,097	16,580	17,077	17,590	18,117
Added client staff costs (1 FTE)	56,250	57,938	59,676	61,466	63,310	65,209	67,165
Total package cost per year	136,115	88,739	90,946	93,219	95,560	97,972	100,455
Discounted annual cost—							
medical center related	136,115	82,165	77,971	74,000	70,240	66,678	63,304
Alternative B: outsourcing costs [b]							
Service fee for 12 months	60,660	62,480	64,354	66,285	68,273	70,322	72,431
Discounted annual cost—outsourcing	60,660	57,852	55,173	52,619	50,183	47,860	45,644

	Alternative A: medical center	Alternative B: outsourcing	Cost–benefit A–B	Savings (%) (A–B) ÷ A
Summary of life cycle costs				
5-Year sum of discounted costs	440,491	276,487	164,004	37.2%
7-Year sum of discounted costs	570,473	369,991	200,482	35.1%

[a]All amounts in U.S. dollars. Assumptions:
1. Annual increase in CPI — 3.0%
2. Discount rate — 8.0%
3. Annual cost of 1 FTE with benefits — $56,250
4. Annual software maintenance percent — 20.0%

[b]Outsourcing pricing formula:
1. Number of adjusted occupied beds (AOB) — 211
2. Volume charge per bed (VOL) — $5
3. Monthly service fee = $4,000 + (VOL × AOB) — $5,055

after; incur annual costs of standards maintenance, starting at $15,628 in the second year and increasing thereafter; and add one new FTE, at an annual cost of $56,250, with increases in subsequent years. Alternative B— outsourcing—requires an initial monthly fee of $5,055 (a base of $4,000 plus a volume charge of $5 per adjusted occupied bed) during the first year, which totals $60,660, with increases in subsequent years.

Table 10.8 shows the cost stream—discounted to present value—for both alternatives with the assumptions that annual inflation measured by the consumer price index will be 3.0%; the discount rate will be 8.0%; and the annual cost standards maintenance will increase 3.0% per year, starting with the second year. Evaluation of the 5- and 7-year sums of discounted costs for both alternatives indicates that outsourcing (Alternative B) is more cost-effective for both time periods. Over a 5-year time period, outsourcing, compared with the in-house alternative, would save $164,004; it would save $200,483 over the 7-year time period. Given this information, it is logical to outsource cost accounting and decision support applications. A nonquantitative consideration is whether the HSO wants to be dependent on an outside vendor for such critical information.

SIMULATION

Simulation is one of the most powerful analytical tools available to health services managers in making resource allocation decisions and in determining whether and how processes can be improved.

It enables managers to ask "what if" questions and review the implications and consequences of alternatives without altering the present situation.

Simulation involves constructing a detailed, computer-based mathematical model that represents situations and variables. The model has detailed rules that each variable follows as it interacts with the "system," which may be a work process such as diagnostic testing or surgery and recovery. The simulation literature uses the term *system* to denote such a process, and that term is used here. The simulation model replicates and reflects variables in the system. It is constructed using mathematical expressions of relationships, attributes, and probability distributions of events derived from empirical observations of the system. The model is activated by use of a random number generator to represent events, such as admission, arrival for service, a particular type of surgical case, and length of stay.

Simulation models are dynamic. When variables, rules, or assumptions are changed, the model produces the consequences of that change. When no change is made in the relationships of variables in the model (static state), simulation can forecast the effect of increased demand on the system and suggest what resource allocation and capacity changes are needed to meet the desired level of quality. In a dynamic state, variable relationships can be changed, "what if" questions can be asked, and the results will indicate whether and how systems can be improved to enhance the quality of a product or service.

Simulation is applicable to any activity that involves scheduling and service rates and capacity constraints, for both physical plant and staffing.[101] Simulation has been applied to admission processes, operating room utilization, emergency departments, diagnostic testing, clinics, ancillary services, bed planning, and nurse staffing.

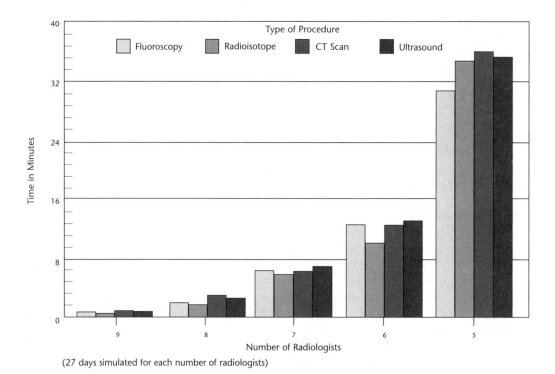

(27 days simulated for each number of radiologists)

Figure 10.9. Patient wait time by procedure (excludes processing time); average wait time for greater than zero. (Based on data from Klafehn, Keith A., Paul J. Kuzdrall, Jonathon S. Rakich, and Alan G. Krigline. "Application of Simulation in Hospital Resource Allocation and Utilization." *Journal of Management Science & Policy Analysis* 8 [Spring/Summer 1991]: 346–356.)

To solve a capacity problem and to increase patient satisfaction, a simulation model for diagnostic testing was designed for a 500-bed acute care hospital. Management was concerned about the quality of patient service, specifically complaints about waiting times in radiology.[102] The simulation model depicted arrival, processing, and waiting times for eight types of inpatients and outpatients. Procedures tracked included fluoroscopy, radioisotope scanning, computerized tomography (CT) scan, and ultrasound. Distributions of arrival rates by type of patient and service times by type of procedure were based on observation of the actual system. The simulation determined the effects of various capacity changes on queues and patient waiting time. Figure 10.9 shows the results of simulating changes in capacity—increasing the number of radiologists (note that the scale is reversed, so the horizontal axis should be read right to left). Patient waiting time before the start of service decreased substantially (approximately 22 minutes for each of the procedures) when capacity was increased from five to six radiologists. Increasing the number of radiologists provided the largest marginal gain for all capacity configurations. Only a modest decrease in waiting time (about 6 minutes) occurred when a seventh radiologist was added.[103] This simulation provided "what if" information useful in deciding whether and how to alter a capacity-bound process. Such information enables managers to make more-informed resource allocation and utilization decisions.

The power of simulation as an analytical technique in resource allocation and utilization and in process improvement is evident. To the extent that health services managers are generally familiar with it and the other techniques presented here, they can positively affect the quality of output, improve the processes that generate it, make more informed resource allocation decisions, and control to ensure that actual results meet or exceed expected results.

▬ DISCUSSION QUESTIONS ▬

1. Define *control*. What are the major elements of control?
2. What are the three monitoring and two intervention points for control? Why is MIS important to control?
3. Review the control model in Figure 10.2, and give examples of situations for each of the control loops. What are the similarities between the control model (Figure 10.2) and the problem-solving model presented in Figure 6.4?
4. How does CQI relate to control? Specifically, what control point is its focus, and how does this affect the control model (see Figure 10.2)?
5. Describe the purpose, structure, and process of RM and QI. From the perspective of control, why are both important to HSOs/HSs?
6. What are the duties of risk managers? How do they fit into the organization of HSOs? HSs?
7. Discuss the concept of insurance. What is the role of insurance in HSO/HS management? How does insurance fit into a RM program?
8. Contrast traditional QA with QI as formulated by W. Edwards Deming (see Chapter 7). How are they complementary? Contradictory?
9. Distinguish Donabedian's conceptualization of quality as a function of and measurable by process and outcome. Provide and discuss a clinical or nonclinical example that shows the application of this conceptualization.
10. Identify control methods presented in this chapter. Why are budgets and ratio analyses so important? How do both relate to the control model in Figure 10.2?
11. Identify the analytical techniques for resource allocation presented in this chapter. Explain how and why they are useful.
12. Define *suboptimization*. Describe how this concept must be incorporated into financial analysis.

▪ Case Study 1: Admitting Department

Shelley York is supervisor of the admitting department at Newhealth, a health maintenance organization. Three clerks—Shemenski, Turner, and Underwood—report to her. All are responsible for processing patients. Using a sampling method for monitoring productivity, York obtained the following data for a 2-hour period:

Shemenski processed 14 patients.
Turner processed 16 patients.
Underwood processed 11 patients.

Each clerk is expected to process 7 patients per hour.

QUESTIONS

1. What should York do?
2. What is the control point (input, process, or output)?
3. What kind of information should York obtain relative to Turner and Underwood? What might be some of the "causes" for the deviations?

▪ Case Study 2: Centralized Photocopying

Carey Snook saw Ted Rath drinking coffee in the cafeteria. "I thought you guys in management services were up to your eyeballs in productivity improvement projects," Snook said as he walked over to sit down with Rath.

"We are," Rath said. "In fact, we have so much work and so many project deadlines coming up that we've had to work Saturdays."

Snook responded, "Then how come you're goofing off by wasting time and drinking coffee?"

"I'm not wasting time," said Rath. "I'm waiting."

"For what?" said Snook.

"For some layout prints to be reproduced. We're in the middle of a systems analysis project. We're redesigning the outpatient department layout and work process flow. I can't continue with the project until I get the template layout drawings copied in central photocopying. Our secretary took them over there 20 minutes ago, and they won't be ready for another 20 minutes. So, I'm waiting. This happens about three times a week to each of the three of us in my department."

Rath continued, "We used to have a photocopier in our department. Well, some people were caught copying personal documents. This probably cost the hospital about $10 a week, so they centralized all photocopying equipment to save money on use and have fewer machines. Now we have to walk our materials way over there to the central building and wait until it's our turn to have them reproduced.

"I guess the biggest gripe I have is with Smith, head of centralized photocopying. Sometimes it takes 10 minutes to convince Smith that the reproduction job is hospital business and is important. Smith really seems to like the authority. Anyway, take this isometric drawing I have here; I bet Smith will think it's my 6-year-old daughter's homework assignment. I wonder how long it will take me to convince Smith it is job related."

"Want some more coffee?" asked Snook.

QUESTIONS

1. What is the focus of control in this situation?
2. What dysfunctional results have occurred from centralizing photocopying?

Case Study 3: Barriers to an Effective QI Effort

District Hospital is a 260-bed, public, general acute care hospital owned by a special tax district. Its service area includes five communities with a total population of 180,000 in a southeastern coastal state in one of the nation's fastest growing counties. It is one of three hospitals owned by the special tax district. The seven other hospitals in District Hospital's general service area make the environment highly competitive.

District Hospital has a wide range of services and a medical staff of 527 representing most specialties. The emergency department (ED) is a major source of admissions. Last year, 26,153 patients visited the ED and 3,745, or 14.3%, were admitted. This was 42% of total hospital admissions. Some admissions were sent to the ED by private physicians, and some came by ambulance, but most were self-referred.

The hospital chief executive officer, W.G. Lester, noted that the number of visits to the ED was decreasing. Over a 3-year period, they had declined from a high of 29,345 to the current low of 26,153. Only part of this reduction seemed attributable to competition. Lester was also concerned about an increasing number of complaints concerning the quality of ED services. The complaints related to waiting time, poor attitudes of physicians, and questions about the quality of care. Investigation found that many complaints were justified, but the causes of these problems were difficult to discern.

Registered nurses (RNs) employed in the ED want a larger role in triaging and treating patients, but the dominance of ED physicians limits the RNs' duties and frustrates other staff, as well. This is manifested among RN staff by high turnover, low morale, and difficulty in recruitment and retention.

Another factor is the emergency medical technician (EMT) program started in the county a few years ago. The EMTs are an important community medical resource and are very influential in deciding the hospital to which patients in ambulances will be transported. It will be necessary for District Hospital, through the ED physicians, to participate actively in training and managing the EMT program if District Hospital is to receive its share of emergency patients. ED physicians have refused to participate in teaching or directing the program, however. In fact, they often alienate the EMTs.

Lester is concerned, too, that the position of full-time director of emergency medicine at District Hospital has been vacant for 4 years. Residency programs in emergency medicine are producing physicians who are seeking positions with higher salaries and better working conditions than those available at District Hospital.

There has been little turnover among the six physicians who staff the ED; they include one general surgeon (retired from private practice), two internists, and three non–U.S.-trained medical graduates with specialties in family practice. The ED physicians seem to lack a clear commitment to District Hospital. All of them contract separately with the hospital to provide ED services. District Hospital bills ED patients and collects the physicians' fees: moneys above the guaranteed minimum are paid to them pro rata. They participate in District Hospital's fringe benefits and are covered by its professional liability insurance policy.

One ED physician, Dr. Balck (the retired surgeon), recognizes the progress being made nationally in emergency medicine. She made several unsuccessful attempts to move District Hospital in the same direction. With great effort, she instituted programs on intradepartmental education and mandatory attendance at approved courses in emergency medicine. Quality-related activities, however, are done perfunctorily. Also, she had tried to obtain full recognition of the ED and its work by other members of the PSO.

The members of the PSO seem satisfied with the situation. Its executive committee does not understand the changing status of emergency medicine. As evidence of its unwillingness to grant full recognition to the department, the PSO has consistently denied the ED's requests for full departmental status.

QUESTIONS

1. Use the problem-solving methodology described in Chapter 6 to define the problem facing Lester. Which alternative solution should be implemented? Why?
2. Describe the relationship between inpatient census and ED admissions. Outline a strategy to educate the members of the ED physician staff as to the relationship and importance of the ED to the financial good health of District Hospital.
3. Use the principles of CQI from Chapter 7 to outline a basic effort to improve quality in the ED.
4. Analyze the role of the EMTs and their relationship with District Hospital. What should be the role of ED physicians and staff at District Hospital in terms of educating the EMTs? What are the negative aspects of this educational activity? Is there a potential conflict of interest?
5. Identify some control measures that could be used by Lester.

■ Case Study 4: State Allocation Decisions—Centralize or Decentralize[104]

The 50 states vary in how much control of operations and funding is delegated to city and county health departments. In Ohio, for instance, the state health department provides very little funding for local health departments and provides little direction as to how they manage public health programs for the state.

In Kentucky, local health departments are generously supported by the state health department and are expected to be its agent in managing programs such as family planning, health education, and well-baby clinics. However, numerous "strings" come with the money in Kentucky. Unlike in Ohio, the Kentucky state health department dictates the local health department's accounting systems, restaurant inspection fee structure, septic tank exception, employee health insurance benefits, and many other decisions that would be left to the local health departments in Ohio.

Still another type of state-local arrangement is that in Virginia. Local health departments in Virginia are staffed solely with state employees and are operated exclusively by policies set in the state capital.

These varied relationships raise a classic management question: centralization or decentralization of operational authority. Each approach has significant advantages and disadvantages. For example, some managers prefer the clarity and fairness of centralized systems. Others want policy setting to be more flexible and responsive—keeping it as close to the delivery site and its clients as possible.

QUESTIONS

1. What risks are present with the Ohio policy that allows local health departments to establish their own bookkeeping systems?
2. Why might some regulated clients, such as home builders and restaurant chains, prefer to have local health department policies and fees determined centrally for the entire state?
3. Why might a decentralized local health department prefer to negotiate its own employees' health insurance package even if it represents a group of smaller size that cannot get as low a premium?
4. Based on considerations of centralization and decentralization, would you prefer to be the *state* health department director in Kentucky, Ohio, or Virginia? Why?

■ Case Study 5: Financial Ratios

General Hospital (GH) is a freestanding 265-bed nongovernmental, not-for-profit HSO. Review the income statement and balance sheet provided here.

GENERAL HOSPITAL INCOME STATEMENT (YEAR ENDING DECEMBER 31, 2007)

Revenues	
Operating revenue	
Inpatient	$38,800,000
Outpatient	49,000,000
Gross patient revenue	$87,800,000
Less contractual allowances & deductions	($23,500,000)
Net patient operating revenue (operating revenue)	$64,300,000
Other income	
Contributions	$ 2,000,000
Misc. income	5,400,000
Total other income	7,400,000
Total operating revenue and income	$71,700,000
Expenses	
Salaries and benefits	$27,000,000
Depreciation and amortization	3,400,000
Interest	300,000
Other expenses	30,000,000
Total operating expenses	$60,700,000
Net income	$11,000,000
Net operating income[a]	$ 3,600,000

[a]Net operating revenue/income = 11,000,000 less $7,400,000 = $3,600,000.

GENERAL HOSPITAL BALANCE SHEET (YEAR ENDING DECEMBER 31, 2007)

Assets	
Current assets	
Cash	$ 4,000,000
Temporary investments	2,700,000
Accounts receivables	11,000,000
(less allowance for uncollectable accounts receivables)	(2,800,000)
Other receivables	1,400,000
Inventory	1,100,000
Prepaid expenses	20,000
Total current assets	$17,420,000
Fixed assets	
Land and improvements	$ 3,000,000
(less accumulated depreciation)	(1,500,000)
Buildings	24,000,000
(less accumulated depreciation)	(10,000,000)
Equipment	45,000,000
(less accumulated depreciation)	(25,000,000)
Total fixed assets	$35,500,000
Other assets (investments long term)	$25,400,000
Total assets	$78,320,000

(continued)

GENERAL HOSPITAL BALANCE SHEET (YEAR ENDING DECEMBER 31, 2007) *(continued)*

Liabilities

Current liabilities

Accounts payable	$ 3,000,000
Wages and salaries payable	4,200,000
Short-term loans	4,000,000
Total current liabilities	$11,000,000

Long-term liabilities

Mortgage payable	$12,000,000
Other long-term debt	4,200,000
Total long-term liabilities	$16,200,000
Total liabilities	$27,200,000

Equity

General fund balance	$51,120,000
Total liabilities and equity	$78,320,000

Use the financial ratio formulas provided in Table 10.6 to calculate the values listed in the following table.

Item	Calculated value	Benchmark value
1. Current ratio		1.95
2. Acid test		0.31
3. Average payment period		60 days
4. Long-term debt to fixed assets		0.70
5. Operating profit margin		4.3%
6. Return on total assets		5.7%
7. Collection period		46.4 days
8. Total asset turnover		0.92
9. Contractual allowances and discounts as percentage of operating patient revenue[a]		41.3%

[a]Contractual allowances and discounts divided by gross patient revenue.

QUESTION

1. What do you conclude when comparing the calculated values for GH with the benchmark values that are supplied by HCIA for hospitals of similar size and type in the same state?

Notes

1. Bartol, Kathryn M., and David C. Martin. *Management,* 3rd ed., 523. Boston: Irwin/McGraw-Hill, 1998.
2. Bartol and Martin, *Management,* 523.
3. Van Fleet, David D. *Contemporary Management,* 444. Boston: Houghton Mifflin, 1991.
4. Pearce, John A., II, and Richard B. Robinson, Jr. *Management,* 584. New York: Random House, 1989.
5. Bartol and Martin, *Management,* 515.
6. Enthoven, Alain C., and Carol B. Vorhaus. "A Vision of Quality in Health Care Delivery." *Health Affairs* 16 (May/June 1997): 48.

7. Brown, Michael S. "Industry Information: Technology Trends." *CARING Magazine* 16 (December 1997): 69.

8. Austin, Charles J., and Stuart B. Boxerman. *Information Systems for Healthcare Management,* 6th ed., 4–5. Chicago: Health Administration Press, 2003.

9. Nilson, Julie T. "How to Hire the Right CIO." *Healthcare Executive* 13 (May/June 1998): 8–13.

10. Austin and Boxerman, *Information Systems for Healthcare Management,* 362.

11. Shaffer, Michael D., and Michael J. Shaffer. "Business Reengineering, Information Technology, and the Healthcare Connection." *Hospital Topics* 74 (Spring 1996): 12.

12. Austin and Boxerman, *Information Systems for Healthcare Management,* 231.

13. Clerkin, Daniel, and Peter J. Fos. "A Decision Support System for Hospital Bed Assignment." *Hospital & Health Services Administration* 40 (Fall 1995): 386.

14. Austin and Boxerman, *Information Systems for Healthcare Management,* 251.

15. "Increased CAD Use Prompts Look at Advantages, Drawbacks." *RSNA News* (February 2007): 10–11.

16. Austin and Boxerman, *Information Systems for Healthcare Management,* 163–167.

17. Kleinke, J.D. "Release 0.0: Clinical Information Technology in the Real World." *Health Affairs* 17 (November/December 1998): 27.

18. SATTELIFE. *Critical Care Medicine: Introduction,* 3–4. December 28, 2002. *http://www.healthnet.org .np/resource/thesis/anes/Introduction.pdf,* retrieved January 9, 2004.

19. Supplemented and adapted from White, Andrea W., and Gloria R. Wakefield. "Developing an Electronic Medical Record for an Integrated Physician Office Practice." In *Information Systems for Healthcare Management,* 6th ed., edited by Charles J. Austin and Stuart B. Boxerman, 326. Chicago: Health Administration Press, 2003.

20. Kleinke, "Release 0.0," 27.

21. Austin, Charles J., Jerry M. Trimm, and Patrick M. Sobczak. "Information Systems and Strategic Management." *Health Care Management Review* 20 (Summer 1995): 31.

22. Austin and Boxerman, *Information Systems for Healthcare Management,* 6th ed., part III.

23. U.S. Department of Labor, Bureau of Labor Statistics. "Occupational Employment and Wages, 2006." *http://www.bls.gov/news.release/pdf/ocwage.pdf,* retrieved August 26, 2007.

24. The Joint Commission. *Comprehensive Accreditation Manual for Hospitals, Refreshed Core,* HR-1. Oakbrook Terrace, IL: Joint Commission on Accreditation of Healthcare Organizations, January 2007.

25. Hernandez, S. Robert, Myron D. Fottler, and Charles L. Joiner. "Integrating Strategic Management and Human Resources." In *Essentials of Human Resources Management in Health Services Organizations,* edited by Myron D. Fottler, S. Robert Hernandez, and Charles L. Joiner, 2. Albany, NY: Delmar Publishers, 1998.

26. Gómez-Mejía, Luis R., David B. Balkin, and Robert L. Cardy. *Managing Human Resources,* 3rd ed., 147. Upper Saddle River, NJ: Prentice-Hall, 1998.

27. Cascio, Wayne F. *Managing Human Resources: Productivity, Quality of Work Life, Profits,* 5th ed., 148. Boston: Irwin/McGraw-Hill, 1998.

28. Mathis, Robert L., and John H. Jackson. *Human Resource Management: Essential Perspectives,* 72. Cincinnati, OH: South-Western Publishing, 1999.

29. Gómez-Mejía, Balkin, and Cardy, *Managing Human Resources,* 153–154.

30. Cascio, *Managing Human Resources,* 134–136.

31. Fottler, Myron D. "Job Analysis." In *Essentials of Human Resources Management in Health Services Organizations,* edited by Myron D. Fottler, S. Robert Hernandez, and Charles L. Joiner, 118. Albany, NY: Delmar Publishers, 1998.

32. Harris, Michael. *Human Resource Management: A Practical Approach,* 120. Fort Worth, TX: Dryden Press/Harcourt Brace, 1997.

33. Mathis and Jackson, *Human Resource Management,* 58.

34. Harris, *Human Resource Management,* 121.

35. Landau, Jacqueline, and Michael Abelson. "Recruitment and Selection." In *Essentials of Human Resources Management in Health Services Organizations,* edited by Myron D. Fottler, S. Robert Hernandez, and Charles L. Joiner, 134–165. Albany, NY: Delmar Publishing, 1998.

36. See Fottler, "Job Analysis," 117–133.

37. See Joiner, Charles L., and John C. Hyde. "Performance Appraisal." In *Essentials of Human Resources*

Management in Health Services Organizations, edited by Myron D. Fottler, S. Robert Hernandez, and Charles L. Joiner, 223–247. Albany, NY: Delmar Publishing, 1998.

38. Drucker, Peter F. *Managing the Non-Profit Organization,* 62. New York: HarperCollins, 1990.
39. Cascio, *Managing Human Resources,* 321.
40. Noe, Raymond A. *Employee Training and Development,* 4. Boston: Irwin/McGraw-Hill, 1999.
41. Smith, Howard L., and Myron D. Fottler. "Training and Development." In *Essentials of Human Resources Management in Health Services Organizations,* edited by Myron D. Fottler, S. Robert Hernandez, and Charles L. Joiner, 197–222. Albany, NY: Delmar Publishing, 1998.
42. Fottler, Myron D. "The Role and Impact of Multiskilled Health Practitioners in the Health Services Industry." *Hospital & Health Services Administration* 41 (Spring 1996): 56.
43. See Joiner, Charles L., Kerma N. Jones, and Carson F. Dye. "Compensation Management." In *Essentials of Human Resources Management in Health Services Organizations,* edited by Myron D. Fottler, S. Robert Hernandez, and Charles L. Joiner, 248–270. Albany, NY: Delmar Publishing, 1998.
44. Noe, Raymond A., John R. Hollenbeck, Barry Gerhart, and Patrick M. Wright. *Human Resource Management: Gaining a Competitive Advantage,* 2nd ed., 463. Boston: Irwin/McGraw-Hill, 1997.
45. Hofrichter, David A., and Gordon W. Hawthorne. "Governing Performance: Examining the Board's Role in Executive Compensation." *Trustee* 50 (June 1997): 7; Keefe, Thomas J., George R. French, and James L. Altman. "Incentive Plans Can Link Employee and Company Goals." *Journal of Compensation and Benefits* 9, 4 (January/February 1994): 27.
46. Kleiman, Lawrence S. *Human Resource Management: A Tool for Competitive Advantage,* 272. Minneapolis-St. Paul, MN: West Publishing, 1997.
47. Fernberg, Patricia. "Substance Abuse Is Risky Business." *Occupational Hazards* 60 (October 1998): 67.
48. Howard, John C., and David Szcerbacki. "Employee Assistance Programs in the Hospital Industry." *Health Care Management Review* 13 (Spring 1988): 74.
49. Kleiman, *Human Resource Management,* 412.
50. Occupational Safety and Health Act of 1970, PL 91-596, 29 U.S.C. sect 651 et seq.; Twomey, David P. *A Concise Guide to Employment Law, EEO & OSHA,* 109. Cincinnati, OH: South-Western Publishing, 1986.
51. Kennedy, Marilyn Moats. "What Managers Can Find Out from Exit Interviews." *Physician Executive* 22 (October 1996): 45.
52. *Risk Management Handbook for Health Care Facilities,* edited by Linda Marie Harpster and Margaret S. Veach, 378. Chicago: American Hospital Association, 1990.
53. Kavaler, Florence, and Allen D. Spiegel. "Risk Management Dynamics." In *Risk Management in Health Care Institutions: A Strategic Approach,* edited by Florence Kavaler and Allen D. Spiegel, 18–19. Sudbury, MA: Jones & Bartlett, 1997. ("At least 10 states [Arkansas, Colorado, Florida, Kansas, Maryland, Massachusetts, New York, North Carolina, Rhode Island, and Washington] have legislative mandates for risk management programs. These state regulations relate to the administration of a risk management program, investigation and analysis of identified risks, education programs, patient grievance procedures, and confidentiality of risk management data." [p. 18])
54. Occupational Safety and Health Act of 1970, PL 91-596, 84 Stat. 1590 (1970).
55. The Joint Commission. *Comprehensive Accreditation Manual,* PI-8.
56. *Risk Management Handbook for Health Care Facilities,* edited by Linda Marie Harpster and Margaret S. Veach, 107.
57. Sedwick, Jeannie. "The Risk Manager Role." In *Risk Management Handbook for Health Care Organizations,* 2nd ed., edited by Roberta Carroll, 4. Chicago: American Hospital Publishing, 1997.
58. Sedwick, "The Risk Manager Role," 17.
59. Nakamura, Peggy L.B. "The Risk Manager's Role in Contract Review." In *Risk Management Handbook for Health Care Organizations,* 2nd ed., edited by Roberta Carroll, 499–513. Chicago: American Hospital Publishing, 1997.
60. *Black's Law Dictionary* defines insurance as "a contract whereby one undertakes to indemnify another against loss, damage, or liability arising from an unknown or contingent event and is applicable only to some contingency or act to occur in the future." Black, Henry Campbell. *Black's Law Dictionary,* 5th ed., 721. St. Paul, MN: West Publishing Company, 1979.

61. Mahaffey, Paul F. "Lawyers' Professional Liability Insurance." *Lawyers' Liability Review Quarterly Journal* (April 1989): 1–3.

62. Ashley, Ruthe Catolico. "Malpractice Insurance: Do I Need it?" National Association of Pediatric Nurse Practitioners. *http://www.napnap.org/index.cfm?page=10&sec=390&ssec=396,* retrieved August 24, 2007; "Do Nurses Need to Carry Personal Liability Insurance?" Nurse Link Up. *http://nurselinkup.com/blogs/articles/archive/2007/03/21/Do-Nurses-Need-to-Carry-Personal-Liability-Insurance_3F00.aspx,* retrieved August 24, 2007.

63. Health Care Quality Improvement Act of 1986, PL 99-660, 100 Stat. 3784 (1986).

64. Sedwick, "The Risk Manager Role," 19.

65. Kellogg, Sarah. "The Art and Power of the Apology." *Washington Lawyer* 21, 10 (June 2007) 20–26.

66. American College of Surgeons. *The Minimum Standard.* Chicago: American College of Surgeons, 1918.

67. Donabedian, Avedis. *Explorations in Quality Assessment and Monitoring. Vol. II. The Criteria and Standards of Quality.* Ann Arbor, MI: Health Administration Press, 1982.

68. Donabedian, Avedis. *Explorations in Quality Assessment and Monitoring. Vol. I. The Definition of Quality and Approaches to Its Assessment,* 81. Ann Arbor, MI: Health Administration Press, 1980.

69. Donabedian, *Explorations,* vol. I, 79–89.

70. Donabedian, *Explorations,* vol. I, 8.

71. Donabedian, *Explorations,* vol. I, 83.

72. Donabedian, *Explorations,* vol. I, 82.

73. The Joint Commission. *A Comprehensive Review of Development and Testing for National Implementation of Hospital Core Measures,* 2. Oak Brook Terrace, IL: Joint Commission on Accreditation of Healthcare Organizations, 2007.

74. Berwick, Donald M., A. Blanton Godfrey, and Jane Roessner. *Curing Health: New Strategies for Quality Improvement,* 11. San Francisco: Jossey-Bass, 1990.

75. The Joint Commission. *Agenda for Change,* 3–4. The Joint Commission on Accreditation of Healthcare Organizations, June 1988.

76. The Joint Commission. *Accreditation Manual for Hospitals,* Appendix D, 225–232. Oakbrook Terrace, IL: Joint Commission on Accreditation of Healthcare Organizations, 1992.

77. The Joint Commission. *A Comprehensive Review of Development and Testing for National Implementation of Hospital Core Measures,* 2. Oak Brook Terrace, IL: Joint Commission on Accreditation of Healthcare Organizations, 2007.

78. The Joint Commission. *Ongoing Activities: 2000 to 2004 Standardization of Metrics,* 1. Oak Brook Terrace, IL: Joint Commission on Accreditation of Healthcare Organizations, 2007.

79. Esmond, Truman H., Jr. *Budgeting for Effective Hospital Resource Management,* 26. Chicago: American Hospital Association, 1990.

80. Neumann, Bruce R., James D. Suver, and William N. Zelman. *Financial Management: Concepts and Applications for Health Care Providers,* 2nd ed., 269. Owings Mills, MD: National Health Publishing/AUPHA Press, 1988.

81. Meeting, David T., and Robert O. Harvey. "Strategic Cost Accounting Helps Create a New Competitive Edge." *Healthcare Financial Management* 20 (December 1998): 43.

82. Finkler, Steven A. "Flexible Budgeting Allows for Better Management of Resources as Needs Change." *Hospital Cost Management and Accounting* 8 (June 1996): 1.

83. Stiles, Renee A., and Stephen S. Mick. "What Is the Cost of Controlling Quality? Activity-Based Cost Accounting Offers the Answer." *Hospital & Health Services Administration* 42 (Summer 1997): 199.

84. Zelman, William N., Michael J. McCue, and Alan R. Millikan. *Financial Management of Health Care Organizations: An Introduction to Fundamental Tools, Concepts, and Applications,* 365. Malden, MA: Blackwell, 1998.

85. Zelman, McCue, and Millikan, *Financial Management,* 365–366.

86. Finkler, Steven A. "Responsibility Accounting in a Dynamic Environment: Activity-Based Cost Management." *Hospital Cost Management and Accounting* 8 (October 1996): 3.

87. Drucker, Peter F. "The Information Executives Truly Need." *Harvard Business Review* 73 (January/February 1995): 14.

88. Baker, Judith J., and Georgia F. Boyd. "Activity-Based Costing in the Operating Room at Valley View Hospital." *Journal of Health Care Finance* 24 (Fall 1997): 2.

89. Upda, Suneel. "Activity-Based Costing for Hospitals." *Hospital & Health Services Administration* 21 (Summer 1996): 84.
90. Meeting and Harvey, "Strategic Cost Accounting," 47.
91. Zelman, McCue, and Millikan, *Financial Management,* 365.
92. Zelman, McCue, and Millikan, *Financial Management,* 32.
93. Those interested in more information about this subject may refer to Zelman, McCue, and Millikan, *Financial Management,* chap. 4.
94. Center for Healthcare Industry Performance Studies. Solucient. *http://www.solucient.com/aboutus/about us.shtml,* retrieved August 24, 2007.
95. "What Is Benchmarking?" *Hospital Cost Management and Accounting* 7 (January 1996): 8; Freeman, James M. "Benchmarking for Success." *Healthcare Executive* 13 (March/April 1998): 51.
96. Cleverley, William O. "Financial Ratios: Summary Indicators for Management Decision Making." *Hospital & Health Services Administration* 26 (Special Issue 1981): 30–31. See also Berman, Howard J., Lewis E. Weeks, and Steven F. Kukla. *The Financial Management of Hospitals,* 6th ed., 664–665. Ann Arbor, MI: Health Administration Press, 1986; Zeller, Thomas L., Brian B. Stanko, and William O. Cleverley. "New Perspectives on Hospital Financial Ratio Analysis." *Healthcare Financial Management* 51 (November 1997): 62–66.
97. Smith-Daniels, Vicki L., Sharon B. Schweikhart, and Dwight E. Smith-Daniels. "Capacity Management in Health Care Services: Review and Future Directions." *Decision Sciences* 19 (Fall 1988): 889–919; "Decision Making and Analytical Techniques: Mind Tools." *http://www.psywww.com/mtsite/page2.html,* retrieved August 20, 2007.
98. Halley, Marc D., and Robin L. Lloyd. "How to Break Even on an Acquired Primary Care Network." *Healthcare Financial Management* (November 2000). *http://findarticles.com/p/articles/mi_m3257/is_11_54ai_66936335/print,* retrieved July 24, 2007.
99. Further reading about the capital budgeting analytical technique in HSOs can be found in Baker, Judith J., and R.W. Baker. *Health Care Finance: Basic Tools for Non-financial Managers,* 2nd ed., chap. 14. Sudbury, MA: Jones and Bartlett Publishers, 2006; Broyles, Robert W., and Michael D. Rosko. *Fiscal Management of Healthcare Institutions,* chap. 13. Owings Mills, MD: National Health Publishing, 1990; and Zelman, William N., Michael J. McCue, and Alan R. Millikan. *Financial Management of Health Care Operations: An Introduction to Fundamental Tools, Concepts, and Applications,* chap. 7. Malden, MA: Blackwell, 1998.
100. AMA Council on Long Range Planning and Development in Cooperation with the Council on Constitution and Bylaws, and the Council on Ethical and Judicial Affairs. *Policy Compendium of the American Medical Association,* E-2.03, E-2.095. Chicago: American Medical Association, 1999. Adopted by the board of trustees November 13, 1997; amendments adopted by the board of trustees, February 21, 2004.
101. An excellent review of the literature concerning the application of simulation and other operations research techniques to health care is found in Smith-Daniels, Schweikhart, and Smith-Daniels, "Capacity Management." For classic reviews of applications, see Stimpson, David H., and Ruth H. Stimpson. *Operations Research in Hospitals: Diagnosis & Prognosis,* chap. 2. Chicago: Hospital Research and Educational Trust, 1972; and Valinsky, David. "Simulation." In *Operations Research in Health Care: A Critical Analysis,* edited by Larry J. Shuman, R. Dixon Speas, Jr., and John P. Young, 114–176. Baltimore: The Johns Hopkins University Press, 1975. A recent example using simulation in healthcare is Jun, J.B., S.H. Jacobson, and J.R. Swisher. "Application of Discrete-Event Simulation in Health Care Clinics: A Survey." *The Journal of the Operational Research Society* 50, 2 (February 1999): 109–123.
102. Klafehn, Keith A., Paul J. Kuzdrall, Jonathon S. Rakich, and Alan G. Krigline. "Application of Simulation in Hospital Resource Allocation and Utilization." *Journal of Management Science & Policy Analysis* 8 (Spring/Summer 1991): 346–356.
103. Klafehn, Kuzdrall, Rakich, and Krigline, "Application of Simulation," 351.
104. Written by Gary E. Crum, Ph.D., M.P.H., Executive Director, Graduate Medical Education Consortium, The University of Virginia at Wise (Past Director, Northern Kentucky Health Department). Used with permission.

11

Designing

Designing and redesigning is a vital management activity in all organizations. How well managers carry out design is critical to how well their organizations perform. Organizing is necessary to achieve cooperation. The complexity of work done in health services organizations/health systems (HSOs/HSs), and the variety of the professional, technical, and support people who perform it, requires a high degree of cooperation. In fact, the need for cooperation may be more prevalent and important in HSOs/HSs than in any other type of organization. For example, even within a single unit, such as imaging or finance, a wide range of work is performed at many skill levels, and organizing this work is vital to success.

As illustrated in Figure 11.1, designing begins by designating individual positions. It then progresses through workgroups to clusters of workgroups to HSOs, and to HSs for some HSOs, and finally to a set of interorganizational relationships (IORs) with other organizations in the environment. Effective designs require attention to all these levels of organization design.

▨ The Ubiquity of Designing ▬▬▬▬▬▬▬▬▬

Managers at all levels of HSOs/HSs, as presented in Figure 11.1, are involved in organization design. Senior-level managers are concerned more with broad aspects of organizing, such as authority and responsibility relationships, establishment of departments and other subunits so that the components can be effectively coordinated, perhaps formation of systems of organizations, and establishing and maintaining workable interorganizational relationships with other organizations in the external envi-

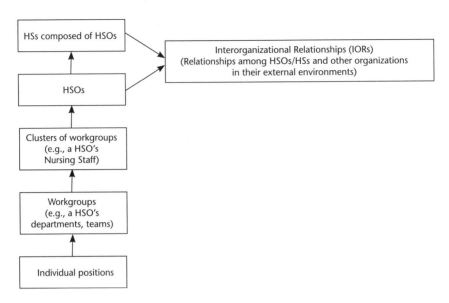

Figure 11.1.   Levels of organization design in HSOs/HSs, including interorganizational relationships (IORs).

ronment. In essence, they are concerned with how effectively the entity is structured to fulfill its mission and meet its objectives. Middle-level managers are more concerned with organizing clusters of workgroups into divisions or other groupings such as nursing service. First-level managers are more directly concerned with organizing individual positions into workgroups such as departments and teams; their organizing tasks include job design, work process flow, and work methods and procedures.

Although organizing is ubiquitous and continuous, involving not only initial design but also routine redesign, there are a number of specific instances and circumstances in which managers are likely to find design changes especially likely. Examples include situations in which HSOs/HSs face operational problems that must be corrected by redesign, such as inadequate performance found through an accreditation review. Sometimes, changes in an HSO's/HS's external environment stimulate urgent redesign. For example, an environmental change in reimbursement levels can lead to changes in individual positions, groups, departments, or entire organizations. Similarly, the development and implementation of a new program, as well as decisions to drop or modify existing programs, products, or services, can trigger significant redesign. Finally, changes in senior-level management positions almost always bring redesign in parts of organizations and systems.[1]

▬ Formal and Informal Aspects of Organization Design ▬▬▬▬

Through organization design, managers build the *formal* organization, the structure conceptualized and sanctioned by senior-level managers and governing bodies (GBs). Coexisting within the formal organization, however, are its *informal* aspects, which exist because people working together invariably establish relationships and interactions outside the formal structure. Thus every HSO/HS has a formal structure developed by management and informal aspects that reflect the wishes and preferences of the staff.

The formal organization is a planned and prescribed effort to establish relationships, and a great deal of management time and effort is spent establishing and maintaining it. The results of organizing activity include development of formal organization structures, such as those depicted in Figures

2.5 and 2.6, and related job descriptions, formal rules, operating policies, work procedures, control procedures, coordinating mechanisms, compensation arrangements, and other ways to guide employee behavior. However, many interactions among members of an organization are not prescribed by the formal structure.

Interactions and relationships that arise spontaneously from activities of members but that are not set forth in the formal structure make up the informal aspects of an organization. Formal and informal aspects of organizations coexist. Interest in the informal aspects of organization design was stimulated by the famous Hawthorne studies conducted in the 1930s.[2] These studies showed that informal aspects of organizations, which arise from the social interactions of people in them, are integral to all work settings. These studies also showed that informal aspects of organizations can improve or detract from organization performance, depending in part on how managers react to the informal aspects.

Together, the formal and the informal aspects of organizations constitute the organizational setting in which work is performed. The formal organization is characterized by prescribed authority—responsibility relationships, division of work and departmentation, and the hierarchical structure. The formal organization is the planned interrelationships of people, things, and activities. By contrast, the informal aspects of organization are characterized by dynamic behavior and activity patterns that occur within the formal organization structure as a result of the activity of people working with other people—their interaction and fraternization across formal structural lines.

The informal relationships and arrangements that exist within the formal design are a fact of organizational life. Formal and informal aspects of organizations must be balanced to achieve optimal performance and objectives of individuals and entire organizations. Attempts by managers to suppress informal relationships and arrangements can create destructive and dysfunctional situations. To protect themselves and to make their work situations acceptable, people typically resist what they perceive as autocratic management. The resistance often takes place within the context of informal relationships and arrangements and might exhibit itself in the form of such undesirable outcomes as work restriction, insubordination, disloyalty, and other manifestations of an antiorganization attitude.

The optimum situation occurs when the formal organization design maintains suitable progress toward organizational objectives but simultaneously permits a well-developed pattern of informal relationships to exist. Attaining a balance between formal and informal aspects of organization design may be difficult, but managers can do two things to help achieve it. First, they can seek to understand the informal relationships within their designs and demonstrate their acceptance by minimizing the negative effect of their actions on these often fragile informal relationships. Second, managers can integrate the interests of the formal and informal aspects of organization design to the maximum extent. In so doing, managers should avoid actions through the formal organization that unnecessarily threaten or diminish the quality of informal relationships. In effect, blending the informal relationships and arrangements with their formal design elements helps establish the culture within the organization.

Organizational culture is the pattern of shared values and beliefs that becomes ingrained over time in the members of an organization or system and helps influence behaviors and decisions. An HSO/HS can nurture an organizational culture that values excellence in patient care, for example. Strong organizational cultures invariably are built through both formal and informal organization design elements. Furthermore, understanding the informal relationships that people establish at work reflects the manager's recognition that people in organizations are not mechanistic—they are, instead, changing, complex, and social beings.

Indeed, managers must pay careful attention to both formal and informal aspects of organization design. Both have deep roots in what have come to be described as the classical concepts of organization design. As will be seen in the following sections, these classical concepts may be somewhat less relevant to the IORs that form the top level of organization design illustrated in Figure 11.1. However, they do have relevance to that level as well as to the establishment of individual positions, formation of workgroups, clustering of workgroups, and the design of HSOs and HSs involving some of them.

Classical Design Concepts in Building Organization Structures

Because of their natural affinity for contemporary things and ideas, it is difficult for some to recognize the importance of old ideas and concepts. It would be a serious mistake, however, to overlook the historical roots of what is known about organization design. Although they have been modified over the years, many key organization design concepts that guide the structures of contemporary HSOs/HSs were developed by a group of general administrative theorists early in the 20th century.

Most influential among these classical theorists were Max Weber, a German sociologist, and Henri Fayol, a French industrialist. The writings of Weber[3] and Fayol,[4] and their colleagues and contemporaries, including other early management theorists such as Luther Gulick and Lyndall Urwick,[5] James Mooney and Alan Reiley,[6] and Fritz Roethlisberger,[7] remain relevant to the design of modern organizations, including HSOs/HSs. These published findings and ideas are now widely viewed as the classical concepts of organization design, and their durability strongly influences the designs of contemporary HSOs/HSs.

WEBER'S CONTRIBUTION TO ORGANIZATION DESIGN: BUREAUCRACY

The best example of an early theorist with abiding influence is Weber (1864–1920), who is associated with the organizational form he termed bureaucracy. Weber thought that bureaucracy, in its pure form, represented an ideal or completely rational form of organization. The term *bureaucracy,* usually associated with large public-sector organizations, is now used frequently to disparage such undesirable characteristics as duplication, delay, waste, low morale, and general frustration (characteristics sometimes termed *red tape*) found in many large organizations. In Weber's conceptualization, however, the term meant something very different—an organization structure based on the sociological concept of rationalization of collective activities.

Weber abstracted the concept of an "ideal" organization from observing many actual organizations and combining them into his model of an ideal bureaucracy. This model became the basis for his theories about how work should be done in large organizations. The key features that Weber believed were necessary for an organization to achieve the maximum benefits of ideal bureaucracy included the following:[8]

- A clear division of labor ensures that each task performed by employees is systematically established and legitimized by formal recognition as an official duty.
- Positions are arranged in a hierarchy so that each lower position is controlled and supervised by a higher one. The effect of this arrangement is a chain of command.
- Formal rules and regulations uniformly guide the actions of employees. In Weber's view, a system of rules ensures a rational approach to organization design and a degree of uniformity and coordination that could not exist otherwise. The basic rationale for rules in Weber's model is that the manager uses them to eliminate uncertainty in the performance of tasks resulting from differences among individuals. Beyond this, he believed that rules and regulations provide continuity and stability to an organization.
- Managers should maintain impersonal relationships and should avoid involvement with employees' personalities and personal preferences. Weber believed this practice ensured that the bureaucrat did not permit emotional attachments or personalities to interfere with rational decisions.

- Employment should be based entirely on technical competence and protection against arbitrary dismissal. Employees in the ideal bureaucracy are selected using rigid criteria that apply uniformly and impersonally to each candidate. Criteria are based on objective standards for the job established by the officials of the organization. Promotions in the ideal bureaucracy are awarded on the basis of seniority and achievement.

Originally published in 1916, these characteristics of Weber's ideal bureaucracy continue to provide many important aspects of the design prototype for large contemporary organizations, including HSOs/HSs.[9] However, to be most useful, Weber's concept of bureaucracy and all of the classical concepts must be updated to reflect how organizations are best structured to meet the present and future needs of society as well as the needs of workers.

The following sections present the most important and relevant classical concepts of organization design, along with a contemporary perspective on each concept. The key classical concepts that remain relevant and important to managers as they design and redesign their HSOs/HSs are 1) division of work, 2) authority and responsibility relationships, 3) departmentation, 4) span of control, and 5) coordination.

Division of Work

The classical theorists—and before them, the economist Adam Smith, author of *The Wealth of Nations,* published in 1776[10]—recognized the potential benefits of division of work. Fayol, for example, considered division of work to be the most important design concept.[11] He and other classical theorists considered the division of work—or, as it is also known, the specialization of work—to be an important source of certain economic benefits. These economic benefits derived from the fact that division of work enhanced individuals' proficiency in performing their work and thus improved the efficiency and effectiveness with which work could be performed. For example, in a contemporary context, a liver transplant team reflects a careful division of work among a group of people. Each member performs specialized work and becomes proficient in it. The team is excellent because the work of individual members is marked by excellence. The team is efficient because individual members are proficient at their work and contribute to the team's overall efficiency.

Technically, division of work means dividing the work of an organization into specific jobs, each consisting of specified activities.[12] The content of a job is determined by what the person doing it is to accomplish. For example, the job of pharmacist in a healthcare organization is defined by the activities a person in this position is expected to accomplish. These activities are different from those expected of someone with the job of nurse, vice president for professional affairs, dietitian, or chief information officer.

Much of the world's work, and certainly that performed in HSOs/HSs, is performed by people who are specialized in particular work through education and experience. Specialization of workers is a common way to divide work in these organizations, because licensure and accreditation rules and policies require HSOs/HSs to employ people who have met specific licensure and certification requirements—in other words, to employ people who are properly credentialed for the work they do. The work of health professionals is to some extent defined and to a large extent prescribed by licensure and certification requirements. Specialization, including but not limited to that which is documented by licensure or certification, implies expertise based on education and experience in the activities of a job. HSOs/HSs, more so than most organizations, are structured to accommodate the specialties of the people who work there.

Organizations, through the division of work, also encourage job or work specialization. Much specialization has a functional basis.[13] *Functionalization* means division of the organization's work based on functions to be performed. Division of work means that entities are organized into numerous departments or units within which work is functionally similar but among which work is functionally dissimilar. For example, work in the dietary department is dissimilar from that in admitting. Within these departments, however, the work is functionally similar. Specializing has several advantages, including enhancing the HSO's/HS's ability to select, train, and equip people to do work by matching their activities with functions. In functionally specialized work, people often learn the job more quickly, and managers can standardize functionally specialized work to achieve greater levels of control.

CONTEMPORARY VIEW

The classical theorists who developed the concept of the division of work saw it as an important, and at the time largely untapped, source of increased productivity. Potential economic benefits of work division and specialization abounded at the beginning of the 20th century. However, increased division of work has a negative side—people who perform specialized work may find it repetitive, monotonous, and unfulfilling. The proficiency and efficiency benefits of the division or specialization of work are real, and they can be significant, but they must be balanced against negative consequences. Taken too far, the division of work can become dysfunctional.

In response, such contemporary developments as programs in cross-training (equipping people with skills and tools that permit them to perform more than one job), job enlargement (combining tasks to create a new job with broader activities), and job enrichment (expanding responsibilities so that work becomes more challenging and satisfying) are increasingly important in all types of organizations, including HSOs/HSs. For example, integrated patient care teams formed through job enrichment efforts involve each member in team decisions and the total care of patients. Cardiac rehabilitation teams work together to diagnose, treat, rehabilitate, and provide extended care, as a team, from the point of patients' initial incidents through satisfactory recoveries.

Many jobs in HSOs/HSs include work that is tedious and narrow in scope; transportation, food preparation, and laundry are good examples. Such jobs can be enlarged readily and to good effect. Similarly, however, health professionals with relatively broad duties in their work also can benefit from job enlargement. Nurses with enlarged responsibilities often enjoy the new challenges. The best job enlargement and enrichment programs are consistent with the widely popular quality-of-work-life (QWL) movement. Organizations initiate QWL programs to make the work environment more compatible with their employees' physical, social, and psychological needs at work.[14] The central purpose of QWL programs is to make work meaningful for people and to create an environment in which they can be motivated to perform and derive satisfaction from the results of their work.

▬ Authority and Responsibility Relationships ▬

Another important classical organization design concept relevant for contemporary HSOs/HSs is the establishment of the relationships of authority over and responsibility for performance of work. Growing directly out of the division of work is the need to assign responsibility for and authority over the performance of the work. *Authority* is the power derived from a person's position in an organization. Sometimes called legitimate power, organizational authority permits managers to give orders and to expect them to be carried out as managers fulfill their directing function. *Responsibility* is the obligation to perform certain functions or achieve certain objectives and, like authority, is derived from one's position in the organization. Persons with responsibility are accountable for results.

Classical theorists were obsessed with the concept of authority in organizations, viewing it as the glue that held organizations together. Furthermore, they believed that the rights attached to one's position were the only important sources of power or influence in the organization and that managers were all-powerful. This might have been true 100 years ago, but no longer. Now, authority is seen as just one element in the larger concept of power in organizations.[15]

Authority and responsibility are delegated downward in organizations or systems from higher levels of management to lower levels, resulting in a scaling or grading of levels of authority and responsibility. The authority and responsibility of an HSO/HS chief executive officer (CEO) are different from those of vice presidents, department heads, and individual employees. Vertical layers in an organization are the clearest evidence of this scalar process. As Higgins noted,

> The scalar chain simply defines the relationships of authority from one level of the organization to another. In the scalar chain, individuals higher up on the chain have more authority than those below them. This is true of all succeeding levels of management from top management to the first-level employee. The scalar chain helps define authority and responsibility and, thus, accountability.[16]

Classical theorists distinguished two forms of authority relationships: line authority and staff authority. As organization design concepts, *line* and *staff* are best understood as a matter of relationships. A line relationship is one in which a superior exercises direct authority over a subordinate. This is command authority and is represented by the chain of command in an organization. The chain of command in an HSO/HS is illustrated by the relationships of nurses on a unit to the nurse manager of the unit, to the nursing supervisor, to the vice president for nursing, and eventually to the CEO of the HSO, and from there on up the ladder if the organization is part of an HS. Each person in this chain has the authority, by virtue of organizational position, to issue directives to and expect compliance from people who are lower in the chain.

Staff authority, in contrast, is advisory authority. Staff authority is expressed in the form of counsel, advice, and recommendations. An HSO's/HS's in-house attorney occupies a staff position. This means that the attorney cannot dictate the terms of a sales contract between the HSO/HS and another organization acquiring it. However, based on expertise, the in-house attorney is expected to advise the line managers (CEO and other senior-level managers involved in the sales decision, along with the GB, in this instance) about language and terms in the contract.

CONTEMPORARY VIEW

The most important contemporary developments in how authority and responsibility are viewed in organizations derive from broader views of power in organizations than the narrow perspective held by the classical theorists. There are numerous sources of power and influence in organizations (discussed more fully in Chapter 12 in relationship to the power of leaders). The authority that derives from one's formal position is only one source of power. French and Raven[17] conceptualized interpersonal power with five distinct bases in organizations: legitimate, reward, coercive, expert, and referent. Only the first three bases derive from the manager's formal position in the organization.

Power that is derived from position in an organization is legitimate power. This formal authority resides in managers and exists because organizations find it advantageous to assign power to certain individuals so that they can do their jobs effectively. All managers have some legitimate power or formal authority based on position. Managers also have reward power, based on their ability to reward desirable behavior, which stems from the legitimate power granted to managers. Because of their position, managers control rewards such as pay increases, promotions, and work schedules, and this buttresses legitimate power. Managers also have coercive power because of their position. It is the opposite of reward power and is based on the ability to punish employees or prevent them from obtaining desired rewards. By definition, these sources of power in organizations are restricted to managers. However, other sources of power that are not restricted to managers are quite important in HSOs/HSs, and the existence of these other sources often means that power and influence are spread beyond the organization's managers.

One of the most important sources of power in healthcare organizations and systems is expert power, which derives from possessing knowledge that is valued by the HSO/HS. Expert power is personal to the individual with the expertise. Thus it is different from legitimate, reward, and coercive power, which are prescribed by the organization, even though people may be granted such power because they possess expert power. For example, people with expert power often rise to management positions in their areas of expertise. It is also noteworthy that, in healthcare settings where work is highly technical or professional, expert power alone makes people powerful. For example, the power of physicians and other licensed independent practitioners is based on clinical knowledge and skills. Physicians with scarce expertise, such as transplant surgeons, have more expert power than do physicians whose expertise is more readily replaceable.

Some individuals arouse admiration, loyalty, and emulation to the extent that they gain the power to influence others. This referent power, sometimes called charismatic power, certainly is not limited to managers. In HSOs/HSs, charismatic individuals wield considerable influence. As with expert power, referent power cannot be given by the organization as legitimate, reward, and coercive powers can.

The contemporary view of authority and responsibility in HSOs/HSs is that they remain key concepts, heavily influencing the organization design. In addition, the contemporary view expands on the classical idea and views authority as only one of several sources of power. In this larger context, power is not limited to managers.

Another important contemporary development in the concept of authority and responsibility pertains to delegation. Almost without exception, classicists thought decisions should be made at the lowest possible level in the organization and that this was compatible with good decisions. This meant higher-level managers should not make decisions on routine matters that could be handled at lower levels. A viewpoint typical of the classicists was this:

> One of the tragedies of business experience is the frequency with which men [business in 1931 was an almost exclusively male domain], always efficient in anything they personally can do, will finally be crushed and fail under the weight of accumulated duties that they do not know and cannot learn how to delegate.[18]

The importance and logic of delegation was first expounded by the classicists and is now considered by contemporary managers as an integral part of centralized or decentralized decision making in HSOs/HSs.[19] Decentralization is closely related to delegation, but it is also a philosophy of management that requires more than simply handing authority or responsibility to subordinates. Decentralizing authority and responsibility requires carefully selecting at what levels which decisions should be made.

It is relatively simple to assess the degree of decentralization in an organization or system. For example, the more decisions made in the lower management hierarchy, the greater the degree of decentralization. Also, if important decisions are made in the lower management hierarchy, the degree of decentralization is greater. For example, an HSO/HS manager's ability to commit to capital expenditures indicates the degree to which authority has been delegated. Another indication of decentralization is that checking or gaining clearance is not required for decisions made at lower levels. Decentralization is greatest when no check at all is required; decentralization is less when organizational superiors must be informed of the decision after it has been made; it is still less if superiors must be consulted before the decision is made. The fewer people consulted and the lower they are in the management hierarchy, the greater the degree of decentralization.

▬ Departmentation

Every organized human activity—from sandlot baseball to the U.S. Army or the Human Genome Project—has two fundamental and opposing requirements: division of work performed on the one hand, and integration and coordination of the divided work on the other. Classical management theorists recognized the relationship of dividing work and subsequently coordinating divided work to achieve satisfactory results. They developed the concept of departmentation (sometimes called departmentalization) as an organization design concept to partially address these dual concerns. Departmentation, the grouping of work and workers into manageable units or departments, still heavily influences the design of modern organizations.

The classical view of departmentation is a natural consequence of division and specialization of work that also rationally groups similar workers into workgroups, which in turn are grouped into larger and larger clusters until a superstructure is formed (see Figure 11.1). The classicists Gulick and Urwick[20] noted four reasons for departmentation: purpose, process, persons and things, and place. New bases for departmentation have emerged since their time, but the basic concept is largely unchanged. Mintzberg,[21] for example, suggested six bases for grouping workers into units and units into larger units:

1. *Knowledge and skills:* Grouping by specialized knowledge and/or skills; for example, surgeons in one department and pediatricians in another
2. *Work process and function:* Grouping by processes or functions performed; for example, departments of marketing or finance or laboratories
3. *Time:* Grouping by when work is done; for example, day, evening, and night shifts in 24-hour-a-day healthcare organizations
4. *Output:* Grouping by services or products; for example, production of inpatient or outpatient services
5. *Client:* Grouping by age or gender of clients or patients served; for example, geriatric and women's health programs
6. *Physical location*: Grouping by where work is done; for example, operating ambulatory clinics in downtown locations as well as in the city's suburbs

A single HSO/HS may use all six of these bases for grouping workers to design an effective entity. No matter which basis is used, the act of grouping workers helps establish the means by which their work can be coordinated within the groups and with other workgroups. Mintzberg[22] suggested that grouping (or departmentation) has at least four important implications for workers and their organizations:

1. *Grouping sets up a system of common supervision.* Once workers are grouped, a manager can be appointed to coordinate and control the work of the group.
2. *Grouping facilitates sharing resources.* People in workgroups share a common budget, facilities, and equipment.
3. *Grouping typically leads to common measures of performance.* Shared resources on the input side and group-level objectives on the output side permit group members to be evaluated by common performance criteria. Common performance measures encourage group members to coordinate work.
4. *Grouping encourages communication.* Shared input resources and output objectives and close physical proximity encourage communication, which facilitates coordinating the work of group members.

Departmentation by function was the basis most favored by the classical theorists. Reinforced by the specialized knowledge and skills of many workers, this basis is clearly visible in contemporary HSOs/HSs. Nurses are in nursing service, pharmacists in the pharmacy, and so forth. Even within departments, the departmentation concept is evident. For example, a large clinical laboratory (a result of functional departmentation) comprises even more functionally specialized workgroups, such as blood bank, chemistry, and hematology.

CONTEMPORARY VIEW

One important contemporary development in the organization design of many HSOs/HSs is the increased focus on patients as the basis for departmentation or grouping, a result of the increased competition for patients. A direct outgrowth of this phenomenon is a significant increase in grouping workers on the basis of patients. Geriatric and women's health programs abound, as do comprehensive cardiac care programs marketed specifically to corporate executives as HSOs/HSs seek to hold or build market share.

Another important contemporary development in organization design is that rigidly departmented organizational structures, no matter what the basis for departmentation, face significant problems of coordination across departments and other divisions of workers. The bureaucratic form, which stresses departmentation and hierarchy, works well in some circumstances but not in others. The bureaucratic form is effective in stable circumstances, but it is a disadvantage when flexibility in response to changing circumstances is more important. Organization designs that are more flexible—or, as some prefer to call them, more organic—work better in dynamic circumstances.

A good example of organic design occurs in the context of how HSOs/HSs respond to difficulties encountered in managing large-scale projects that require the skills of people in different departments or in situations in which patient care is enhanced by multidisciplinary teams. Project teams can use groups of workers drawn from different departments to carry out specific projects or programs. Project teams do not replace the departmental structure. They are organic complements to the more mechanistic and bureaucratic functional departmental structure and eliminate some of its rigidity in certain circumstances. Figure 11.2 illustrates such a design.

A project team might be used to organize services for a comprehensive home health program for the chronically ill. Team members would be drawn from nursing, social services, respiratory therapy, occupational therapy, pharmacy, and physicians specializing in chronic disease. To market

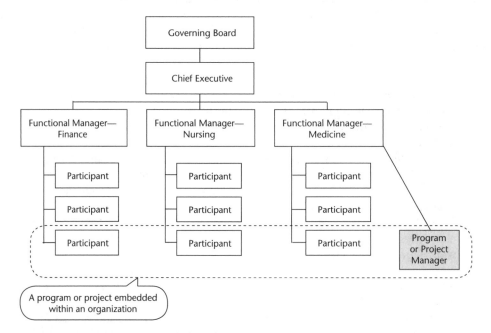

Figure 11.2. Matrix organization design. (From Beaufort B. Longest, Jr., *Managing Health Programs and Projects,* p. 103. San Francisco: Jossey-Bass, 2004. Copyright © 2004 John Wiley & Sons, Inc. Reprinted with permission of John Wiley & Sons, Inc.)

the program and to handle finance and reimbursement issues, expertise would be provided by team members drawn from the HSO's/HS's administration. A project manager would be named.

Project organization has many positive attributes. It permits flexibility, enhances skill development, and enriches jobs for team participants, but it also has a negative side. Project organization can cause ambiguity for workers who participate in a project with its own manager while holding positions in their home departments, which have different managers. Project organization is time-consuming because it relies on extensive communication, often in face-to-face team meetings. Managers accustomed to working in a departmented structure must adopt a new approach to the job to successfully manage projects.

HSOs/HSs can utilize project organization designs by superimposing these designs on their existing functionally departmented design. This can be done in a few areas, such as the home health program noted earlier, or for the whole organization. Figure 11.3 is a matrix design for a psychiatric hospital in which functional managers head departments, and program or product line managers head

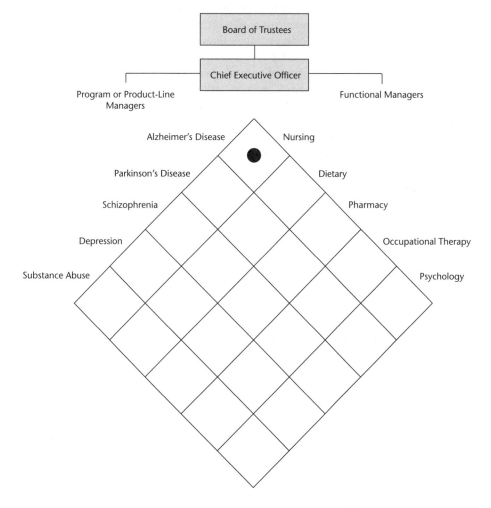

Figure 11.3. A matrix design: a psychiatric center. (From Leatt, Peggy, Ross Baker, and John R. Kimberly. "Organization Design." In *Health Care Management: Organization Design and Behavior,* 5th ed., edited by Stephen M. Shortell and Arnold D. Kaluzny, 332. Clifton Park, NY: Thomson Delmar Learning, 2006. Reprinted with permission of Delmar Learning, a division of Thomson Learning (www.thomsonrights.com). Fax 800-730-2215.)

major clinical programs or product lines. Notice that the worker depicted is a member of the nursing department and the Alzheimer's disease program.

Span of Control

An organization design question of fundamental concern to classical theorists was how large to make groupings of workers. How many people should be grouped in a department, and on what basis was the decision made? In considering these questions, classical theorists developed the span-of-control concept, which remains important in the design of HSOs/HSs. Span of control is defined as the number of subordinates reporting directly to a superior.

Classical theorists generally agreed that managers should have a limited number of subordinates reporting directly to them, a pragmatic conclusion based on the need for managers to exercise control. Some theorists even specified numbers for the optimum span. For example, Urwick[23] specified six as the maximum span for the manager to maintain close control. Davis[24] distinguished two types of span of control: executive and operative. Executive span refers to senior- and middle-level management positions; operative span refers to first-level management positions. Davis judged that an effective executive span of control could vary from three to nine, while the operative span could have as many as 30 employees reporting directly to a first-level manager.

How an organization answers the span-of-control question significantly affects its design. As seen in Figure 11.4, narrower spans of control produce "tall" organizations, and wider spans produce "flat" organizations. The tall and flat structures in Figure 11.4 have equal numbers of positions, but the tall structure has five levels and the flat one has three.

Most complex HSOs have tall patterns. The shape of an HS depends on whether it is horizontally or vertically integrated. The tall patterns of HSOs result from differentiation and specialization of numerous and varied departments (e.g., from the dietary department to the department of surgery) and consequently the need for limited spans of control. Less complex HSOs, such as clinics or small nursing facilities, have flatter structures. More important, even large HSOs have begun to flatten

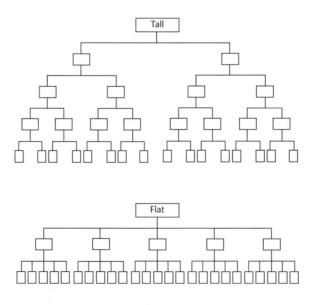

Figure 11.4. Contrasting spans of control.

their structures as they seek efficiencies and cost reductions by reducing work forces, cuts that often have been concentrated in the middle-management ranks.

CONTEMPORARY VIEW

In contemporary thinking, several factors have been recognized to determine the appropriate spans of control in an organization or system's design, including[25]

- *Level of professionalism and training of subordinates:* Professionalized and highly trained workers (prevalent in HSOs/HSs) require less close supervision, which permits wider spans of control.
- *Level of uncertainty in the work being done:* Complex and varied work requires close supervision, compared with simple and repetitive work. Close supervision requires narrow spans of control.
- *Degree of standardization of work:* Standardized and routinized work—whether professional, such as in a pharmacy or laboratory, or work such as food preparation—requires less direct supervision; thus spans of control can be wider.
- *Degree of interaction required between managers and workers:* Work situations in which more interaction is needed between managers and workers require narrower spans of control because effective interaction takes time. Increasing the number of subordinates reporting to a manager exponentially increases the number of possible interactions between managers and subordinates because managers can interact with individuals and/or groups. The number of possible interactions between a manager and two subordinates, individually or in combination, is 6. If the number of subordinates is five, potential interactions increase to 100; six subordinates mean 222 possible interactions between manager and subordinates.
- *Degree of task integration required:* If work done in a group is integrated or interdependent, a narrower span of control may be needed.

The contemporary view is that the classical concept of span of control is highly relevant to HSO/HS design. However, several contingencies must be recognized when applying it. Senior levels in an HSO/HS typically have narrow spans of control (e.g., a president may have 5 or 6 vice presidents). At levels at which work is more standardized and routinized, the spans can be much wider. Another factor is the nature of the work. It is easier to supervise 10 file clerks than 5 nurses. Also, the abilities and availability of managers must be taken into account. Training and personal qualities of some managers enable them to manage more subordinates, thus facilitating a wider span of control. Similarly, better training and higher potential for self-direction of subordinates reduce the need for relationships with management and increase the number of subordinates a manager can effectively supervise.

▬ Coordination ▬

Chester Barnard, an influential classical theorist, went so far as to say that, in most circumstances, "the quality of coordination is the crucial factor in the survival of the organization."[26] Fayol's conceptualization was representative of how classicists viewed coordination in that a well-coordinated organization had distinct characteristics: Each department worked in harmony with other departments, each department knew the share of common tasks it must assume, and work schedules of all departments were integrated as required.[27] Early theorists saw coordination as consciously assembling and synchronizing different work efforts to function harmoniously in attaining organization objectives. This view remains valid.[28]

Some authors use the term *integration* to express the coordination concept. Lawrence and Lorsch, for example, define integration as the process of achieving unity of effort among the various parts of an organization.[29] *Coordination* and *integration* have similar meanings and may be used interchangeably.

CONTEMPORARY VIEW

The classicists' perspective on coordination has an important limitation when applied to coordination in contemporary HSOs/HSs. It focuses only on coordination within an HSO—an intraorganizational perspective. Increasingly important, with the development of HSs, is the issue of coordination among and between organizations—an interorganizational perspective. Much of what is known about intraorganizational coordination as conceptualized by the classicists applies to interorganizational coordination. However, important differences are examined in this section. It is important to note that the definition of *coordination* applies both to intraorganizational coordination within HSOs and to interorganizational coordination among HSOs in an HS. Thus, coordination in contemporary HSOs/HSs can be described as activity that is intended to achieve unity and harmony of effort in pursuit of missions and shared organizational objectives within HSOs or among the organizations participating in HSs.

The contemporary view of coordination as an organization design concept is that it is vital to effective HSO/HS operation and performance and that managers can select from a lengthy menu of coordinating mechanisms *contingent* upon circumstances. Many of the available coordination mechanisms are described in the next section—including administrative systems; committees; customs; practice guidelines (also discussed in Chapter 7); critical pathways (also known as clinical pathways, care maps, and critical paths); direct supervision; feedback; hierarchy; integrators; linking pins in matrix designs; mutual adjustment; outcomes assessments and planning; programming; project management through teams; report cards; standardization of work processes, outputs, or workers' skills; QITs; and voluntary action. Managers in HSOs/HSs use various combinations of these mechanisms to achieve coordination; usually several are used concurrently.

Coordination remains a critical task for all managers in contemporary HSOs/HSs. It differs with the organizational levels of managers. Senior-level managers are concerned with coordination or integration of an entire HSO, and with interorganizational coordination among their organizations and others in the external environment. This latter responsibility is especially important when an HSO is part of an HS. Middle-level managers face significant challenges as they seek to coordinate various clusters of workgroups that compose HSOs. First-level managers focus on coordination within their departments and, along with the middle-level managers to whom they report, between their departments or units and other parts of their HSO. Appropriate coordinating mechanisms differ from one organizational level to another, but their selection and use are important for all managers.

Depending on the circumstances inherent in different situations, various packages of coordination mechanisms can be appropriately tailored contingent upon the circumstances. For example, a senior-level manager concerned about how responsibilities, roles, and performance of the departments in an HSO are coordinated might select one package of coordination mechanisms. The vice president for nursing services in the same organization, concerned about coordination within nursing service, might select a somewhat different set of mechanisms. The pharmacy director, concerned about coordination issues involved in the proper dispensing of pharmaceuticals, might select yet another set of mechanisms. A different package of coordinating mechanisms might be selected by the president of an HS who is concerned about coordinating the set of HSOs in the system.

MECHANISMS OF COORDINATION

A wide variety of mechanisms is available to coordinate within and among HSOs/HSs. As noted above, the success of these mechanisms varies with the situations in which they are applied. That is, the choices managers make from the menu of coordinating mechanisms are *contingent* on the situations in which coordination is pursued. Among the mechanisms, an early dichotomy was developed by March and Simon.[30] They identified two primary types of coordination: *programming* and *feedback*.

Programming approaches to coordination seek to clarify work responsibilities and activities in advance of the performance of work, as well as specify outputs of the work process and skills required. Programming approaches essentially standardize work activities for all expected requirements. By contrast, *feedback* approaches to coordination entail the exchange of information among staff, usually while the work is being carried out. These approaches permit staff to change or modify work activities in response to unexpected requirements and rely extensively on effective communication (discussed in Chapter 13).

Litterer[31] argued that managers have three mechanisms available to achieve coordination. They can coordinate by using the organization's hierarchy or its administrative system or through voluntary activities. An HSO's/HS's *hierarchy* links various activities by placing them under a central authority. In a simple HSO, this form of coordination is often sufficient. In larger, more complex HSOs and HSs, hierarchical coordination is more difficult. The chief executive officer is a focal point of authority, but one person cannot solve all of the coordinating problems in the hierarchy. Therefore, coordination through the hierarchical structure must be supplemented by other mechanisms.

The *administrative system* is a second mechanism used to coordinate activities. Litterer noted that "a great deal of coordinative effort in organizations is concerned with a horizontal flow of work of a routine nature. Administrative systems are formal procedures designed to carry out much of this routine coordinative work automatically."[32] Work procedures such as memoranda with routing slips help coordinate operating units. For nonroutine and nonprogrammable events, administrative systems or techniques such as coordinating committees also may provide integration.

A third type of coordination, according to Litterer, is accomplished through *voluntary action* when individuals or groups perceive a need for coordination, develop a method, and implement it. In HSOs/HSs, much of the coordination depends on willingness and ability of individuals or groups to voluntarily integrate their activities with other organizational participants. Achieving voluntary coordination is one of the most important yet difficult problems for the manager. Voluntary coordination requires that individuals possess sufficient knowledge of organizational objectives, information about specific problems of coordination, and the motivation to do something about the problems. Fortunately, voluntary coordination is motivated by the professionalism of many of the staff. Their value systems, which are supportive of patients' welfare, facilitate voluntary coordination. Managers can further facilitate voluntary coordination by providing individuals with knowledge of the objectives and information concerning specific problems of coordination. Voluntary coordination can easily occur if knowledge of objectives and information about the problems are coupled with motivation.

Mintzberg[33] illustrates one of the most extensive and useful conceptual frameworks for categorizing the mechanisms of coordination available to managers. The categories are mutual adjustment, direct supervision, standardization of work processes, standardization of work outputs, and standardization of workers' skills. Figure 11.5 illustrates these coordinating mechanisms.

- *Mutual adjustment*—This mechanism provides coordination by informal communications among those whose work must be coordinated. As with Litterer's voluntary actions, noted earlier, work is coordinated by those performing it (see Figure 11.5a).

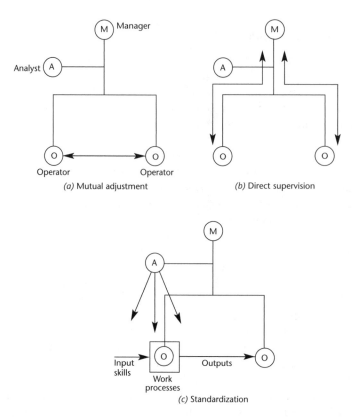

Figure 11.5. Mintzberg's five coordinating mechanisms. (From *Structure in Fives: Designing Effective Organizations,* 2nd edition, 5. Mintzberg, Henry, 1992. Reprinted by permission of Pearson Education, Inc., Upper Saddle River, NJ.)

- *Direct supervision*—Like Litterer's hierarchical coordination, this mechanism coordinates work when someone takes responsibility for the work of others, including issuing instructions and monitoring actions (see Figure 11.5b).
- *Standardization of work processes*—This mechanism is an alternative coordinating mechanism that programs or specifies the content of work. HSOs/HSs can rather easily standardize many work processes through such actions as establishing standard admission and discharge procedures or standard methods of performing laboratory tests. Other standardization efforts are more complicated, such as those involving development of patient care protocols (see Figure 11.5c, work processes).
- *Standardization of work outputs*—This mechanism specifies the product or expected performance, with the process of how to perform the work left to the worker (see Figure 11.5c, outputs).
- *Standardization of workers' skills*—Standardization of workers' skills occurs when neither work processes nor output can be standardized. If standardization is to occur in such situations, it must be through worker training (see Figure 11.5c, input skills). This form is frequently found in HSOs/HSs, in which complexity does not allow standardization of work processes or outputs. Standardization of workers' skills and knowledge is an excellent coordinating mechanism. For example, according to

Mintzberg, "When an anesthesiologist and a surgeon meet in the operating room to remove an appendix, they need hardly communicate; by virtue of their respective training, they know exactly what to expect of each other. Their standardized skills take care of most of the coordination."[34]

In Hage's[35] framework of coordinating mechanisms, the inclusion of a new mechanism, *customs,* plays a prominent role. Customs are a frequently overlooked mechanism, yet many managers rely heavily on them to help achieve coordination. For example, it may be customary in a particular nursing facility to use the holiday season as an occasion to invite the families of residents into the facility for a meal and social interaction. Knowing of this custom permits departments to begin their preparations well in advance and facilitates coordination of their contributions to its success. Customs based on a history of trial and error represent a distillation of good practice, but in complex HSOs/HSs, they are not sufficient to meet the coordination challenge.

In addition to the coordination mechanisms identified by March and Simon, Litterer, Mintzberg, and Hage, there are a number of other effective mechanisms available to HSO/HS managers. In certain circumstances, *committees* can be very effective coordination mechanisms. Committees are frequently composed of members from a number of departments or functional areas for the specific purpose of coordination among them. Of course, committees serve purposes other than coordination; they may act in a service, advisory, informational, or decision-making capacity.

In contrast to committees, a single person can sometimes be an effective mechanism of coordination. Lawrence and Lorsch[36] found that well-coordinated organizations often rely on individuals, whom they term *integrators,* to achieve coordination. Successfully playing an integrator role depends more on having relevant expertise than occupying a particular formal position; integrators represent a central source of information. Examples of effective integrators are found among individual nurses who provide significant coordination among various departments and subunits, particularly as they relate to patient care. Others have referred to individuals who link units together for purposes of coordination as *linking pins*[37] between the various organizational units.

Coordination may be especially difficult in managing large-scale programs or projects requiring skills of people from several different units or that incorporate multidisciplinary approaches to patient care. For example, in the earlier discussion about using matrix designs to organize services into a comprehensive home health program for the chronically ill, the project manager would coordinate the work of the entire team. This person would play an important integrator role and would be crucial to achieving effective coordination within the project and between it and other parts of the HSO in which it was embedded. When entire HSOs use the project organization design—creating a matrix design as shown in Figure 11.3—program and product line managers play integrator roles. This coordination mechanism will be increasingly important as HSOs/HSs continue to utilize product line management orientations.

Other structural devices or organization design features also can help with problems of coordination. Cross-functional quality improvement teams (QITs) are useful mechanisms through which HSOs/HSs achieve coordination. Originally developed in Japan, QITs have gained widespread acceptance as a means of coordinating, especially at the operational level, in organizations and systems. This mechanism features small-group, problem-oriented meetings in which organizational participants focus on ways to improve quality and work processes. The result of improved communication inspires more effective teamwork and contributes directly to enhanced coordination. Cross-functional QITs rely on flow diagrams, nominal group processes, multicriteria decision making, cause-and-effect diagrams, and related problem identification and problem-solving tools to improve communication, coordination, and ultimately the quality of work. QITs received further attention in Chapter 7.

Coordinating Direct Patient Care Activities

One of the most important recent developments in coordinating work in HSOs/HSs is the movement toward increased standardization of direct patient care activities.[38] Studies of intensive care units, for example, have demonstrated that effective coordination among clinical staff results in more efficient and better quality of care.[39] Recent studies of surgical services also show that effective coordination of staff leads to better clinical outcomes.[40]

For HSOs/HSs, coordination is also related to their compliance with requirements of regulatory bodies such as The Joint Commission on Accreditation of Healthcare Organizations (The Joint Commission) and accreditation standards that address staff coordination specifically.[41] Similarly, other accrediting bodies, such as the National Committee for Quality Assurance (NCQA), which accredits managed care organizations, also have standards addressing staff coordination. "While setting standards obviously cannot ensure good coordination, it does symbolize the growing recognition among accrediting and other oversight bodies that coordination is highly important to the performance of healthcare organizations."[42]

HSOs/HSs have been reluctant to seek better coordination of patient care activities through standardizing because historically these activities have not been good candidates for standardization.[43] This is due to the high levels of uncertainty in patient care, professional independence, variation among patients' responses to medical intervention, and difficulty defining outputs of patient care. Today, in contrast, significant efforts are being made to standardize work activities, as well as outputs of direct patient care, in response to pressures on HSOs/HSs to reduce utilization and to clearly demonstrate the value of patient care activities.[44]

Mechanisms available to standardize patient care activities include practice guidelines and critical pathways (also known as clinical pathways, care maps, and critical paths), which are "management plans that display goals for patients and provide the corresponding ideal sequence and timing of staff actions to achieve those goals with optimal efficiency."[45] Practice guidelines for specific diagnoses or conditions specify the work activities to be done in advance and are typically used for high-volume, high-cost conditions such as coronary bypass graft procedures and dementia. Practice guidelines, or protocols, address the appropriateness of care by specifying the clinical indications for either tests or treatments.[46] "Thus, whereas critical pathways standardize the treatment approach for a given clinical condition, clinical [or practice] guidelines standardize the decision process for adopting a treatment approach."[47] As noted in Chapter 3, the Agency for Healthcare Research and Quality (*www.ahrq.gov*) maintains a National Guideline Clearinghouse (*www.guideline.gov*), which contains practice guidelines for most common diseases and conditions, as well as for a number of prevention activities.

Yet another mechanism for standardizing direct patient care is outcomes assessment. Using this mechanism, which was further discussed in Chapter 7, managers systematically collect, monitor, and report performance results in an effort to standardize the outputs of patient care by focusing on such variables as mortality or complications rates for inpatient care and the percentage of enrollees in a managed care plan who receive cholesterol screening or other basic preventive services. Outcomes assessments also can be conducted at the level of the populations for which an HSO/HS is accountable by utilizing such outcomes as general health status of the population or incidence of specific clinical conditions, such as heart disease or diabetes. Some regulatory bodies have used outcomes assessment to develop profiles of the outcomes of HSOs/HSs called *report cards,* although the experience has been mixed.[48] Through these assessments "managers from different organizations or units can detect and attend to undesirable variations in outputs (over time or relative to competitors) by changing or modifying work activities as needed."[49]

Concerns that patient care quality may be compromised and flexibility of providers limited through standardized patient care[50] have been negated by new studies indicating that patient care can be improved by standardization efforts accompanied by well-developed feedback mechanisms. One important study of 44 surgical departments found that those with a relatively high emphasis on standardizing patient care activities, combined with a similar emphasis on feedback-type approaches, had better surgical outcomes than their counterparts that did not.[51] For example, one surgical department in the study developed and implemented a protocol that nurses used to identify patients at high risk for pressure sores. This would trigger a conference to develop effective prevention strategies involving nurses, the attending surgeon, and a consulting physician from the department of medicine. The protocol was a form of standardization of work, while the conference served as a feedback mechanism.

Application of the Classical Organization Design Concepts

The relationship of classical design concepts to the actual organizational structure of an HSO/HS is readily seen in the schematic representation known as an organization chart. For example, the prototype organization chart in Figure 2.3 shows the basic nature of the application of the classical design concepts. Of course, organizational structures built on the classical design concepts, such as the one shown in Figure 2.3, do not show the entire organizational structure. Coexisting within this formal organization are informal aspects of the structure not visible in the organization chart, except through imagining how many people might be involved in such an organization and the interactions among them.

This chart does, however, reflect the concept of division of work. Each unit in the chart represents a subdividing of work and suggests that staff in each unit specialize. The chart also suggests authority and responsibility relationships. The vertical dimension generally suggests who has authority over and responsibility for whom. People who are higher in the chart generally have authority over those who are lower in it. People on the same level have similar authority and responsibility. The chart also depicts groupings into units in the departmentation process. The chart permits easy assessment of a span of control, simply by counting the people with a direct reporting relationship to a manager, and suggests who is responsible for coordinating parts of the HSO, although the coordinating mechanisms they might use are not apparent. With some variation, the application of these classical design concepts also helps explain the structures of systems comprising sets of organizations. For example, Figure 2.2 shows an HS comprising a number of HSOs, both hospitals and long-term care facilities.

Designing Interorganizational Relationships (IORs)

The top level of organization design depicted in Figure 11.1 is composed of the myriad relationships among HSOs/HSs and other organizations in their external environments. Healthcare entities invariably establish relationships with other entities outside their boundaries. Because no HSO/HS can exist and function as an "island unto itself," the design of IORs is quite important. Every HSO/HS is interdependent with many other entities, that is, with other entities that can affect it or that can be affected by it. Figure 11.6 shows interdependent relationships with many other entities.

In Chapter 2, an HS was defined as a formal linkage of HSOs, which may include financing arrangements, to provide more coordinated and comprehensive health services. Beyond the linking of HSOs into HSs, however, are other forms of IORs utilized by HSOs/HSs to manage their interdependencies with other entities. Three distinct forms of IORs are discussed here.

As is generally true for organizations, the most prevalent type of IOR for HSOs/HSs involves the market transactions between them and other entities. HSOs/HSs use market transactions to secure needed resources from suppliers and to ensure markets for their outputs. For example, an HSO/HS maintains an IOR with a supplier, such as Baxter International, Inc. (*www.baxter.com*),

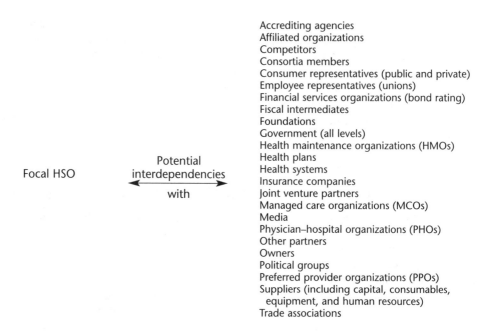

Figure 11.6.   Interdependencies among HSOs and other entities.

through which it purchases medical supplies. The HSO/HS can help ensure markets for its services through IORs with insurance companies, managed care plans, employers, or groups of employers joined together in purchasing coalitions.

A second type of IOR occurs because HSOs/HSs *must* participate in linkages with certain entities such as federal or state regulatory agencies, fiscal intermediaries, bond rating services, utilization management companies, and unions with which they have collective bargaining agreements. Because the HSO/HS has no choice but to participate in these IORs, they can be labeled *involuntary IORs*. An example is the IOR that must be maintained between an HSO/HS operating in Pennsylvania and the Pennsylvania Department of Health's Bureau of Facility Licensure and Certification. Such departments license and verify compliance with state and federal health and safety standards in supervised healthcare facilities as mandated by law. The Pennsylvania Department of Health (*www.dsf.health.state.pa.us/health*), like other state health departments, conducts regular on-site surveys to ensure health, safety, sanitation, fire, and quality-of-care requirements. These surveys identify deficiencies that may affect state licensure or eligibility for federal reimbursements under the Medicaid and Medicare programs.

The third type of IOR in which HSOs/HSs engage—the type through which HSOs establish HSs as well as accomplish other purposes—is *voluntary IORs*. These occur when HSOs/HSs voluntarily enter into a variety of linkages and relationships with other entities that are different from their market transactions. Voluntary IORs are established between or among entities for purposes of mutual benefit or gain and are used by HSOs/HSs to accomplish purposes such as enhancing their competitive positions by better meeting consumer expectations for delivery and coordination of care. Such linkages among HSOs are pervasive in health services. For example, most hospitals are now "allied with other hospitals in their markets through . . . organizational linkages."[52]

Voluntary IORs, ranging from the simplest to the most complex and extensive linkages, are generally referred to as alliances, or strategic alliances (SAs), as they are called in this chapter.

STRATEGIC ALLIANCES

SAs are defined as "any formal arrangements between two or more organizations for purposes of ongoing cooperation and mutual gain/risk."[53] The arrangements are established through a variety of mechanisms, including but not limited to the formation of HSs.[54] By definition, all HSs are SAs, although HSs range from simple to very complex; not all SAs, however, are HSs.

A taxonomy developed by Stein[55] suggests that SAs form in three ways: Participants in a SA can pool resources, they can ally for some shared purpose, or they can link together through bonds of ownership or contractual relationships. The acronym PAL (pool, ally, link) is used by Stein to identify the three possibilities. Important structural attributes and characteristics of SAs can be described more fully in terms of participants, purposes, and form.

The concept of integration[56] is vital to understanding the formation of SAs, including HSs. In this context, integration can be thought of as bringing together component parts to make a whole. A SA can involve little integration or a great deal of integration. For example, in a SA established between a single HSO and members of its professional staff organization, there is integration, but it is limited. In contrast, Partners HealthCare, based in Boston, is an integrated health system involving extensive integration. Founded by Brigham and Women's Hospital and Massachusetts General Hospital in 1994, it is a SA with an extensively integrated system built around these two academic medical centers. The Partners system also includes "community hospitals, specialty hospitals, community health centers, a physician network, home health and long-term care services, and other health-related entities."[57]

SAs in their rich variety and diversity can be usefully examined from three interrelated perspectives: participants, purpose, and form. Each approach is considered in the following sections, along with examples demonstrating how each perspective contributes to understanding SAs. Among the most important aspects of SAs, however, is that no matter who participates in them or for what purposes or their specific form, alliances are established for strategic purposes, and they are entered into voluntarily. Senior-level managers and GBs of HSOs/HSs voluntarily enter into SAs because they believe that they can better achieve some organizational objective or improve some aspect of organizational performance.

SAs CATEGORIZED BY PARTICIPANTS

Although integration in health services frequently is considered in terms of HSOs linking into HSs, the integrative activity through which SAs are established can begin with individuals. Individual physicians engage in integration when they form a group practice, which is "a formal association of three or more physicians, dentists, podiatrists, or other health professionals providing services, with income from the medical practice pooled and redistributed to the members of the group according to a prearranged plan."[58] Group practices, which are SAs, can in turn participate in many other alliances.[59] The extent and variety of integrative activity forming SAs, categorized by participants, is explained in the following interactions between and among physicians, HSOs, and HSs.

Physician–Physician SAs

In addition to group practices, physicians can form other SAs, one of which is an independent practice association, a "legal entity composed of physicians who have organized for the purpose of negotiating contracts to provide medical services."[60] They also can form a physician-owned management services organization (MSO), a "legal corporation formed to provide practice management services to physicians."[61]

Physician–HSO/HS SAs

SAs are formed when individual physicians or groups of physicians are employed by, when their practices are owned by, or when they contract with HSOs/HSs. The popularity of HSO/HS ownership of physician practices as a SA—typically in the context of a highly integrated HS—has been mixed. Still, as Orlikoff and Totten noted,

> A fully integrated health system model is often achieved by purchasing physician practices (and subsequent employment of those physicians) or by establishing a staff-model health maintenance organization, or HMO. This model promises the greatest opportunity for hospitals and physicians to respond together to the market, manage outcomes and rationalize resource allocation. While doctors still tend to favor a degree of autonomy over total integration with hospitals, continuing market pressure for effective cost control and the ability to demonstrate quality and performance are moving hospitals and physicians closer together.[62]

Other relationship models include HSOs/HSs and physicians forming HSO/HS-based MSOs, in contrast to those that are physician-only. The services that are provided to physicians by such MSOs typically include billing, information system acquisition and installation, staffing, staff training and development, managed care contract negotiation and compliance, and other office management functions.[63]

Physicians and a hospital can form a physician-hospital organization (PHO), defined as a "legal entity formed by a hospital and a group of physicians to further mutual interests and to achieve market interests."[64] PHOs play important roles in many other SAs because each combines physicians and a hospital into a single entity, making it easier to obtain contracts with health plans, employers, or purchasing coalitions.[65] PHOs form SAs with the entities with whom they contract. For example, SAs are routinely established between PHOs and HMOs.

MSOs and PHOs involving HSOs/HSs and physicians typically are organized as joint ventures. A joint venture is "a legal entity characterized by two or more parties who work on a project together, sharing profits, losses, and control."[66] Joint ventures between HSOs/HSs and members of their professional staff organizations, including ventures in which they set up diagnostic imaging facilities or establish surgicenters or urgicenters, are commonplace.[67] Joint ventures, which are widespread in health services, are discussed in more detail in a subsequent section.

HSO–HSO SAs

Very important SAs arise in the form of voluntary interorganizational relationships developed between and among HSOs. HSOs that are alike, such as groups of community hospitals or nursing facilities, can form horizontally integrated HSs (see Figure 2.7A). Alternatively, joining with dissimilar or other types of HSOs, they can form vertically integrated HSs (see Figure 2.7B).

Horizontal integration is the formation of lateral relationships among like entities performing at the same functional level. Its primary purpose is to improve the efficiency with which resources are utilized and to improve purchasing power, as well as to enhance marketing and management capacity. It "occurs when two or more separate firms, producing either the same services or services that are close substitutes, join to become either a single firm or a strong interorganizational alliance."[68] Vertical integration, in contrast, is the formation of vertical relationships, within a single organization, among entities at different stages of a production process.[69] In this context, the production process is the production and delivery of patient care or of health services.

As discussed more fully in Chapter 2 in the section on health systems, vertical integration may involve as few as two entities at different stages of the process of producing and delivering health services, or it may involve more entities at different stages. The phrase *highly integrated HS* is increasingly used to refer to situations in which an HS has integrated to the extent that it includes at least three stages of health services production and delivery and at least one systemwide contract with a payer.

To summarize, SAs can usefully be considered in terms of their *participants*. Physician-physician SAs are commonplace. Physician-HSO/HS alliances are another category, as are those that are HSO-HSO. SAs also can be categorized and usefully considered according to their *purpose,* as is discussed next.

SAs CATEGORIZED BY PURPOSE

When HSOs/HSs participate in SAs, they do so for one or more purposes. Two common, although not exclusive, purposes for alliance activity are cost reduction and revenue enhancement. Group purchasing organizations (GPOs), for example, are SAs formed for the purpose of gaining purchasing power as a means of reducing the participants' costs of certain supplies. An example of such a SA is Amerinet, a national GPO founded by a consortium of regional GPOs. This alliance is one of the nation's largest GPOs, with a membership including about 2,000 acute care hospitals and about 1,800 long-term care facilities.[70] It negotiates on behalf of its members to obtain volume discount contracts with suppliers to provide its members with favorable pricing, terms, and conditions. Its product and service agreements include administrative services, diagnostic imaging, environmental services, information and technical services, IV solutions and supplies, laboratory supplies, medical supplies, nutrition supplies, pharmacy supplies, plant engineering, office supplies, and surgical supplies.

A typical example of a SA that is formed for the purpose of revenue enhancement is a PHO, a legal entity formed by a hospital and members of its professional staff to further their mutual interests. The typical purposes of forming PHOs are to seek contracts with managed care plans or to sponsor surgery centers, imaging centers, or other business ventures.[71]

Other purposes, or at least contibuting purposes, for which SAs can be formed include the ability of alliances to enhance participants' capacity to innovate and adapt to environmental threats, to experience organizational learning, and to make quality improvements.[72] For example, SAs such as Harvard Pilgrim Health Care[73] in Massachusetts, Henry Ford Health System[74] in Michigan, and Lovelace Health System[75] in New Mexico have been cited for their ability to help HS participants make quality improvements.[76] Kraatz has shown that organizations that face threatening environmental changes, as many HSOs/HSs do, may significantly increase their chances of successfully adapting by forging SAs that provide informational benefits and opportunities for mutual learning among participants.[77]

SAs, as noted earlier, also can be formed as ways for participants to stabilize themselves in uncertain environments or to maintain and enhance their competitive positions. Hospitals, for example, have been especially prone to pursue SAs as a means of positioning themselves to compete more effectively for managed care contracts. Luke, Olden, and Bramble pointed out that hospitals, by aligning with other hospitals in their local markets, gain certain advantages in a managed care environment.[78] They argued that many hospital SAs provide their members with important advantages because the alliances are able to negotiate for contracts that cover whole communities. SAs also give participants greater "mass and leverage,"[79] providing them with strength in their negotiations with managed care companies that might otherwise pit one hospital against others in negotiations based on price.

To summarize, in addition to being considered in terms of who participates in them, SAs can be usefully considered in terms of their purposes, including cost reduction and revenue enhancement; increased capacity to innovate and adapt to environmental threats; the advantages of organizational learning that can accompany participation in an alliance; opportunities to enhance quality; and the increased likelihood that participants might stabilize themselves, enhance their competitive positions, or both in uncertain environments. These are important purposes from the viewpoint of HSOs/HSs, and some SAs have more than one.

Although considerations of SA participants and the purposes for which SAs are pursued are important in understanding them, neither fully explains the forms that the alliances might take. Thus, form can be used as a third basis for categorizing and considering SAs and is discussed in the next section.

SAs CATEGORIZED BY FORM

No matter who participates in them or what their purpose, SAs can take many different organizational forms. Choice of form is related to participants and purposes but also to dimensions of SAs such as their importance and the need for permanence of the IORs that they are established to serve. Some IORs are of critical importance to participants; others are of less importance. Some IORs are intended to be of short duration; others are entered into for the long term. Often, enduring relationships are necessary if SA participants are to achieve important shared strategic objectives. Form also is shaped in part by whether SA participants adopt limited, or what are called loose, coupling arrangements or whether they develop more extensive, tightly structured arrangements.

HSO/HS managers considering a SA have options about form in a continuum from simple to complex. The options described in this section include co-opting, loose coupling or coalescing, and mergers and consolidations.

Co-opting

At the simplest end of the continuum, an HSO/HS can absorb limited elements or components of interdependent entities into itself. Thompson labeled such arrangements *co-opting*.[80] Other than market transactions, co-opting is the most flexible and easiest to implement of all SAs, two advantages that make it a pervasive form of alliance.

The most basic form of co-opting occurs when one entity appoints a representative from another interdependent entity to a position within itself. For example, an HSO/HS that wishes to improve ties to the community it serves might add community representatives to an advisory panel to help guide decision making and gain support. Similarly, an HMO that is concerned about quality may find advantages in adding members of the clinical staff to its GB.

A somewhat more complex but still relatively simple co-opting form through which to establish a SA is contract management. Also known as outsourcing, contract management is an administrative arrangement whereby an HSO/HS arranges for a firm that specializes in a particular area, such as dialysis, clinical equipment maintenance, waste management, housekeeping, laundry, or food service, to manage its corresponding department under contract.[81] In these arrangements, contractors perform the day-to-day management of departments or other units or functions of an HSO/HS under terms specified in the contract.

Loose Coupling or Coalescing

Moving along the continuum of organizational forms for SAs from relatively simple to more complex, one finds IORs in which participants "coalesce"[82] or couple themselves loosely[83] into SAs in forms such as joint ventures, partnerships, or consortia. The central feature of these coalesced or loosely coupled SAs is the partial pooling of resources by two or more entities to pursue defined objectives.

Loosely coupled or coalesced SAs link interdependent and mutually responsive organizations and systems in ways that preserve their legal identities and most of their functional autonomies. These relationships are bound by ties that are stronger than those in market transactions or in the simplest IORs, such as co-opting or contract management, but are less binding and extensive than those in ownership arrangements.

When SAs are not based on formal ownership arrangements but behave as if they are, they are called *virtual SAs*. Such alliances exhibit many of the characteristics of a true organization (shared goals, mutual dependency, task subdivision and specialization, bureaucratic structures, and formal coordinating and control mechanisms), but they lack ownership linkages among participants. They rely instead on contractual relationships.

For example, a virtual SA can be formed by an acute care hospital, a large multispecialty group practice, a nursing facility, and an insurance carrier creating IORs among themselves based on con-tractual agreements to collaborate in designing, producing, and marketing a managed care product. This is an example of a virtual vertically integrated HS. In such an arrangement, the four organiza-tions forming the SA continue to operate independent of one another in accomplishing other, perhaps mutually exclusive, objectives. However, the collaborative activity may have significant strategic importance to the participating organizations. In this example, the interdependencies among partic-ipants in the SA are managed through IORs that avoid the restrictions and diminution of autonomy and identity associated with such ownership arrangements as acquiring or merging with other inter-dependent entities.

Joint ventures are a prevalent type of loosely coupled SA for HSOs/HSs. As noted earlier, a joint venture is an IOR that is characterized by the presence of a contract or agreement and a legal entity through which participants pursue some activity in which they share costs, revenues, and control. Some joint ventures are organized as limited liability companies (LLCs), as discussed in Chapter 2. However, joint ventures involving HSOs/HSs and physician members of their clinical staff typically are limited partnerships, a different type of legal entity. The HSO/HS is the general partner, and physi-cians are limited partners. The general partner usually invests the bulk of the capital and usually is the managing partner. Limited partners invest far less capital, sometimes insignificant amounts, a fact that has caused problems with the Internal Revenue Service for some not-for-profit HSOs/HSs. The pri-mary reason to involve physicians in joint ventures, however, is not the capital they bring to the enter-prise. The key reasons are that this ties them more closely to the HSO/HS and that they provide referrals to the health services delivery activity that is the purpose of the joint venture; or, in the case of a medical office building (usually on the HSO's/HS's campus), physicians rent space from the lim-ited partnership and locate their practices there. Efforts to tie physicians who are independent con-tractors into the HSO/HS are known as bonding. Well-conceived and well-executed joint ventures may help HSOs/HSs improve their profitability or market position, and perhaps even physician relations.

Mergers and Consolidations

Extensive ownership arrangements are found at the most complex end of the continuum of forms that alliances can take. Some involve changes in ownership of entire HSOs/HSs through mergers or consolidations. A merger results when one or more HSOs/HSs are absorbed by another, which retains its name and identity. Consolidation occurs when two or more HSOs/HSs dissolve and are unified in a new legal entity.

The most complex SAs are formed through the establishment of ownership-based highly inte-grated HSs. As noted earlier, these SAs seek to link the components of health services delivery, and in some cases the financing, in ways that more efficiently and effectively meet the health services needs of the populations they serve. The specific forms that HSs take are idiosyncratic; each is unique. However, the objectives of the integrative activity involved in forming highly integrated HSs—whether through ownership, contract, or a combination—are rather uniformly established as[84]

- Acceptance of financial risk and the ability to contract based on a single signature
- Capability to manage the different components of risk among the different providers
- Development of a strong central GB (discussed later) that has earned support from all HS components
- Increased physician leadership and participation in management

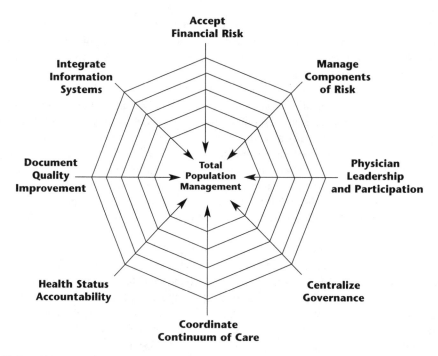

Figure 11.7.   Objectives of integration. (Adapted from *Sanofi-Aventis Managed Care Digest Series®: Hospitals Systems Digest 2007,* 2. Bridgewater, NJ: Sanofi Aventis, 2007. Used with permission from Sanofi-Aventis Managed Care Digest Series® Hospital/Systems Digest and Verispan LLC.)

- Information systems capable of integrating financial, operational, clinical, and management data and delivering them in an appropriate and timely manner
- Coordination to ensure a smooth transition of patients along the continuum of care
- Improvements in outcomes of care and quality of services
- Accountability for the health status of enrollees
- Assumption of responsibility for managing the total health of the enrolled population

These interconnected objectives are shown in Figure 11.7. As this figure illustrates, the process of integration can begin at any of a number of points—either one at a time or several simultaneously—as objectives for integration are pursued. The figure also shows that a particular HS may be closer to achieving effective integration in one objective than in others. For example, an HS may be quite far along in centralizing governance but at the same time have made relatively little progress toward the goal of involving physicians in leadership roles.

Figure 11.7 does not rank the objectives of integration by importance. However, other investigators argue that clinical integration is the most important aspect of integration.[85] Clinical integration, whether vertical or horizontal, is defined by Shortell and colleagues as "the extent to which patient care services are coordinated across people, functions, activities, processes, and operating units so as to maximize the value of services delivered."[86]

Clinical integration, at the operational level, includes concern for continuity and coordination of care as well as "disease management, good communication among caregivers, smooth transfer of information and patient records, elimination of duplicate testing and procedures, and efficient use and management of resources."[87] Conrad noted that "administrative and organizational-managerial integration is a necessary complement to the clinical integration of patient care, but it is the latter that is crucial to achieve a viable vertically integrated regional health system."[88]

Voluntary IORs or, as they have been called in this chapter, SAs can begin as simply as one HSO/HS appointing a representative from another to a position within itself, perhaps to a seat on its GB. The continuum of SA forms, with increasing complexity, moves from this relatively simple form to contract management or outsourcing to IORs in which participants coalesce or couple themselves loosely into alliances based on the partial pooling of their resources to pursue common objectives. These SAs might be more virtual than real in the sense that they are based more on contractual relationships than ownership. They move through joint ventures, which are SAs that are characterized by the presence of contracts or agreements and a legal entity that pools only limited interests through ownership, to SAs in which the ownership of entire HSOs/HSs is involved. Going back for a moment to Figure 11.1, it can be seen that design runs from the creation of individual positions up to the most complex IORs. At the IOR level, whether examined from the perspective of participants, purposes, or forms, the trend is toward increased formation of highly integrated HSs, the most extensive form of integration in health services. However, HSOs/HSs participate in a variety of IORs—those involving market transactions, involuntary IORs, and voluntary IORs or SAs—because they relate to many different interdependent entities, as shown in Figure 11.6.

▬ An Integrated Perspective on Organization Design ▬▬▬▬

HSOs/HSs, from the simplest enterprise to large, complex systems, have five interrelated parts. Mintzberg[89] labeled them the strategic apex, the operating core, the middle line, the technostructure, and the support staff.

- The *strategic apex* consists of those who set the strategic direction of an organization. In HSOs/HSs, this typically includes the GB, the president, and perhaps the vice presidents.
- The *operating core* is composed of those who do the basic work of the organization or system. They convert inputs to outputs, the products and services of the organization or system. Physicians, nurses, technologists, therapists, and others who provide health services in an HSO/HS are examples.
- The *middle line* is made up of middle- and first-level managers who are located between the senior-level managers in the strategic apex and the people in the operating core. They are the middle of the organization's or system's chain of command. Included are department heads and heads of other units and subdivisions. Examples include nurse managers, nursing supervisors, and directors of pharmacy, laboratory, and dietetics.
- The *technostructure* consists of workers who help plan and control the basic work of the organization or system. The people in the technostructure affect the work of others; their role is to help standardize the work of the organization. Workers in the technostructure are removed from direct operations—from the operating work flow—but "they may design it, plan it, change it, or train the people who do it."[90] The technostructure in HSOs/HSs varies with size and complexity but can include industrial engineers, risk managers, and those who support efforts for continuous quality improvement, because they help standardize work processes; strategic planners, budget analysts, and accountants, because they help standardize outputs; and people who recruit and train workers, because they help standardize the skills in the organization's or system's work force.
- *Support staff* are those who provide indirect services. In Mintzberg's conceptualization, they provide support to the organization's or system's basic work, but they do not do the basic work. In HSOs/HSs, these staff support the provision of health ser-

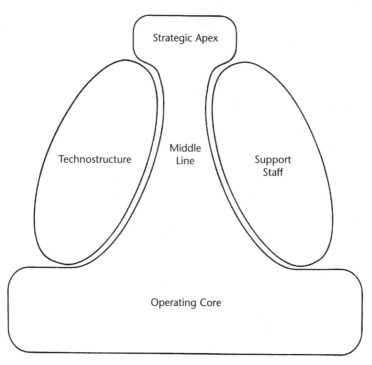

Figure 11.8.   Mintzberg's five basic parts of organizations. (From *Structure in Fives: Designing Effective Organizations,* 2nd edition, 5, by Henry Mintzberg, © 1992. Reprinted by permission of Pearson Education, Inc., Upper Saddle River, NJ.)

vices but do not directly provide these services. Examples of support staff include people involved in fund-raising and development, legal counsel, marketing, public relations, finance, and human resources management. Support staff differ from people in the technostructure primarily in that support staff do not focus on work standardization.

Mintzberg diagrammed the five parts of organizations or systems as shown in Figure 11.8 and described that structure:

> [It] shows a small strategic apex connected by a flaring middle line to a large, flat operating core. These three parts of the organization are shown in one uninterrupted sequence to indicate that they are typically connected through a single line of formal authority. The technostructure and the support staff are shown off to either side to indicate that they are separate from this main line of authority, and influence the operating core only indirectly.[91]

FIVE BASIC ORGANIZATION DESIGNS

In Mintzberg's view, the structures of almost all organizations or systems can be included in one of five basic designs based on various configurations of the strategic apex, operating core, middle line, technostructure, and support staff. He labeled these design alternatives the simple structure, the machine bureaucracy, the professional bureaucracy, the divisionalized form, and the adhocracy.[92] They are shown in Figure 11.9.

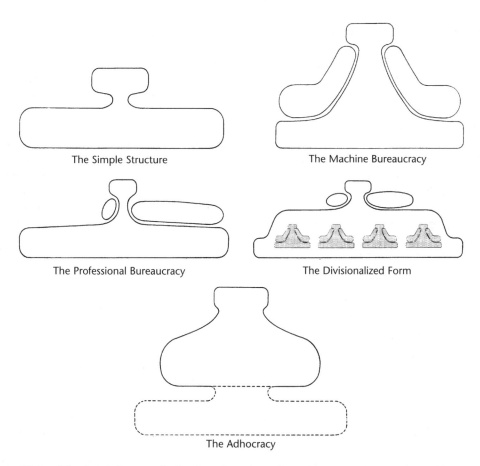

The Simple Structure

The Machine Bureaucracy

The Professional Bureaucracy

The Divisionalized Form

The Adhocracy

Figure 11.9. Mintzberg's five organizational configurations. (From *Structure in Fives: Designing Effective Organizations,* 2nd edition, 5, by Henry Mintzberg, © 1992. Reprinted by permission of Pearson Education, Inc., Upper Saddle River, NJ.)

Simple Structure

As this design's name implies, it represents the simplest organization design. It has a strategic apex, which may be one person, such as the owner of a small enterprise, a physician in private practice, or the director of a small ambulatory care center. In addition, it has an operating core consisting of a group of workers. The middle line, technostructure, and support staff components are very small or missing.

Machine Bureaucracy

This design is characterized by a large, well-developed technostructure and support staff because there is great emphasis on work standardization and a focus on marketing and financial and operational control systems. Major decisions are made in the strategic apex, which features rigid patterns of authority. Spans of control are narrow, decision making is centralized, and the organization is functionally departmentalized. This design typifies manufacturing organizations, although some hospitals also exhibit elements of this design.

Professional Bureaucracy

More typically, hospitals and other large HSOs, as well as universities and other professionally dominated organizations such as public accounting firms, are organized as professional bureaucracies.

This form is characterized by an operating core composed primarily of professionals that form the heart of the organization; authority is decentralized. The technostructure is underdeveloped because work is done largely by professionals who do not need—indeed, do not permit—others to do their work. In larger professional bureaucracies, such as hospitals, support staff may be highly developed and diverse. This staff is needed to support the professionalized operating core.

Divisionalized Form

The divisionalized form of organization design has independent units joined by a shared administrative overlay. In contrast to other designs, this form is characterized by a large, well-developed middle line of division managers responsible for their divisions and who may be given considerable decision-making latitude. Examples of divisionalized forms include corporations such as IBM, federal and large state governments, and HSs. Such HSs have become prevalent through corporate restructuring (creating several corporate entities to perform medical and nonmedical functions previously carried out by one corporation) and through active programs of merger and consolidation within the healthcare industry.

Adhocracy

The adhocracy, the fifth of Mintzberg's organization designs, is the most difficult of the five to describe or understand. It is both complex and nonstandardized. This form contradicts much of what is dictated by the classical design concepts described earlier—hierarchical authority and control, standardization of work and workers, and strategic direction from the top level of the organization. Instead, adhocracies have "a tremendously fluid structure in which power is constantly shifting and coordination and control are by mutual adjustment through the informal communication and interaction of competent experts."[93]

The adhocracy form is complicated by the existence of two variations of this configuration: the operating adhocracy and the administrative adhocracy. In the operating adhocracy, "the operating and administrative work blend into a single effort. That is, the organization cannot easily separate the planning and design of the operating work—in other words, the project—from its actual execution."[94] As shown in the solid-line portion of the adhocracy diagram in Figure 11.9, "the organization emerges as an organic mass in which line managers, staff, and operating experts all work together on project teams in ever-shifting relationships."[95] By contrast, administrative work in an administrative adhocracy is sharply separated from operating work. This is shown by the dotted-line operating core in the adhocracy diagram.

The adhocracy often takes the form of a matrix structure or project team (see Figure 11.3), with emphasis on activities in both the operating core and technostructure. The power in adhocracies shifts between professionals and technical experts. This design can be a free-form structure with frequently changing job descriptions and a flexible concept of authority. HSOs/HSs might use adhocracy in multidisciplinary programs for the elderly, chronically ill, or women or in the research-oriented departments (e.g., oncology, genetics) in academic health centers.

CHOOSING AN ORGANIZATION DESIGN

There is no magic formula by which managers choose an organization design. Furthermore, typical HSOs/HSs have many different designs embedded in them as various parts try to match structure to objectives, management philosophies, the preferences of their workers, and environmental pressures.

In a large and complex HSO, such as a teaching hospital, the dental clinic may have a simple structure, the clinical laboratory may be structured as a machine bureaucracy, and the medical and surgical nursing units may be professional bureaucracies. The hospital might be one of several hospitals that form an HS, with the system using the divisionalized form. Simultaneously, the hospital may have a project team of administrative experts in strategic management, marketing, finance, and information systems that, parallel to the team members' regular staff positions and structured as an adhocracy, operates as a consulting firm selling expertise to clients such as smaller hospitals and physician groups.

A leading management theorist, Peter Drucker, suggested that managers selecting an organization design evaluate the options against the following criteria:

- *Clarity,* as opposed to simplicity. Just as the Gothic cathedral is not a simple design, but your position inside it is clear and you know where to stand and where to go, in contrast to a modern office building, which is exceedingly simple in design but very easy to get lost in
- *Economy of effort* to maintain control and minimize friction
- *Direction of vision* toward the product rather than the process, the result rather than the effort
- *Understanding* by each individual of his or her own task, as well as that of the organization as a whole
- *Decision making that focuses on the right issues,* is action oriented, and is carried out at the lowest possible level of management
- *Stability,* as opposed to rigidity, to survive turmoil, and adaptability to learn from it
- *Perpetuation and self-renewal,* requiring that an organization be able to produce tomorrow's leaders from within, helping each person develop continuously, and that the structure be open to new ideas[96]

DISCUSSION QUESTIONS

1. What are the major characteristics of Weber's ideal bureaucracy as an organization form?
2. Discuss the concept of departmentation, and apply it to a hospital, a nursing facility, and a small freestanding ambulatory center.
3. Why is coordination so important for HSOs/HSs, and what are the mechanisms of coordination?
4. Discuss the relationships among span of control, delegation, and centralization-decentralization.
5. Discuss the characteristics of a matrix organization and how it differs from the "classical" functionally departmented organization.
6. Is decentralization better than centralization of authority and decision making?
7. Compare and contrast Mintzberg's five basic organizational configurations.
8. Briefly distinguish among market transactions, involuntary interorganizational relationships, and strategic alliances as categories of mechanisms through which HSOs/HSs link with interdependent entities.
9. Discuss strategic alliances in terms of who participates in them. Discuss strategic alliances in terms of the purposes for which they are formed.
10. Discuss strategic alliances in terms of their forms.

Case Study 1: Is the Matrix the Problem or the Solution?

A number of problems existed at Horizon Hospital, a large psychiatric facility. Turnover among nursing personnel was much higher than is typical for psychiatric hospitals, and relationships between the nursing service and members of the professional staff organization (PSO) were unusually poor. Psychiatrists and clinical psychologists often complained that their patients received inadequate attention from nurses and that their orders were not fully and promptly followed.

The hospital president asked the vice president for nursing to recommend a course of action to resolve the problems. The vice president developed a plan to restructure the nursing units, using a matrix design (as in Figure 11.3). His plan included a new structure, reporting relationships, authority and responsibility relationships, and a timetable for implementing the matrix design.

The president was impressed with the plan and believed it might improve the situation. However, when she showed the plan to the chief of professional staff and several members of the PSO, she was told in no uncertain terms that they would oppose it and would do nothing to implement the change.

Puzzled by their reaction, the president called the vice president into her office to discuss the next step.

QUESTIONS

1. Why do you think the PSO members reacted as they did?
2. Is there anything inherently wrong with the matrix design? Is it inappropriate for psychiatric hospitals?
3. What should the president and vice president for nursing do now?

■ Case Study 2: Trouble in the Copy Center

Janice Arnold, the new and ambitious administrative resident at the central office of Eastern Rehabilitation System, an HS comprising 22 rehabilitation hospitals in the eastern United States, was eager to make improvements in the organization of the system's central office. She found what she thought was a likely candidate for improvement in the system's copy center. She rolled up her sleeves when she found out by talking with the center's supervisor that, although turnover was very low, there was a great deal of dissatisfaction among the personnel in the copy center. The six people who ran the copying equipment were very close in age (mid-40s), were all women, socialized with one another after working hours, and frequently discussed personal matters at work. Arnold regarded Ms. Kelly, the center's supervisor, as very capable, although she complained frequently that the center's employees were overworked and underpaid.

Arnold checked with other employers in the area and found that, among copy centers, Eastern Rehabilitation System had one of the lowest rates of pay for such employees in the region. When she approached the HS's vice president for administration on the matter of higher pay for the center's personnel, she was told it would be impossible to increase their pay at the present time.

Arnold set about to do what she could to help the center's employees in other ways. In order to even out the work, she proposed changing their work schedule. Instead of all six employees working the day shift, Arnold proposed having three of them work a night shift when many of the larger copying jobs could be run without too much interruption. To her surprise, neither the center's supervisor nor the six employees liked this idea. As a second idea, Arnold actually convinced the vice president for administration to hire a receptionist so that the center's employees could concentrate on running the copying machines. However, the receptionist was not given any cooperation by the center's other employees and soon resigned. Arnold felt certain that the center's supervisor was responsible for the other employees' not accepting the new receptionist. She requested that the vice president for administration terminate the supervisor.

The vice president not only refused to do so but also told Arnold that things were worse in the copy center than when she started "reforming" it.

QUESTIONS

1. What do you think about Arnold's decisions and behavior?
2. Why did the copy center's employees react as they did?
3. Why did the center's employees not help the receptionist?
4. If you were the vice president for administration, what would you do?

■ Case Study 3: "I Cannot Do It All!"

When Harold Brice was named president of Healthcare, Inc., a health maintenance organization (HMO), he inherited a staff including vice presidents for marketing, finance, medical affairs, and professional services. Each executive was capable in many ways, and Healthcare, Inc., was on a solid financial footing with bright prospects. It was located in an expanding community; a 15%–20% annual growth rate was projected for the next 5 years.

Within a few weeks of joining Healthcare, Inc., Brice perceived a serious flaw in his vice presidents: None of them would make a decision, not even on rather routine matters such as personnel questions, choice of marketing media, or changing suppliers. This troubled him. Before long, the situation seriously impeded his efforts to give thought to strategic plans for the HMO. To make matters worse, he found that the vice presidents routinely discussed their own problems among themselves, to the extent that a great deal of time was consumed in doing so. Yet even with all of this activity, the vice presidents frequently presented him with issues in their areas of responsibility and requested that he make the decision.

At a regular staff meeting, when every member of his staff had an issue requiring a decision, Brice finally lost his temper. Waving his arms in exasperation, he shouted (which was very uncharacteristic for him), "I cannot do it all! You are going to have to make these decisions yourselves."

The meeting broke up with the vice presidents looking very puzzled and with Brice realizing that he had to do something besides shout at them.

QUESTIONS

1. Is this an organization problem? What factors might be contributory?
2. In terms of organization design, what can Brice do?

■ Case Study 4: Somebody Has to Be Let Go[97]

Ken was a senior vice president of one of the nation's leading quality consulting firms. In 4 years, the makeup of the company had expanded from the founder, a secretary, 2 full-time trainers, and 4 part-time trainers to 125 full-time employees. Of these, 15 were full-time account executives, trainers with limited sales and customer service responsibility. About 70% of the company's revenues came from offering training courses on continuous quality improvement to clients. Revenues and profits had grown substantially, but early in the 4th year, revenues dropped drastically as managed care cost-cutting pressures were felt throughout the health sector and expected sales to the company's largest client, an HS, failed to materialize.

Ken was assigned the task of determining what to do in design changes. Losses were projected for this quarter, and the president and chairman of the board—the firm's founder—had decreed that members of the work force who were not productive had to be let go. A target number of 25 people had been set. Ken had been placed in charge of a three-person task force and given 1 week to develop a plan, including the names of those to be fired and the timing of these personnel actions. The firings had to be completed within 3 weeks.

The company had grown so rapidly that it had not had time to complete job descriptions for any of the jobs in the company. It was common knowledge that a lot of people, including some account executives, were sitting around doing nothing a lot of the day. There had never been any evaluations of employees, other than those of the training staff.

At the end of the briefing session in which Ken was assigned this task, the president commented: "Good luck! You are going to need it."

QUESTIONS

1. If you were Ken, where would you start? How would you proceed?
2. How can you rationally make these choices?
3. What kind of organization design does this company need?

Notes

1. Leatt, Peggy, Ross Baker, and John R. Kimberly. "Organization Design." In *Healthcare Management: Organization Design and Behavior,* 5th ed., edited by Stephen M. Shortell and Arnold D. Kaluzny, 318. Albany, NY: Thomson Delmar Learning, 2006.
2. Roethlisberger, Fritz J., and William J. Dickson. *Management and the Worker.* Cambridge, MA: Harvard University Press, 1939.
3. Weber, Max. *The Theory of Social and Economic Organization.* Translated by A.M. Henderson and Talcott Parsons. New York: The Free Press, 1947.
4. Fayol, Henri. *General and Industrial Management.* Translated by Constance Storrs. London: Sir Isaac Pitman & Sons, 1949.
5. *Papers on the Science of Administration,* edited by Luther Gulick and Lyndall Urwick. New York: Institute of Public Administration, 1937.
6. Mooney, James D., and Alan C. Reiley. *Onward Industry: The Principles of Organization and Their Significance to Modern Industry.* New York: Harper & Brothers, 1931.
7. Roethlisberger, Fritz J., and William J. Dickson. *Management and the Worker.* Cambridge, MA: Harvard University Press, 1939.
8. Weber, *The Theory of Social and Economic Organization.*
9. Robbins, Stephen P., and Mary K. Coulter. *Management,* 9th ed. Upper Saddle River, NJ: Prentice-Hall, 2007.
10. Smith, Adam. *The Wealth of Nations.* London: Dent, 1910.
11. Fayol, Henri. *General and Industrial Management.* Translated by Constance Storrs. London: Sir Isaac Pitman & Sons, 1949.
12. Newstrom, John W., and Keith Davis. *Organizational Behavior: Human Behavior at Work,* 12th ed., chap. 11–12. New York: McGraw-Hill, 2006.
13. Newstrom and Davis, *Organizational Behavior,* chap. 11–12; Leatt, Baker, and Kimberly, "Organization Design," 328.
14. Schermerhorn, John R., Jr. *Management,* 9th ed.. New York: John Wiley & Sons, 2007.
15. Clegg, Stewart, David Courpasson, and Nelson Philips. *Power and Organizations.* Thousand Oaks, CA: Sage Publications, 2006.
16. Higgins, James M. *The Management Challenge: An Introduction to Management,* 42. New York: Macmillan, 1991.
17. French, John R.P., and Bertram H. Raven. "The Basis of Social Power." In *Studies of Social Power,* edited by Dorwin Cartwright, 150–167. Ann Arbor, MI: Institute for Social Research, 1959.
18. Mooney and Reiley, *Onward Industry,* 39.

19. Leatt, Baker, and Kimberly, "Organization Design," 322.
20. Gulick and Urwick, *Papers on the Science,* 15.
21. Mintzberg, Henry. *Structuring of Organizations,* 108–111. Englewood Cliffs, NJ: Prentice-Hall, 1979.
22. Mintzberg, *Structuring of Organizations,* 106.
23. Urwick, Lyndall. *The Elements of Administration.* New York: Harper & Row, 1944.
24. Davis, Ralph C. *Fundamentals of Top Management.* New York: Harper & Row, 1951.
25. Barkdull, Charles W. "Span of Control—A Method of Evaluation." *Michigan Business Review* 15 (May 1963): 27–29; Steiglitz, Harry. *Organizational Planning.* New York: National Industrial Conference Board, 1966.
26. Barnard, Chester I. *The Functions of the Executive,* 256. Cambridge, MA: Harvard University Press, 1938.
27. Fayol, *General and Industrial,* 104.
28. Schermerhorn, John R., Jr. *Management,* 9th ed. New York: John Wiley & Sons, 2007.
29. Lawrence, Paul R., and Jay W. Lorsch. "Differentiation and Integration in Complex Organizations." *Administrative Science Quarterly* 11 (June 1967): 1–47.
30. March, James G., and Herbert A. Simon. *Organizations.* New York: John Wiley & Sons, 1958.
31. Litterer, Joseph A. *The Analysis of Organizations,* 223–232. New York: John Wiley & Sons, 1965.
32. Litterer, *Analysis of Organizations,* 227.
33. Mintzberg, *Structuring of Organizations;* Mintzberg, *Structure in Fives.*
34. Mintzberg, *Structuring of Organizations,* 6–7.
35. Hage, Jerald. *Theories of Organizations: Forms, Processes, and Transformations.* New York: Wiley-Interscience, 1980.
36. Lawrence and Lorsch, "Differentiation and Integration."
37. Likert, Rensis. *The Human Organization,* 156. New York: McGraw-Hill, 1967.
38. Longest, Beaufort B., Jr., and Gary J. Young. "Coordination and Communication." In *Healthcare Management: Organizations Design and Behavior,* 5th ed., edited by Stephen M. Shortell and Arnold D. Kaluzny, 237–275. Albany, NY: Thomson Delmar Learning, 2006.
39. Shortell, Stephen M., Jack E. Zimmerman, Denise M. Rousseau, Robin R. Gillies, Douglas P. Wagner, Elizabeth A. Draper, William A. Knaus, and Joanne Duffy. "The Performance of Intensive Care Units: Does Good Management Make a Difference?" *Medical Care* 32, 5 (1994): 508–525.
40. Young, Gary J., Martin P. Charns, Jennifer Daley, Maureen G. Forbes, William Henderson, and Shukri F. Khuri. "Best Practices for Managing Surgical Services: The Role of Coordination," *Healthcare Management Review* 22, 4 (1997): 72–81; Young, Gary J., Martin P. Charns, Kamal Desai, Shukri F. Khuri, Maureen G. Forbes, William Henderson, and Jennifer Daley. "Patterns of Coordination and Surgical Outcomes: A Study of Surgical Services," *Health Services Research* 33 (December 1998): 1,211–1,223.
41. The Joint Commission. *Accreditation Manual for Hospitals, Continuum of Care.* Chicago: Joint Commission on Accreditation of Healthcare Organizations, 1997.
42. Longest and Young, "Coordination and Communication," 241.
43. Flood, Anne B. "The Impact of Organizational and Managerial Factors on the Quality of Care in Healthcare Organizations." *Medical Care Review* 51, 4 (1994): 381–428.
44. Longest and Young, "Coordination and Communication," 244.
45. Pearson, Steven D., Dorothy Goulart-Fischer, and Thomas H. Lee. "Critical Pathways as a Strategy for Improving Care: Problems and Potential." *Annals of Internal Medicine* 123 (December 1995): 941–948.
46. Pearson, Goulart-Fischer, and Lee, "Critical Pathways as a Strategy for Improving Care: Problems and Potential."
47. Longest and Young, "Coordination and Communication."
48. General Accounting Office. *Healthcare Reform: Report Cards Are Useful but Significant Issues Need to Be Addressed.* Report to the Chairman, Committee on Labor and Human Resources, U.S. Senate, September 1994. GAO/HEHS-94-219; Kapp, Marshall B. "Cookbook Medicine: A Legal Perspective." *Archives of Internal Medicine* 150 (March 1990): 496–500.
49. Longest and Young, "Coordination and Communication," 246.
50. Kapp, "Cookbook Medicine: A Legal Perspective"; Flood, "The Impact of Organizational and Managerial Factors on the Quality of Care in Healthcare Organizations."

51. Young, Charns, Daley, Forbes, Henderson, and Khuri, "Best Practices for Managing Surgical Services: The Role of Coordination"; Young, Charns, Desai, Khuri, Forbes, Henderson, and Daley, "Patterns of Coordination and Surgical Outcomes: A Study of Surgical Services."

52. Barton, Phoebe Lindsey. *Understanding the U.S. Health Services System,* 218. Chicago: Health Administration Press, 1999.

53. Zajac, Edward J., Thomas A. D'Aunno, and Lawton R. Burns. "Managing Strategic Alliances." In *Healthcare Management: Organization Design and Behavior,* 5th ed., edited by Stephen M. Shortell and Arnold D. Kaluzny, 358. Clifton Park, NY: Thomson Delmar Learning, 2006.

54. *The Grand Alliance: Vertical Integration Strategies for Physicians and Health Systems.* Washington, DC: The Advisory Board Company, 1993; Kaluzny, Arnold D., and Howard S. Zuckerman. "Strategic Alliances: Two Perspectives for Understanding Their Effects on Health Services." *Hospital & Health Services Administration* 37 (Winter 1992): 477–490; Longest, "Interorganizational Linkages"; Luke, Roice D., James W. Begun, and Dennis D. Pointer. "Quasi-Firms: Strategic Interorganizational Forms in the Healthcare Industry." *Academy of Management Review* 14 (January 1989): 9–19; Provan, Keith G. "Interorganizational Cooperation and Decision Making Autonomy in a Consortium Multihospital System." *Academy of Management Review* 9 (1984): 494–504; Sofaer, Shoshanna, and Robert C. Myrtle. "Interorganizational Theory and Research: Implications for Healthcare Management, Policy, and Research." *Medical Care* 48 (Winter 1991): 371–409.

55. Stein, Barry A. "Strategic Alliances: Some Lessons from Experience." In *Partners for the Dance: Forming Strategic Alliances in Healthcare,* edited by Arnold D. Kaluzny, Howard S. Zuckerman, and Thomas C. Ricketts, III, 19–62. Ann Arbor, MI: Health Administration Press, 1995.

56. Coddington, Dean C., Keith D. Moore, and Elizabeth A. Fischer. *Making Integrated Healthcare Work.* Englewood, CO: Center for Research in Ambulatory Healthcare Administration, 1996.

57. Partners Healthcare. "Welcome to Partners Healthcare." *www.partners.org,* retrieved on October 7, 2006.

58. O'Leary, Margaret R. *Lexikon,* 337. Oakbrook Terrace, IL: Joint Commission on Accreditation of Healthcare Organizations, 1994.

59. Coddington, Moore, and Fischer, *Making Integrated,* 14–21.

60. Ginter, Swayne, and Duncan, *Strategic Management,* 6.

61. Ginter, Swayne, and Duncan, *Strategic Management,* 6.

62. Orlikoff, James E., and Mary K. Totten. "New Relationships with Physicians: An Overview for Trustees." *Trustee* 50 (July/August 1997 [workbook insert]).

63. Orlikoff and Totten, "New Relationships."

64. O'Leary, *Lexikon,* 614.

65. Burns, Lawton R., and Darrell P. Thorpe. "Physician-Hospital Organizations: Strategy, Structure, and Conduct." In *Integrating the Practice of Medicine: A Decision Maker's Guide to Organizing and Managing Physician Services,* edited by Ronald B. Connors, chap. 17. Chicago: AHA Press, 1997.

66. O'Leary, *Lexikon,* 413.

67. Blair, John D., Charles R. Slaton, and Grant T. Savage. "Hospital-Physician Joint Ventures: A Strategic Approach for Both Dimensions of Success." *Hospital & Health Services Administration* 35 (Spring 1990): 3–26.

68. Conrad, Douglas A., and Stephen M. Shortell. "Integrated Health Systems: Promise and Performance." *Frontiers of Health Services Management* 7 (Fall 1996): 3–40.

69. Dowling, William L. "Strategic Alliances as a Structure for Integrated Delivery Systems." In *Partners for the Dance: Forming Strategic Alliances in Healthcare,* edited by Arnold D. Kaluzny, Howard S. Zuckerman, and Thomas C. Ricketts, III, 141. Chicago: Health Administration Press, 1995; Conrad, Douglas A., and William L. Dowling. "Vertical Integration in Health Services: Theory and Managerial Implications." *Healthcare Management Review* 14 (Fall 1990): 9–22.

70. Amerinet. "Our Network." *www.amerinet-gpo1.com/Amerinet.aspx?tabid=148&NavId=2#members,* retrieved October 9, 2006.

71. Dowling, William L. "Strategic Alliances as a Structure for Integrated Delivery Systems." In *Partners for the Dance: Forming Strategic Alliances in Healthcare,* edited by Arnold D. Kaluzny, Howard S. Zuckerman, and Thomas C. Ricketts, III, 140. Chicago: Health Administration Press, 1995.

72. Kraatz, Matthew S. "Learning by Association? Interorganizational Networks and Adaptation to Environmental Change." *Academy of Management Journal* 41 (December 1998): 621–643; Zajac, Edward J., Brian R. Golden, and Stephen M. Shortell. "New Organizational Forms for Enhancing Innovation: The Case of Internal Corporate Joint Ventures." *Management Science* 37 (1991): 170–184.

73. Harvard Pilgrim Healthcare. "About Harvard Pilgrim Healthcare." *www.harvardpilgrim.org,* retrieved October 10, 2006.

74. Henry Ford Health System. "About Henry Ford." *www.henryford.com,* retrieved October 10, 2006.

75. Lovelace Health System. "About Us." *www.lovelace.com,* retrieved October 10, 2006

76. Satinsky, Marjorie A. *The Foundations of Integrated Care: Facing the Challenges of Change,* vii. Chicago: American Hospital Publishing, 1998.

77. Kraatz, "Learning by Association?"

78. Luke, Roice, Peter C. Olden, and James D. Bramble. "Strategic Hospital Alliances: Countervailing Responses to Restructuring Healthcare Markets." In *Handbook of Healthcare Management,* edited by W. Jack Duncan, Peter M. Ginter, and Linda E. Swayne, 86. Malden, MA: Blackwell, 1998.

79. Luke, Olden, and Bramble, "Strategic Hospital Alliances," 86.

80. Thompson, James D. *Organizations in Action.* New York: McGraw-Hill, 1967.

81. Sunseri, Reid. "Outsourcing Loses Its 'Mo.'" *Hospital & Health Networks* 72, 22 (November 20, 1998): 36–40.

82. Thompson, *Organizations in Action.*

83. Weick, Kenneth. "Educational Organizations as Loosely Coupled Systems." *Administrative Science Quarterly* 21 (March 1976): 1–19; Zuckerman, Howard S., and Thomas A. D'Aunno. "Hospital Alliances: Cooperative Strategy in a Competitive Environment." *Healthcare Management Review* 15 (1990): 21–30.

84. Adapted from "Introduction and Methodology." *Managed Care Digest Series* 2007: *Hospitals/Systems Digest* 2 (2007): 2–3. Provided by Sanofi-Aventis at *http://www.managedcaredigest.com/resources/hosp2007/hosp2007.pdf.*

85. Shortell, Stephen M., Robin R. Gillies, David A. Anderson, Karen Morgan Erickson, and John B. Mitchell. *Remaking Healthcare in America: The Evolution of Organized Delivery Systems,* 2nd ed., 129. San Francisco: Jossey-Bass, 2000.

86. Shortell, Gillies, Anderson, Erickson, and Mitchell, *Remaking Healthcare,* 28.

87. Satinsky, *The Foundations of Integrated Care,* 15.

88. Conrad, Douglas A. "Coordinating Patient Care Services in Regional Health Systems: The Challenge of Clinical Integration." *Hospital & Health Services Administration* 38, 4 (Winter 1993): 492.

89. Mintzberg, Henry. "Organization Design: Fashion or Fit?" *Harvard Business Review* 59 (January/February 1981): 103–116; Mintzberg, Henry. *The Structuring of Organizations.* Englewood Cliffs, NJ: Prentice-Hall, 1979; Mintzberg, Henry. *Structure in Fives: Designing Effective Organizations.* Englewood Cliffs, NJ: Prentice-Hall, 1983.

90. Mintzberg, *Structuring of Organizations,* 29.

91. Mintzberg, *Structuring of Organizations,* 20.

92. Mintzberg, *Structuring of Organizations;* Mintzberg, "Organization Design"; Mintzberg, *Structure in Fives.*

93. Mintzberg, "Organization Design," 111.

94. Mintzberg, "Organization Design," 112.

95. Mintzberg, "Organization Design," 112.

96. Drucker, Peter F. "New Templates for Today's Organizations." *Harvard Business Review* 52 (January/February 1974): 51.

97. Adapted from Higgins, James M. *The Management Challenge: An Introduction to Management,* 2nd edition, 311. New York: Macmillan, 1994; reprinted by permission of Pearson Education Inc., Upper Saddle River, NJ.

12

Leading

classic writer

The quality of leading in health services organizations/health systems (HSOs/HSs) affects the work accomplished by individuals and groups, as well as performance of organizations and systems in pursuing their missions and objectives.[1] Burns, in a classic work, established that leading in organizations is of two distinct types: transactional and transformational.[2] Both are relevant to performance and considered in this chapter.

Transactional leading occurs throughout organizations because managers relate directly to people. A transactional process, leading in these relationships permits some of the needs of followers to be met if they perform to the leader's expectations; leaders and followers undertake transactions through which each receives something of value. Good leadership skills and techniques facilitate transactions that are essential if these pervasive relationships are to function well.

In the second type of leading—more likely to be practiced in organizations and systems by senior-level managers—the purpose is significant change in the status quo. In practicing transformational leadership, managers are more focused on creating change than on exchanges. In their transformational leadership roles, managers focus on changes that are organizationwide or system-wide in scope and relate to such things as

- Vision, mission, objectives, and values
- Attaining or modifying the level of support for the mission among internal and external stakeholders
- Allocating responsibility for the HSO's/HS's operation and performance
- Developing new strategies or implementing existing ones differently
- Altering the balance among the economic, professional, and social interests of the HSO/HS and those who work in it
- Establishing new, or discarding existing, relationships with other organizations or systems with which interdependencies are shared

In contrast to the transactional leading process that occurs between managers and other individuals, a transformational leader must have a vision for the entire entity and must lead followers both inside and outside the entity if the vision is to be realized.[3] Often, when people speak of leadership, they mean transformational leadership. When an organization's perceived success is attributed to strong and effective leadership, this means generally that leaders have made good decisions regarding mission, objectives, structure, service mix, quality, and new technologies, not that its leaders (managers) have only been good at transactional leadership. Transactional leadership, through which better performance from people is achieved as leaders help them plan their tasks, coordinate their work, or learn new skills, is important but is not the only determinant of senior-level managers' success in their transformational leader roles.[4]

Senior managers lead in part by managing organizational culture, which focuses on decisions and activities that affect the entire organization or system, including those that are intended to ensure its survival and overall good health.[5] They lead by providing strategic direction and vision to the entity, ensuring that its mission and objectives are achieved. Effective organization- or system-level leaders also lead by inculcating certain values; building intraorganizational and interorganizational coalitions; and interpreting and responding to various challenges and opportunities from the external environment, which includes taking steps to alter the environment.

Before a discussion of the extensive research and various theories about both transactional and transformational leadership roles, it is necessary to first define *leading* precisely and to model it as a process, to discuss power and influence as central to leading, and to consider the role of motivation in effective leading.

Leading Defined and Modeled

Leading is defined in different ways, although most definitions have common elements. Adapting well-known definitions[6] of leading by managers to a healthcare setting produces the definition that *leading* is influencing others to understand and agree about what needs to be done in order to achieve the mission and objectives established for the HSO/HS *and* facilitating the individual and collective contributions of others to achieve these desired results. Influencing is the most critical element of this definition and is central to success in leading; it is the means by which "people successfully persuade others to follow their advice, suggestion, or order."[7]

Taking these definitions into account gives a comprehensive perspective of this complex, multidimensional activity—that leading is a process of one individual influencing another individual or a group to achieve particular objectives. *Leader* can be defined as one who leads, that is, an individual who influences other individuals or groups to achieve particular objectives. These perspectives of leaders and leading apply to transformational organizational or system-level leading as well as transactional leading at the level of managers interacting with individuals and groups. In both situations, leadership means determining what is to be accomplished and influencing others to contribute to its accomplishment. Figure 12.1 shows a simplified model of this process.

The processes of transactional and transformational leading differ. For example, managers at the level of leading individuals and groups often work with people who tend to be relatively homo-

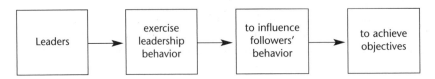

Figure 12.1.   The process of leadership.

geneous in terms of their work. This stands in contrast to the transformational leadership of an entire organization or system, in which there is likely to be great diversity and heterogeneity. Another very important difference in leading roles of managers at different organizational levels is the amount and sources of power available to them. As is discussed in the next section, power is crucial to the ability to exert influence, and the ability to influence is essential to the ability to lead.

Power and Influence in Leading

The essence of leading is influencing followers; therefore, influence is central to the leading process and to success in the leader role. To have influence, however, one also must have power. Power is the potential to exert influence. More power means more potential to influence others. To understand influence, one must first understand interpersonal power and its sources.

SOURCES OF POWER

Those who wish to exert influence must first acquire power by utilizing the various sources of power available to them. The classic scheme for categorizing the bases of interpersonal power identified by French and Raven[8] includes legitimate, reward, coercive, expert, and referent power. Building on this earlier work, Yukl[9] extended the understanding of the sources of interpersonal power to include information power and ecological power, and he divided the expanded set of sources of interpersonal power into position and personal power types,[10] as shown in Figure 12.2.

Legitimate power is derived from a person's position in an organization. It also is called formal power or authority and exists because organizations find it advantageous to assign certain powers to individuals so that they can do their jobs. Based on their position, all managers have some degree of legitimate power or authority, but amounts fluctuate with levels.

Reward power is based on the leader's ability to reward desirable behavior. Reward power stems partly from legitimate power granted to the leader by the organization. In other words, managers, by virtue of their positions, are given control over certain rewards to buttress their legitimate, or positional, power. Rewards include pay increases, promotions, work schedules, recognition of accomplishments, and status symbols such as office size and location.

Coercive power is the opposite of reward power and is based on the leader's ability to punish people or prevent them from obtaining desired rewards. As described below, rewards and punishments are powerful motivational tools, although managers playing their leader roles are, in general, better served by reward power than coercive power.

Expert power derives from having knowledge valued by the organization or system, such as expertise in problem solving or critical tasks. Expert power is personal to the individual who pos-

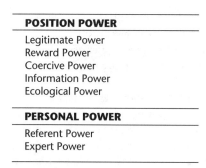

POSITION POWER

Legitimate Power
Reward Power
Coercive Power
Information Power
Ecological Power

PERSONAL POWER

Referent Power
Expert Power

Figure 12.2. Different types of power. (From *Structure in Fives: Designing Effective Organizations,* 2nd edition, 5, by Henry Mintzberg, © 1992. Reprinted by permission of Pearson Education, Inc., Upper Saddle River, NJ.)

sesses the expertise. Thus it is different from legitimate, reward, and coercive power, which are prescribed by the organization or system, even though people may be granted these forms of power because they possess expert power. For example, certain health professionals enter management positions because of their superior levels of expertise. When they make this shift, they acquire legitimate, reward, and coercive power in addition to their expert power. It also is noteworthy that, in organizations where work is highly technical or professional, expert power alone makes some people very powerful. For example, the power of the professional staff is based on clinical knowledge and skills. Physicians with scarce expertise, such as in transplant surgery, gain more power than physicians whose expertise is readily replaceable. Expert power is not reserved for those with clinical or technical skills, however. The ability to effectively manage complex HSOs/HSs is a source of power for those with the expertise.

Referent power results when individuals engender admiration, loyalty, and emulation to the extent that they gain the power to influence others. This is sometimes called charismatic power. Charismatic leaders typically have a vision for groups or organizations they lead, strong convictions about the integrity of the vision, and great self-confidence in their ability to realize the vision. They are perceived by their followers as agents of change.[11] It is rare for a leader, whether transactional or transformational, to gain sufficient power to heavily influence followers simply from referent or charismatic power. As with expert power, referent power cannot be given by the organization or system as legitimate, reward, and coercive power can.

Information power depends on the leader's (or manager's) having access to vital information and some degree of control over its distribution. Ecological power stems from the leader's control over the physical environment in the workplace, as well as some degree of control over technology and organization designs used in the workplace.

EFFECTIVE USE OF POWER

The seven sources of interpersonal power considered in the previous section are not necessarily independent and, in fact, can be complementary. Leaders who use reward power wisely strengthen their referent power. Conversely, leaders who abuse their coercive power will quickly weaken or lose referent power. Effective leaders are those who can translate power into influence and who understand the sources of their power and act accordingly. Good interpersonal and political skills distinguish individuals who effectively use and translate power into influence as they lead others. However, access to power is not enough. One must know how to use power effectively to influence others. Politics in organizations and systems have been defined as "activities to acquire, develop, and use power and other resources to obtain a preferred outcome."[12] Mintzberg attributes the successful use of power in organizations largely to leaders' political skills, which he defines as

> The ability to use the bases of power effectively—to convince those to whom one has access, to use one's resources, information, and technical skills to their fullest in bargaining, to exercise formal power with a sensitivity to the feelings of others, to know where to concentrate one's energies, to sense what is possible, and to organize the necessary alliances.[13]

As noted earlier, people in organizations derive power, in part, from their positions in the organizational design. Position or legitimate power (see Figure 12.2) includes the authority that is granted to managers by the organization and its inherent control over certain resources, processes, and information. However, power in organizational settings also depends on interpersonal relationships between leaders and followers. Personal power includes relative task expertise, friendship and the loyalty that some people engender in others, and sometimes the leader's charismatic qualities. Finally, power also depends on certain political processes and skills. Political power derives from the leader's control over key decisions, ability to form coalitions, ability to co-opt or diffuse and weaken the influence of rivals in the organization, and ability to institutionalize the leader's power by exploiting ambiguity to interpret events in a manner that is favorable to the leader.[14]

Depending on circumstances, power of the types shown in Figure 12.2 is available in different degrees to leaders in HSOs/HSs. For example, at the departmental level, where leadership occurs primarily through transactions taking place in manager-subordinate relationships, first-level managers have the power to influence or lead because they have formal authority. First-level managers also have some control over resources, rewards, punishments, and information (position power), and they may have more expertise in the work than others in the department (personal power derived from expertise). Such managers may have little political power, but this is not a problem if position and personal power sources are sufficient to lead the department.

In contrast, senior-level managers, who lead at the organization or system level, derive power from the same menu of sources but in a different mix. For example, the chief executive officer (CEO) possesses political power by virtue of the authority to control decision processes, form coalitions of key decision makers, or co-opt opponents. The CEO may have charisma, extremely loyal assistants, and deep friendships with key physicians and governing body members, all of which provide the CEO with personal power. The CEO's position power can be great in terms of control over resources and information. Finally, the CEO may be in a strong position to control access to the sources of power in the organization or system.[15] This is an important source of power in itself.

What is known about power and influence is pertinent to understanding leadership. By definition, leadership involves one person influencing others, and power is the ability to influence others. Power and influence alone, however, do not fully explain leadership effectiveness or the success or failure of leaders. Supporting and assisting others to be motivated to perform well also is key to successfully leading.

Motivation Defined and Modeled

Motivation is a crucial concept in effectively managing and leading. Understanding the motivations and behaviors of people employed in HSOs/HSs is important because these organizations and systems benefit from several specific types of behaviors. First, however, people must be motivated to enter the work force. Then they must be motivated to continue their employment or contractual relationship, and they must be motivated to attend work regularly, punctually, and predictably. These behaviors are motivated behaviors. People also must be motivated to perform their work at acceptable levels, in terms of both the quantity and quality of work. Finally, organizations need certain good citizenship behaviors from its work force.[16] People can be motivated to exhibit such behaviors as cooperation, altruism, protecting fellow workers and property, and generally going above and beyond the call of duty. The presence of good citizenship behaviors invariably makes the manager's job easier and contributes directly to organizational performance. Leaders must help motivate people to practice all these behaviors.

In concept, motivation is at once simple and complex. Motivation is simple because it is now known that behavior is goal directed and is induced by increasingly well understood forces, some of which are internal to the individual, others external. Motivation is complex because mechanisms that induce behavior include very complicated and individualized needs, wants, and desires that are shaped, affected, and satisfied in different ways.

Why does one person work harder than another? Why is one more cooperative than another? In part, these differences occur because people have varying needs and act differently to satisfy them. People's needs are deficiencies that cause them to undertake patterns of behavior intended to fill the deficiencies. For example, at a very simple level, human needs are physiological. A hungry person needs food, is driven by hunger, and is motivated to satisfy the need or, stated another way, to over-

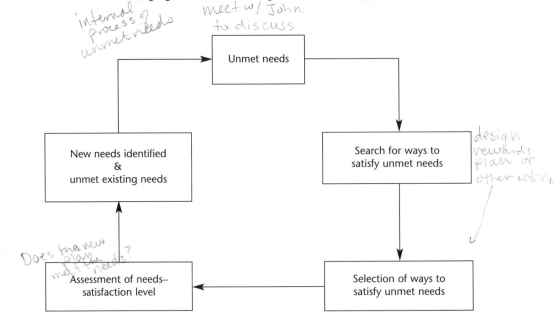

Figure 12.3.   The motivation process. (From Longest, Beaufort B., Jr. *Health Professionals in Management,* 247. Stamford, CT: Appleton & Lange, 1996; reprinted by permission.)

come the deficiency. Other needs are more complex; some are psychological (e.g., the need for self-esteem) and some are sociological (e.g., the need for social interaction). In short, unmet needs trigger and energize human behaviors. This fact is the basis for a model of the motivation process.

As shown in Figure 12.3, the motivation process is cyclical. It begins with an unmet need and cycles through the individual's assessment of the results of efforts to satisfy the need, which may confirm the continuation of an unmet need or identify a new need. Meanwhile, the person searches for ways to satisfy the unmet need and chooses a course of action, exhibiting goal-directed behavior intended to satisfy the unmet need.

The model is oversimplified, but it contains the essential elements of the process by which human motivation occurs. Motivation is driven by unsatisfied needs and results in goal-directed behaviors in the person experiencing it, although it also can be influenced by factors that are external to the individual. This model also suggests a definition of motivation: an internal drive that stimulates behavior that is intended to satisfy an unmet need. Most contemporary definitions include these terms or express the same concept. For example, motivation has been defined as "a goal-directed, internal drive which is always aimed at satisfying needs"[17] or as "a state of feeling or thinking in which one is energized or aroused to perform a task or engage in a particular behavior."[18] It is important to note that the direction, intensity, and duration of this state can be influenced by factors outside the individual experiencing the state, including the ability of leaders and HSOs/HSs to contribute to or impede the satisfaction of the individual's needs. Thus it may be concluded that motivation

- Is driven by unsatisfied or unmet needs
- Results in goal-directed behaviors
- Is influenced by factors that may be internal or external to the individual experiencing motivation

Motivation is a key determinant of individual performance in work situations and is of obvious importance in achieving the missions and organizational objectives of HSOs/HSs. However, motivation alone does not fully explain performance. It is only one of many variables affecting performance. Intelligence, physical and mental abilities, previous experiences, and the nature of the work environment also determine performance. Good equipment and pleasant surroundings facilitate high levels of performance. The variables affecting performance can be conceptualized as follows:

$$\text{Performance} = \text{Ability/Talent/Experience} \times \text{Environment} \times \text{Motivation}$$

This equation shows that performance is a function of, or results from, an interaction of variables, an interaction that goes beyond being merely additive.[19] Without motivation, no amount of ability or talent, and no environmental conditions, can produce acceptable performance.

HOW MOTIVATION OCCURS

Understanding motivation and applying knowledge of how it occurs are critical to effectively leading others; therefore, a great deal of attention is given to determining the mechanisms of human motivation. To motivate participants, managers need to know the answers to such questions as What energizes or causes participants to behave in contributory ways? What variables help direct their energies into particular behaviors? Can the energized state be intensified or made to last longer?

It is important to note at the outset when seeking answers to questions about motivation that researchers have not established an undisputed and comprehensive theory about motivation or about how leaders affect it in the workplace. Instead, many competing theories have been posited to explain motivation. These varied approaches to motivation can be divided into two broad categories: *content* and *process* perspectives on motivation (see Table 12.1). Each of the perspectives contributes something to understanding motivation and has implications for leading.

The content perspective on motivation focuses on the internal needs and desires that initiate,

TABLE 12.1. COMPARISON OF CONTENT AND PROCESS PERSPECTIVES ON MOTIVATION

Content Perspective

Focus:
  Identifying factors within individuals that initiate, sustain, and terminate behaviors

Key studies:
  Maslow's five levels of human needs in hierarchy
  Alderfer's three levels of human needs in hierarchy
  Herzberg's two sets of factors
  McClelland's three learned needs

Implication for managers in leading:
  Managers must pay attention to the unique and varied needs, desires, and goals of participants

Process Perspective

Focus:
  Explaining how behaviors are initiated, sustained, and terminated

Key studies:
  Vroom's expectancy theory of choices
  Adams' equity theory
  Locke's goal-setting theory

Implication for managers in leading:
  Managers must understand how the unique and varied needs, desires, and goals of participants interact with their preferences, and with rewards and accomplishments to affect their behavioral choices

Source: Beaufort B. Longest, Jr. *Managing Health Programs and Projects.* 116. San Francisco: Jossey-Bass, 2004. Reprinted by permission.

sustain, and eventually terminate behavior. The focus is on *what* motivates. In contrast, the process perspective seeks to explain *how* behavior is initiated, sustained, and terminated. Combined, these perspectives on motivation define variables that explain motivated behavior and show how they interact and influence one another to produce certain behavior patterns. Key theories that underpin contemporary thought about human motivation in the workplace are noted in Table 12.1 and are briefly described below, beginning with four theories that fall within the content perspective.

Maslow's Hierarchy of Needs

Perhaps the most widely recognized theory about what motivates human behavior—certainly the one with the most enduring impact—was advanced by Abraham Maslow in the 1940s. A psychologist, Maslow formulated a theory of motivation that stressed two fundamental premises.[20] First, he argued that human beings have a variety of needs and that *unmet* needs influence behavior; an adequately fulfilled need is not a motivator. His second premise was that people's needs are arranged in a hierarchy. Maslow stressed the idea of needs existing in a hierarchy, with "higher" needs becoming dominant only after "lower" needs are satisfied. Figure 12.4 illustrates Maslow's needs hierarchy, with an example for each category of need and how it can be fulfilled in an HSO/HS.

From lowest to highest order, the five categories of needs in Maslow's hierarchy begin with basic physiological needs, such as air, water, food, shelter, and sex, which are necessary for survival. Participants can satisfy many of these needs through resources that their paychecks provide. Then come safety and security needs. Once survival needs are met, attention can be turned to ensuring continued survival by protecting oneself against physical harm and deprivation. Participants seek to meet their safety and security needs through assuring job security, having adequate life and health insurance, and other benefits. The third level of needs is for social activity, which relates to people's

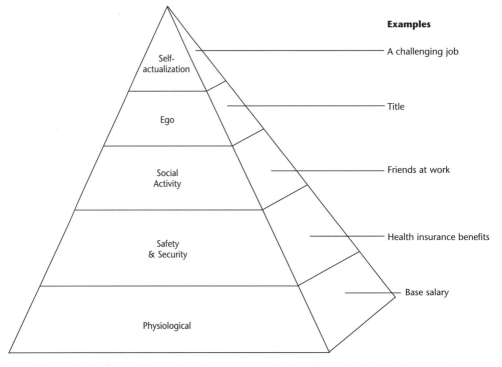

Figure 12.4. Maslow's needs hierarchy. (From Longest, Beaufort B., Jr. *Health Professionals in Management*, 251. Stamford, CT: Appleton & Lange, 1996; reprinted by permission.)

social and gregarious nature and includes their needs for belonging, friendship, affection, and love. The ability to have friendships with other participants and to engage in social activity within the workplace helps satisfy these needs.

It is important to note that third-level needs are something of a breaking point in the hierarchy because these needs are removed from the physical or quasi-physical needs of the first two levels. This level reflects people's needs for association or companionship, belonging to groups, and giving and receiving friendship and affection.

The fourth level, ego needs, includes two different types of needs: the need for a positive self-image and self-respect, and the need for recognition and respect from others. Examples of ego needs include independence, achievement, recognition from others, self-esteem, and status. Opportunities for advancement within programs or projects, or within the larger organizations within which they may be embedded, can help participants fulfill these needs.

The top level of the Maslow hierarchy is self-actualization needs. These fifth-level needs include realizing one's potential for continued growth and development; they represent the need to become everything a person is capable of being. Self-actualization needs are evidenced by a need to be creative and to have opportunities for self-expression and self-fulfillment. A challenging and satisfying job is a primary pathway to satisfying such needs in contemporary society.

Managerial Implications of Maslow's Model

In part because of its great intuitive appeal, Maslow's concept of what motivates human behavior has been widely adopted. However, in a remarkable bit of candor, he once wrote of his concern that the theory was "being swallowed whole by all sorts of enthusiastic people, who really should be a little more tentative."[21] Although this view of what motivates human behavior has limitations, it makes a crucial and valid point that people have numerous needs that they seek to fulfill. In this way, Maslow contributes important insight into the nature of motivation and especially how unmet needs influence behaviors. Maslow's views on motivation provided a conceptual framework that was used to build and test more sophisticated theories about needs and how they affect human behavior. Two of these theories are described next.

Alderfer's ERG Theory

In another theory of what motivates human behavior, Clayton Alderfer[22] advanced the idea that the hierarchy of needs is more accurately conceptualized as having only three distinct categories, not five as in Maslow's formulation.[23] This theory is known as the ERG theory for the three categories of needs: existence, relatedness, and growth. Existence needs include material and physical needs that can be satisfied by such things as air, water, money, and working conditions. Relatedness needs include all needs that involve other people—needs satisfied by meaningful social and interpersonal relationships. Growth needs, in Alderfer's scheme, include all needs involving creative efforts— needs satisfied through an individual's creative or productive contributions.

Alderfer's ERG theory is obviously similar to Maslow's. His existence needs are similar to Maslow's physiological and safety needs; his relatedness needs parallel Maslow's affection and social activity category; and his growth needs are similar to the esteem and self-realization needs identified by Maslow. The theories differ, however, in a very important aspect; the manner in which needs influence behavior.

Maslow theorized that unfulfilled lower-level needs are predominant and that the next higher level of needs is not activated until the predominant (unmet lower-level) need is satisfied. He called this the satisfaction-progression process. In contrast, Alderfer argued that the three categories of needs form a hierarchy only in the sense of increasing abstractness, or decreasing concreteness: As an individual moves from existence to relatedness to growth needs, the means to satisfy the needs become less and less concrete.

In Alderfer's theory, people focus first on needs that are satisfied in relatively concrete ways; then they focus on needs that are satisfied more abstractly. This is similar to Maslow's idea of satisfaction-progression. However, Alderfer proposed that a "frustration-regression process" is also present in determining which category of needs predominates at any time. By this he meant that someone frustrated in efforts to satisfy growth needs may regress and focus on satisfying more concrete relatedness or even more concrete existence needs. In Alderfer's view, the coexistence of the satisfaction-progression and the frustration-regression processes leads to a *cycling* between categories of needs.

Managerial Implications of Alderfer's Theory

A case example from an HSO will help to clarify Alderfer's concept of cycling. Consider the case of Jennifer Smith, a 32-year-old registered nurse who works in a women's health program sponsored by a major hospital. Ms. Smith, a single parent of two young children, is appropriately concerned about the security of her position and her pay and benefits, although she finds the social interactions with co-workers rewarding. Clinically, she is an excellent nurse who enjoys her work.

When a vacancy occurred in a nurse manager position in the HSO, Ms. Smith considered the opportunities this presented for professional growth and development, as well as for a higher salary. She applied for the position and looked forward to the challenges she would face if selected.

However, a more experienced and equally qualified nurse was promoted. Ms. Smith's disappointment showed, and she also became quite concerned about her future in the program. Several other participants in the program noticed her reaction and made special efforts to ease her disappointment. They told her that other opportunities would arise and that with more experience, she would be promoted.

The newly promoted nurse manager was sensitive to this situation and made a point of telling Ms. Smith what a valuable contribution she was making to the success of the program in which she worked. After a few weeks, Ms. Smith returned to the level of enjoyment of her work she had felt before this episode. In terms of predominant needs, she had *cycled* from existence and relatedness needs to the growth needs represented by the promotion and then back to relatedness needs, all in a few weeks. In other words, Ms. Smith had experienced a satisfaction-progression process and a frustration-regression process.

An important part of Alderfer's ERG theory that differs from Maslow's formulation lies in Alderfer's view that when individuals satisfy their existence and relatedness needs, these needs become less important. The opposite is true for growth needs, however. In Alderfer's view, as growth needs are satisfied, they become increasingly important. As people become more creative and productive, they raise their growth goals and are not satisfied until the new goals are reached. In the case of Jennifer Smith described above, this means that when she becomes a nurse manager, she will likely raise her goals, anticipating further growth and development in her career.

An important element of the ERG theory for managers is the assumption that all employees have the potential for continued growth and development. Recognizing this fact leads naturally to the "desirability of offering ongoing opportunities for training and development, transfer, promotion, and career planning to all employees."[24]

Herzberg's Two-Factor Theory

Frederick Herzberg took a different approach to the study of what motivates human behavior in the workplace. He began with questions about what satisfies or dissatisfies people at work and assumed the answers would contribute to understanding what motivates people.[25]

Herzberg and his associates found one set of factors associated with satisfaction and high levels of motivation and a different set of factors associated with dissatisfaction and low motivation. In the "two-factor theory" of motivation, they argued that "satisfiers" or "motivators" are factors that result in satisfaction and high motivation when they are present in adequate levels or form. These factors are achievement, recognition, advancement, the work itself, possibility of growth, and responsibility. The other set of factors, labeled "dissatisfiers" or "hygiene factors," causes dissatisfaction and low motivation when they are not present in adequate levels or form. These factors include organizational policy and administration, supervision, interpersonal relations, and working conditions.

Managerial Implications of Herzberg's Theory

The most important contribution of Herzberg's formulation lies in the fact that it has caused managers to carefully consider factors that contribute to motivation and what managers can do to enhance opportunities to achieve intrinsic satisfaction from work. If managers are to help motivate participants, they must be concerned with one set of factors to minimize dissatisfaction *and* another to help them achieve satisfaction and be motivated in their work.

McClelland's Learned Needs Theory

Another important contributor to the content perspective of motivation was David McClelland, who developed the learned needs theory.[26] McClelland posited that people learn their needs through life experiences; they are not born with them. This theory builds on the much earlier work of Murray,[27] who theorized that people acquire individual profiles of needs by interacting with their environment. McClelland was also influenced by the work of Atkinson[28] and Atkinson and Raynor.[29]

Both McClelland and Atkinson argued that people have three distinct sets of needs: 1) the need for achievement, including the need to excel, achieve in relation to standards, accomplish complex tasks, and resolve problems; 2) the need for power, including the need to control or influence how others behave and to exercise authority over others; and 3) the need for affiliation, including the need to associate with others, form and sustain friendly and close interpersonal relationships, and avoid conflict.

McClelland hypothesized that people are not born with these needs. Instead, they are *learned* or acquired as people grow and develop. For example, children learn the need to achieve through encouragement and reinforcement of autonomy and self-reliance from adults who influence their early years.

McClelland also posited that people typically have these three sets of needs, although one predominates and most strongly affects each individual's behavior. This point is important because it relates to how well people fit particular work situations. In fact, the most useful aspect of McClelland's formulation is the importance of matching people, considering their particular dominant needs, with the work situation. If this is done carefully, participants will be more motivated and their performance will reflect this.

Transition from Content to Process Theories and Models of Motivation

The content perspective on motivation—as reflected in the four theories or models discussed above—emphasizes that human motivation originates from the needs of people and their search to satisfy them. The common thread running through the content models is their focus on needs that motivate human behavior. Each theory defines human needs differently, but all support the concept that managers can motivate participants in their programs and projects by helping them identify their specific needs and can, at least in part, meet the needs in the workplace.

These models emphasize the importance of managers' roles in helping participants understand their needs and the extraordinarily complex task of finding ways to satisfy these unique and constantly changing needs within the workplace. Managers can help participants identify and meet their needs by empathizing with them. Combining empathy with effective two-way communication, as discussed in Chapter 13, about needs and the potential to satisfy them within the context of the workplace usually results in progress toward identifying and fulfilling needs.

The content perspective on motivation, with its singular focus on *what* motivates behavior, provides many useful insights for managers. However, other models are needed to provide insight into the *process* of motivation—to explain the mechanisms through which motivation occurs. The process perspective focuses on *how* an individual's performance is influenced by expectations and preferences for outcomes. A central element in the process perspective on motivation is that people are decision makers who weigh the personal advantages and disadvantages of their behaviors.

As outlined in Table 12.1, there are three models that fall within the process perspective on motivation: Vroom's expectancy model, Adams's equity model, and Locke's goal-setting model. Each of these major models of the processes by which motivation occurs seeks to explain *how* motivation occurs in human beings.

Vroom's Expectancy Model

Victor Vroom's formulation of how motivation occurs is based on the idea that although people are driven by their unmet needs, they make decisions about how they will and will not behave in attempting to fulfill their needs. Their decisions are affected by three conditions: 1) people must believe that through their own efforts, they are more likely to achieve desired levels of performance, 2) people must believe that achieving the desired level of performance will lead to some concrete outcome or reward, and 3) people must value the outcome.[30] Figure 12.5 shows the three central components and the relationships in the expectancy theory model.

In this model, *expectancy* is what individuals perceive to be the probability that their efforts will lead to desired levels of performance. If a person believes that more effort will lead to improved performance, expectancy will be high. If, in a different situation, the same person believes that trying harder will not improve performance, the expectancy will be low.

Instrumentality is the probability perceived by individuals that their performance will lead to desired outcomes or rewards. If a person believes that better performance will be rewarded, the instrumentality of performance to reward will be high. Conversely, if the person believes that improved performance will not be rewarded, the instrumentality of improved performance will be low.

Outcomes are listed only once in Figure 12.5, but they play two important roles in the expectancy model. Level of performance (in the center of Figure 12.5) actually represents an outcome of the "individual effort to perform" component of the figure. Vroom calls this a first-order outcome. Examples of first-order outcomes include productivity, creativity, absenteeism, quality of work, and other behaviors that result from an individual's effort to perform. The outcomes component shown on the right side of Figure 12.5 is a second-order outcome that results from attainment of first-order outcomes. That is, these second-order outcomes are the rewards (or punishments) associated with

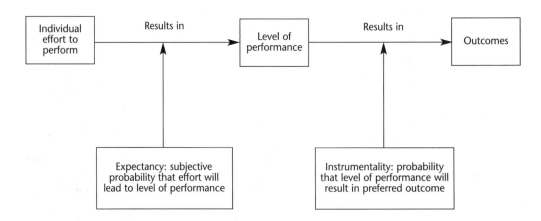

Figure 12.5. Simplified model of expectancy theory.

performance. Examples include merit pay increases, esteem of co-workers, approval of managers, promotion, and flexible work schedules.

Crucial to Vroom's expectancy model is the concept that people have preferences for outcomes. Vroom termed the value an individual attaches to a particular outcome its *valence*. When an individual has a strong preference for a particular outcome, it receives a high valence; similarly, a lower preference for an outcome yields a lower valence. People have valences for both first- and second-order outcomes. For example, a participant might prefer a merit pay increase to a flexible work schedule, while another participant might prefer the flexibility (second-order outcomes). A participant might prefer to produce quality work (a first-order outcome) because this person believes this will lead to a merit pay increase (a second-order outcome).

The three components of the expectancy theory (expectancy, instrumentality, and valence for outcomes) can be combined into an equation to express the motivation to work:

$$Motivation = Expectancy \times Instrumentality \times Valence$$

or

$$M = E \times I \times V$$

It is important to note that because the equation is multiplicative, a low value assigned to any variable will yield a low result. For example, if a person is certain that effort will lead to performance (an expectancy value of 1.0 is assigned), is certain that performance will lead to reward (an instrumentality value of 1.0 is assigned), but does not have a very high preference for the reward involved (a valence value of 0.5 is assigned), when the components are multiplied ($1.0 \times 1.0 \times 0.5 = 0.5$), the result is low, indicating that motivation is low. For motivation to be high, expectancy, instrumentality, and valence values all must be high.

Managerial Implications of the Expectancy Model

For managers and leaders, the expectancy model explains a great deal about motivated behavior. By applying the expectancy model, managers and leaders can focus on leverage points that help them influence the motivation of other participants. For motivated behavior to occur, three conditions must be met by the participant: 1) a high expectancy that effort and performance are actually linked; 2) a high expectancy that performance will lead to outcomes or rewards; and 3) a preference (which assigns a high valence value) for the outcomes that result from effort, including both first- and second-order outcomes.

Managers who know what participants prefer in terms of second-order outcomes for their efforts and performance have an advantage in developing effective approaches to their motivation. It is important to remember that implicit in Vroom's model is the fact that individuals have different preferences about outcomes. The design of approaches to motivation must reflect this fact—the approaches must be flexible enough to address differences in individual preferences regarding the rewards of work.

Bateman and Zeithaml identify three crucial implications for management work inherent in expectancy theory.[31] First, they argue that managers should take steps to increase expectancies by providing a work environment that facilitates work performance and by establishing realistic performance objectives. It also means providing training, support, and encouragement to give participants confidence to perform their work at levels expected of them.

Second, they urge managers to identify positive-valence outcomes for participants they seek to motivate. This means thinking about what it is that jobs provide to those who perform them, as well as what is not provided by these jobs, but could be. Managers must consider how and why participants assign valences to outcomes and what this means for motivating behavior. In considering outcomes with positive valences for participants, managers must think about the needs participants seek to fulfill through work.

Third, Bateman and Zeithaml stress that managers should make performance instrumental to positive outcomes by making certain that good performance is followed by such positive results as praise and recognition, favorable performance reviews, pay increases, or other positive results. Conversely, managers should make certain that poor performance has fewer positive outcomes and more negative ones. Instrumentality, in the context of expectancy theory, means that there is a perceived relationship between performance and outcome, positive or negative.

Adams's Equity Model

Equity is an important extension of the expectancy theory. In addition to preferences of outcomes or rewards associated with performance, individuals also assess the degree to which potential rewards will be equitably distributed. Equity theory posits that people calculate the ratios of their efforts to the rewards they receive and compare them to ratios they believe exist for others in similar situations. They do this because they have a strong desire to be treated fairly. J. Stacy Adams argues that people judge equity with the following equation:[32]

$$\frac{O_P}{I_P} = \frac{O_o}{I_o}$$

where

O_P is the person's perception of the outcomes received.

I_P is the person's perception of personal inputs.

O_O is the person's perception of the outcomes that a comparison person (or comparison other) is receiving.

I_O is the person's perception of the inputs of the comparison person (or comparison other).

This formula suggests that participants believe equity exists when they perceive that the ratio of inputs (efforts) to outcomes received (rewards) is equivalent to that of some "comparison other" or "referent." Conversely, inequity exists when the ratios are not equivalent.

It is noteworthy that perception, not reality, is considered in this equation. Furthermore, there are options as to the "comparison others" or "referents" in the equation. These options include people in similar circumstances (e.g., co-workers or those whose circumstances are thought to be similar), a group of people in similar circumstances (e.g., all registered nurses working in the HSO/HS), or the perceiving person under different circumstances (e.g., earlier in the person's present position or in a previous position). Choice of referent is a function of information available as well as perceived relevance. Finally, it is important to note that in the equation, there may be many different inputs and outcomes. Inputs are what people believe they contribute to their jobs—things such as experience, time, effort, dedication, and intelligence. Outcomes are what they believe they get from their jobs—things such as pay, promotion, status, esteem, monotony, fatigue, and danger.

Equity theory recognizes that people are concerned both with the absolute rewards they receive for their efforts and with the relationship of these rewards to what others receive. Participants in programs and projects routinely make judgments about the relationship between their inputs and outcomes and the inputs and outcomes of others. In effect, equity theory recognizes that people are interested in distributive fairness—getting what they believe they deserve for their work. Extensive research supports the fact that, even with all the variables involved in making comparisons, people consider equity regularly.[33]

When faced with situations they perceive to be inequitable, people seek to restore equity in a number of alternative ways. They may use some or all of the following alternatives simultaneously or in sequence before a feeling of equity is restored or attained. For example, people who feel an inequity about their pay (i.e., feel that it is too low or that they work harder than others with the same pay) may decrease their input by reducing effort, to compensate for this perceived inequity. Alternatively, they may seek to change their total compensation package as a means to reduce the perceived pay inequity. They may seek to modify their comparisons or referents. For example, they may try to persuade low performers who are receiving equal pay to increase their efforts, or they may try to discourage high performers from exerting so much effort.

Others, feeling an inequity in their pay, perhaps in desperation, may distort reality and rationalize that the perceived inequities are somehow justified. Finally, as a last resort, people may choose to leave an inequitable situation. This action, as a response to perceived inequities, usually occurs only when people cannot resolve the inequities and conclude that they will not be resolved. Thus, participants can attempt to restore equity by changing the reality or the perception of the inputs and outcomes in the equity equation, which can create serious problems for managers.

Managerial Implications of the Equity Model

Equity theory's important contribution to understanding human motivation shows that motivation is significantly influenced by both absolute *and* relative rewards. It also shows that if people perceive inequity, they act to reduce it. Thus, it is important that managers minimize inequities—real and perceived—in their programs and projects. This means helping participants understand differences among jobs and associated rewards and making certain that rewards accurately reflect different performance requirements.

The bottom-line implication of equity theory for managers is that people who feel equitably treated in their workplaces are more satisfied. Although satisfaction alone does not ensure high levels of work performance, dissatisfaction, especially when many participants feel it in a work situation, has very negative consequences: higher absenteeism and turnover rates, fewer citizenship behaviors, more work-related grievances and lawsuits, stealing, sabotage, vandalism, more job stress, and other costly negative consequences for health programs and projects and the participants in them. The equity theory emphasizes the importance of managers' treating fairly those they manage and lead.

Locke's Goal-Setting Theory

A third model within the process perspective on motivation, one now enjoying increased popularity, derives from the work of Edwin Locke.[34] Building on the goal directedness of human behavior, Locke viewed goal setting as a cognitive process through which conscious goals, as well as intentions about pursuing them, are developed and become primary determinants of behavior.[35]

In Locke's view, an important part of an individual's motivation is the intent to work toward his or her goals. The central premise in this perspective on the process of motivation is that people focus their attention on the concrete tasks related to attaining their goals, and they persist in the tasks until the goals are achieved.[36]

In general, studies affirm the importance of goals in motivation.[37] Locke's original theory that goal specificity (the degree of quantitative precision of the goal) and goal difficulty (the level of performance required to reach the goal) are important to motivation has been affirmed by other studies.[38] It is also well established that goals that are specific lead to improvement in individuals' performance because they understand what is to be done.[39] Finally, understanding the role of goals in motivation has been enhanced by research that shows the positive relationship of goal acceptance by a person to that person's performance.[40] Other studies show that people are more likely to accept goals (other than those they set for themselves), especially difficult goals, when they participate in establishing them.[41]

Goals that can effectively motivate desirable behaviors in the workplace have certain characteristics that should be kept in mind as managers and leaders set goals or encourage participants in their domains or areas of responsibility to set goals for themselves. The most important characteristic of goals, in terms of their ability to motivate, is that they be acceptable. Acceptability is increased when work-related goals do not conflict with personal values and when people have clear reasons to pursue the goals. It is also important that goals be challenging but attainable, specific, quantifiable, and measurable.[42] In addition, managers and leaders must provide participants with timely and specific feedback on their progress toward achieving established goals.

Managerial Implications of Goal-Setting Theory

Locke's original work and resulting studies have important implications for managers and leaders. Significant challenges of leading and helping motivate participants in the workplace arise because managers do not clearly define and specify the desired results—outputs, outcomes, and impacts.

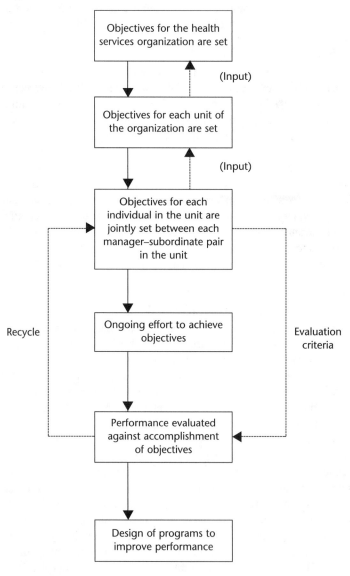

Figure 12.6. The MBO process in HSOs/HSs. (From Longest, Beaufort B., Jr. *Health Professionals in Management*, 226. Stamford, CT: Appleton & Lange, 1996; reprinted by permission.)

Leading effectively, and using motivation to support this, depends upon clear statements of desired results, to which participants can link work-related goals they establish, have established for them, or establish in consultation with managers. Statements of desired results are especially useful in motivating behaviors, and in leading in general, when those who will be influenced by them participate in and agree with their formulation.[43]

Timely and specific feedback from managers and leaders on progress toward achieving goals also is important. The most widely adopted method of goal setting to enhance the contributions of people in organizations is management by objectives (MBO). The MBO process involves participation in developing specific, attainable, and measurable personal objectives (goals) and works when individual objectives mesh with and support the attainment of organizational objectives.[44]

Figure 12.6 shows MBO applied in HSOs/HSs and illustrates how manager-participant or leader-follower pairs jointly establish objectives (goals). Jointly developed goals provide the desired degrees of specificity and difficulty needed to maximize their usefulness. Participating in the development of objectives increases their acceptability to those trying to achieve the objectives. Finally, it is important that goal achievement serve as a basis for rewards in the workplace.

Conclusions About the Roles of Power, Influence, and Motivation in Leading

As presented above, power and influence are critical to leading, as is the role of motivation. Leading by managers in an HSO/HS is defined above as influencing others to understand and agree about what needs to be done in order to achieve the mission and objectives established for the HSO/HS *and* facilitating the individual and collective contributions of others to achieve these desired results. The essence of leading is influencing followers and is the most critical element of this definition. Influencing is central to the leading process and to success in the leader role. To have influence, however, one also must have power, which is the potential to exert influence.

Motivation, defined above as "a state of feeling or thinking in which one is energized or aroused to perform a task or engage in a particular behavior,"[45] is important to leading successfully. The content and process perspectives on motivation in Table 12.1 and expressed in the discussion above guide researchers in their search for answers to what motivates human behaviors and how motivation occurs. Understanding motivation supports a manager's core activity of leading effectively and therefore means influencing participants to contribute to achieving desired results established for an HSO/HS or its subparts, including individuals working within it. Motivation is a means to the end results of leading (influencing) participants to make contributions that help accomplish desired results. In combination with effectively using power to influence, motivating others contributes significantly to leading them. Additional variables also explain leadership effectiveness and the success or failure of leaders. The three broad approaches to effective leadership described next build toward an integrative framework for understanding leading.

Approaches to Understanding Leadership

The study of leadership has followed several paths but has not produced a definitive theory of effective leadership. Much of the theorizing about leadership and many of the studies of the subject can be classified into one of three basic approaches. One approach has been based on the proposition that inherent traits, skills, abilities, or characteristics explain why some people are better leaders. Theories and studies developed around this assumption belong to the "traits and skills approach" to understanding leadership and leaders. The failure of traits to fully explain leadership effectiveness led to another approach, based on the assumption that particular behaviors might be associated with successful leaders. A third approach, an integrative approach to understanding leadership, focuses on how leaders, followers, and the situations in which they find themselves interact and work.

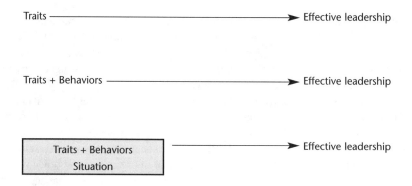

Figure 12.7.   Comparing three approaches to leadership.

These approaches to an explanation of how leadership is practiced successfully (trait, behavior, and situational perspectives) contribute to understanding leadership; the key theories, findings, and conceptualizations that are developed in each approach are examined. Figure 12.7 illustrates the evolutionary relationships these approaches bear to one another.

One can best understand leading by integrating all three conceptual approaches or perspectives, rather than by thinking of them as competing approaches. Each approach is discussed, and the chapter concludes with an integrative model of the leadership process that incorporates elements of trait, behavior, and situational perspectives.

LEADER TRAITS AND SKILLS

The link between interpersonal and political skills, added to the fact that some personal characteristics such as expertise and personal charisma are important bases of power, suggests that certain traits and skills are associated with effective leaders. Most studies of leading in the first half of the 20th century sought to find leader traits in physical characteristics, personality, and ability. Researchers theorized that it was possible to identify traits that distinguished leaders and followers, or successful and unsuccessful leaders. These studies focused on the traits that are associated with effective leaders in business, but they also looked at leaders in government, military, and religious organizations. Of course, to prove that traits explained leadership, it was necessary to find traits that all leaders had in common. The many different traits studied included physical characteristics such as height, weight, appearance, and personality traits such as alertness, originality, integrity, and self-confidence, as well as intelligence or cleverness.

None of the studies conducted in search of universal leader traits was successful. A landmark review of the subject by Stogdill analyzed all the major studies of leader traits and concluded that "a person does not become a leader by virtue of the possession of some combination of traits . . . the pattern of personal characteristics of the leader must bear some relevant relationship to the characteristics, activities, and goals of the followers."[46] This conclusion was useful in later research that studied leadership in the context of specific situations.

Stogdill's conclusion discouraged additional research to identify universal leader traits. However, people interested in the selection of effective managers through the identification of people with leadership potential continued to search for traits that might at least be associated with successful leaders. They used improved methodologies and added administrative and technical abilities to the traits of intelligence and personality studied earlier. Many of these studies, in fact, showed associations between

TABLE 12.2.   TRAITS AND SKILLS FOUND IN SUCCESSFUL LEADERS

Traits	Skills
Adaptable to situations	Clever (intelligent)
Alert to social environment	Conceptually skilled
Ambitious, achievement oriented	Creative
Assertive	Diplomatic and tactful
Cooperative	Fluent in speaking
Decisive	Knowledgeable about the work
Dependable	Organized (administrative ability)
Dominant (power motivation)	Persuasive
Energetic (high activity level)	Socially skilled
Persistent	
Self-confident	
Tolerant of stress	
Willing to assume responsibility	

In Mintzberg, Henry, *Structure in Fives: Designing Effective Organizations,* 2nd edition, 5. Upper Saddle River, NJ: Pearson, 1992. Reprinted by permission of Pearson Education, Inc., Upper Saddle River, NJ.

certain traits and leader effectiveness. In a later review of these newer, more sophisticated studies, Stogdill confirmed his original negative assessment of efforts to identify universal leader traits. He concluded, however, that it is possible to develop a trait profile that characterizes successful leaders:

> The leader is characterized by a strong drive for responsibility and task completion, vigor and persistence in pursuit of goals, venturesomeness and originality in problem solving, drive to exercise initiative in social situations, self-confidence and sense of personal identity, willingness to accept consequences of decision and action, readiness to absorb interpersonal stress, willingness to tolerate frustration and delay, ability to influence other persons' behavior, and capacity to structure social interaction systems to the purpose at hand.[47]

The idea that traits—whether intelligence, personality, or ability—are associated with leader effectiveness continues to be assessed. Although there is no longer a search for universal leader traits, the traits that are associated with leader effectiveness continue to be refined. Table 12.2 lists traits and skills that frequently characterize successful leaders. Kirkpatrick and Locke summarize contemporary thought about the role of traits in determining leadership effectiveness as follows:

> Although research shows that the possession of certain traits alone does not guarantee leadership success, there is evidence that effective leaders are different from other people in certain key respects. Key leader traits include drive (a broad term that includes achievement, motivation, ambition, energy, tenacity, and initiative), leadership motivation (the desire to lead but not to seek power as an end in itself), honesty and integrity, self-confidence (which is associated with emotional stability), cognitive ability, and [expert] knowledge. There is less clear evidence for traits such as charisma, creativity, and flexibility. We believe that the key leader traits help the leader acquire necessary skills; formulate an organizational vision and an effective plan for pursuing it; and take the necessary steps to implement the vision in reality.[48]

Goleman has made an important contribution to understanding the role of "emotional intelligence" in leadership success.[49] He identifies five components of emotional intelligence: self-awareness, self-regulation, motivation, empathy, and social skill. These components are defined in Table 12.3, and the hallmarks of their presence in leaders are given. Goleman concludes that successful leaders vary in many ways, but notes,

TABLE 12.3.   THE FIVE COMPONENTS OF EMOTIONAL INTELLIGENCE AT WORK

Component	Definition	Hallmarks
Self-awareness	The ability to recognize and understand your moods, emotions, and drives, as well as their effect on others	Self-confidence Realistic self-assessment Self-deprecating sense of humor
Self-regulation	The ability to control or redirect disruptive impulses and moods The propensity to suspend judgment—to think before acting	Trustworthiness and integrity Comfort with ambiguity Openness to change
Motivation	A passion to work for reasons that go beyond money or status A propensity to pursue goals with energy and persistence	Strong drive to achieve Optimism, even in the face of failure Organizational commitment
Empathy	The ability to understand the emotional makeup of other people Skill in treating people according to their emotional reactions	Expertise in building and retaining talent Cross-cultural sensitivity Service to clients and customers
Social skill	Proficiency in managing relationships and building networks An ability to find common ground and build rapport	Effectiveness in leading change Persuasiveness Expertise in building and leading teams

From Goleman, Daniel. "What Makes a Leader?" *Harvard Business Review* 76 (November–December 1998): 95; reprinted by permission of *Harvard Business Review*. Copyright 1998 by the Harvard Business School Publishing Corporation; all rights reserved.

> The most effective leaders are alike in one crucial way: they all have a high degree of what has come to be known as emotional intelligence. It's not that IQ and technical skills are irrelevant. They do matter, but mainly as "threshold capabilities"; that is, they are the entry-level requirements for executive positions. But my research, along with other current studies, clearly shows that emotional intelligence is the sine qua non of leadership. Without it, a person can have the best training in the world, an incisive, analytical mind, and an endless supply of smart ideas, but still won't make a great leader.[50]

Because the search for universal leader traits was unsuccessful, researchers began to expand their views on the role of leader traits in leadership effectiveness. They came to view traits as predispositions to behaviors, adopting the view that "a particular trait, or set of them, tends to predispose (although does not cause) an individual to engage in certain behaviors that may or may not result in leadership effectiveness."[51] They began to appreciate that traits had an impact, but not in the way imagined in the earlier search for the universal traits of leaders. These researchers came to understand that what appears to be most important is not a set of traits but rather how they are expressed in the behaviors and styles of leaders.[52]

LEADER BEHAVIORS AND STYLES OF LEADING

Studies of the relationships between the exhibited behaviors and styles of leaders and their effectiveness were premised on the exciting possibility that if especially successful behaviors or styles could be identified, then people could be *taught* how to be leaders. Leaders would not have to be born with certain traits or attributes. The ensuing studies in leader behavior focused on describing leader behaviors, developing concepts and models of styles of leading (styles being thought of as combinations of behaviors), and examining the relationships between styles and effectiveness in leading. These studies added an important dimension to the understanding of leading and new insights into effectiveness in leading.

The most important early studies of leader behaviors were conducted in the late 1940s at Ohio State University and the University of Michigan. In fact, most studies of leader behavior are based, at least in part, on this pioneering work. The Ohio State University studies identified two dimensions of leader behavior—consideration and initiating structure.[53]

Consideration was defined as the degree to which a leader acts in a friendly and supportive manner, shows concern for followers, and looks out for their welfare. *Initiating structure* was defined as the degree to which a leader defines and structures the work to be done by followers and the extent to which attention is focused on achieving desired results established by the leader. These dimensions were not viewed as ends of a spectrum of behavior, but as two distinct and separate dimensions.

Other researchers at the University of Michigan paralleled the studies at Ohio State University. Based on extensive interviews of leaders and followers in a variety of organizations, Likert and his colleagues at Michigan identified two distinct styles of leader behavior, *job centered* and *employee centered*.[54] In these studies, leaders who were employee centered emphasized interpersonal relations, took a personal interest in the needs of their subordinates, and readily accepted differences among work group members. These leaders were considerate, supportive, and helpful with followers.

In contrast, job-centered leaders emphasized technical or task aspects of the job, were most concerned with participants' accomplishing their tasks, and regarded participants as a means to this end. These leaders spent their time planning, scheduling, coordinating, and closely supervising the work of participants.

Studies conducted in a variety of settings found that effective leaders were employee centered and focused on their needs. These studies also demonstrated that, in addition to being employee centered, effective leaders established high performance objectives and encouraged participants to participate in establishing the objectives.[55]

Likert, who was especially influenced by the findings on employee-centered behaviors, came to believe that a key element in effective leadership was the degree to which leaders allow followers to influence the leader's decisions. He believed that participation encourages acceptance of decisions and commitment to them, both of which contribute directly to productivity and to follower satisfaction.[56] His views on the benefits of participatory leadership stimulated substantial research on its effects. Miller and Monge[57] provide a good meta-analytic review of studies of the value of participatory leadership. The relevance of these studies to managing and leading in HSOs/HSs can be summarized as follows:

- *Participation encourages followers to identify with the HSO/HS more closely.* This enhances motivation, especially in such citizenship behaviors as cooperation, protecting fellow employees and organizational property, avoiding waste, and in general, going beyond the call of duty. If people have some voice in their jobs, they tend to be more enthusiastic.
- *Participation can be a means to overcome resistance to change.* Those who participate in decisions that cause change will understand the changes and be less likely to resist.
- *Participation enhances personal growth and development of employees.* By participating in decisions, followers gain experience and become more proficient in decision making.
- *Participation enables a wider range of ideas and experiences to be brought to bear on a problem.* Often, followers familiar with a situation can solve related problems better than the leaders.
- *Participation increases organizational flexibility;* therefore, followers gain a wider range of work experience about the job situation.

In general, HSO/HS managers rely heavily on participative decision making,[58] which is critical to the success of continuous quality improvement (CQI) activities. The professional employees of HSOs/HSs will not tolerate being left out of CQI decisions that are related to patient care. A participative leadership style is facilitated by adherence to the following managerial guidelines:

- *Participants in decisions should have relevant expertise and skill,* or expertise must be developed before they can participate effectively.
- *The consequences of error should be considered.* When others participate, do they raise or lower the risk of mistakes?
- *Avoid abrupt shifts in leadership style.* Steps should be taken to prepare followers for any change in style, to reduce skepticism and build confidence.
- *Followers must be willing participants.* Some people do not want the responsibility that participation entails. Furthermore, the climate of respect between manager/ leader and subordinates/followers should be such that followers are not afraid to voice opinions.
- *A participative style of leadership must be used with sincerity and integrity.* Specifically, the manager/leader who frequently asks subordinates/followers to participate but who has no intention of following their recommendations will soon lose support and acceptance. Once mistrust arises, followers may cease viewing the participative style as legitimate. This does not mean that leaders can never reject followers' recommendations; however, if recommendations are rejected, then the manager must explain the decision.

The behavioral studies provided the intellectual foundation for subsequent efforts to identify effective styles of leading (i.e., particular combinations of behaviors) by identifying the optimal mix of leader behaviors to achieve effectiveness. One such effort useful for depicting variations in leadership styles was undertaken by Blake and Mouton[59] and subsequently expanded by Blake and McCanse.[60] Their model of leading styles uses two variables—concern for people and concern for production—as the axes of a diagram.

The concern-for-people orientation focuses on enhancing the leader's relationships with followers. The concern-for-production orientation focuses on tasks and objectives in relation to performing work. The two orientations can be used to create a diagram to help visualize the variation in possible styles of leading. For example, using a scale from 1 (minimum concern) to 10 (maximum concern), a style characterized by minimum concern for both people and production would be located at the bottom left side of the diagram. Similarly, a maximum concern for both people and production would be located at the top right of the diagram. Different levels of concern for these two variables permit plotting of various styles of leading.

A Turning Point in the Study of Leaders' Behaviors and Styles

Tannenbaum and Schmidt[61] developed a model in which several alternative styles of leading are arrayed as a continuum (see Figure 12.8) based on the degree of participation leaders permit in their decision making. The resulting styles of leading, with labels given by Tannenbaum and Schmidt, are as follows:

- *Autocratic leaders* make decisions and announce them to other participants. The role of other participants is to carry out orders without an opportunity to materially alter decisions already made by the manager.
- *Consultative leaders* convince other participants of the correctness of the decision by carefully explaining the rationale for the decision and its effect on other participants and on the program or project. A second consultative style is practiced when managers permit slightly more involvement by other participants—the manager presents

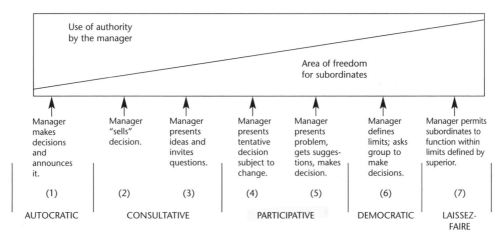

Figure 12.8. Continuum of leader decision-making authority. (Tannenbaum, Robert, and Warren H. Schmidt. "How To Choose a Leadership Pattern." *Harvard Business Review* 51 (May–June 1973): 162–180; reprinted by permission of *Harvard Business Review.* Copyright 1973 by the Harvard Business School Publishing Corporation; all rights reserved.)

decisions to other participants but invites questions to enhance understanding and acceptance.

- *Participative leaders* present tentative decisions that will be changed if other participants can make a convincing case. A second participative style is practiced when a manager presents a problem to participants, seeks their advice and suggestions, but then makes the decision. This style of leading makes greater use of participation and less use of authority than do autocratic and consultative styles.
- *Democratic leaders* define the limits of the situation and problem to be solved and permit other participants to make the decision.
- *Laissez-faire leaders* permit participants to have great discretion in decision making. The manager bears no more influence than other participants in decision making. The leader's and other participants' roles in decision making are indistinguishable in this style.

The importance of the Tannenbaum and Schmidt model to understanding leading lies in their conclusion that the best style of leading depends on the circumstances. In their view, the choice of a style should be based on forces internal to the manager (e.g., the manager's value system, confidence in other participants, and tolerance for ambiguity and uncertainty), forces within the other participants in a situation (e.g., their expectations, need for independence, ability, knowledge, and experience), and forces in the particular situation (e.g., type of organization, nature of the problem to be solved or the work to be done, and time pressure).

Tannenbaum and Schmidt made a significant leap forward in understanding leading by arguing that no single style of leading is correct all the time or in all situations. Leaders must adapt and change styles to fit different situations. An autocratic style might be appropriate in certain clinical situations in programs and projects where work frequently involves a high degree of urgency. However, this style could be disastrous in other situations. The Tannenbaum and Schmidt model identifies a set of relatively discrete styles of leading but couples this with the concept that certain factors dictate choosing one style over the others. In this way, their model represents a turning point between the early trait and behavioral studies of leading and the contemporary—and much more sophisticated—situational or contingency models of leading described in the next section.

SITUATIONAL OR CONTINGENCY MODELS OF LEADING

When traits, behaviors, or styles could not fully explain effectiveness in leading, and especially when behaviors and styles appropriate and effective in one situation produced failure in others, researchers turned their attention to incorporating situational influences, or contingencies, into models of leading. From among the many resulting models that seek to explain how situational variables help to determine the relative effectiveness of leading styles, three of the most important are described briefly.

Fiedler's Contingency Model

Fred Fiedler sought to identify situations in which certain leader styles are especially effective. His hypothesis was that effective leading is contingent upon whether the elements in a particular leading situation fit the specific style of the leader. Complex theories have ample room for criticism, and Fiedler's is no exception. Considerable research, however, supports the model.[62]

The *contingency* model refers to Fiedler's theory that effective leadership is contingent on whether the elements in a particular leadership situation fit the style of the leader.[63] He sought to identify leader styles that fit particular situations and that could be used to improve leader effectiveness by 1) changing leader styles to fit situations, 2) selecting leaders whose styles fit particular situations, 3) moving leaders to situations that fit their styles, or 4) changing situations to better fit leader styles.

Fiedler's leadership model is complex, but the underlying theory can be appreciated by understanding the leader styles he examined and the way in which he assessed situations. He was interested in whether a leader was more task or relations motivated or oriented. The task-motivated leader is more concerned about task success and task-related problems. Such leaders are motivated primarily by achieving task objectives and are not motivated to establish good relationships with followers unless the work is going well and there are no serious task-related problems.

In contrast, the relations-motivated leader is more concerned with good leader-follower relations, is motivated to have close interpersonal relationships, and will act in a considerate, supportive manner when relationships need to be improved. For such leaders, the achievement of task objectives is important only if the primary affiliation motive is adequately satisfied by good personal relationships with followers.

Fiedler considered the two orientations to be polar. He measured these two orientations in leaders by using the least preferred co-worker (LPC) score. The LPC questionnaire asked leaders to think of the present or past co-worker with whom they least liked to work. The LPC questionnaire has a number of attribute sets, such as pleasant/unpleasant, with an eight-point rating scale. The LPC score is the sum of the ratings for the attribute sets. A high score reflects a leader who is primarily relations motivated; a low score reflects a leader who is primarily task motivated. In effect, the score reflects the degree of regard a leader holds for the least preferred co-worker. Leaders with low LPC scores, interpreted as reflecting disregard for the least preferred co-worker, are considered to have a task-motivated leadership style. Leaders with high LPC scores, interpreted as reflecting favorable assessments of the co-worker they least prefer, are considered to have a relations-motivated leadership style.

According to Fiedler's theory, the relationship between a leader's LPC score and leadership effectiveness depends on a complex situational variable that he called situational favorability. Favorability is determined by three aspects of a situation:

1. Leader-follower relations can be good or poor (good leader-follower relations imply that the leader is able to obtain compliance with minimum effort, whereas poor relations imply compliance with reservation and reluctance, if at all).
2. Task structure can be structured (specific instructions and standard procedures provide for task completion) or unstructured (the task has only vague and inexplicit procedures without step-by-step guidelines).

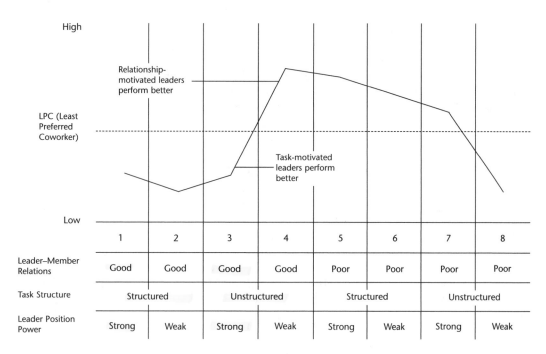

Figure 12.9. How the style of effective leadership varies with the situation. (Adapted from Fiedler, Fred E. "Engineer the Job to Fit the Manager." *Harvard Business Review,* [Sept/Oct 1965]: 118. Reprinted by permission of *Harvard Business Review.* Copyright 1974 by the Harvard Business School Publishing Corporation; all rights reserved.)

3. Leader position power can be strong or weak and refers to the extent to which the leader has authority (including reward, coercive, and legitimate power) to evaluate the performance of followers (workgroup members) and reward or punish them.

Figure 12.9 shows that the style of effective leadership varies with the situation, and it illustrates information relevant to the Fiedler contingency theory of leadership. The bottom portion shows combinations of the three situational favorability aspects: leader-follower relations (good/poor), the task structure (structured/unstructured), and the leader's position power (strong/weak). The result is eight unique combinations that Fiedler calls octants.

Octant 1 shows good leader-follower relations, a structured task, and a leader with strong position power. Octant 8 shows poor leader-follower relations, an unstructured task, and a leader with weak position power. An intermediate octant, Octant 4, shows good leader-follower relations, an unstructured task, and a leader with weak position power. Octant 1 is most favorable and Octant 8 least favorable in Fiedler's schema to measure the favorability of particular situations for leaders.

With a method established to measure certain leader traits and to scale the favorability of the situations faced by leaders, Fiedler tested the relationships. His results, in the upper portion of Figure 12.9, show that relationship-motivated leaders (with high LPC scores) do well (relative to task-motivated leaders) in moderately favorable situations. Conversely, task-motivated leaders (with low LPC scores) do relatively well in situations that are either very favorable or very unfavorable.

Fiedler[64] attributes success of relationship-motivated leaders in situations with intermediate favorability to the leader's nondirective, permissive approach; a more directive approach could cause anxiety in followers, conflict in the workgroup, and lack of cooperation. He attributes success of the task-motivated leader in very favorable situations to the fact that because the leader has power, formal backing, and a well-structured task, followers are ready to be directed in their tasks. He attributes success of the task-motivated leader in very unfavorable situations to the fact that without the leader's active and aggressive intervention and control, the group might fall apart.

Fiedler's work is important because it represents the first comprehensive attempt to incorporate situational variables directly into a model of leading, a new dimension refined in many subsequent studies. The contingency model has utility in management practice, emphasizing to managers the importance of systematically assessing their relationships with participants and the organization designs and processes utilized, in relationship to their leading styles and, in turn, how these affect their effectiveness as leaders.

Hersey and Blanchard's Situational Leadership® Model

Hersey and Blanchard developed a leadership model that attempts to explain effective leadership as interplay among 1) the leader's relationship behavior, defined as the extent to which a leader engages in two-way (or multi-way) communication, listening, facilitating behaviors and supportive behaviors with followers through open communication and actions toward them; 2) the leader's task behavior, which is the extent to which the leader organizes, defines roles, and guides and directs followers; and 3) the followers' readiness level, which Hersey and Blanchard define as readiness to perform a task or function or pursue an objective.[65] This model focuses on followers, specifically their readiness to perform, as the key situational variable. The central premise is that the most effective leadership style is determined by the readiness level of the people whom the leader is attempting to influence. Even though their model focuses on only one situational variable, Hersey and Blanchard call it the Situational Leadership® model.

Appreciation of the Situational Leadership® model requires an understanding of how it incorporates leadership styles, as well as a concept called "performance readiness." Hersey and Blanchard contend that the relative presence (high/low) of task and relationship behaviors can be used to identify four distinct leadership styles (S1–S4) as follows:

- *S1, or telling (high task, low relationship):* The leader makes the decision. The leader defines roles and tells followers what, how, when, and where to do various tasks, emphasizing directive behavior.
- *S2, or selling (high task, high relationship):* The leader makes the decision and then explains it to followers. The leader provides both directive behavior and supportive behavior.
- *S3, or participating (low task, high relationship):* The leader and followers share decision making. The main role of the leader is to encourage and assist followers in contributing to sound decisions.
- *S4, or delegating (low task, low relationship):* The followers make the decision. The leader provides little direction or support.

Follower readiness in the Situational Leadership® model refers to a person's readiness to perform a particular task. Readiness is assessed by two factors, ability and willingness. Ability refers to knowledge, experience, and skill that an individual or group possesses. Willingness is the extent to which an individual or group has the motivation, confidence, and commitment needed to accomplish a specific task.[66]

Hersey and Blanchard used followers' abilities and their willingness (divided into commitment/motivation and confidence) to develop a four-stage continuum of follower readiness, from low (R1) to high (R4):

- *R1:* Followers are unable and unwilling to take responsibility for performing a task (i.e., they do not possess the necessary ability, and they feel insecure about taking responsibility).

- *R2:* Followers are unable but willing to do job tasks (i.e., they do not possess the necessary ability, but they are motivated and feel confident if the leader provides guidance).
- *R3:* Followers are able but unwilling to do what the leader wants (i.e., they possess the necessary ability, but they feel insecure about doing what the leader wants).
- *R4:* Followers are able and willing to do what is asked of them (i.e., they possess the necessary ability, and they feel confident about their ability to do what is asked of them).

In the Hersey and Blanchard model of situational leadership, the four leadership styles (telling, selling, participating, and delegating) are best used with specific levels of follower readiness (see Figure 12.10). Leadership effectiveness results when the leader's style matches followers' readiness. The model suggests that as followers reach high levels of readiness (R4), the leader should respond by decreasing task and relationship behaviors. At R4, the leader need do very little because followers are willing and able to take responsibility. At the lowest level of follower readiness (R1), followers need explicit direction because they are unable and unwilling to take responsibility. At moderate or intermediate levels (R2 and R3), different leadership styles are needed. At R2, the followers are unable but willing, and the leader must exhibit high levels of task and relationship behaviors. High-level task behavior compensates for followers' lack of ability, and high-level relationship behavior may help them to psychologically "buy into" the leader's wishes. At R3, followers are able

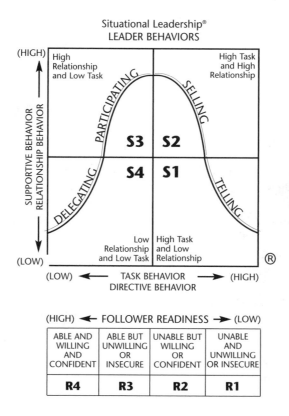

Figure 12.10.   The Situational Leadership® model. (© Copyright 2006. Reprinted with permission of the Center for Leadership Studies, Inc. Escondido, CA 92025. All rights reserved.)

but unwilling or insecure; therefore, a leadership style that incorporates high levels of relationship behaviors may help overcome unwillingness or insecurity among followers.

Although there has been almost no research confirming the relationships theorized in the Situational Leadership® model, it is widely used by managers because it is intuitively appealing.[67] The model clearly illustrates certain important aspects of leader behavior. Leaders must be concerned about the readiness of their followers to be led, and they must recognize that the level of readiness can be affected by leaders' actions. This model also provides a useful and important reminder for leaders to treat followers as distinct individuals. Moreover, the model reminds leaders that individuals change over time in terms of readiness.[68]

House's Path-Goal Model of Leading

Like other situational or contingency models of leading described previously, the path-goal model attempts to predict leader behaviors that will be most effective in particular situations. This model is perhaps the most generally useful situational model of leading effectiveness, named for its focus on how leaders influence participants' perceptions of their work goals and the paths they follow toward attaining these goals. Robert House, in the original conception of this model, posited that the leader's functions are to increase personal payoffs to followers for attaining their work-related goals and to make the path to these payoffs smoother.[69] As House and Terence Mitchell, who helped develop the theory further, note:

> According to this theory, leaders are effective because of their impact on subordinates' motivation, ability to perform effectively, and satisfaction. The theory is called path-goal because its major concern is how the leader influences the subordinates' perceptions of their work goals, personal goals and paths to goal attainment. The theory suggests that a leader's behavior is motivating or satisfying to the degree that the behavior increases subordinate goal attainment and clarifies the paths to these goals.[70]

This model of leading relies on the results of the Ohio State University and the University of Michigan leadership studies and on the expectancy theory of motivation, described previously in this chapter. In this context, expectancy is the perceived probability that effort will affect performance; instrumentality is the perceived probability that performance will lead to outcomes; and the value attached to an outcome by a person is its valence. The expectancy model of motivation focuses on describing the relationships among expectancy, instrumentality, and valence. The path-goal model of leadership focuses on the factors that affect expectancy, instrumentality, and valence. Leaders can increase the valences associated with work-goal attainment, the instrumentalities of work-goal attainment, and the expectancy that effort will result in work-goal attainment.

The path-goal model is situational because its basic premise is that the effect of leader behavior on follower performance and satisfaction depends on the situation, specifically on follower characteristics and characteristics of the work to be performed. Stated in another way, different leader behaviors work better for different situations. There are four categories of leader behavior, according to House and Mitchell,[71] each of which is best suited to a particular situation:

1. *Directive leading:* The leader tells followers what they must do and how to do it, requires that they follow rules and procedures, and schedules and coordinates the work.
2. *Supportive leading:* The leader is friendly and approachable and exhibits consideration for the well-being and needs of followers.
3. *Participative leading:* The leader consults with followers, asks for opinions and suggestions, and considers them.
4. *Achievement-oriented leading:* The leader establishes challenging goals for followers, expects excellent performance, and exhibits confidence they will meet expectations.

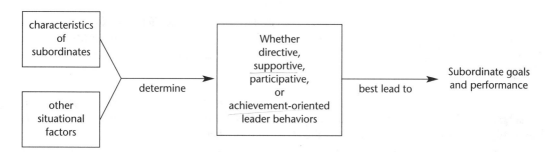

Figure 12.11. Path–goal model of leadership. (From Longest, Beaufort B., Jr. *Health Professionals in Management,* 236. Stamford, CT: Appleton & Lange, 1996; reprinted by permission.)

House believes all four styles of leader behavior can and should be used by leaders as the situation dictates and that effective leaders match styles to situations, which can vary along two dimensions. One dimension is the nature of the people being led. Followers may or may not have the ability to do the job. They differ, too, as to the perceived degree of control they have over their work. The second dimension is the nature of the task, which may be routine and one with which followers have prior experience; or it may be new and ambiguous, and help will be needed if followers are to perform it well.

Figure 12.11 illustrates how to produce leader effectiveness by matching the four leader behavior styles to subordinate characteristics and the nature of the task. Leaders face different situations, and the path-goal model suggests that effective leaders diagnose the situation and match behavior to it. For example, directive leadership could be used when followers are not well trained and the work they do is partly routine and partly ambiguous. Supportive or participative leadership would be most appropriate if followers do routine work and have experience. Achievement-oriented leadership is most effective if followers do innovative and ambiguous work and have a high level of related knowledge and skill.

The path-goal model of leadership suggests that the functions of effective leaders include 1) making the path to achieving work goals easier by providing coaching and direction when needed, 2) removing or minimizing frustrating barriers that interfere with followers' abilities to achieve work goals, and 3) increasing payoffs for followers when they achieve work-related goals.

House and Mitchell intend the path-goal theory to be a partial explanation of the motivational effects of leader behavior, and they do not include all relevant variables. Despite limited validation of much of the path-goal theory, it is a useful construct because it merges leadership and motivation theories. It also provides a valuable pragmatic framework to managers who try to match their leader behavior to subordinate/follower characteristics and task characteristics.

Furthermore, path-goal theory is useful in illustrating substitutes for leadership. For example, if being an effective leader means clarifying the path to a follower's goal, then the existence of clear organizational rules and plans that clarify the path partially substitute for leadership. Substitutes for leader behaviors are anything that clarifies role expectations, motivates employees, or satisfies employees. This phenomenon is significant for HSOs/HSs, with their highly professional work force and possession of a body of knowledge with standard practices to guide their work. These factors reduce the need for leaders to guide the work; they are a substitute for leadership.

▬ Toward an Integrative Approach to Effective Leading ▬▬▬▬

Clearly, managers' effectiveness at leading contributes to the performance of individual participants, teams and work groups, departments, and larger units, as well as to entire HSOs/HSs.

Each of the three main approaches to understanding leading—traits, behaviors, and situational or contingency approaches (again, see Figure 12.7)—has something to offer in understanding leaders and their effectiveness. Studies utilizing these different approaches have resulted in numerous models, each seeking to explain the phenomenon of effective leading. Individually, however, none of the models fully explains how a leader is effective. Levey suggests, "We will probably never be able to achieve a truly elegant and rigorous general theory of leadership."[72] This view reflects the complexity and variety of variables involved in leading. Leading is a dynamic process "that does not reside solely within a given person or a given situation; rather, situations create an interplay of needs, and effective leaders work to continually identify and meet them."[73]

It is possible, however, to integrate portions of the different models into a useful approach to effective leading. Leading effectiveness results from interactions among variables, including leader traits and behaviors selected to fit situations, all of which are mediated or influenced by intervening variables such as participants' efforts and abilities, organization design features, and the availability of appropriate inputs/resources. Furthermore, in HSOs/HSs, participative styles of leading work best most of the time.

Above all else, it is important for managers to realize that because leading is a matter of influencing participants to contribute to achieving the desired results established for an organization or system, they must help participants be motivated to make their contributions. Motivation is a means to the end of leading participants to contributions that help accomplish the desired results established for an HSO/HS.

In terms of using motivation in leading, the simplest, and perhaps best, advice is to select motivated participants to fill the positions in an organization. People who have demonstrated appropriate levels of performance in the past are motivated to perform and will likely continue to perform well under favorable conditions. Leading them to contribute to accomplishment of desired results is rather straightforward. This aside, however, some of the most significant challenges of leading and helping motivate participants in the workplace arise because managers do not clearly define and specify the desired results toward which they want participants to contribute. Being an effective leader, and utilizing motivation to support this, begins with clear statements of desired results. These statements are especially useful when those who will be influenced by them have participated in their formulation and agree with them.

The models of how motivation occurs show the powerful and direct connections among participants' efforts, performance, and rewards. A critical step in motivating people is choosing appropriate ways to reward desired performance, remembering that rewards can be intrinsically derived from the work itself or extrinsically provided by managers.

It is also important to remember that people have different valences or preferences about rewards. Reward selection is made more difficult because of individual tastes and preferences. Some people would rather have more challenging assignments, or more vacation time, than more money. For others, the reverse may be true. The point for managers to remember is that rewards must be important to the person receiving them if they are to be effective motivators. Often, valences can be determined simply by discussing the matter with participants. Viewed broadly, managers' responsibilities to provide suitable rewards can lead them into areas such as job redesign and job enrichment, changes in their leading styles, and changes in the degree to which they permit others to participate in decisions, as well as concerns about pay levels and benefits.

Selecting suitable rewards is only part of the process of using rewards to motivate. Managers must link rewards to suitable job performance; that is, rewards must be made contingent upon performance, and the linkage must be explicit. The more a person is told about the relationship between performance (with clearly established expectations about performance) and rewards, the more likely the rewards will help motivate desired performance.

The performance-reward linkage is strengthened by following desirable performance with rewards as soon as possible and by providing extensive feedback. Finally, it is important to remember that people have a strong preference for being treated fairly or equitably. Their perceptions about linkage between performance and rewards are fundamental to their sense of fairness. Managers must pay careful attention to the equity implications of their use of rewards.

It has been seen that motivation, alone, does not fully account for participants' performance or for their contributions to accomplishing the established desired results. A participant's performance also is determined, in part, by the person's abilities and by constraints in the work situation, such as uncoordinated work flow or inadequate budgets for technology or training. This means it is important for managers, in their efforts to motivate and lead, to remove or minimize barriers to performance. Inability to perform can be addressed through increased education and training and in some cases by more careful matching of people with positions. Situational constraints, such as inadequate inputs/resources or organization designs that impede performance, can be addressed once they are identified as constraints.

Managers' capacities to lead effectively, including utilizing motivation to support leading, are greatly enhanced in work situations in which there is concern for the overall quality of work life (QWL). HSOs/HSs can approach QWL from several specific dimensions or foci of attention: 1) adequate and fair compensation; 2) a safe and healthful work environment; 3) a commitment to the full development of participants; 4) a social environment that fosters personal identity, freedom from prejudice, and a sense of community; 5) careful attention to the rights of personal privacy, dissent, and due process; 6) a work role that minimizes infringement on personal leisure and family needs; and 7) commitment to socially responsible organizational actions.[74]

DISCUSSION QUESTIONS

1. Distinguish between the roles of leaders in transactional and transformational leadership.
2. Define *leadership,* and model it.
3. Describe the relationships between influence and leadership and between power and influence.
4. Compare the three basic conceptual approaches to the study of leadership (traits and skills, leader behavior, and situational or contingency approaches), and explain why different approaches to the study of leadership have been taken.
5. How do process theories of motivation differ from content theories of motivation?
6. Use the motivation process model in Figure 12.3 to identify an example of an unmet need you have experienced. Review the goal you established and pursued to correct this deficiency. Was the goal attained? Was the need fulfilled? If it was not fulfilled, what was your response or reaction?
7. Some have argued that leaders are born, not made, and that all great leaders have certain common traits. Discuss this viewpoint about leadership.
8. Draw a general model of expectancy theory. Use this model to discuss how expectations relate to performance.
9. Define *equity theory*. How are people in the workplace likely to react to perceived inequities?
10. Briefly describe three situational models of leadership presented in this chapter.

Case Study 1: Leadership on the West Wing

Anne Harrison, the vice president of nursing at Wildwood Community Hospital (300 beds), had felt comfortable with the leadership provided by Harriet Mur, the unit manager, to the nurses working in the hospital's west wing. From Harrison's perspective, the unit ran smoothly and had done so for 5 years under Mur's leadership. Problems had rarely surfaced from the unit, and they were more operational than managerial when they did surface. However, a recent increase in the census on the unit, due to the closure of a competitor hospital in the community, meant the nurses in Mur's unit, and throughout the hospital, were experiencing the pressure of increased demand.

In a meeting with Harrison, requested by Mur, Mur expressed her concern and disappointment with what she described as "a problem of worker morale in the west wing." Mur also reported that all of the unit's nurse managers were complaining about the problem to her, so "this is not a figment of my imagination." The primary concern expressed by Mur to Harrison was her general feeling that many of the nurses in the west wing were "unhappy about the new work demands" and that some of them seemed "less concerned about quality."

Mur emphasized to Harrison that she thought many of the nurses were "poorly motivated." In this part of the conversation, Mur expressed her opinion that "nurses, as professionals, come to work either motivated or not, and there isn't much I can do to change that." The meeting ended with Harrison telling Mur that she would think about the problem and would get back to her shortly with her thoughts and suggestions. Both women went on to their normal duties. However, the meeting left Harrison troubled about the problem in the west wing.

QUESTIONS

1. Describe the leadership at Wildwood Community Hospital in general and in the west wing in particular.
2. Is this a leadership problem? Motivation problem? Both? What would you recommend to Harrison? To Mur?
3. Do the leadership problems in the west wing require application of any of the process or content theories of motivation? Which and why?

■ Case Study 2: Charlotte Cook's Problem

Charlotte Cook is a registered nurse (RN) who has three certified nursing assistants (CNAs)—Sally, John, and Betty—reporting to her at Longview Nursing Facility. Cook is 48 years old and has worked for Stanley George, the CEO, for 10 years.

Cook is confronted with a leadership problem. Sally, who has worked for Cook for 5 years, is 40 years old, cooperative, dependable, skilled, and an excellent performer. John, who is 28, transferred from another nursing unit 2 months ago after working there for 1 year. The CEO told Cook that he was transferring John because John could not get along with his RN supervisor on that unit. The RN supervisor there is 2 years younger than John, and they had a personality clash. In fact, rumors circulated that John disliked his RN supervisor because she was not satisfied with either his performance or his attitude. Furthermore, the RN supervisor's predecessor and John had been very close socially, she was not demanding of John, and she often made exceptions for him. This had made the other CNAs on that unit resent John, and they had nothing to do with him. The third CNA, Betty, is 30 years old and has worked for Cook for the year she has been at Longview. Her performance is acceptable, although she requires some direct supervision. She and Cook have a good work relationship.

Four weeks ago, John began complaining to Sally and Betty. He has criticized Mr. George and Ms. Cook and has generally been "anti-everything" about Longview and its staff, especially the RN supervisor on his previous unit and Cook. He has been uncooperative, often doing his job poorly, and has gossiped constantly with the patients. Cook has noticed that John always seems to be with Betty during their free time and that Betty tends to agree with him about things on the unit. Cook feels that, if the situation is ignored, matters could get worse.

Presume that CNAs are difficult to recruit and retain and that Cook does not want to discharge John, at least for the present.

QUESTIONS

1. What leadership style should Cook use with Sally? With John?
2. How should Cook approach and interact with Betty?
3. What should Cook do if John does not change?
4. Did Mr. George do the correct thing in transferring John?
5. What could Mr. George have done to remedy the situation at the time he transferred John?

■ Case Study 3: The Presidential Search

Memorial Hospital is a 500-bed teaching hospital located in a thriving, mid-size city in the mid-Atlantic region. In recent years, other hospitals in the area have reduced Memorial's market share. The outgoing president had been preoccupied with issues of a deteriorating physical plant and loss of professional staff to other area hospitals and systems.

The governing body formed an ad hoc search committee to find a new hospital president. The committee plans to use a national executive search firm but wants to develop a clear picture of the person who will lead the HSO back to preeminence in the city before talking with the search firm.

Mr. Adams, a hospital trustee and president of a large financial services company, is chair of the ad hoc committee. He has convened the committee to develop a list of capabilities the president should possess so that this information can be provided to the search firm.

Assume that you are a member of this committee.

QUESTIONS

1. What capabilities should the new president possess? Rank them in order.
2. Should this person be more skilled at the supervisor-subordinate interface or at organization-level leadership? How will the committee distinguish between skill at the two types of leadership?
3. Some committee members point out that the situation at Memorial is unique and that, therefore, finding a person who was successful at another hospital will not guarantee success at Memorial. What would be your position on this issue?

■ Case Study 4: The Young Associate's Dilemma

Jane O'Hara faced a serious choice. Five years after receiving her master of health services administration degree from a prestigious midwestern university, she was advancing quickly in a large consulting firm. She was receiving assignments with some of the firm's most important clients, and her salary had increased steadily. She was certain that she made at least $15,000 more per year than classmates working in hospitals. The only thing that bothered her about her position, besides the travel, was a nagging feeling that she wanted to become the CEO of a large hospital.

One of O'Hara's clients is a large eastern teaching hospital that has a vice president for finance who is about 5 years from retiring. He is set in his ways; O'Hara judges him to be about a decade behind the sophisticated financial management techniques in her "bag of tools." She was surprised when he offered her a position as his assistant—with a strong hint that he wanted to groom a replacement. The salary is about what she makes with the consulting firm, and the hospital position has slightly better fringe benefits.

When she discussed the offer with her managing partner, he showed a resigned interest in learning what it would take to retain her. Over the next several weeks, the firm developed a counteroffer that included an $8,000 salary increase and a clear indication that she was "pegged" for a partnership position in a few years.

O'Hara took a long weekend to consider her choice.

QUESTIONS

1. Identify and describe the motivation variables present in this case.
2. Would these two positions permit O'Hara to fulfill different needs? If so, what are they?
3. What would you do if you were O'Hara? Why?

Notes

1. Ross, Austin, Frederick J. Wenzel, and Joseph W. Mitlyng. *Leadership for the Future: Core Competencies in Healthcare*. Chicago: Health Administration Press, 2002; and also see the readings in "Leadership and Competitive Advantage." In *Contemporary Issues in Leadership,* edited by William E. Rosenbach and Robert L. Taylor, 121–194. Boulder, CO: Westview Press, 1998.
2. Burns, James M. *Leadership*. New York: Harper & Row, 1978.
3. Longest, Beaufort B., Jr., Kurt Darr, and Jonathon S. Rakich. "Organizational Leadership in Hospitals." *Hospital Topics* 71 (1993): 11–15.
4. Tichy, Noel M., and Mary A. Devanna. *The Transformational Leader*. New York: John Wiley & Sons, 1990.
5. Deal, Terrence E. "Healthcare Executives as Symbolic Leaders." *Healthcare Executive* 5 (March/April 1990): 24–27; Nutt, Paul C. "How Top Managers in Health Organizations Set Directions that Guide Decision Making." *Hospital & Health Services Administration* 36 (Spring 1991): 57–75.
6. Yukl, Gary A. *Leadership in Organizations,* 5th ed. Upper Saddle River, NJ: Prentice Hall, 2002; Pointer, Dennis D. "Leadership: A Framework for Thinking and Acting." In *Healthcare Management: Organization Design and Behavior,* 5th ed., edited by Stephen M. Shortell and Arnold D. Kaluzny, 125–147. Clifton Park, NY: Thomson Delmar Learning, 2006.
7. Keys, Bernard, and Thomas Case. "How to Become an Influential Manager." *Executive* 4 (November 1990): 38.
8. French, John R.P., and Bertram H. Raven. "The Bases of Social Power." In *Studies of Social Power,* edited by Dorwin Cartwright, 150–167. Ann Arbor, MI: Institute for Social Research, 1959.
9. Yukl, Gary A. *Leadership in Organizations,* 5th ed. Upper Saddle River, NJ: Prentice Hall, 2002.
10. Yukl, Gary A. *Leadership in Organizations,* 5th ed., 144–153. Upper Saddle River, NJ: Prentice Hall, 2002.
11. Longest, Beaufort B., Jr., *Managing Health Programs and Projects,* 129. San Francisco: Jossey-Bass, 2004.
12. Pfeffer, Jeffrey. *Managing with Power: Politics and Influence in Organizations*. Boston: Harvard Business School Press, 1992; Alexander, Jeffrey A., Thomas G. Rundall, Thomas J. Hoff, and Laura L. Morlock. In *Healthcare Management: Organization Design and Behavior,* 5th ed., edited by Stephen M. Shortell and Arnold D. Kaluzny, 276–310. Clifton Park, NY: Thomson Delmar Learning, 2006.
13. Mintzberg, Henry. *Power In and Around Organizations,* 26. Englewood Cliffs, NJ: Prentice-Hall, 1983.
14. Yukl, Gary A., *Leadership in Organizations,* 5th ed., 141–174.
15. Mintzberg, Henry, *Power In and Around Organizations.*
16. Sun, Li-Yun, Samuel Aryee, and Kenneth S. Law. "High-Performance Human Resource Practices, Citizenship Behavior, and Organizational Performance: A Relational Perspective." *The Academy of Management Journal* 50, 3 (2007): 558–577.
17. O'Connor, Stephen J. "Motivating Effective Performance." In *Handbook of Healthcare Management,* edited by W. Jack Duncan, Peter M. Ginter, and Linda E. Swayne, 431. Malden, MA: Blackwell, 1998.

18. Fottler, Myron D., Stephen J. O'Connor, Mattia J. Gilmartin, and Thomas A. D'Aunno. "Motivating People." In *Healthcare Management: Organization Design and Behavior,* 5th ed., edited by Stephen M. Shortell and Arnold D Kaluzny, 81. Clifton Park, NY: Thomson Delmar Learning, 2006.

19. O'Connor, Stephen J. "Motivating Effective Performance." In *Handbook of Healthcare Management,* 438.

20. Maslow, Abraham H. "A Theory of Human Motivation." *Psychological Review* 50 (July 1943): 370–396; Maslow, Abraham H. *Motivation and Personality,* 2nd ed. New York: Harper & Row, 1970.

21. Maslow, Abraham H. *Eupsychian Management,* 56. Homewood, IL: Dorsey-Irwin, 1965.

22. Alderfer, Clayton P. "A New Theory of Human Needs." *Organizational Behavior and Human Performance* 4 (May 1969): 142–175.

23. Alderfer, Clayton P. *Existence, Relatedness, and Growth: Human Needs in Organizational Settings.* New York: Free Press, 1972.

24. Fottler, Myron D., Stephen J. O'Connor, Mattia J. Gilmartin, and Thomas A. D'Aunno. "Motivating People." In *Healthcare Management: Organization Design and Behavior,* 5th ed., edited by Stephen M. Shortell and Arnold D Kaluzny, 89. Clifton Park, NY: Thomson Delmar Learning, 2006.

25. Herzberg, Frederick. "One More Time: How Do You Motivate Employees?" *Harvard Business Review* 87 (September/October 1987): 109–117; Herzberg, Frederick, Bernard Mausner, and Barbara Snyderman. *The Motivation to Work.* New York: John Wiley & Sons, Inc., 1959.

26. McClelland, David C. *The Achieving Society.* Princeton, NJ: Van Nostrand, 1961; McClelland, David C. *Power: The Inner Experience.* New York: Irvington Publishers, 1975; McClelland, David C. *Human Motivation.* Glenview, IL: Scott Foresman, 1985.

27. Murray, Henry A. *Explorations in Personality.* New York: Oxford University Press, 1938.

28. Atkinson, John W. *An Introduction to Motivation.* New York: Van Nostrand, 1961.

29. Atkinson, John W., and Joel O. Raynor. *Motivation and Achievement.* Washington, DC: Winston, 1974.

30. Vroom, Victor H. *Work and Motivation.* New York: Wiley, 1964.

31. Bateman, Thomas S., and Carl P. Zeithaml. *Management: Function and Strategy,* 2nd ed. Burr Ridge, IL: McGraw-Hill Higher Education, 1992.

32. Adams, J. Stacy. "Toward an Understanding of Inequity." *Journal of Abnormal and Social Psychology* 67 (November 1963): 422–436; Adams, J. Stacy. "Inequity in Social Exchanges." In *Advances in Experimental Social Psychology,* edited by Leonard Berkowitz, vol. 2. New York: Academic Press, 1965.

33. Walster, Elaine H., G. William Walster, and Ellen Berscheid. *Equity: Theory and Research.* Boston: Allyn & Bacon, 1978; Mowday, Richard T. "Equity Theory Predictions of Behavior in Organizations." In *Motivation and Work Behavior,* edited by Richard M. Steers and Lyman W. Porter, 4th ed., 89–110. New York: McGraw-Hill Book Company, 1987.

34. Locke, Edwin A. "Toward a Theory of Task Motivation and Incentives." *Organizational Behavior and Performance* 3 (May 1968): 157–189; Locke, Edwin A. "Purpose without Consciousness: A Contradiction." *Psychological Reports* 24 (June 1969): 991–1,009; Locke, Edwin A. "The Ubiquity of the Technique of Goal Setting in Theories of and Approaches to Employee Motivation." In *Motivation and Work Behavior,* edited by Richard M. Steers and Lyman W. Porter, 4th ed., 111–120. New York: McGraw-Hill Book Company, 1987.

35. Locke, Edwin A., and Gary P. Latham. *A Theory of Goal Setting and Task Performance.* Englewood Cliffs, NJ: Prentice Hall, 1990; Wood, Robert E., and Edwin A. Locke. "Goal Setting and Strategy Effects on Complex Tasks." In *A Theory of Goal Setting and Task Performance,* edited by Edwin A. Locke and Gary P. Latham, 293–319. Englewood Cliffs, NJ: Prentice Hall, 1990.

36. Latham, Gary P., and Edwin A. Locke. "Goal-Setting—A Motivational Technique that Works." In *Motivation and Work Behavior,* edited by Richard M. Steers and Lyman W. Porter, 4th ed., 120–134. New York: McGraw-Hill Book Company, 1987; Locke, Edwin A., and Gary P. Latham. *A Theory of Goal Setting and Task Performance.* Englewood Cliffs, NJ: Prentice Hall, 1990; Muchinsky, Paul M. *People at Work: The New Millennium.* Pacific Grove, CA: Brooks/Cole Publishing Company, 2000.

37. Mento, Anthony J., Robert P. Steel, and Ronald J. Karren. "A Meta-Analytic Study of the Effects of Goal Setting on Task Performance: 1966–1984." *Organizational Behavior and Human Decision Processes* 39 (February 1987): 52–83.

38. Naylor, James C., and Daniel R. Ilgen. "Goal Setting: A Theoretical Analysis of a Motivational Technique." In *Research in Organizational Behavior,* edited by Barry M. Staw and Larry L. Cummings, vol. 6, 95–140. Greenwich, CT: JAI Press, 1984.

39. Latham, Gary P., and J. James Baldes. "The Practical Significance of Locke's Theory of Goal Setting." *Journal of Applied Psychology* 60 (February 1975): 122–124.

40. Erez, Miriam, and Frederick H. Kanfer. "The Role of Goal Acceptance in Goal Setting and Task Performance." *Academy of Management Review* 8 (July 1983): 454–463.

41. Erez, Miriam, P. Christopher Earley, and Charles L. Hulin. "The Impact of Participation on Goal Acceptance and Performance: A Two-Step Model." *Academy of Management Journal* 28 (March 1985): 50–66; Schwartz, Robert H. "Coping with Unbalanced Information About Decision-Making Influence for Nurses." *Hospital & Health Services Administration* 35 (Winter 1990): 547–559.

42. Bateman, Thomas S., and Carl P. Zeithaml. *Management: Function and Strategy,* 2nd ed. Burr Ridge, IL: McGraw-Hill Higher Education, 1993.

43. Bateman, Thomas S., and Carl P. Zeithaml. *Management: Function and Strategy,* 2nd ed. Burr Ridge, IL: McGraw-Hill Higher Education, 1993.

44. Drucker, Peter F. *The Practice of Management.* New York: Harper & Brothers, 1954; Duncan, W. Jack. *Great Ideas in Management.* San Francisco: Jossey-Bass, 1989.

45. Fottler, Myron D., Stephen J. O'Connor, Mattia J. Gilmartin, and Thomas A. D'Aunno. "Motivating People." In *Healthcare Management: Organization Design and Behavior,* 5th ed., edited by Stephen M. Shortell and Arnold D Kaluzny, 81. Clifton Park, NY: Thomson Delmar Learning, 2006.

46. Stogdill, Ralph M. "Personal Factors Associated with Leadership." *Journal of Psychology* 25 (January 1948): 35–71.

47. Stogdill, Ralph M. *Handbook of Leadership: A Survey of the Literature.* New York: The Free Press, 1974.

48. Kirkpatrick, Shelly A., and Edwin A. Locke. "Leadership: Do Traits Matter?" *Executive* 5 (May 1991): 48.

49. Goleman, Daniel. *Emotional Intelligence.* New York: Bantam Books, 1995; Goleman, Daniel. "What Makes a Leader?" *Harvard Business Review* 76 (November/December 1998): 93–102.

50. Goleman, "What Makes," 94.

51. Pointer, Dennis D. "Leadership: A Framework for Thinking and Acting." In *Healthcare Management: Organization Design and Behavior,* 5th ed., edited by Stephen M. Shortell and Arnold D. Kaluzny, 132. Clifton Park, NY: Thomson Delmar Learning, 2006.

52. Van Fleet, David D., and Gary A. Yukl. "A Century of Leadership Research." In *Contemporary Issues in Leadership,* 2nd ed., edited by William E. Rosenbach and Robert L. Taylor, 65–90. Boulder, CO: Westview Press, 1989.

53. *Leadership Behavior: Its Description and Measurement,* edited by Ralph M. Stogdill and Alvin E. Coons. Research Monograph No. 88. Columbus: Bureau of Business Research, Ohio State University, 1957.

54. Likert, Rensis. *New Patterns of Management.* New York: McGraw-Hill, 1961.

55. Katz, Daniel, and Robert L. Kahn. "Some Recent Findings in Human Relations Research." In *Readings in Social Psychology,* edited by Guy E. Swanson, Theodore M. Newcomb, and Raymond E. Hartley. New York: Holt, Rinehart & Winston, 1952; Katz, Daniel, and Robert L. Kahn. *The Social Psychology of Organizations.* New York: Wiley, 1978.

56. Likert, Rensis. *Past and Future Perspectives on System 4.* Ann Arbor, MI: Rensis Likert Associates, 1977.

57. Miller, Katherine I., and Peter R. Monge. "Participation, Satisfaction, and Productivity: A Meta-Analytic Review." *Academy of Management Journal* 29 (December 1986): 727–753.

58. Nutt, Paul C. "How Top Managers in Health Organizations Set Directions that Guide Decision Making." *Hospital & Health Services Administration* 36 (Spring 1991): 57–75.

59. Blake, Robert R., and Jane S. Mouton. *The Managerial Grid III: The Key to Leadership Excellence.* Houston: Gulf Publishing Company, 1985.

60. Blake, Robert R., and Anne Adams McCanse. *Leadership Dilemmas—Grid Solutions.* Houston: Gulf Publishing Company, 1991.

61. Tannenbaum, Robert, and Warren H. Schmidt. "How to Choose a Leadership Pattern." *Harvard Business Review* 51 (May/June 1973): 162–180.
62. Peters, Lawrence H., Darnell D. Hartke, and John T. Pohlman. "Fiedler's Contingency Theory of Leadership: An Application of the Meta-Analysis Procedures of Schmidt and Hunter." *Psychological Bulletin* 97 (March 1985): 274–285.
63. Fiedler, Fred E. "A Contingency Model of Leadership Effectiveness." In *Advances in Experimental Social Psychology,* edited by Leonard Berkowitz. New York: Academic Press, 1964; Fiedler, Fred E. *A Theory of Leadership Effectiveness.* New York: McGraw-Hill, 1967.
64. Fiedler, Fred E. *A Theory of Leadership Effectiveness.* New York: McGraw-Hill, 1967.
65. Hersey, Paul, and Kenneth H. Blanchard. *Management of Organizational Behavior,* 7th ed. Upper Saddle River, NJ: Prentice Hall, 1996.
66. Hersey, Paul, and Kenneth H. Blanchard. *Management of Organizational Behavior,* 7th ed. Upper Saddle River, NJ: Prentice Hall, 1996.
67. Yukl, Gary A. *Leadership in Organizations,* 5th ed. Upper Saddle River, NJ: Prentice Hall, 2002.
68. Bateman, Thomas S., and Carl P. Zeithaml. *Management: Function and Strategy,* 2nd ed. Burr Ridge, IL: McGraw-Hill Higher Education, 1993.
69. House, Robert J. "A Path–goal Theory of Leader Effectiveness." *Administrative Science Quarterly* 16 (September 1971): 321–339.
70. House, Robert J., and Terence R. Mitchell. "Path–goal Theory of Leadership." *Journal of Contemporary Business* 3 (Autumn 1974): 81–98.
71. House, Robert J., and Terence R. Mitchell. "Path–goal Theory of Leadership." *Journal of Contemporary Business* 3 (Autumn 1974): 81–98.
72. Levey, Samuel. "The Leadership Mystique." *Hospital & Health Services Administration* 35 (Winter 1990): 479–480.
73. Druskat, Vanessa Urch, and Jane V. Wheeler. "Managing from the Boundary: The Effective Leadership of Self-Managing Work Teams." *Academy of Management Journal* 46, 4 (August 2003): 435–457.
74. Bateman, Thomas S., and Carl P. Zeithaml. *Management: Function and Strategy,* 2nd ed. Burr Ridge, IL: McGraw-Hill Higher Education, 1993.

13

Communication

Management activities in all settings rely on effective communication—which is the creation or exchange of understanding between sender(s) and receiver(s), not restricted to words alone. Communication includes all verbal and nonverbal methods utilized to convey meaning and achieve understanding between or among those involved in communicating.

Without good communication in organizations and systems, decision making would take place in an information vacuum; missions, objectives, and the strategies and plans to achieve them would be understood by only those who originate them; entities would be organized and staffed only as a conglomeration of isolated people and departments or organizations; leading people as to what, when, how, or why to do their work would be impossible; and control and evaluation would be a meaningless exercise without communication about performance results to influence future performance.

▬ Communicating Is Key to Effective Stakeholder Relations ▬

All health services organizations/health systems (HSOs/HSs) have a variety of stakeholders, individuals or groups with a *stake,* or significant interest, in performance and results.[1] Managers need to communicate effectively with the *internal* stakeholders within their domains *and* ensure effective communication between their organizations and systems and a wide variety of their *external* stakeholders. Internal stakeholders are the participants in an entity, whether employees or volunteers. External stakeholders include all existing and potential patients/customers, as well as accrediting agencies, competitors, government (as both payer and regulator), insurance plans, media, and suppliers, among many others. In a commentary on the role of the manager, Kovner and Neuhauser[2] state:

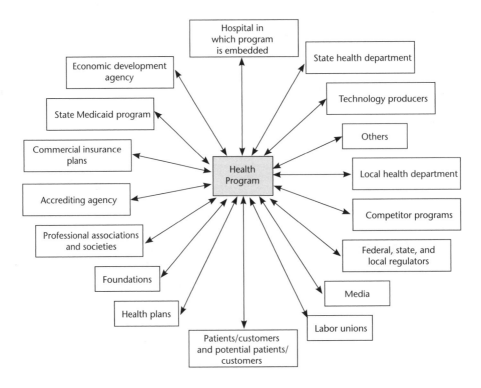

Figure 13.1. External stakeholder map for a health program.

Healthcare managers should ask themselves: Who are the dominant stakeholders affecting goal implementation? What do these stakeholders really want? How satisfied are they with current performance? How do I effectively communicate what I am trying to achieve, and by what means?

Figure 13.1 is an external stakeholder map for a health program operating within an HSO/HS. Such a map can be tailor-made for any HSO/HS or any of its organizational units and programs.

Typically, the relationships and interactions in which managers in HSOs/HSs are involved with internal and external stakeholders are highly information dependent and thus depend on good communication. In short, the degree to which understanding is transmitted and received effectively through communication plays a critical part in successful managing. People communicate facts, ideas, feelings, and attitudes while working. If communication is adequate, then work is done more effectively. In any organized activity, communication is essential and permits people to influence and react to one another.

When managers communicate effectively, four things may be accomplished: Information is transmitted, someone becomes more motivated, something is controlled, or emotions and feelings are expressed.[3] Some communication provides information that people need in order to understand what they are to do. Information about an HSO's/HS's mission and objectives, operating plans and activities, resources, and alternatives are necessary for people to contribute their best to organizational performance. Managers also must provide a great deal of information to external constituencies, especially potential customers, third-party payers, and regulators, if their organizations are to function effectively within their environments.

Although motivation is a process internal to the person (see Chapter 12), managers can affect motivation by informing others about rewards based on performance, by providing information that builds commitment to the HSO/HS and its objectives, and by helping employees understand and fulfill their personal needs. Managers also communicate with external stakeholders to motivate or influence them to act in beneficial ways. Examples include motivating consumers to select an organization as a provider of medical services, motivating health plans to pay adequate rates for services, and influencing public policy makers to establish fair regulations (see Chapter 3). Communication provides a path by which managers can influence behavior, and it serves as a motivation function.

Many kinds of communications facilitate the control of performance in HSOs/HSs. Activity reports, policies to establish standard operating procedures, budgets, and face-to-face directives are examples. Such communications enhance control (see Chapter 10) when they clarify duties, authorities, and responsibilities.

Finally, permitting participants to express emotions and feelings, such as satisfaction, dissatisfaction, happiness, or anger, permits necessary venting or emotive communication to occur. Emotive communication helps managers increase acceptance of the HSO/HS and its actions internally and with external stakeholders and constituencies.

Communication Process Model

Whether communicating with internal or with external stakeholders, managers utilize a process of communication modeled in Figure 13.2. As noted above, managers must be concerned with two types of communication: internal to the organization or system, and external with stakeholders. Communication with internal participants depends on the effectiveness of formal channels and networks to transmit understandable information throughout the organization or system. These channels and networks carry communications multidirectionally—downward, upward, horizontally, and diagonally.

In addition to vital communication within HSOs/HSs, managers—especially senior-level managers—must be concerned with communication with external stakeholders.[4] Examples of communication with external stakeholders include marketing services and products, maintaining good community relations, influencing (lobbying) political constituencies, and building alliances. An

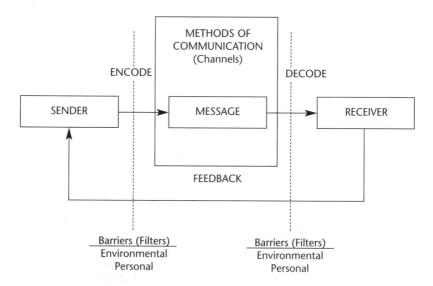

Figure 13.2. The basic mechanism of communication.

important aspect of communication with external stakeholders, discussed more fully later in this chapter, is receiving information from them. No HSO/HS can be well managed unless its managers know a great deal about the external environment. The best way to acquire such information is by systematically communicating with the relevant actors in that environment.

Because communications with internal and external stakeholders involve the creation or exchange of understanding between sender(s) and receiver(s), both types use the mechanisms shown in Figure 13.2. Understanding is the objective in communication, unless, of course, the objective is obfuscation. Unfortunately, complete understanding seldom results, because of the many environmental and personal barriers to effective communication. These barriers and how to overcome them are discussed later in this chapter.

SENDERS AND RECEIVERS

In Figure 13.2, the sender—which be can an individual, a department, a unit of an HSO, an HSO, an HS, or a group of any of these—has ideas, intentions, and information it wishes to convey. A sender uses words and symbols to encode ideas and information into a message for its intended receiver.

Words alone may be insufficient to ensure that the message is understood. Because words may have different meanings for people, or people may not understand certain words, it is often useful to augment the message with symbols. In HSOs/HSs, symbols such as objects, pictures, or actions play a role in communication. For example, uniforms frequently permit the quick identification of staff. Pictures or visual representations are another type of symbol and are efficient and helpful in communication. Consider how many words would be needed to explain an HSO's/HS's organization structure in lieu of the information in an organization chart. Or imagine the difficulty of communicating the information in a magnetic resonance image using only words. Finally, action or inaction communicates. A smile or a hearty handshake has meaning. A promotion or pay increase conveys a great deal to the recipient and to others. Lack of action also has symbolic meaning. As has been noted,

> Failure to act is an important way of communicating. A manager who fails to praise an employee for a job well done or fails to provide promised resources is sending a message to that person. Since we send messages both by action and inaction, we communicate almost all the time at work, regardless of our intentions.[5]

Actions or inactions that are inconsistent with words or other symbols transmit contradictory messages. The manager who tells an employee "I have confidence in your ability, your performance is excellent, and I want to expand your duties by delegating more to you" acts inconsistently by becoming angry if a small error occurs. The receiver who says "I am listening" to the sender and then looks at the clock impatiently or starts to walk away during the conversation sends a mixed message.

CHANNELS OF COMMUNICATION

The channels or methods of communication are the means by which messages are transmitted. Channels include face-to-face or telephone conversations, e-mail, faxes, letters, memoranda, policy statements, operating room schedules, reports, electronic message boards, video teleconferences, newspapers, television and radio commercials, and newsletters for internal or external distribution.

The selection of channels is important in the communication process. Effective communication often involves multiple channels to transmit a message. For example, a major change in human resources policy, such as modifying the benefits package, may be announced in a letter from the vice president of human resources to all employees, graphically illustrated by posters in key locations, and then reinforced in group meetings in which managers explain the policy and answer questions.

A decision to lobby the state legislature for more generous Medicaid reimbursement might result in messages transmitted through channels such as letters to legislators, direct contact between managers/trustees and legislators, and newspaper advertisements stating the organization's position. Other HSOs/HSs might participate through an association to produce and distribute television commercials or use other channels to increase support for their position.

MESSAGES ENCODED AND DECODED

Messages transmitted over any channel must be decoded by the receiver. Decoding means interpreting the words and symbols in the message. The decoding that is done by receivers is affected by their prior experiences and frames of reference. Decoding involves the receiver's perceptual assessment of the content of the message, the sender, and the context in which the message was transmitted. The fact that messages must be decoded (interpreted) by the receiver raises the possibility that the message the sender intends is not the message the receiver gets. The closer the decoded message is to that intended by the sender, the more effective the communication.

The most effective way to determine whether messages are received as intended is through feedback. "Without feedback, you have a one-way communication process. Feedback makes possible a two-way process, reversing the sender and receiver roles so that information can be shared, recycled, and fine-tuned to achieve an unambiguous mutual understanding."[6] In intraorganizational communication, in which interdependencies among individuals and units of an HSO/HS are significant, the feedback loop is very important in ensuring that enough information is exchanged to effectively manage these interdependencies. Similarly, communication with external stakeholders is improved greatly by feedback to senders, who can adjust the message if it is not received as intended. When a sender encodes and transmits a message to a receiver, who decodes the message and indicates understanding by giving feedback, effective two-way communication occurs.

Feedback can be direct or indirect. Direct feedback is the receiver's response to the sender regarding a message. Indirect feedback is more subtle and involves the consequences of a message. Internally, indirect feedback on a policy to change a benefit package might include higher levels of employee satisfaction if the change is liked or increased turnover if the change is disliked. Externally, indirect feedback on attempts to change Medicaid reimbursement might include an increase in rates if the legislature agrees with the HSO/HS, no action if they disagree, or even hostile action if the legislature disagrees with the message or is upset by the methods used to communicate it.

Shortell identified some key elements in effective communication in a study involving hospitals and physicians.[7] The following list summarizes these elements:

- An effective communicator must have a desire to communicate that is influenced by both personal values and the expectation that the communication will be received in a meaningful way.
- An effective communicator must have an understanding of how others learn, including how others perceive and process information. For example, is the receiver analytical or intuitive? Does the receiver prefer abstract or concrete information? Is the receiver better able to interpret information received verbally or in writing?
- The receiver of the message should be cued as to the purpose of the message, that is, whether the message is to provide information, elicit a response or reaction, or help make a decision.
- The content, importance, and complexity of the message should be considered in determining the channels through which the message is communicated.
- The achieved or ascribed credibility of the sender affects how the message will be received; "trust" (an achieved credibility) is most significant.

- The time frame (long versus short) associated with the content of the message must be considered in choosing the channels through which and the manner in which the message is communicated. That is, faster channels and more precise cues are needed with shorter time frames.

Applying these elements can improve a manager's communication, especially in conjunction with the process model described in Figure 13.2. However skillfully one communicates, there are almost always barriers to effective communication within an HSO/HS or between it and external stakeholders.

Barriers to Effective Communication

The environmental and personal barriers illustrated in Figure 13.2 are ubiquitous in the communication process within HSOs/HSs and between them and external stakeholders. These barriers can block, filter, or distort messages as they are encoded, sent, decoded, and received.

ENVIRONMENTAL (OR CONTEXTUAL) BARRIERS

Environmental barriers are created by certain characteristics of an organization and its environmental context. Two common barriers to effective communication are competition for attention and competition for time on the part of senders and receivers. Multiple and simultaneous demands requiring attention may cause the sender to inappropriately package a message, or they may cause the message to be incorrectly decoded by a receiver not giving the message complete attention. Similarly, time constraints may be a barrier to effective communication, prohibiting the sender from thinking through and properly structuring the message to be conveyed or giving the receiver too little time to determine its meaning.

Other environmental barriers that can filter, distort, or block a message include the HSO's/HS's managerial philosophy, multiplicity of hierarchical levels, and power/status relationships between senders and receivers. Managerial philosophy can inhibit or promote effective communication. Managers disinterested in promoting intraorganizational communication upward or disseminating information downward will establish procedural and organizational blockages. Requirements that all communication "flow through channels"; inaccessibility; lack of interest in employees' frustrations, complaints, or feelings; and insufficient time allotted to receiving information are symptoms of a philosophy that retards communication. Furthermore, managers who fail to act on complaints, ideas, and problems signal to those wishing to communicate upward that the effort is unlikely to have much effect, so they discourage information flow.

Managerial philosophy has a significant impact on an HSO's/HS's communications with external stakeholders as well. This topic is addressed more fully in a later section, but suffice it to say here that philosophy leads managers to react in particular ways of communicating with external stakeholders in a crisis. For example, if there is a chance that patients could have been exposed to a dangerous infection while hospitalized, because of improper handling of contaminated material, then managers might react by covering up the incident or by contacting all who may have been exposed so that they can be tested. Varying reactions to events reflect different managerial philosophies and ethical values about communicating.

Multiple levels in an HSO's/HS's hierarchy, and other organizational complexities such as size or scope of activity, present barriers that tend to cause message distortion. As messages are transmitted up or down, people interpret them according to their personal frames of reference and vantage points. When the communication chain has multiple links, information can be filtered, dropped, or added, and emphasis can be rearranged as the message is retransmitted, distorting or even totally blocking the message. For example, a message sent from the chief executive officer (CEO) to employees through several layers of an organization is received in a different form than that originally sent. Or a report prepared for the CEO that passes through the hierarchy may not reach its destination because it is lying on a desk and is, in essence, blocked.

Power/status relationships also can present barriers to effective communication by distorting or inhibiting the transmission of messages. A discordant superior-subordinate relationship can dampen the flow and content of information. Furthermore, an employee's past experiences may inhibit communication because of fear of reprisal, negative sanctions, or ridicule. For example, a subordinate may not inform a superior that something is wrong or that a plan will not work, as a result of poor superior-subordinate rapport. Power/status communication barriers are prevalent in healthcare settings in which many professionals interact and status relationships create a complex situation. Does the nurse with 20 years of experience tell a new medical resident that a procedure or treatment about to be ordered is not efficacious? How is the nurse's message encoded—bluntly or obliquely?

A final environmental or contextual barrier occurs when messages require the use of specific terminology that is unfamiliar to the receiver or when messages are especially complex. Each profession has its own jargon. Managers may use terminology in a different way from those responsible for direct care. Both may use terminology that is unfamiliar to external stakeholders. Communications between people who use different terminology can be ineffective simply because people attribute different meanings to the same words. When a message is complex and also contains terminology that is unfamiliar to the receiver, misunderstanding is likely. This barrier is widespread in communication within HSOs/HSs, as well as between them and many of their external stakeholders.

PERSONAL BARRIERS

Another set of potential barriers—personal barriers—always are present when people communicate. They arise from people's natures, especially in their interactions with others, and apply to communication both within HSOs/HSs and between them and external stakeholders. When people encode and send messages or decode and receive them, they do so according to their frames of reference or beliefs. They may consciously or unconsciously engage in selective perception, and communications may be influenced by emotions such as fear or jealousy.

Socioeconomic background and previous experiences that are an individual's frame of reference shape how messages are encoded and decoded, or even whether communication is attempted. For example, someone whose cultural background includes "don't speak unless spoken to" or "never question elders" may be inhibited in communicating. Naive people tend to accept communication at face value without filtering out erroneous information or observing gaps in information that they receive. Self-aggrandizing people may disseminate information in which messages are distorted for personal gain. Furthermore, unless individuals have experience with the subject of a message, they may not completely understand it. People who have health insurance may have difficulty understanding the concerns of people without health insurance. Those who have never experienced pain or childbirth or witnessed death may be unable to fully understand messages about these experiences.

Closely related to one's frame of reference are beliefs, values, and prejudices that can cause messages to be distorted or blocked in either transmission or reception. This occurs because people's personalities and backgrounds differ; they have preconceived opinions and prejudices in areas such as politics, ethics, religion, equity in the workplace, and lifestyle. These biases, beliefs, and values filter and distort communication.

Selective perception is one of the most difficult personal barriers to overcome for both the sender and the receiver. People tend to screen derogatory information and amplify words, actions, and meanings that flatter them—there is a tendency to filter out the "bad" of a message and retain the "good." Selective perception can be conscious or subconscious. It is conscious when one fears the consequences and intentionally distorts the truth. This happens frequently when patients receive bad news about their conditions, but it also occurs in management situations. For example, supervisors whose units have high turnover may fear the consequences of their superiors' noticing it. They might amplify the argument that turnover is the result of low wages, over which they have no control (or responsibility), or they might delete, alter, or minimize the importance of this information in reports to their superiors.

Sometimes jealousy, especially when coupled with selective perception, may result in conscious efforts to filter and distort incoming information, transmit misinformation, or both. For example, the manager with an able assistant who routinely makes that manager look good may block or distort information that would reveal the truth to superiors. Sometimes petty personality differences, the feeling of professional incompetence or inferiority, or greed can lead to jealousy, resulting in communication distortion.

Two additional personal barriers to communication arise because people receiving messages tend to evaluate the source (the sender) and because people often prefer the status quo. Both of these personal barriers to effective communication are common in HSOs/HSs. Receivers often evaluate the source to decide whether to filter out or discount some of the message. However, this can bias communicators. For example, a hostile union-management atmosphere or one in which employees do not trust management may cause employees to ignore messages from management, or managers may ignore messages from physicians with whom they frequently disagree. Source evaluation may be necessary to cope with the barrage of communication received, but one must recognize the risk that legitimate messages may be misunderstood.

The preference for the status quo can be a barrier when it results in a conscious effort by the sender or receiver to filter out information—in sending, receiving, or retransmitting—that would upset the present situation. Internally, conditions that promote fear of sending bad news, or a lack of candor among participants, can lead to the erection of this barrier. Externally, communicators in an HSO/HS do not want to upset important stakeholders and may react by transmitting messages designed to protect the status quo.

A final personal barrier to effective communication is a lack of empathy—being insensitive to the frames of reference or emotional states of others in the communication relationship. Sensitivity promotes understanding. Empathy helps the sender encode a message for maximum understanding and helps the receiver correctly interpret it. For example, subordinates who empathize with superiors may discount an angry message because they are aware that extreme pressure and frustration can cause such messages to be sent even when they are not warranted.

Similarly, a sender who is sensitive to the receiver's circumstance may decide how best to encode a message or that it is better left unsent. For example, if the receiver is having a difficult day, a reprimand may be interpreted as stronger than it is intended. Or if a receiver has just had a traumatic experience, such as a family illness or financial setback, the empathetic sender may delay bad news until later. Managers concerned about an entity's community image might delay announcing a generous across-the-board wage increase or a large price increase just after a major local employer announces a plant closing because of adverse economic conditions.

MANAGING BARRIERS TO EFFECTIVE COMMUNICATION

Awareness of environmental and personal barriers to effective communication is the first step in minimizing their impact. Positive actions are needed to overcome the barriers, and depending on circumstances, several general guidelines can be suggested.

Environmental barriers are reduced if receivers and senders ensure that attention is given to their messages and that adequate time is devoted to listening. In addition, a management philosophy that encourages the free flow of communications is constructive. Reducing the number of links (levels in the organizational hierarchy or steps between the HSO/HS as a sender and external stakeholders as receivers) reduces opportunities for distortion. The power/status barrier is more difficult to eliminate because it is affected by interpersonal and interprofessional relationships. However, consciously tailoring words and symbols so that messages are understandable and reinforcing words with actions significantly improve communication among different power/status levels. Finally, using multiple channels to reinforce complex messages decreases the likelihood of misunderstanding.

Personal barriers to effective communication are reduced by conscious effort to understand another's frame of reference and beliefs. Recognizing that people engage in selective perception and may be prone to jealousy and fear is a first step toward eliminating or at least diminishing these barriers. Empathy may be the surest way to increase the likelihood that the messages will be received and understood as intended.

Effectively communicating among component organizations in an HS can be especially demanding, as barriers resulting from organizational complexity can be formidable. Adapting Porter's approach to achieving effective linkages among business units in a diversified corporation suggests ways in which managers can overcome some of these barriers:[8]

- Use devices or techniques that cross organizational lines, such as partial centralization and interorganization task forces or committees, to actively facilitate communication. At the governance level, HSs can enhance communication through interlocking boards, defined as boards with overlapping membership. Interlocking boards can enhance communication among components in an HS.
- Use management processes that are cross-organizational to enhance communication in areas such as planning, control, incentives, capital budgeting, and management information systems.
- Use human resource practices that facilitate cooperation among the HSOs in an HS, such as cross-organizational job rotation, management forums, and training, because these increase the likelihood that managers in one part of the HS will understand their counterparts elsewhere in the system and that they will communicate more effectively.
- Use management processes that effectively and fairly resolve conflicts among HSOs in an HS to enhance communication. The key to such processes is that corporate management installs and operates a process that fairly settles disputes among component organizations in the system. Equitable settlement of disputes facilitates effective communication.

Both environmental and personal barriers can be overcome or minimized by effective *listening* within the communication process. The following are especially useful listening habits: clear away physical distractions such as noise or interruptions, express your interest in listening, maintain your focus while listening, ask questions as you listen, listen with your mind as well as your ears, take notes whether you need to or not, and listen early and often.[9]

■ Flows of Intraorganizational Communication

Intraorganizational communication flows downward, upward, horizontally, and diagonally. Each direction has its appropriate uses and unique characteristics, as illustrated in Figure 13.3. Typically, downward flow is communication from superiors to subordinates in organizations; upward flow uses the same channels but in the opposite direction. Horizontal flow is manager to manager or worker to worker. Diagonal flow cuts across functions and levels. Although this violates an organization's chain of command, it may be permitted in situations in which speed and efficiency of communication are particularly important.

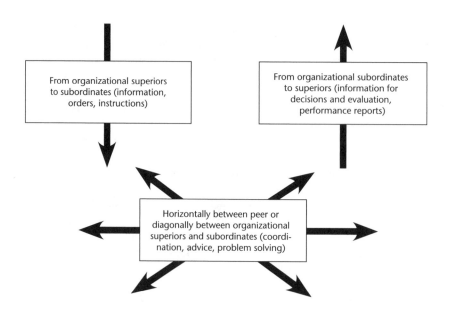

Figure 13.3. Communication flows in organizations.

DOWNWARD FLOW

Downward communication in HSOs/HSs primarily involves passing on information from superiors to subordinates through verbal orders, one-to-one instructions, speeches to employee groups, or meetings. Myriad written methods such as handbooks, procedure manuals, newsletters, bulletin boards, the ubiquitous memorandum, and computerized information systems contribute greatly to downward flow in HSOs/HSs.

UPWARD FLOW

Objectives of upward communication include providing managers with decision-making information, revealing problem areas, providing data for performance evaluation, indicating the status of morale, and in general, underscoring the thinking of subordinates. Upward communication in HSOs becomes more important with increased organizational complexity and scale and with their participation in HSs. Managers rely on effective upward communication and encourage it by creating a climate of trust and respect as integral to the organizational culture.[10]

In addition to being directly useful to managers, upward communication flow helps employees satisfy personal needs. It permits those in positions of lesser authority to express opinions and perceptions to those with greater authority; as a result, they feel a heightened sense of participation. The hierarchical chain of command is the main channel for upward communication in HSOs/HSs, but this may be supplemented by grievance procedures, open-door policies, counseling, employee questionnaires, exit interviews, participative decision-making techniques, and ombudsmen.

HORIZONTAL AND DIAGONAL FLOWS

In HSOs/HSs, which are frequently subject to abrupt demands for action and reaction, horizontal flow also must occur, as in the coordinated work of interdependent patient care units. The matrix designs, as described in Chapter 11, illustrate the value of horizontal communication and coordination in organizations and systems. Committees, task forces, and cross-functional project teams are all useful mechanisms of horizontal communication.

The least common communications in HSOs/HSs are diagonal flows. Diagonal flows, however, are growing in importance. For example, diagonal communication occurs when the director of a hospital pharmacy alerts a nurse in medical intensive care about a potential adverse reaction between two medications. Diagonal flows violate the usual pattern of upward and downward communication flows by cutting across departments, and they violate the usual pattern of horizontal communication, because the communicators are at different levels in the organization. Yet, such communication is essential.

Committees, task forces, quality improvement teams, and cross-functional project teams composed of members from different levels or component areas of the organization or system all can serve as mechanisms of diagonal communication as well as vertical and horizontal communications. The prevalence of such groups in healthcare settings can be attributed to a need for communication in all directions. They encourage representatives of different organizational units to discuss common concerns and potential problems face-to-face and to coordinate activities. Committees and other groupings of participants are useful boundary-spanning devices. However, they tend to be time-consuming and expensive, and their decisions often are compromises that may be ineffectual solutions to problems. Fortunately, there is abundant guidance available in the literature on developing effective groups by taking advantage of their positive potential while avoiding the negative.[11]

COMMUNICATION NETWORKS

Downward, upward, horizontal, and diagonal communication flows can be combined into patterns called communication networks, which are communicators interconnected by communication channels.[12] Figure 13.4 illustrates the five common networks: chain, Y, wheel, circle, and all-channel. The chain network is the standard format for communicating upward and downward, and it follows

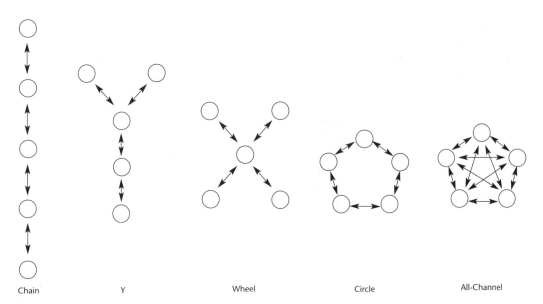

Chain   Y   Wheel   Circle   All-Channel

Figure 13.4. Common communication networks.

line authority relationships. An example is a staff nurse who reports to a nurse manager, who reports to a nursing supervisor, who reports to the vice president for nursing, who reports to an HSO's CEO.

The Y pattern (inverted) shows two people reporting to a superior who reports to another. An example is two staff pharmacists who report to the pharmacy director, who reports to the vice president for professional affairs, who reports to the president. The wheel pattern shows four subordinates reporting to one superior; subordinates do not interact, and all communications are channeled through the manager at the center of the wheel. This pattern is rare in HSOs/HSs, although elements can be found where four vice presidents report to a president and the vice presidents have little interaction. Even though this network pattern is not routinely used, it may be used when urgency or secrecy is required. For example, in an organizational emergency, the president might communicate with vice presidents in a wheel pattern because time does not permit using other modes. Similarly, if secrecy is important, such as when investigating possible embezzlement, the president may require that all relevant communication with the vice presidents be confidential.

The circle pattern allows communicators in the network to communicate directly with only two others, but because each communicates with another communicator in the network, the effect is that everyone communicates with everyone, and there is no central authority or leader. The all-channel network is a circle pattern except that each communicator may interact with all other communicators in the network.

Communication networks vary along several dimensions, and none is best in all situations. The wheel and all-channel networks tend to be fast and accurate compared with the chain or Y-pattern networks, but the chain and Y pattern promote clear lines of authority and responsibility. The circle and all-channel networks enhance morale among those in the networks better than other patterns because everyone is equal in the communication activity, but these patterns result in relatively slow communication. Managers in HSOs/HSs must choose communication networks to fit various communication situations.

INFORMAL COMMUNICATION

Coexisting with formal communication flows and networks within HSOs/HSs are informal communication flows, which have their own networks resulting from interpersonal relationships in organizations and systems. The common name for informal communication flows is "the grapevine," a term that arose during the American Civil War, when telegraph lines were strung between trees, much like a grapevine.[13] Messages transmitted over those flimsy lines were often garbled. As a result, any rumor was said to have come from the grapevine.

Informal communication flows in an organization are as natural as the patterns of social interaction that develop in all organizational settings. Informal communication coexists with the formal flows established by management. No doubt, informal communication channels can be and routinely are misused in HSOs/HSs, especially in transmitting rumors. For example, in times of crisis, organizations and systems are rife with rumors; frequently they are wrong. However, informal communication can be useful. Downward flows move through the grapevine much faster than through formal channels. In an HSO/HS, much of the coordination among units occurs through informal give-and-take in informal horizontal and diagonal flows. In the case of upward flow, informal communication can be a rich source of information about performance, ideas, feelings, and attitudes. Because of the potential usefulness and pervasiveness of informal communication, managers should understand and use it to advantage.

Similar in concept to formal communication flows, informal flows follow predictable patterns and form identifiable networks. Figure 13.5 illustrates four common patterns that the grapevine can take. The single-strand pattern shows the way many people think the grapevine works. Instead, it is more likely to be a cluster pattern.

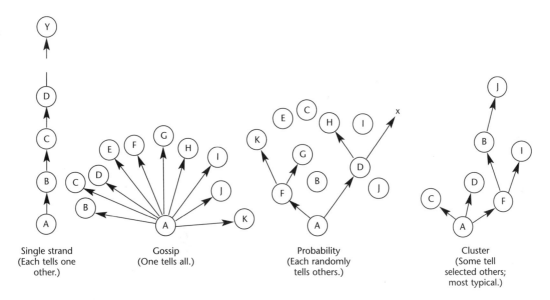

Figure 13.5. Grapevine networks. (From Newstrom, John W., and Keith Davis. *Organizational Behavior: Human Behavior at Work,* 9th ed., 445. New York: McGraw-Hill, 1993. Reproduced with permission of the McGraw-Hill Companies, Inc.)

Managers occasionally get the impression that the grapevine operates like a long chain in which A tells B, who tells C, who then tells D, and so on, until Y finally receives the information—very late and very incorrect. (See the single-strand network in Figure 13.5.) Sometimes the grapevine operates this way, but it generally follows a different pattern. Employee A tells three or four others, such as C, D, and F. (See the cluster network in Figure 13.5.) Only one or two of these receivers pass the information forward, usually to more than one person. Then as the information grows older and the proportion of those knowing it is greater, it gradually dies out because not all those who receive it repeat it. This network is a cluster chain because each link in the chain tends to inform a cluster of others instead of only one person.[14]

Informal communication present in every organization can either aid or inhibit effectiveness. Managers can achieve some organization objectives by paying attention to informal communication (even inaccurate rumors reflect some aspects of employees' feelings and views) and by occasionally and selectively using informal communication, especially when speed is critical.

To summarize, each of the multidirectional communication flows and the networks they form within HSOs/HSs have a purpose, and each is an important tool for managers. These flows are planned and designed as parts of an HSO's/HS's formal organization design, and they represent formal communication channels and networks. Natural informal communication channels and networks arise between and among people outside the formal design. The flow of understandable messages, whether through formal channels or informal ones, is as crucial to the life of an HSO/HS as the circulation of blood is to human life. Figure 13.3 summarizes the key uses of downward, upward, horizontal, and diagonal communication.

Communicating with External Stakeholders

HSOs/HSs typically maintain relationships with a large number of external stakeholders.[15] As defined earlier, stakeholders include individuals, groups, or organizations interested in the perfor-

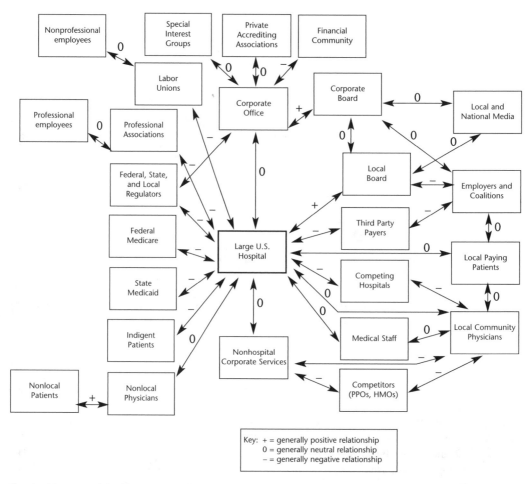

Key: + = generally positive relationship
     0 = generally neutral relationship
     − = generally negative relationship

Figure 13.6.   Stakeholders in a large hospital. (From Fottler, Myron D., John D. Blair, Carlton J. Whitehead, Michael D. Laus, and Grant T. Savage. "Assessing Key Stakeholders: Who Matters to Hospitals and Why?" *Hospital & Health Services Administration* 34 [Winter 1989]: 530; reprinted by permission. Copyright 1989, Health Administration Press.)

mance of and results achieved by the organization or system, and they attempt to influence them. See Figure 13.1 for the diversity of stakeholders in one small healthcare setting.

HSOs/HSs are affected, sometimes quite dramatically, by external stakeholders. The relationship and communication between them can be complex. HSOs/HSs are dynamic, open systems in complex and turbulent external environments, as discussed in Chapter 8. In most cases, the sheer number and variety of external stakeholders complicates communication with them.

Communication with stakeholders also is complicated by the varying natures of the relationships. Communication with external stakeholders tends to be more effective in positive relationships. Figure 13.6 uses a large hospital to illustrate the extraordinary diversity of stakeholders with which relationships must be maintained. Some of the relationships in Figure 13.6 are positive (shown by the plus [+] symbol), some are negative (shown by the minus [−] symbol), and some are neutral (shown by zero [0]). It is important to note that the arrows connecting the hospital with its stakeholders go in both directions, illustrating that managers must be concerned about communication to and from external stakeholders.

Boundary spanning is another name for the process through which an organization's managers communicate with external stakeholders. Boundary spanners carry out this process by obtaining information from external stakeholders that can be useful to the organization. Strategizing and marketing in HSOs/HSs are examples of boundary spanning. On the other hand, boundary spanners also represent the entity to its external stakeholders. This activity includes marketing, public relations, guest or patient relations, government relations, and community relations. Because information is the object of boundary-spanning activities, communication is critical to success. An entity's ability to glean useful information from external stakeholders or to be effectively represented to them depends on effective communication.

LISTENING TO EXTERNAL STAKEHOLDERS

When managers in HSOs/HSs listen to external stakeholders, they act as good receivers in the communication process, systematically and analytically using stakeholder analysis in a way that increases the chances of acquiring useful or necessary information.[16]

Approaches for systematically listening to external stakeholders vary; in general, however, these efforts include a set of interrelated activities akin to the environmental assessments that HSOs/HSs make in the context of strategic management (see Chapter 8). In conducting environmental assessments, managers scan their entity's environment to identify strategically important issues, monitor the issues, forecast trends in the issues, assess the importance of the issues, and diffuse information obtained to those in the organization or system who need it.[17] In stakeholder analyses, managers in HSOs/HSs also scan to identify important stakeholders, forecast or project the trends in stakeholders' views or positions, assess the implications of the stakeholders' views and positions, and diffuse this information to those who need it.

Scanning activities involve acquiring and organizing important information about an HSO's/HS's external stakeholders. In most instances, this is a straightforward task that readily leads to the development of a stakeholder map, such as that shown in Figure 13.6 for a large hospital in the United States.

Determining who are an HSO's/HS's external stakeholders is frequently a matter of judgment. To ensure quality judgments, it is useful to utilize ad hoc task forces, committees, or outside consultants. Several expert-based techniques used to help determine the stakeholders are the delphi technique, the nominal group technique, brainstorming, focus groups, and dialectic inquiry.[18]

Scanning is followed by monitoring that tracks the stakeholders' views and positions on matters important to the HSO/HS. Monitoring is critical when views and positions are dynamic, not well structured, or ambiguous as to strategic importance. Monitoring stakeholder views and positions clarifies degrees of importance or the rates at which they are becoming strategically important. Expert opinions as used in scanning can help managers determine which stakeholders to monitor, while consultants may do the actual monitoring.

Effective scanning and monitoring cannot provide managers with all the information they need about the views and positions of external stakeholders. Because these views, positions, and perspectives are frequently dynamic, managers will benefit from forecasts of likely changes in stakeholders' views and perceptions. Such forecasts give managers time to factor these views and preferences into their decisions.

Scanning and monitoring the views and positions of external stakeholders, and even accurately forecasting trends in their views and positions, do not ensure good stakeholder analysis. Managers also must be concerned about the importance of the information. That is, they must assess and interpret the strategic importance and implications of this information. At a minimum, this means characterizing stakeholders as positive, negative, or neutral, as shown in Figure 13.6. Although the determination of positive, negative, or neutral positions is relatively easy to make, assessment of stakeholders' importance is not an exact science. Intuition, common sense, and best guesses all play a role. Beyond the difficulties of collecting and analyzing enough information to make an informed assessment, other problems arise from the personal prejudices and biases of those judging external stakeholders and their relative importance. This can result in assessments that fit preconceived notions about which stakeholders are strategically important rather than the realities of a situation.[19]

The final step in conducting stakeholder analyses involves diffusing the results to those in the HSO/HS who need the information. This step frequently is undervalued in the process and sometimes overlooked. Unless diffusing the results is done effectively, however, it does not matter how well the other steps are performed.

There are two basic ways that information about external stakeholders can be diffused into the organization or system. One is to rely on the power of senior-level managers to dictate diffusion and use of the information. Alternatively, reason can be used to persuade or educate those involved in decision making to use the information. Combinations of power- and reason-based approaches work best.

Diffusion of strategically important information obtained from external stakeholders completes the process of stakeholder analysis. Given the vital linkage between an entity and its external stakeholders such as customers, payers, and regulators, it is unlikely that any organization or system can succeed without an effective process through which its managers listen to the stakeholders and respond to their communication.

■ Special Circumstances in Communicating with Certain External Stakeholders

Although the communication process with all external stakeholders is the creation of understanding between sender and receiver, each stakeholder must be considered in terms of its unique dimensions if effective communication is to occur. This is especially true of four important sets of external stakeholders of the typical HSO/HS:

- Those to whom the HSO/HS wishes to market its products and services
- The geographic community in which the organization or system is located
- The public sector with which the organization or system interacts
- The stakeholder groups that form when something goes wrong in the HSO/HS

Communicating with these important external stakeholders is examined in the following sections.

COMMUNICATING IN MARKETING[20]

Marketing is discussed in depth in Chapter 9. Suffice it to say here that the central purpose of marketing is to support the voluntary exchange of something of value between buyers and sellers.[21] Successful HSOs/HSs produce and make available services or products that are of value to certain individuals, groups, or organizations (e.g., individual patients/customers, health plans, or government). In turn, individuals, groups, or organizations seek out and choose the services or products. Communication is vital to how this process occurs; indeed, communicating effectively is necessary for the exchanges to occur at all.

Marketing can help ensure an adequate supply of patients/customers, that their needs are identified and met, and that the HSO/HS receives value in return.[22] The major activities in commercial marketing include

- Determining what groups of potential patients/customers (or markets) exist, determining their needs, and identifying which of these groups of potential patients/customers the HSO/HS wishes to serve. In essence, these activities determine target markets. If there are competitors, it is also necessary to determine what they are doing or may do in regard to the target markets.

- Assessing current service mix or product line relative to the identified target market's needs. This is done in order to determine what products or services can be provided in response or that can be developed and then provided.

- Deciding how to facilitate exchanges between the HSO/HS or its various units and its target markets, and implementing these decisions. Prerequisites to mutually satisfactory exchanges between an entity and its target markets include responding to how and where customers prefer to gain access to and use the products and services, as well as developing pricing structures that both attract patients/customers and provide the necessary financial resources. Accomplishing both requires communicating information effectively to the target markets.

- Carrying out all of the activities involved in commercial marketing. This depends on exchanging information through effective communication. Similarly, as can be seen in the discussion of the topic in Chapter 9, effective communication is essential in the use of social marketing techniques.

COMMUNICATING WITH THE COMMUNITY OR SERVICE AREA

HSOs/HSs consider their communities to be external stakeholders requiring intensive communication. All effective communication between healthcare organizations and their communities or service areas involves the creation of understanding between senders and receivers, as well as identification of the communities in different ways. Effective communication also depends on the sender's identifying the receiver in the exchange. Therefore, the first step in an HSO's/HS's effective communication with its community is to identify the community or service area.

The meaning of *community* usually implies physical location, although for some organizations or systems, it is not straightforward. For example, community may be a function of specialized services provided (such as pediatrics or psychiatric services) or of cohorts of patients served (patients needing rehabilitation services). The impact of some HSOs/HSs extends far beyond their immediate geographic locations, as they attract international patients, draw students widely and return graduates to serve their own communities, or conduct research that influences diagnosis and treatment without respect to physical boundaries. HSs may have numerous and broadly dispersed physical locations. All HSOs/HSs are concerned to some extent with their relationships with the people and other organizations in their immediate geographic locations. However, physical location is not the only way an entity identifies its community. For most HSOs/HSs, physical location is their "community of first loyalty,"[23] and relationships between them and their geographic communities require a great deal of communication.

In addition to identifying communities and service areas, another important aspect of communicating with them is the nature of the relationship with them. Perhaps more with communities than with other external stakeholders, effective communication is the basis for clear understanding and acceptance of the expectations each has of the other and of the responsibilities each bears for the other. Communities anticipate contributions from organizations and systems to community life, while managers ponder their entities' roles in the community as well as what the community provides in the way of customers or patients, employees, infrastructure, or resources. Until such questions are answered, effective communication flows may be hampered by misunderstanding relationships, responsibilities, and expectations.

Managers need to consider carefully the nature of the relationship that their organization or sys-

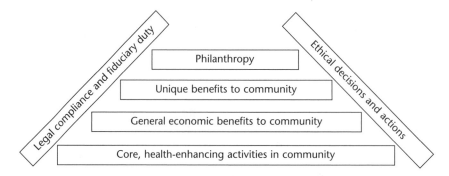

Figure 13.7.   The benefits HSOs/HSs can provide to their communities.

tem has with the community as a foundation on which to build effective communication. As Figure 13.7 suggests, these organizations and systems can do much more for their communities than provide healthcare services. In building the foundational relationship with its community, an HSO's/HS's managers can be guided by the answers to several questions:[24]

- Do we enhance health in our community across a broad front of efforts reflecting the determinants of health?
- Do we fulfill our core, health-enhancing mission by providing unique benefits to our community?
- Are our economic contributions broadly defined and fully met?
- Are our philanthropic activities established broadly and generously and collaboratively pursued?
- Are we in compliance with legal requirements and obligations?
- Are our fiduciary and ethical obligations met?

COMMUNICATING WITH THE PUBLIC SECTOR

HSOs/HSs are affected by public policies such as laws and regulations. The fact that these entities are targets of much public policy stems from their fundamental contributions to the physical and psychological well-being of people, as well as their role in the nation's economy. In view of these important contributions, government at all levels is keenly interested in their performance. This interest is reflected in the numerous public policies that directly affect HSOs/HSs, including policies affecting the provision and financing of healthcare services as well as the production of inputs (e.g., the education of health professionals, the development of health technology) to those services.[25] The importance of public policy to healthcare organizations and systems makes effective communication with the public sector a high priority. A public policy issues life cycle model and suggested ways for managers to affect such issues are discussed in Chapter 8.

Managers in healthcare settings have two important categories of communication responsibilities regarding their public sector environment.[26] First, they must analyze this environment to acquire sufficient information and data to understand the strategic consequences of events and forces in the public policy environment. Such analysis yields an assessment of the effects of public policies on the HSO/HS, in terms of opportunities and threats, and permits managers to make strategic adjustments that reflect planned responses.

Second, managers are responsible for influencing the formulation and implementation of public policies. This responsibility derives from the fact that effective managers seek to make the external environment, including the public policy component, favorable to the HSO/HS. Inherent in this

---

Managers can influence the formulation or modification of policy by doing the following:

- Helping shape the policy agenda by defining and documenting problems that need to be addressed, developing and evaluating solutions to the problems, and shaping the political circumstances affecting problems and solutions

- Helping develop specific legislation by participating in the drafting of legislation or testifying at legislative hearings

- Documenting the case for modification of policies by sharing operational experiences and formal evaluations of the impact of policies

---

Managers can influence the implementation of policy by doing the following:

- Providing formal comments on draft rules and regulations

- Serving on and providing input to rulemaking advisory bodies

- Interacting with policy implementers

Exerting influence on public policy through each of the means listed previously requires effective and persuasive communication.

Figure 13.8. Influencing public policy. (*Source:* Adapted from Longest, Beaufort B., Jr., *Health Policymaking in the United States,* 4th edition. Used with permission. Chicago: Health Administration Press, 2005, p. 146.)

responsibility are requirements to identify public policy objectives consistent with their organization's or system's values, mission, and objectives and to help meet those objectives through appropriate and ethical means, such as lobbying and advocating individually or through associations and trade groups. As Figure 13.8 indicates, managers have many available avenues through which to help shape public policies.

Advocacy, defined as the effort to influence public policy through various forms of communicating persuasively, is a primary mechanism through which program and project managers can influence public policy. It has been argued that every manager involved in health services is an advocate and that success at advocacy depends directly on communicating effectively.[27]

COMMUNICATING WHEN THINGS GO BADLY

Occasionally, things go badly even in a well-managed healthcare setting. Entities in which this happens may face threats of losing their accreditation by The Joint Commission on Accreditation of Healthcare Organizations or perhaps their state licensure because of fire code violations. An entity may encounter serious financial difficulties, perhaps threatening its continued operation or raising the specter of major layoffs or closure of some of its component HSOs. Serious clinical errors may occur, perhaps causing a patient's death. Based on a large-scale study of medical errors,[28] Figure 13.9 indicates the types of things that can go wrong in clinical settings. One of the verities of life for managers is that on occasion, even in well-managed entities, something will go wrong.[29] After all, HSOs/HSs employ, under fallible human direction, dangerous drugs, devices, and procedures in their battles against disease and injury. This is complicated by the fact that these technologies are employed on behalf of people at vulnerable stages or moments in their lives, people who often have an inflated and unrealistic expectation of what can be done for them or their loved ones.

Diagnostic

> Error or delay in diagnosis
> Failure to employ indicated test
> Use of outmoded tests or therapy
> Failure to act on results of monitoring or testing

Treatment

> Error in the performance of an operation, procedure, or test
> Error in administering the treatment
> Error in the dose or method of using a drug
> Avoidable delay in treatment or in responding to an abnormal test
> Inappropriate (not indicated) care

Preventive

> Failure to provide prophylactic treatment
> Inadequate monitoring of condition or progress or inadequate follow-up
> treatment

Other

> Failure of communication
> Equipment failure
> Other system failure

Figure 13.9. Types of errors in clinical settings. (*Source:* Adapted with permission from Leape, Lucian L., Ann G. Lawthers, Troyen A. Brennan, and William G. Johnson, "Preventing Medical Injury," *Quality Review Bulletin,* Vol. 19, No. 5 (May 1993): 144–149. Copyright © Joint Commission Resources.)

For example, suppose a diabetic patient being treated in a hospital for complications of that disease dies unexpectedly, and results of blood tests taken several hours before death show insulin levels 200 times normal. There are several possible explanations, including a fatal overdose of insulin given accidentally or intentionally in a criminal act committed by any of several people. How should the hospital handle this situation? Whose interests are to be protected? What information is to be communicated? To whom? By whom? There are few hard-and-fast rules to guide managers in such circumstances, but relevant ethical guidelines in Chapter 4 will help managers communicate with those within the hospital and with its external stakeholders.

When things go wrong, internal and external communications take on greater importance. How managers communicate in such circumstances affects resolution of the problem and the internal and external perception of the HSO/HS after the problem is resolved. Actions and communications in response to serious problems can be characterized along a continuum from reactive to proactive. Reactive responses, at one end of the continuum depicted in Figure 13.10, include concealing a problem—doing and saying nothing. Less extreme, but highly reactive, is to admit that a problem may exist but deny any wrongdoing and take no action to find the cause of the problem or resolve it. Such an obstructionist position could be taken by the HSO/HS regarding further communication about a problem.

A similar reaction to a problem is one that is best labeled defensive. The HSO's/HS's managers and spokespeople act and communicate in a way that complies with the letter of the law. Such actions and communications are intended to minimize legal liability, reflecting in part the expensive liability for serious problems involving human health and life. However, some managers take defen-

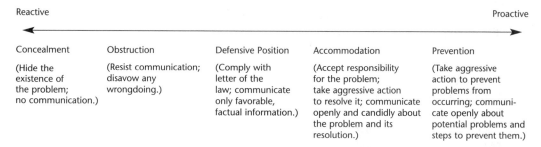

Figure 13.10. Continuum of action and communication to stakeholders in difficult times.

sive positions with internal and external communications whenever problems arise. They may communicate defensively about layoffs, mergers, closures, or problems in which many stakeholders have a legitimate interest.

Figure 13.10 illustrates these reactive responses and two that are more proactive: accommodation and prevention. Accommodation involves accepting responsibility for a problem and aggressively resolving it. Communications are characterized by openness and candor about the problem, its causes, and the actions being taken to resolve it. Prevention is further along the continuum and focuses on taking concerted actions to prevent problems.

In attempting to prevent the occurrence of negative events, managers are increasingly turning to integrated sets of activities aimed at making certain that the right things are done, that they are done correctly, and that they are done correctly the first time.[30] These sets of activities go by various names. A popular one is *continuous quality improvement,* or CQI. James[31] suggests that the essence of CQI is to answer three questions: Are we doing the right things? Are we doing things right? How can we be certain that we do things right the first time, every time? Each of these sets of activities relies heavily upon communications.

Continuous quality improvement (see Chapter 7) is an important approach in prevention, as are risk management and performance improvement (see Chapter 10). Communications, as in the case of accommodation, are open and candid, but they focus on the existence and probabilities of potential problems and steps taken to prevent them.

HSOs/HSs are better served in managing difficult situations by actions and communications that are proactive rather than reactive. Reactive responses (concealment, obstruction, and defensive positions) imply crisis management and invite the scrutiny of those affected by the problem. Technically, managers who choose accommodation also are reacting to a problem, but their response is positive and proactive as they take responsibility, actively seek to resolve the problem, and communicate openly and candidly about the problem and their actions. Prevention involves focused action to avoid problems. Here, managers communicate to interested parties that problems might occur but that actions have been taken to prevent them or minimize their impact. Problems in HSOs/HSs are inevitable, but many can be prevented. Furthermore, the consequences of problems can be managed far more effectively if managers have established a foundation of understanding and trust with stakeholders by communicating potential problems and their actions to prevent problems or prepare for them.

DISCUSSION QUESTIONS

1. Draw a model of the communication process. Describe the interrelationships of its parts.
2. Discuss the importance of feedback in communicating.

3. Discuss the various types of communication networks, and describe the advantages and disadvantages of each.
4. Discuss the purpose of the downward communication flow in an HSO/HS.
5. Discuss the purpose of the upward communication flow in an HSO/HS.
6. Discuss the role of committees in relation to communication in an HSO/HS.
7. What are barriers to communication? How can they be overcome?
8. Discuss the role of symbols in communication.
9. Think of a situation in which an HSO/HS receives bad press. How might the HSO/HS respond along the reactive-proactive continuum? How should it respond to stakeholders? What are the basic differences between formal and informal communication channels?

■ Case Study 1: Apple Orchard Assisted Living

As the manager in charge of several important projects at Apple Orchard Assisted Living, Janelle Wilkins has been confronted by some behavior and leadership problems with the project team leader, Emilio Jones, whom she assigned to develop a new staffing plan for the nursing service. Jones has been on the job approximately 6 months, and Wilkins has had several meetings with him. He is leading a team of six people drawn from the assisted-living facility staff.

Wilkins recently sent Jones this memorandum:

> Mr. Jones:
>
> You mentioned to me that you have had a difficult time getting people to work as a team on the staffing project I assigned to you. You also mentioned that you feel frustrated because I haven't given you enough direction or backed you up in trying to replace two of the team's members.
>
> The purpose of this memorandum is to strongly suggest that you look to yourself as a source of these problems, rather than elsewhere. It is important that you avoid complaining about things that aren't being done for you and start doing things on your own. Don't always look to others as the source of your problems. Working with people is a difficult challenge.
>
> You have to stand or fall on your own. You cannot expect me to settle all of the problems that arise. You have to develop confidence in yourself and learn to work with the people on the team you are leading. If your problems persist, it will be necessary to replace you.

QUESTIONS
1. What was communicated in the memorandum?
2. What effect will the memorandum have?
3. How else might Wilkins have communicated with Jones?

■ Case Study 2: Information Technologies in Rural Florida Hospitals

The use of information technologies (IT) is experiencing widespread growth in hospitals as a means to improve operations, including patient outcomes. These expensive technologies appear to be utilized differently in rural settings, depending upon whether a rural hospital is a stand-alone or a system-affiliated hospital. The authors of one study of this phenomenon, conducted in Florida, found the following differences in use of IT between stand-alone rural hospitals and system-affiliated rural hospitals.[32] System-affiliated hospitals were statistically more likely to have information systems in

- Laboratory (93% versus 39%)
- Pharmacy (87% versus 46%)
- Pharmacy dispensing (53% versus 8%)
- Chart deficiency (60% versus 15%)
- Order communication results (60% versus 23%)

Furthermore, 20% of system-affiliated facilities reported financial barriers to successful IT implementation, and 69% of stand-alone hospitals reported these barriers.

QUESTIONS

1. What else might account for some of this difference in IT utilization?
2. How might these differences affect patient care?
3. What might be done to offset the negative effect of lower IT usage in rural stand-alone hospitals?

◼ Case Study 3: "You Didn't Tell Me!"

Metropolitan Hospital has 500 beds with 1,500 full-time employees and a professional staff organization of 400. As part of a comprehensive analysis of communication at Metropolitan, a consulting firm called Management Strategies, Inc., surveyed all of the employees. The results of one question troubled the CEO. The question was, Does your immediate superior tell you about changes well in advance of their implementation so that you are prepared for them?

The responses (in percentages) were as follows:

	Always	Often	Sometimes	Seldom	Never
Senior-level managers	90	8	2		
Middle-level managers (department heads)	78	12	10		
First-level managers	65	25	10		
Nonmanagers	40	20	18	12	10

QUESTIONS

1. What do these results show? Why?
2. What reasons could explain these results?
3. What steps should the CEO take based on these results?

◼ Case Study 4: How Much Should We Say?

The executive committee of the governing body and the senior management team of a large midwestern HS were meeting to decide how much information to release to the media about the system's financial condition. Following an extensive period of growth and aggressive acquisition of hospitals and physician practices, the HS experienced serious financial difficulties, leading to a chapter 11 filing (bankruptcy protection).

A key decision linked to the bankruptcy filing had been to separate the HSOs in the system into geographic clusters and include only some in the filing. Other HSOs in the system were not included. The stakeholders of the HS itself and of its various component HSOs were very concerned about the financial condition of the system and its future prospects. Many were interested in exactly how this disastrous situation had come about.

QUESTIONS

1. Draw a stakeholder map of this HS.
2. Discuss the options available for how communication with external stakeholders can be undertaken. Which option would be best?
3. Consider the relationship that this HS had previously established with its community, and discuss the effect it would have on the HS's communication with this important external stakeholder in this crisis situation.

Notes

1. Fottler, Myron D. "Strategic Human Resources Management." In *Human Resources in Healthcare: Managing for Success,* edited by Bruce J. Fried and James A. Johnson, 1–18. Chicago: Health Administration Press, 2002; Blair, John D., and Myron D. Fottler. "Effective Stakeholder Management: Challenges, Opportunities and Strategies." In *Handbook of Healthcare Management,* edited by W. Jack Duncan, Peter M. Ginter, and Linda E. Swayne, 20. Malden, MA: Blackwell, 1998.
2. Kovner, Anthony R., and Duncan Neuhauser. *Health Services Management: Readings, Cases, and Commentary,* 8th ed., 6. Chicago: Health Administration Press, 2004.
3. Scott, William G., Terence R. Mitchell, and Philip H. Birnbaum. *Organization Theory: A Structural and Behavioral Analysis,* 4th ed., 3. Homewood, IL: Irwin, 1981.
4. Longest, Beaufort B., Jr., and Wesley M. Rohrer. "Communications Between Public Health Agencies and Their External Stakeholders."*Journal of Health and Human Services Administration* 28, 2 (Fall 2005): 189–217.
5. Newstrom, John W., and Keith Davis. *Organizational Behavior: Human Behavior at Work,* 9th ed., 102. New York: McGraw-Hill, 1993.
6. Holt, David H. *Management: Principles and Practices,* 3rd ed., 483. Englewood Cliffs, NJ: Prentice-Hall, 1992.
7. Shortell, Stephen M. *Effective Hospital–Physician Relationships,* 70–92. Chicago: Health Administration Press, 1991.
8. Porter, Michael E. *Competitive Advantage: Creating and Sustaining Superior Performance.* New York: The Free Press, 1985.
9. Rice, James A. *Leadership Insights.* La Jolla, CA: The International Health Summit, 2003.
10. Robbins, Stephen P., and Mary K. Coulter. *Management,* 6th ed. Englewood Cliffs, NJ: Prentice-Hall, 1998.
11. Hackman, J. Richard. *Leading Teams: Setting the Stage for Great Performance.* Boston: Harvard Business School Press, 2002; Harris, Thomas E., and John C. Sherblom. *Small Group and Team Communication.* Boston: Allyn and Bacon, 2002.
12. Scott, William G., Terence R. Mitchell, and Philip H. Birnbaum. *Organization Theory: A Structural and Behavioral Analysis,* 4th ed., 165. Homewood, IL: Irwin, 1981.
13. Newstrom, John W., and Keith Davis. *Organizational Behavior: Human Behavior at Work,* 9th ed., 441. New York: McGraw-Hill, 1993.
14. Newstrom, John W., and Keith Davis. *Organizational Behavior: Human Behavior at Work,* 9th ed., 444–445. New York: McGraw-Hill, 1993.
15. Longest, Beaufort B., Jr. "Interorganizational Linkages in the Health Sector." *Healthcare Management Review* 15 (Winter 1990): 17–28.

16. Fottler, Myron D., John D. Blair, Carlton J. Whitehead, Michael D. Laus, and Grant T. Savage. "Assessing Key Stakeholders: Who Matters to Hospitals and Why?" *Hospital & Health Services Administration* 34 (Winter 1989): 525–546.

17. Fahey, Liam, and V.K. Narayaman. *Macroenvironmental Analysis for Strategic Management.* St. Paul, MN: West Publishing, 1986; Ginter, Peter M., Linda M. Swayne, and W. Jack Duncan. *Strategic Management of Healthcare Organizations,* 3rd ed., 53–58. Malden, MA: Blackwell, 1998; Longest, Beaufort B., Jr., *Seeking Strategic Advantage Through Health Policy Analysis,* 63–79. Chicago: Health Administration Press, 1996.

18. Ginter, Peter M., Linda M. Swayne, and W. Jack Duncan. *Strategic Management of Healthcare Organizations,* 3rd ed., 60–64. Malden, MA: Blackwell, 1998.

19. Thomas, James B., and Reuben R. McDaniel, Jr. "Interpreting Strategic Issues: Effects of Strategy and the Information-Processing Structure of Top Management Teams." *Academy of Management Journal* 33 (1990): 288–298.

20. This section is adapted from Longest, Beaufort B., Jr., *Managing Health Programs and Projects,* 205–206. San Francisco: Jossey-Bass, 2004.

21. Kotler, Philip. *Social Marketing,* 2nd ed. Thousand Oaks, CA: Sage Publications, 2002.

22. Berkowitz, Eric N. *Essentials of Healthcare Marketing.* Gaithersburg, MD: Aspen Publishers, Inc., 1996; American Organization of Nurse Executives. *Market-Driven Nursing: Developing and Marketing Patient Care Services.* San Francisco: Jossey-Bass, 1999.

23. Friedman, Emily. *The Right Thing,* 228. San Francisco: Jossey-Bass, 1996.

24. Longest, Beaufort B., Jr. "The Civic Roles of Healthcare Organizations." *Health Forum Journal* 41 (September/October 1998): 40–42.

25. Longest, Beaufort B., Jr. *Health Policymaking in the United States,* 4th ed., chap. 1. Chicago: Health Administration Press, 2006.

26. Longest, Beaufort B., Jr. *Seeking Strategic Advantage Through Health Policy Analysis.* Chicago: Health Administration Press, 1997.

27. Filerman, Gary L., and D. David Persaud. "Advocacy." In *Government Relations in the Healthcare Industry,* edited by Peggy Leatt and Joseph Mapa, 77. Westport, CT: Praeger, 2003.

28. Brennan, Troyen A., Lucian L. Leape, Nan M. Laird, A. Russell Localio, Ann G. Lawthers, Joseph P. Newhouse, Paul C. Weiler, and Howard H. Hiatt. "Incidence of Adverse Events and Negligence in Hospitalized Patients: Results of the Harvard Medical Practice Study." *New England Journal of Medicine* 324, 6 (February 7, 1991): 370–376.

29. *To Err Is Human: Building a Safer Health System,* edited by Linda T. Kohn, Janet M. Corrigan, and Molla S. Donaldson. Washington, DC: National Academy Press, 2000.

30. Deming, W. Edwards. *Out of the Crisis.* Cambridge, MA: Massachusetts Institute of Technology, Center for Advanced Engineering Study, 1986; Juran, Joseph M. *On Leadership for Quality: An Executive Handbook.* New York: Free Press, 1989; Griffith, John R., and Kenneth R. White. *The Well-Managed Healthcare Organization,* 6th ed. Chicago: Health Administration Press, 2007.

31. James, Brent C. *Quality Management for Healthcare Delivery.* Chicago: The Health Research and Educational Trust of the American Hospital Association, 1989.

32. Menachermi, Nir, Darrell Burke, Art Clawson, and Robert G. Brooks. "Information Technologies in Florida's Rural Hospitals: Does System Affiliation Matter?" *The Journal of Rural Health* 21, 3: 263–268.

Author Index

Page references followed by *f* and *t* indicate figures and tables, respectively. References followed by *n* indicate notes.

Subject Index

Page references followed by *f* and *t* indicate figures and tables, respectively. References followed by *n* indicate notes.